BREAST CANCER - FROM BIOLOGY TO MEDICINE

Edited by **Phuc Van Pham**

Breast Cancer - From Biology to Medicine
http://dx.doi.org/10.5772/62922
Edited by Phuc Van Pham

Contributors

Hiba Al-Amodi, Hanan Mohamed AbdElmoneim, Hala Fawzy Mohamed Kamel, Thuan Duc Lao, Phuong Kim Truong, Huyen Ai Thuy Le, Jeffrey Johnson, William Audeh, Hisashi Tanaka, Farin Amersi, Armando Giuliano, Xiaojiang Cui, Mohamed Kamal, Wajeeha Razaq, Macall Leslie, Takemi Tanaka, Maria Del Pilar Camacho Leal, Shahid Ahmed, Nilufer Bulut, Stefan Krämer, Michael Friedrich, I-Hsuan Lin, Ming-Ta Hsu, Yasemin Bolukbasi, Ugur Selek, Yunbao Pan, Francois X Claret, Peng-Fei Qiu, Bin-Bin Cong, Yong-Sheng Wang, Khalid Dafaallah Awadelkarim, Moawia Mohammed Ali Elhassan, Gitana Aceto, Ahmed Abdalla Mohamedani, Renato Mariani Costantini, Felipe Da Luz, Rogério De Araújo, Alberto Moraes, Marcelo Silva, Diego Aguilera Braico, Gabriela Balogh, Muntaser Ibrahim, Joanna Zarzynska, Sudhakar Jha, Ajda Coker-Gurkan, Damla Arisan, Narcin Palavan-Unsal, Pinar Obakan-Yerlikaya, Ming-Shen Dai, Natalia Chaves, Marcia Oliveira Da Rocha, Sônia Nair Báo, Saverio Gentile, Joel Monárrez-Espino, Anna Riegel, William Kietzman, Virginie Ory, Letícia Rangel, Yashomati Patel

Published by InTech
Janeza Trdine 9, 51000 Rijeka, Croatia

Notice

Statements and opinions expressed in the chapters are these of the individual contributors and not necessarily those of the editors or publisher. No responsibility is accepted for the accuracy of information contained in the published chapters. The publisher assumes no responsibility for any damage or injury to persons or property arising out of the use of any materials, instructions, methods or ideas contained in the book.

Publishing Process Manager Iva Simcic
Technical Editor SPi Global
Cover InTech Design team

First published April, 2017
Printed in Croatia
Legal deposit, Croatia: National and University Library in Zagreb

Additional hard copies can be obtained from orders@intechopen.com

Breast Cancer - From Biology to Medicine, Edited by Phuc Van Pham
p. cm.
Print ISBN 978-953-51-2999-8
Online ISBN 978-953-51-3000-0

For EU product safety concerns:
IN TECH d.o.o., Prolaz Marije Krucifikse Kozulić 3, 51000 Rijeka, Croatia,
info@intechopen.com or visit our website at intechopen.com.

Meet the editor

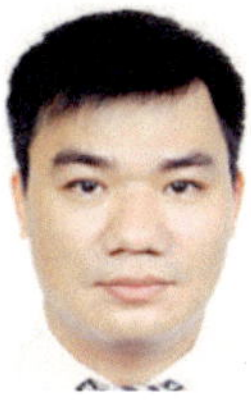

Phuc Van Pham received his PhD in Human Physiology in 2007. He is currently a professor of Biology, director of the Laboratory of Stem Cell Research and Application, and vice-director of the Laboratory of Cancer Research at the University of Science, Vietnam National University in Ho Chi Minh City, Vietnam. He is a long-standing lecturer and translational scientist at the University and is a member of several societies and journal editorial boards focused on cancer and regenerative medicine. Dr. Pham and his colleagues have established one of the first multidisciplinary cancer and regenerative medicine centers in Vietnam, and he has successfully launched an array of technologies in stem cell isolations and immunotherapies for cancer, especially breast cancer stem cells. After many years of experience as an embryologist, cell biologist, and molecular biologist, collaborating with leading researchers in Singapore, Japan, and the United States, Dr. Pham is a student again, keen to reach beyond the traditional boundaries of biology.

Contents

Preface

The term "breast cancer" refers to a malignant tumor that has developed from cells in the breast. The types of cells that most commonly give rise to breast cancers are the milk-secreting *cells* and duct cells, which drain milk from the lobules to the nipple. The past 20 years have seen a significant worldwide reduction in mortality from breast cancer, largely due to improved early detection methods and development of more effective therapies, including adjuvant therapies. However, to date, more than 50% of breast tumors do not respond to these therapies and more than 70% of patients relapse after 5 years. Recently, studies in molecular and cellular biology explored some novel mechanisms of breast cancer that can be used in prognosis, diagnosis, treatment, as well as monitoring. With these useful supports from molecular and cellular biology tools, breast cancer diagnosis and treatment will become more efficient in the near future.

Breast Cancer - From Biology to Medicine thoroughly examines breast cancer from basic definitions, to cellular and molecular biology, to diagnosis and treatment. This book also has some additional focus on preclinical and clinical results in diagnosis and treatment of breast cancer. The book begins with introduction on epidemiology and pathophysiology of breast cancer in Section 1. In Section 2, the subsequent chapters introduce molecular and cellular biology of breast cancer with some particular signaling pathways, the gene expression, as well as the gene methylation and genomic imprinting, especially the existence of breast cancer stem cells. In Section 3, some new diagnostic methods and updated therapies from surgery, chemotherapy, hormone therapy, immunotherapy, radiotherapy, and some complementary therapies are discussed.

This book provides a succinct yet comprehensive overview of breast cancer for advanced students, graduate students, and researchers as well as those working with breast cancer in a clinical setting.

Many people have contributed to making our involvement in this project possible. We are extremely thankful to all of the contributors to this book and to people having a hand in the preparation of this book. We thank our readers, who have made our hours putting together this book worth it.

Prof. Phuc Van Pham, PhD
Laboratory of Cancer Research
Laboratory of Stem Cell Research and Application
University of Science, Vietnam National University
Ho Chi Minh City, Vietnam

Section 1

Introduction

Chapter 1

Epidemiology, Pathology, Management and Open Challenges of Breast Cancer in Central Sudan: A Prototypical Limited Resource African Setting

Renato Mariani-Costantini,
Moawia Mohammed Ali Elhassan,
Gitana Maria Aceto,
Ahmed Abdalla Mohamedani and
Khalid Dafaallah Awadelkarim

Additional information is available at the end of the chapter

http://dx.doi.org/10.5772/67175

Abstract

Little is known about breast cancer in Sudan. According to the recent data published by the Khartoum Cancer Registry, breast cancer was the most common cancer among Sudanese women. Generally, breast cancer in native African women is characterized by young age at onset, occurrence in multiparous premenopausal patients, advanced stage at diagnosis, large tumor size, high-grade and triple-negative phenotype, with correspondingly poor prognosis. In Sudan, it was reported that about 70% of the women diagnosed with breast cancer were younger than 50 years old. We present here data from local and international publications as well as primary information from the National Cancer Institute in Wad Medani (one of the only two cancer hospitals of the country, both located in Central Sudan in Khartoum and Wad Medani). We provide an up-to-date situation analysis of breast cancer in Central Sudan as an example for an African reality and the various open challenges of breast cancer in a limited resource setting. A better understanding of breast cancer in black African women is of global relevance, as there is an alarming increase in breast cancer among young black women worldwide, and these patients have the lowest survival rates.

Keywords: breast cancer, epidemiology, pathology, management, Sudan, Africa, limited resource setting

1. Introduction

Worldwide breast cancer is the most frequent cancer in women. Breast cancer is considered a biologically heterogeneous disease that is influenced by complex and still incompletely understood interactions between multiple genetic and environmental risk factors. These interactions could play an important role in the marked geographical variation of breast cancer incidence rates [1, 2]. Incidence rates are higher in the developed countries than in the developing countries and in urban versus rural areas [1–3]. In sub-Saharan Africa, low incidence of breast cancer has been documented [1–8]. This could be explained by the fact that high parity and prolonged breast-feeding, which act as protective factors [9, 10], are prevalent [9]. However, the estimated mortality rates for breast cancer in Africa are not greatly inferior to those registered in Europe. Another interesting observation is that in Africa, breast cancer tends to affect younger women [1, 2, 8, 11, 12]. A woman's age is one of the strongest risk factors for breast cancer. Its incidence rates increase steadily between 25 and 50 years of age, after which continue to rise at slower rate. In women under 20 years of age, the risk of breast cancer is very low [2, 13]. In parts of the world including sub-Saharan Africa, where life expectancy is shorter, the median age at diagnosis is 10–15 years younger than in the developed world, that is, Europe and the USA [2, 4, 11, 12, 14].

In any case, breast cancer is the most commonly diagnosed cancer among African women [15]. It has been noted that breast cancer overtook cervical cancer as the most commonly diagnosed cancer in several countries in sub-Saharan Africa, including Nigeria, Chad, Sudan, Cameroon, Central African Republic, Niger, Namibia, Congo, Kenya and Somalia [15, 16]. This was attributed to increase in the prevalence of breast cancer risk factors associated with urbanization and economic development, such as earlier menarche, later childbearing, having fewer children, obesity and increased awareness and detection [15].

Little is known about breast cancer in Sudan [17]. According to the recent data published by the Khartoum Cancer Registry, breast cancer was the most common cancer among Sudanese women [16]. During 2009–2010, the incidence rate of breast cancer was substantially higher than that of any other type of cancer in adults, males and females combined. The age-standardized rate (ASR) of breast cancer for women living in Khartoum was 66.8 per 100,000, which was higher than what was reported for women in East Africa and North Africa, but similar to those reported for Nigerian women living in Abuja or in Ibadan [16].

In the Sudan, breast cancer was the most frequent hospital-treated malignancy, accounting for about 16% (4005/25,064) of all reported cancer cases between the years 1959 and 2007 [17]. As in many African countries, this probably represents a gross underestimation due to incomplete case ascertainment and reporting [18]. In fact, accurate data are difficult to obtain in Africa because cancer registries cover only 11% of the population [19], and the quality of information about cancer types is poor [6, 20]. Mortality statistics for cancer are also inadequate. Since 1995, only three African countries (Mauritius, Egypt and South Africa) have contributed to the cancer mortality database. However, even in South Africa, death registrations for cancer were estimated to be incomplete [6]. In Sudan, precise anagraphic and clinical data are lacking, rendering it difficult, if not impossible, to make clinicopathologic correlations and to compile databases and registries. The problematic referral system has been previously described by Dafaallah et al. in the Wad Medani area, Sudan [21].

2. Major clinicopathological features of breast cancer in Sudan

Generally, breast cancer in native African women is characterized by young age at onset, occurrence in multiparous premenopausal patients, advanced stage at diagnosis, large tumor size, high-grade and triple-negative phenotype, with correspondingly poor prognosis. The median age at diagnosis among women with breast cancer in developed countries is 61 years [22, 23]. Interestingly, a recent overview of female breast cancer statistics in the United States showed that the median age at diagnosis was somewhat younger for black women (58 years) than for white women (62 years) [24]. In Sudan, it was reported that about 70% of the women diagnosed with breast cancer were younger than 50 years (**Figure 1**) [25].

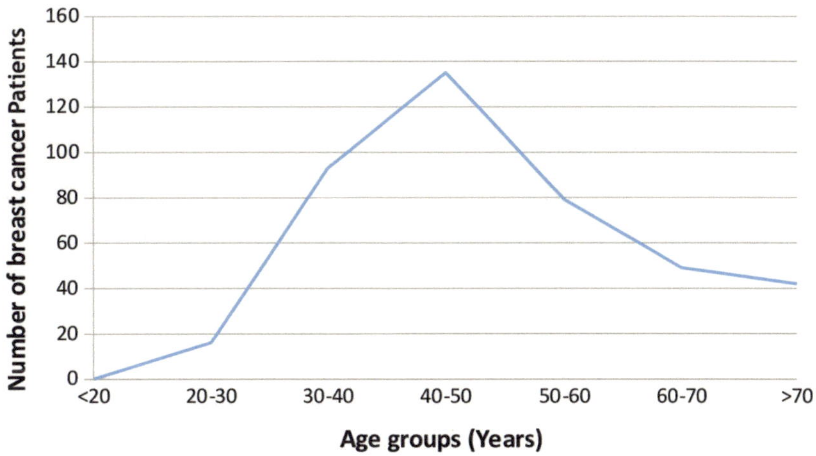

Figure 1. Age distribution of breast cancer patients treated at the NCCI-UG (Data from NCI-UG cancer registry, 2010–2011).

This could be related to the fact that Sudan has a young population structure, with 44% of the Sudanese population under 15 years of age, in addition to a relative, but significant, increase in life expectancy [26, 27]. Previous studies from other sub-Saharan countries reported that the average age of diagnosis of breast cancer among African women tends to be low. This is may be partially due to the short-life expectancy and young population structure of African women. However, the full spectrum of this phenomenon could reflect complex gene-environment interactions associated with both traditional and new lifestyles in Africa [6, 17, 19, 28–32].

Young age at breast cancer presentation in Sudanese women (**Figure 1**) appears to be contributed in minor part by genetic predisposition [13, 33, 34]. It is worth mentioning that breast cancer at a young age is generally associated with aggressive behavior, advanced stage at presentation and poorer prognosis [35].

The clinical stage of the disease at presentation is the most important factor for the outcome of the patient with breast cancer. In limited resource countries, breast cancer is typically characterized by a relatively advanced stage at presentation [33, 36–40].

Data from National Cancer Institute, University of Gezira (NCI-UG) confirm that the patients with breast cancer present in small proportion with localized disease and in large proportion with regionally diffuse and metastatic disease, as shown in **Table 1**.

Stage	Number	Percent
I	11	3
II	128	31
III	179	44
IV	93	23
Total	411	100

Source: NCI-UG cancer registry 2010–2011.

Table 1. Distribution of breast cancer patient according to clinical stage at diagnosis at NCI-UG.

It has been reported that about 80% of the breast cancer cases in Sudanese patients were diagnosed at locally advanced or metastatic stage [39]. Similar high proportions of advanced stage at diagnosis of breast cancer have been reported by several studies from other sub-Saharan African countries [36–38]. The contrary was reported from high resource countries, where 38% of the European and 30% of the US breast cancer cases have either locally advanced or metastatic disease at diagnosis [41]. Several factors may contribute to the delayed presentation of patients with breast cancer. These include lack of education, poverty, limited access to medical care and the fear of being perceived as a burden to caregivers. Other likely factors are fear of mastectomy and misconceptions about the nature or curability of the disease, which can lead women to seek alternative care instead of standard treatment [31]. About 60–75% of women in Central Sudan who develop breast cancer live in rural areas [39] and many of these women go untreated, mostly due to lack of access (financial and geographical) to health care (**Figure 2**).

Typically, in our setting, cases with breast lumps are referred by the attending physician to surgical facilities in governmental hospitals or private clinics for tissue biopsy. The average time to get the histopathology result is about 2–3 weeks [42, 43]. In Sudan, there are only two specialized treatment centers for cancer, both located in Central Sudan, that is, the Radiation and Isotopes Center, Khartoum (RICK) and the National Cancer Institute (NCI-UG) of Gezira University in Wad Medani, Gezira State, Central Sudan. Given the size of the country, this situation by itself could lead to the above-mentioned delayed presentation in which most of cancer patients come after traveling long distances from different parts of the country (**Figure 2**). Therefore, the financial aspects of investigations and treatment, alongside with the availability of boarding and lodging close to the oncology centers, represent a huge burden for the patients and their caregivers [17, 42].

Molecular profiling indicates that breast cancer is a constellation of partially diverse and clinically relevant tumor subtypes whose prevalence across populations could be influenced by ethnicity, a complex variable combining genetic, environmental and other discriminating factors. Moreover, different breast cancer subtypes may progress along partially independent molecular pathways, which could reflect etiological and biological differences (i.e. luminal A, luminal B, Her-2/neu overexpressing, basal like, etc.) [44–46]. However, little is known about the molecular subtypes of breast cancer associated with high multiparity and lactation in non-contracepting populations, such as African populations. The molecular portrait(s) of breast tumors in Africa might be different compared to those of breast cancer in Western women [47]. Studies conducted in the USA suggest that black ethnicity adversely influences breast cancer phenotype [48]. Indeed, African Americans have been reported to manifest a higher rate of the most aggressive breast cancer subtype, that is, the basal-like subtype, associated with high grade, poor prognosis and younger age [48]. Data on the molecular subtypes of breast cancer among Sudanese patients are scarce. The basal cytokeratins, markers of the basal-like breast cancer subtype, were expressed in a fraction of cases from Central Sudan comparable to those reported for East and West African case series [49]. Lack of associations with age and tumor size may represent a special feature of basal-like breast cancer in Sudan [49].

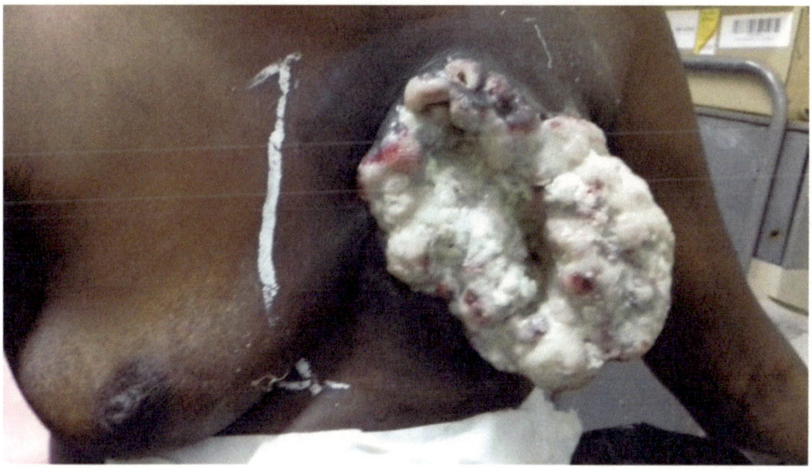

Figure 2. A 25-year-old female with locally advanced breast cancer treated at NCI-UG. This shocking presentation demonstrates how far our patients are in term of early detection. On the other hand, the biological features of such advanced primary tumors, since several decades exceedingly rare in developed countries, are almost unknown. Hence, treatment options do not rely on scientific evidence.

Very few studies assessed the clinical and pathological characteristics of breast cancer in Sudan. One study investigated in parallel series of patients the possible differences between breast cancer in indigenous sub-Saharan African (i.e., Sudanese) versus European (i.e., Italian) women. Compared with the Italian patients, the Sudanese patients were younger and their tumors were larger, more advanced in stage, higher in grade and more frequently positive for nodal metastases. Estrogen receptor (ER) expression varied between the two series, but no significant differences were found for PgR, combined hormone receptors, Her-2/neu, CK5/6, CK17, combined basal CK status or breast cancer subtypes [33]. The study concluded that the differences between the Sudanese and the Italian breast cancer series reflected stage at diagnosis rather than intrinsic biological characteristics [33]. This was in accordance with data reported for a breast cancer series from Nigeria, where Adebamowo and collaborators reported a high frequency of hormone receptor-positive cases, when the histopathology samples were collected under rigorous control for appropriate fixation [50]. On the contrary, studies that compared extensive series of African-American and European-American breast cancer patients found associations between aggressive estrogen receptor (ER)-negative breast cancer and both younger age at diagnosis and black ethnicity [19, 40, 48]. This suggests the possible contribution of ethnic factors to a higher burden of aggressive ER-negative breast cancer in African women. Huo et al. (2009) found that hormone receptor-negative breast cancer was predominant in a large series of 507 patients with invasive breast cancer from Nigeria and Senegal, in which only 25% of the studied cases were ER positive [40].

Similar findings were reported in studies comparing Nigerian and UK breast cancer patients. In this regards, the immunoprofile of 308 breast tumors from Nigeria, together with the patients' outcomes, was compared with a tumor grade-matched UK control group. The Nigerian women presenting with breast cancer were more frequently premenopausal, and their tumors were characterized by large primary tumor size, high tumor grade, advanced lymph node stage and higher rate of vascular invasion compared with the tumors in the UK women. In the grade-matched groups, the Nigerian breast cancers showed over representation of triple-negative and basal phenotypes and *BRCA1*-deficient breast cancer compared with the UK women, but no difference was found regarding Her-2/neu expression between the two series. The Nigerian patients showed significantly poorer outcome compared with the UK patients [47].

Elgaili et al. evaluated the clinicopathological features of breast cancer in Central Sudan and reported that estrogen and progesterone receptors expression were performed on a limited number of samples and that the majority of the tested cases resulted negative [39]. This finding was in accordance with data from other African countries, such as Tanzania, Nigeria and Kenya, where the majority of the studied breast cancers were negative for estrogen and progesterone receptors [51–54].

Huo et al. suggested that the reported high frequency of hormone receptor negativity should be interpreted with caution, as false-negative results might be introduced by antigen degradation of archival materials, besides referral, which may generate a bias towards a lower proportion of ER-positive tumors [40]. Suboptimal assays most likely contribute to the low positive estrogen and/or progesterone receptors status reported for breast cancer in Africa [55]. Moreover, the high fractions of receptors-negative cases could reflect early age at breast cancer diagnosis, in Sudan as well as elsewhere in Africa, since young breast cancer patients are more likely to have tumors with negative estrogen and/or progesterone receptors status [56, 57].

Eng et al. conducted a meta-analysis and a systematic review of the publications reporting on the frequency of breast cancer receptor-defined subtypes in indigenous populations in North and Sub-Saharan Africa and found that there was marked between-study heterogeneity in the ER+ estimates in both regions, with the majority reporting proportions between 0.40 and 0.80 in North Africa and between 0.20 and 0.70 in sub-Saharan Africa. Similarly, large between-study heterogeneity was observed for PR+ and HER2+ estimates [58]. This meta-analysis showed that the proportion of ER+ disease was lower for studies based on archived tumor blocks compared to prospectively collected specimens and lower for series enriched in grade 3 tumors. For prospectively collected samples, the pooled proportions for ER+ and triple negative tumors were 0.59 (0.56–0.62) and 0.21 (0.17–0.25), respectively, regardless of region. This suggests that two-thirds of the African women with breast cancer have a less aggressive disease (ER+), for which targeted endocrine treatment could improve survival rates [58]. Thus, the data suggest the distribution of receptor-defined subtypes in African patients may not dramatically differ from that found in non-African patients, given the younger age structure and late presentation [58].

Nonetheless, the diversity of the African breast cancer patient population was not comprehensively represented in the case series studied thus far [40]. As a result, the impact of breast cancer with hormone receptor negativity in sub-Saharan Africa needs to be further verified, under stringent quality control, in larger and more specific studies involving different African populations [40, 58, 59].

The Ki-67 labeling index, which has been linked to patient outcome in breast cancer, is not routinely performed in Sudan and very few published reports have examined Ki-67 labeling index in African breast cancer patients. In a pilot study, the association(s) between Ki-67 labeling index and individual, pathological, clinical and immunohistochemical characteristics were investigated in 62 patients diagnosed with primary invasive breast cancer at RICK, Sudan. The results suggested a correlation with tumor differentiation and not with tumor size or any other tested marker [60].

3. Male breast cancer in Sudan

Data from Central Sudan show that to 2.3% (34/1505) of all breast cancer patients registered at NCI-UG between 1999 and 2010 are males [61], which is over two-fold higher than the proportion reported worldwide [62]. In this regard, the incidence of male breast cancer (MBC) is reportedly higher in sub-Saharan Africa [63]. In Central Sudan, the mean age at diagnosis for MBC was 56 years [61], about a decade younger than the mean age seen in developed countries [63]. The mean period between complaint awareness and MBC diagnosis was 25.3 ± 46 months. Most patients presented with a large lump (mean size, 6.8 + 3.0 cm) or with metastatic disease (stages III/IV, 21/34, 61.8%) [61]. Because MBC is a matter of stigma in Africa, this could be a reason for late presentation, together with the same issues that apply to breast cancer in females.

4. Breast cancer genetics in Sudan

As in industrialized countries, strong genetic factors contribute to a subset of breast cancer cases in the Sudan. The germline status of the two major breast cancer susceptibility genes, *BRCA1* and *BRCA2*, was investigated in an NCI-UG breast cancer series selected based on diagnosis within 40 years of age (34 cases) or male gender (1 case). A total of 60 sequence variants, including 5 deleterious truncating mutations (2 in *BRCA1,* 3 in *BRCA2*) and 55 variants (30 in *BRCA1,* 25 in *BRCA2*) presumed to be neutral or of little clinical significance were detected. The data suggest that in Sudan BRCA1/2 could represent an important etiological factor of breast cancer in males and young women less exposed to pregnancy and lactation [64]. Biunno et al. found 33 BRCA1 point mutations, one of which of pathogenetic relevance, in 59 Central Sudanese premenopausal breast cancer patients. The high fractions of mutations with both intercontinental and uniquely African distribution were in agreement with the high genetic diversity expected in an African population [65]. Thus, genetic variation and frequency of unique or rare mutations of uncertain clinical relevance pose significant challenges to BRCA1 testing in Sudan, as it might happen in other African contexts [34]. It is worth mentioning that a determination of BRCA1 and BRCA2 genetic mutational status will go a long way towards an effective advice on prophylaxis for breast cancer [66].

Masri et al. studied 20 unselected breast cancer patients in Sudan. They analyzed exon 11 of the BRCA2 gene and exons 5–9 of the p53 gene. They found only one somatic mutation and one polymorphism in BRCA2, without any further elaboration [67].

Hereditary breast cancer is more likely to manifest with synchronous or metachronous bilateral disease. A study from the Khartoum Teaching Hospital assessed the frequency and features of bilateral breast cancer among the patients treated during the 5-year period from 1994 to 1999. Of 521 patients treated for breast cancer, only seven (1.3%) were diagnosed with bilateral breast cancers [68].

Susceptibility to breast cancer could be predisposed by low penetrance gene polymorphisms. A single nucleotide polymorphism in the estrogen receptor gene (ESR1), C325G, implicated in breast cancer susceptibility, was genotyped in breast cancer patients and in age- and sex-matched Sudanese controls. Overall, there was a trend in the direction of an association between the CC genotype and breast cancer, which became significant in the subgroup within 50 years of age [69]. The association of the Her-2/neu Ile655Val polymorphism with breast cancer in the Sudan was also investigated [70]. Val/Val and Ile/Ile genotype frequencies were similar in patients and controls; Ile/Val had a borderline-significant association with breast cancer, not confirmed when the genotypic and allelic frequencies were stratified by age and menopausal status. Possible joint effects of Her-2/neu Ile655Val and ESR1 C325G on breast cancer risk were also investigated. The frequency of the polymorphic variants varied with ethnic origin. A significantly higher risk of breast cancer was observed among carriers of homozygous ESR1 325 CC and heterozygous Her-2/neu 655 Ile/Val [70]. These results suggest that an interaction between the ESR1 325C and Her-2/neu Ile655Val variants could contribute to breast cancer risk in Sudanese women [70].

Oncogenic viruses, such as Epstein-Barr virus (EBV), could play a role in breast carcinogenesis in Sudan. EBV genomic sequences were detected in a large fraction of tested Sudanese breast cancer specimens, suggesting an association between EBV and breast carcinoma in Sudanese patients [71].

http://dx.doi.org/10.5772/67175

5. Current status of breast cancer screening in Sudan

International policies recommend screening mammography for women aged 50–69 years [72]. Other imaging modalities, such as MRI and ultrasound, are not recommended for screening in the general population. According to an analysis from the 2003 World Health Survey, only 2.2% of women age 40–69 years in limited resource settings had received any breast cancer screening. Mammography screening programs have also been estimated to cost from US$16,000 to US$37,000 per life saved, which exceeds by a significant margin the per capita health care budgets in many limited resource settings [73, 74]. Therefore, International guidelines recommend clinical breast examination (CBE) as a preferred approach to screening in settings in which mammography screening is not available [75, 76].

In Sudan, the health care system is significantly weakened by limited resources and human capacity. Resources available for health care are predominantly spent on infectious disease care, such as malaria, diarrheal diseases and tuberculosis. In our setting, the challenges of establishing national cancer screening programs include limited financial resources, shortage in trained health care professionals and social barriers that impede population enrollment into cancer screening program. In our setting, mammography machines are few. In addition, the target population is mostly young women and the available traditional film mammography machines are not efficacious for breast cancer detection in young women with dense breast.

In 2000, medical students from the Faculty of Medicine, University of Gezira, performed a breast self-examination (BSE) intervention project in "Um-Alghora," one of the poorest localities in Gezira State. During one academic semester, the students covered 200 families by training on competences of BSE. Four breast lumps were detected (two of which were fibroadenomas and two carcinomas). This project revealed that medical students, through relevant community based educational activities in preventive medicine, could have a significant effect on early detection of breast cancer by BSE [77, 78].

Given that breast cancer is the most commonly observed cancer in Sudan, an initiative for breast cancer awareness and early detection was launched in 2008, led by the National Cancer Institute, University of Gezira. Abuidris and colleagues conducted a pilot study in two localities in Gezira State, Sudan (**Figure 3**). Approximately 10,000 rural women aged 18 years or older were screened for breast cancer by using trained volunteers (**Figure 4**). Seventeen of those screened had carcinoma in situ or breast cancer, including eight with carcinoma in situ and nine with early breast cancer. In control villages, only four women self-referred for breast symptoms, three of whom had advanced-stage breast cancer [79]. Therefore, in our setting, the implementation of a cancer awareness and breast examination program that uses local volunteer women might be better used to raise awareness and encourage more women with palpable breast lumps to seek and receive early medical care.

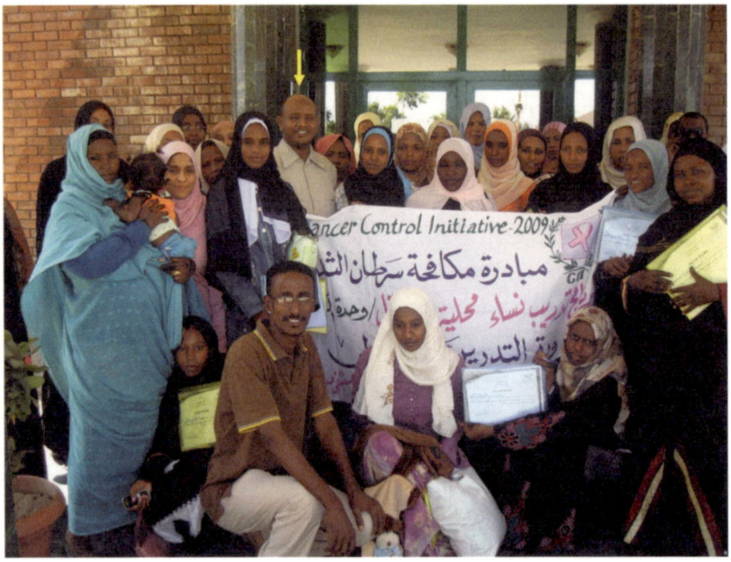

Figure 3. Volunteers participants to the intensive training course of the breast cancer awareness and early detection initiative (March 1–5, 2009). This image shows Dr. Dafalla Abuidris, indicated by the yellow arrow, a clinical oncologist and the initiative leader. Blue arrows indicate some of the NCI-UG team members involved the in the training activities. The other women are some of the volunteers who attended the course and conducted the screening.

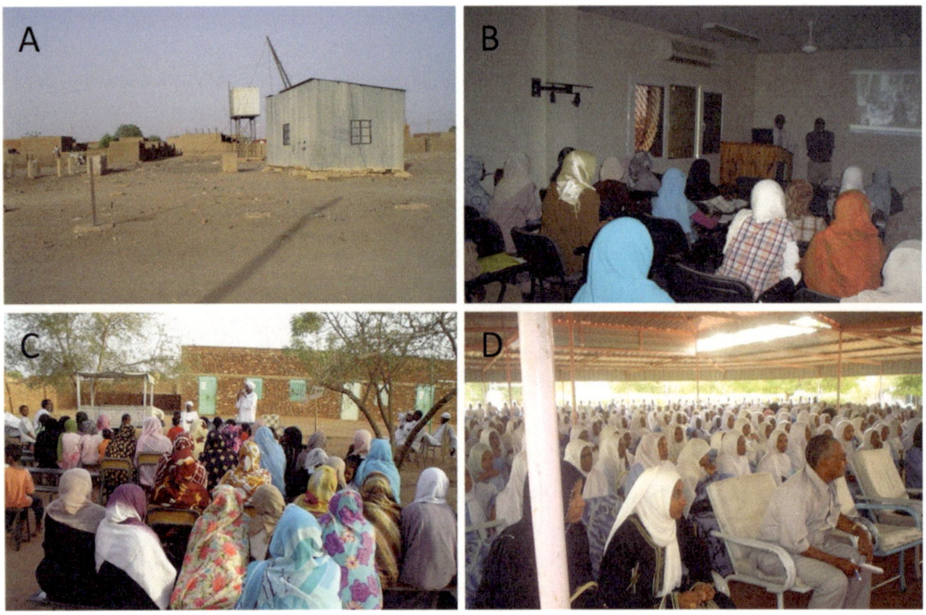

Figure 4. This set of images shows the context and some of the activities of the breast cancer initiative. (A) One of the poor villages in the Keremet locality, El Managil District, Gezira State, where the breast cancer initiative was launched. (B) Educational lectures conducted for the training of the volunteers at NCI-UG during March 1–5, 2009. (C) and (D) Awareness activities performed at the community level in 33 villages at the Keremet locality during 2009–2010 with the participation of the target women of the community.

6. Breast cancer management in Central Sudan

The management of patients with breast cancer requires a multidisciplinary approach to treatment (MDT). The MDT team includes a surgeon, a clinical oncologist, a pathologist, a clinical radiologist, a social worker, a nurse and a counselor. These specialists are lacking in limited-resource countries, and where they exist they tend to work in isolation, rather than in team. Therefore, almost all patients with breast cancer are treated without been seen in an MDT context. Practice guidelines that outline the optimal approach to breast cancer management have been developed by several international organizations and scientific committees, such as National Comprehensive Cancer Network (NCCN) guidelines. However, these guidelines may be inappropriate in limited resource countries for many reasons, including the extreme limitation of resources for diagnosis and treatment and the extreme shortage in trained health care providers.

The NCI-UG has a multidisciplinary breast clinic for management decisions. This clinic, established in 2002 (**Table 2**), is hosted by the Oncology Department of the NCI-UG and is attended by surgeons, oncologists, pathologists, psychologists, social workers and oncology nurses. The Gezira guidelines for the management of breast cancer, developed in 2004 and updated in 2006, are oriented towards the limited financial resources of the Sudan [80]. These guidelines represent a milestone for the improvement of breast cancer medical care in Central Sudan and are the first application of the MDT concept to patient's management in Sudan. Thus, the activities related to Gezira guidelines for management of breast cancer are part of an overall progress of the local oncology services in Central Sudan (**Table 2**). Cancer treatment is free of charge for all citizens in Sudan. Furthermore, boarding and lodging facilities close to the oncology center (NCI-UG) are available free of charge for cancer patients.

Year	Achievement
1999	Establishment of NCI-UG—formerly Institute of Nuclear Medicine & Oncology (INMO), the first center outside Khartoum (the capital city), offering radiotherapy and systemic therapy for cancer and nuclear medicine services for diagnosis
2002	Establishment of the Gezira multidisciplinary breast cancer clinic
2004	Installation of a mammography machine
2004	Development of the Gezira guidelines for management of breast cancer
2006	Update of the Gezira guidelines for management of breast cancer
2009	Establishment of hormone receptors testing using immunohistochemistry at the Department of Pathology, Faculty of Medicine, University of Gezira
2010	Development of the Sudan guidelines for management of breast cancer

Table 2. Timeline showing the overall progress of the oncology services at the NCI-U, Central Sudan.

In the next sections of diagnosis and treatment, we present and discuss the currently adopted Gezira guidelines for management of breast cancer patients [80].

6.1. Breast cancer diagnosis in Central Sudan

6.1.1. Clinical assessment

All referred breast cancer cases should undergo a thorough clinical assessment to provide guidance about the extent of the disease and the patient's fitness to tolerate cancer treatment.

6.1.2. Breast imaging

Breast ultrasound with diagnostic mammography should be part of triple assessment for all patients with breast lump. In Sudan, diagnostic breast ultrasound is often used to make a diagnosis of breast cancer, whereas diagnostic mammography is available only in few centers in Khartoum and Wad Medani (capital of the Gezira state). Therefore, triple assessment cannot be done in most parts of the country.

6.1.3. Histopathological investigations

Pathology practice in Sudan, like in other limited resource countries, has suffered from lack of funding, making it difficult for practicing pathologists to develop and apply recent technologic advances in their everyday practice [42, 43].

In Central Sudan, histopathology services are provided by the Department of Pathology, Faculty of Medicine, University of Gezira, located in Wad Medani (capital of the Gezira state), and serving the population of the Gezira state (about four million people living in an area of about 26,075 km^2; 10% of the total Sudanese population). This laboratory was established in 1978 and was the first of its kind outside Khartoum (the capital city). The average annual load during the years 2005–2009 at the above-mentioned laboratory was 5749 ± 476 and 1052 ± 128 specimens per year for histopathology and cytopathology, respectively; the overall annual load average was 6802 ± 494 [42]. There is a gross shortage of pathologists outside the capital, Khartoum. Currently, there are approximately eight anatomic pathologists serving the population of Central Sudan. Generally, there is a very poor logistic system for delivering the specimens to the laboratories. Surgical specimens are brought to the laboratory by the care givers of the patients. Buffered 10% formalin is rarely used, sometimes the specimens are received in normal saline and, rarely, in absolute ethanol [42]. Histopathologists mainly use hematoxylin-eosin routine stains. Pathologists in Gezira State depend largely on their skills in morphology (with its limitations) to classify tumors on routine stains.

According to the Gezira guidelines for management of breast cancer, the standard pathology report must include information on tumor size, lymph node status, histologic type, tumor grade, lymphovascular invasion and margin status [80]. Immunohistochemistry stains for estrogen-progesterone receptors, proliferative index (Ki67) and HER2-neu expression statuses are available, but the costs associated with testing for ER, PR and HER2 status are high, therefore these tests are not included in the primary report and are separately requested, added as extras paid by the patients. As a result, not all patients undergo hormonal receptor testing. **Figure 5** shows that 78% of the patients referred to NCI-UG in 2010–2011 had receptor testing. Cost reduction using tissue microarray immunohistochemistry (TMA-IHC), a known cost reduction technique relative to standard whole slide IHC, is problematic when dealing with large tumors in limited resource settings, where quality control in pathology processing may be less than optimal [81]. Frozen section, fluorescence in situ hybridization (FISH) and electron microscopy services are presently not available.

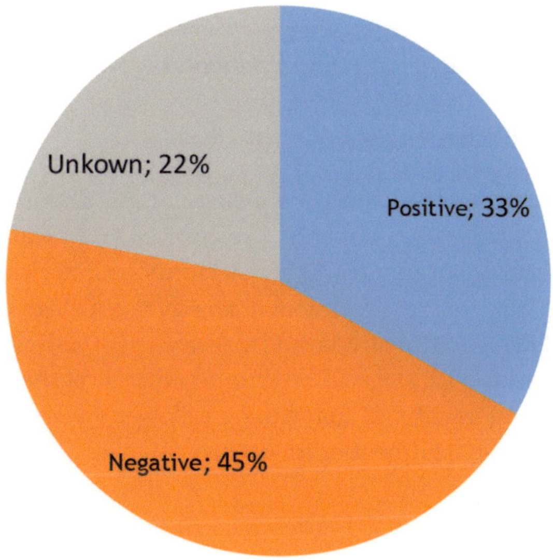

Figure 5. Distribution of breast cancer patients according to hormonal receptor status at NCI-UG (Source: NCI-UG cancer registry 2010–2011).

Because fine needle aspiration cytology (FNAC) is cheap, quick and repeatable, it was used extensively in the initial diagnosis of breast lumps. Fibroadenomas, cysts and abscesses (including antibiomas) are the most commonly diagnosed benign entities. Breast cancer initial diagnosis is usually done by FNAC, especially for late cases with ulcerations, since it is less invasive in such moribund patients with very poor general condition. In the last few years, ultrasound directed true-cut biopsies are been increasingly used initially or more commonly following FNAC.

In short, in Gezira State the preoperative diagnosis of breast cancer is based on FNAC, clinical evidence and excisional or incisional biopsy.

6.1.4. Staging investigations

In Central Sudan, diagnostic staging modalities, such as chest and skeletal radiography and liver ultrasound, are available in most tertiary hospitals. Computed tomography (CT) scans are available in two governmental institutes and in two private centers but are generally cost-prohibitive. The Department of Nuclear Medicine of the NCI-UG is the only provider of nuclear medicine services, such as bone scan, thyroid scan, multigated acquisition (MUGA) scan and renal scan for the population of the Gezira State. Complete blood count, renal function tests and liver function tests are mandatory for newly diagnosed cases as part of staging investigation [80]. Selected blood tests (i.e. CBC, blood chemistry profile) are required for the safe administration of chemotherapy.

Despite the improved availability of pathology, radiology and nuclear medicine services, financial difficulties turn away many women with few financial resources who have breast complaints. Without adequate health insurance coverage, limited personal finances can be a significant barrier to care for many breast cancer patients regarding investigations related costs.

6.2. Treatment workup and challenges in Central Sudan

Treatment of breast cancer is dependent on the stage of the disease, age and medical state of the patient, tumor characteristics, patients' preferences and available resources. Options range from breast-conserving surgery (BCS), mastectomy, axillary clearance, chemotherapy, radiotherapy (RT), to palliative care. Treatment at an advanced stage has poor prognosis with lowest cure rates. Challenges frequently faced by oncologist treating breast cancer in Sudan are (1) most patients present with stage III or IV when they first seek medical treatment and (2) lack of adherence to treatment and inadequate follow-up because patients may have to travel long distance to receive treatment or follow-up.

6.2.1. Surgery

Breast surgery is often the initial treatment for patients who present with operable tumors. In Sudan, breast surgery is mostly performed by general surgeons. The ability to perform modified radical mastectomy (MRM) and breast-conserving surgery (BCS) is considered fundamental for surgical residence training by the Sudan Medical Specialization Board. Therefore, general surgeons in Sudan are generally well trained and have high exposure to breast surgery.

In Sudan, due to the fact that the majority of breast cancer patients present with locally advanced stage, MRM, after or without neoadjuvant chemotherapy, is the predominant surgical procedure. MRM includes removal of breast tissue, axillary tail and clearance of level I and II axillary lymph nodes. The low rate of BCS in our patients reflects the high rate of late presentation. BCS requires (1) breast imaging (mammography and ultrasound) and pathology services to ensure tumor free margins of excision, (2) surgeons experienced in achieving a good cosmetic result with negative pathologic margins of excision and (3) radiotherapy facilities. These requirements are met in our setting. Therefore, BCS is currently used as an alternative option for young patients with early breast cancer, obviously a choice that is cosmetically desirable. BCS could be a choice for patients with large tumors who achieved good response to neoadjuvant chemotherapy. Randomized trials have shown that there are no significant differences in disease-free or overall survival between patients treated by mastectomy and those treated by breast-conserving surgery and whole-breast radiotherapy [82–84]. Breast cancer peaks among Sudanese women in their 30s. Therefore, breast-conserving therapy preserves the body image and may offer better quality of life.

http://dx.doi.org/10.5772/67175

Reconstruction breast surgery is not an option in our setting, due to lack of plastic and reconstructive surgeons. Although sentinel lymph node (SLN) biopsy has become the preferable standard to axillary dissection in breast cancer surgery, this advanced technique is presently not available in Sudan.

6.2.2. Radiotherapy

Radiotherapy (RT) is an essential part of the multimodality treatment of breast cancer. In limited resource countries, and particularly in Sudan, the need for radiotherapy is much greater due to late presentation and inoperability of the tumors. Access to radiotherapy, however, is severely limited. Africa has less than 2% of all radiotherapy centers globally and is home to approximately 15% of the world's population, demonstrating a dire need to improve the availability of radiotherapy [85]. The NCI-UG is a governmental facility with two Co60 machines, linear accelerator machine (Linac) and a treatment planning system (**Figure 6** and **Table 3**) that treats 80–100 patients daily, about 20% of whom are breast cancer patients. Patients from different regions of Sudan are referred to NCI-UG for RT. Radiotherapy is delivered with cobalt-60 units (Co 60). The linear accelerator was installed in 2007 (VARIAN, manufactured in 2005). Energy levels of this machine are 6 and 16 MV-photons and 6, 9, 12 and 15 MeV. The machine was stored for 2 years before installation as the bunker was not constructed in time, but never treated even a single patient because of licensing issues and economic sanctions imposed to Sudan.

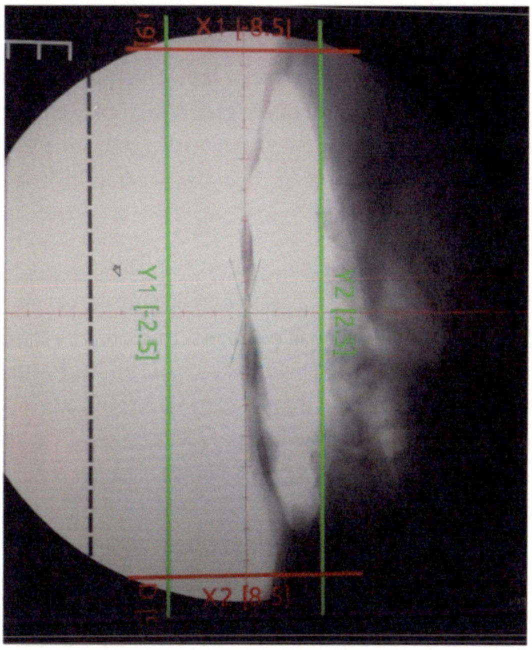

Figure 6. Simulator planning image for a chest wall radiation field at the NCI-UG.

Recourse	Counts
Clinical oncologists	4
Radiographers	10
Medical physicists	3
Engineering technicians	3
Co 60 radiotherapy machines	2
Linear accelerator[a]	1
Simulator[b]	1

[a] Non-functioning since installation in 2007.
[b] Simulator machine includes fluoroscopy and radiography option.

Table 3. Human (Staff) and physical resources (machines) at the NCI-UG.

Although linear accelerator machines (Linac) are considered preferable, cobalt machines represent a reasonable alternative in our setting because Co 60 radiotherapy machines are simpler to operate and much less expensive than Linac machines. Drawbacks of the Co 60 machines are the lower percentage depth dose and the decaying source that reduces the output, resulting in increased treatment time, which in turn reduces the patients outputs. Furthermore, the radioactive components are difficult to procure, because of the current international concerns.

The most common schedule for irradiation is 50 Gy in 25 fractions to the whole breast, administered daily, five times per week. In a large randomized trial, however, a shorter fractionation schedule (42.5 Gy in 22 days or 40 Gy in 3 weeks), more convenient and less costly, proved to be just as safe and effective [86, 87]. Thus, due to the long waiting list, cost and demand for the machine time, we considered hypo-fraction radiotherapy (treatment over 3 weeks) that simplifies the radiotherapy planning process, permitting more efficient use of our limited resources, and thus allowing the treatment of more patients with the existing equipment and personnel.

According to the Gezira guidelines for management of breast cancer, post-mastectomy irradiation is considered for patients with a tumor larger than 5 cm, or a tumor involving the chest wall or skin. It is also considered for patients with more than three positive axillary lymph nodes. Adjuvant radiotherapy is indicated for all patients who underwent BCS. Supraclavicular fossa irradiation is recommended for patients with more than three positive axillary lymph nodes. For patients with locally advanced breast cancer in which mastectomy is still not possible after initial systemic therapy, breast and regional irradiation is given, followed whenever possible by mastectomy. For patients with distant metastases, irradiation may provide relief of symptoms such as pain, bleeding, ulceration and lymphedema.

6.2.3. *Chemotherapy*

Systemic therapy for cancer treatment represents one of the great challenges in cancer control efforts in limited resource countries. The well-established cytotoxic chemotherapy drugs and endocrine therapies available for breast cancer patients in Sudan are shown in **Table 4**. At NCI-UG, a wide variety of chemotherapy regimens is in use. Anthracycline-based combination is the appropriate first-line chemotherapy for most breast cancer patients, based on significant survival benefits of the anthracycline based regimens, that is, 5-flurouracil (5FU), cyclophosphamide, doxorubicine (FAC) or 5-flurouracil (5FU), cyclophosphamide, epirubicine (FEC), when compared with 5-flurouracil (5FU) methotrexate, cyclophosphamide combinations (CMF). The anthracycline-based regimens are associated with a high risk of cardiotoxicity. Thus, CMF is still used for elderly patients with comorbidities. Taxanes-based regimens, such as cyclophosphamide, doxorubicine and taxane, are reserved for patients with extensive axillary lymphadenopathy. Systemic therapies are dispensed by a pharmacist and administered by trained nurses under supervision of a clinical oncologist. Tamoxifen is the most widely used endocrine therapy for breast cancer patients and a large proportion of post-menopausal patients are treated with aromatase inhibitors either alone or sequential with Tamoxifen. Furthermore, Tamoxifen is prescribed empirically for breast cancer patients with unknown hormone receptors.

Drug	Dose
Doxorubicin	60 mg/m^2
Epirubicin	100 mg/m^2
Cyclophosphamide	600 mg/m^2
5FU	600 mg/m^2
Methotrexate	40 mg/m^2
Docetaxel	100 mg/m^2
Paclitaxel	175 mg/m^2
Carboplatin	AUC 6
Cisplatin	50 mg/m^2
Capecitabine	1250 mg/m^2
Gemicitabine	1000 mg/m^2
Novalbine	25 mg/m^2
Tamoxifen	20 mg P.O
Anastrazole	1 mg P.O
Letrozole	2.5 mg P.O
G-CSF	5 mcg/kg

[a]These drugs were included in the 2014 WHO model list for essential medicine.

Table 4. List of available cancer drugs for breast cancer patients at the NCI-UG[a].

The choice of chemotherapy and hormonal therapy for breast cancer depends on the indication in the Gezira guidelines for management of breast cancer.

6.2.4. *Targeted therapy agents*

In our setting, Trastuzumab is the only available targeted therapy. However, the costs to the patients and issues related to insurance coverage limit patient access to this drug. Therefore, Trastuzumab is not included in the WHO model list for essential medicines, and HER2 targeted therapy is not considered as a priority in our limited resource setting by health care policy makers and insurance companies. Another limitation is that HER2 borderline cases (IHC score 2+) cannot be reassessed due to the unavailability of the fluorescence in situ hybridization (FISH) technique [88].

6.2.5. *Palliative care services*

The NCI-UG palliative care service was established in 1999 for pain control, stoma care and wound care. The available pain medications are paracetamol, nonsteroidal anti-inflammatory drugs, tramadol and morphine (both intravenous and oral). These medications are provided free of charge. However, these services remain grossly inadequate and represent a further area of priority, which led to the establishment of the Gezira palliative care program in 2015, to provide palliative care at home for terminal-stage cancer patients.

7. Conclusions, future perspectives and open challenges

Sudan and many other sub-Saharan African countries need to face alarming increases in cancer incidence [19, 28–30, 32, 89]. This situation impacts on the above-mentioned African health care crisis. At the same time, there is a very scarce and often incorrect perception of cancer as a disease in many African communities [13, 19, 28–30, 32, 37, 90–92]. In Sudan, breast cancer, particularly in premenopausal women, is increasingly recognized as an emerging health problem. Overall, the features of breast cancer in the Sudan may reflect population structure and reproductive factors resulting in low postmenopausal breast cancer incidence. On the other hand, the available data indicate that the Sudanese breast cancer series are enriched with cases of male breast cancer and early onset female breast cancer, particularly in parous women, suggesting specific risk factors [17, 64]. Information on breast cancer incidence in our limited resource setting is lacking due to lack of population cancer registry. In Sudan, as suggested by hospital-based case series the burden of disease is clearly increasing and breast cancer may account for large proportion of cancer load. Population-based studies, however, are needed to determine the true incidence of the disease, which, in present contest, is difficult to evaluate. It is probable that the breast cancer cases arising in Sudanese women derive from poorly understood interactions between strong genetic and environmental factors, which may include factors promoted by pregnancy and lactation. Moreover, an understanding of the above-mentioned complex situation is primarily important in view of the need of developing ad hoc designed preventive and therapeutic strategies. This requires local political will, painstaking development of infrastructures, trained personnel and focused international support [33, 43, 93]. Finally, but not lastly, a better understanding of breast cancer in black African women is of global crucial relevance, as there is an alarming increase in breast cancer among young black women worldwide and these patients have the lowest survival rates.

Author details

Renato Mariani-Costantini[1]*, Moawia Mohammed Ali Elhassan[2], Gitana Maria Aceto[3], Ahmed Abdalla Mohamedani[4] and Khalid Dafaallah Awadelkarim[5]

*Address all correspondence to: rmc@unich.it

1 Department of Medicine, Dentistry and Biotechnology, and Unit of General Pathology, Aging and Translational Medicine Research Center (CeSI-MeT), "G. d'Annunzio" University, Chieti, Italy

2 Radiation Oncology Department, National Cancer Institute (NCI-UG), University of Gezira, Wad Medani, Sudan

3 Department of Medicine, Dentistry and Biotechnology, "G. d'Annunzio" University, Chieti, Italy

4 Department of Pathology, Faculty of Medicine, University of Gezira, Wad Medani, Sudan

5 Department of Molecular Biology, National Cancer Institute (NCI-UG), University of Gezira, Wad Medani, Sudan

References

[1] Igene, H., *Global health inequalities and breast cancer: an impending public health problem for developing countries.* Breast J, 2008. **14**(5): 428–34.

[2] Bray, F., P. McCarron, and D.M. Parkin, *The changing global patterns of female breast cancer incidence and mortality.* Breast Cancer Res, 2004. **6**(6): 229–39.

[3] Parkin, D.M., et al., *Global cancer statistics, 2002.* CA Cancer J Clin, 2005. **55**(2): 74–108.

[4] Veronesi, U., et al., *Breast cancer.* Lancet, 2005. **365**(9472): 1727–41.

[5] Ferlay, J., et al., *GLOBOCAN 2002: Cancer Incidence, Mortality and Prevalence Worldwide.* 2004, IARC Press: Lyon.

[6] Parkin, D.M., et al., *Cancer in Africa: Epidemiology and Prevention.* 2003, Lyon: IARC Press.

[7] Parkin, D.M. and C.S. Muir, *Cancer incidence in five continents. Comparability and quality of data.* IARC Sci Publ, 1992(120): 45–173.

[8] Sighoko, D., et al., *Population-based breast (female) and cervix cancer rates in the Gambia: evidence of ethnicity-related variations.* Int J Cancer, 2010. **127**(10): 2248–56.

[9] Huo, D., et al., *Parity and breastfeeding are protective against breast cancer in Nigerian women.* Br J Cancer, 2008. **98**(5): 992–6.

[10] Enger, S.M., et al., *Breastfeeding history, pregnancy experience and risk of breast cancer.* Br J Cancer, 1997. **76**(1): 118–23.

[11] Basro, S. and J.P. Apffelstaedt, *Breast cancer in young women in a limited-resource environment.* World J Surg, 2010. **34**(7): 1427–33.

[12] Baltogiannis, G. and D.H. Roukos, *Letter to the editor: Breast cancer in young women in Africa: are there genetic and clinical differences with European ancestry patients?* World J Surg, 2010. **34**(8): 1982–3.

[13] Awadelkarim, K.D., et al., *Hereditary breast cancer in Sub-Saharan Africa.* Curr Women's Health Rev, 2012. **8**(1): 44–54.

[14] Vorobiof, D.A., F. Sitas, and G. Vorobiof, *Breast cancer incidence in South Africa.* J Clin Oncol, 2001. **19**(18 Suppl): 125S–127S.

[15] Jemal, A., et al., *Cancer burden in Africa and opportunities for prevention.* Cancer, 2012. **118**(18): 4372–84.

[16] Saeed, I.E., et al., *Cancer incidence in Khartoum, Sudan: first results from the Cancer Registry, 2009-2010.* Cancer Med, 2014. **3**(4): 1075–84.

[17] Awadelkarim, K.D., R. Mariani-Costantini, and N.E. Elwali, *Cancer in the Sudan: an overview of the current status of knowledge on tumor patterns and risk factors.* Sci Total Environ, 2012. **423**: 214–228.

[18] Adesunkanmi, A.R., et al., *The severity, outcome and challenges of breast cancer in Nigeria.* Breast, 2006. **15**(3): 399–409.

[19] Porter, P., *"Westernizing" women's risks? Breast cancer in lower-income countries.* N Engl J Med, 2008. **358**(3): 213–6.

[20] Parkin, D.M., *The evolution of the population-based cancer registry.* Nat Rev Cancer, 2006. **6**(8): 603–12.

[21] Dafallah, S.E., E.M. Yousif, and A.A. Idris, *Analysis of documents used in referral system in Wad Medani, Sudan.* Saudi Med J, 2005. **26**(1): 148–50.

[22] Howlader N, N.A., Krapcho M, et al., *SEER Cancer Statistics Review, 1975-2012, based on Nov 2014 SEER data submission.* 2015, National Cancer Institute: Bethesda, MD.

[23] Altekruse, S.F., et al., *SEER Cancer Statistics Review, 1975-2007, http://seer.cancer.gov/csr/1975_2007/.* 2010, National Cancer Institute: Bethesda, MD.

[24] DeSantis, C.E., et al., *Breast cancer statistics, 2015: Convergence of incidence rates between black and white women.* CA Cancer J Clin, 2016. **66**(1): 31–42.

[25] Salim, O.H., et al., *Breast cancer in Africa, are we dealing with a different disease.* Sudan Med J 2014. **50**(1): 1–12.

[26] Sudan Demographic and Health Survey, *Sudan Demographic and Health Survey 1989/1990.* 1991, Department of Statistics, Ministry of Economic and National Planning, Khartoum, Sudan and Institute for Resource Development/Macro International, Inc., Columbia, Maryland, USA: Khartoum, Sudan. p. 1–145.

[27] The Republic of Sudan, *Country Report, The Fourth Meeting of the Follow-up Committee on the Implementation of Dakar/Ngor Declaration and the Programme of Action of the International Conference on Population and Development, 28–31 January*. 2002: 1–16.

[28] Ikpatt, O.F., et al., *Breast cancer in Nigeria and Finland: epidemiological, clinical and histological comparison.* Anticancer Res, 2002. **22**(5): 3005–12.

[29] Morris, K., *Cancer? In Africa?* Lancet Oncol, 2003. **4**(1): 5.

[30] Gondos, A., et al., *Cancer survival in Kampala, Uganda.* Br J Cancer, 2005. **92**(9): 1808–12.

[31] Hamad, H.M., *Cancer initiatives in Sudan.* Ann Oncol, 2006. **17 Suppl 8**: viii32–viii36.

[32] Kerr, F. and D. Kerr, *Do we bear any moral responsibility for improving cancer care in Africa?* Ann Oncol, 2006. **17**(12): 1730–1.

[33] Awadelkarim, K.D., et al., *Pathological, clinical and prognostic characteristics of breast cancer in Central Sudan versus Northern Italy: implications for breast cancer in Africa.* Histopathology, 2008. **52**(4): 445–56.

[34] Biunno, I., et al., *BRCA1 point mutations in premenopausal breast cancer patients from Central Sudan.* Fam Cancer, 2014. **13**(3): 437–44.

[35] Swanson, G.M., and Chen-Sheng Lin., *Survival patterns among younger women with breast cancer: the effects of age, race, stage, and treatment.* J Nat Cancer Inst 1993. **Monographs, 16**: 69–77.

[36] Amir, H., et al., *TNM classification and breast cancer in an African population: a descriptive study.* Cent Afr J Med, 1997. **43**(12): 357–9.

[37] Ekortarl, A., P. Ndom, and A. Sacks, *A study of patients who appear with far advanced cancer at Yaounde General Hospital, Cameroon, Africa.* Psychooncology, 2007. **16**(3): 255–7.

[38] Sarre, B., et al., *Epidemiological, therapeutic and prognostic aspects of breast cancer: about 473 cases collected in Hopital Principal de Dakar.* Dakar Med, 2006. **51**(2): 92–6.

[39] Elgaili, E.M., et al., *Breast cancer burden in central Sudan.* Int J Womens Health, 2010. **2**: 77–82.

[40] Huo, D., et al., *Population differences in breast cancer: survey in indigenous African women reveals over-representation of triple-negative breast cancer.* J Clin Oncol, 2009. **27**(27): 4515–21.

[41] Sant, M., et al., *Breast carcinoma survival in Europe and the United States.* Cancer, 2004. **100**(4): 715–22.

[42] Awadelkarim, K.D., A.A. Mohamedani, and M. Barberis, *Role of pathology in Sub-Saharan Africa: an example from Sudan.* Pathol Lab Med Int, 2010. **2**: 49–57.

[43] Mariani-Costantini, R., et al., *Building Sustainable Capacity for Disease Diagnosis in Sub-Saharan Africa: Case Studies of Cooperation in Diagnostic Pathology*, in *New Knowledge in a New Era of Globalization*, P. Pachura, Editor. 2011, InTech Open Access Publisher Rijeka: Croatia. p. 243–266.

[44] Perou, C.M., et al., *Molecular portraits of human breast tumours.* Nature, 2000. **406**(6797): 747–52.

[45] Sorlie, T., et al., *Gene expression patterns of breast carcinomas distinguish tumor subclasses with clinical implications.* Proc Natl Acad Sci U S A, 2001. **98**(19): 10869–74.

[46] Sorlie, T., et al., *Repeated observation of breast tumor subtypes in independent gene expression data sets.* Proc Natl Acad Sci U S A, 2003. **100**(14): 8418–23.

[47] Agboola, A.J., et al., *Molecular characteristics and prognostic features of breast cancer in Nigerian compared with UK women.* Breast Cancer Res Treat, 2012. **135**(2): 555–69.

[48] Carey, L.A., et al., *Race, breast cancer subtypes, and survival in the Carolina Breast Cancer Study.* Jama, 2006. **295**(21): 2492–502.

[49] Awadelkarim, K.D., et al., *Basal-like phenotype in a breast carcinoma case series from Sudan: prevalence and clinical/pathological correlations.* Pathol Res Int, 2011. **2011 (Article ID: 806831)**: 1–10.

[50] Adebamowo, C.A., et al., *Immunohistochemical and molecular subtypes of breast cancer in Nigeria.* Breast Cancer Res Treat, 2008. **110**(1): 183–8.

[51] Mbonde, M.P., et al., *Expression of estrogen and progesterone receptors in carcinomas of the female breast in Tanzania.* Oncol Rep, 2000. **7**(2): 277–83.

[52] Burson, A.M., et al., *Clinical and epidemiologic profile of breast cancer in Tanzania.* Breast Dis, 2010. **31**(1): 33–41.

[53] Ikpatt, O.F. and R. Ndoma-Egba, *Oestrogen and progesterone receptors in Nigerian breast cancer: relationship to tumour histopathology and survival of patients.* Cent Afr J Med, 2003. **49**(11-12): 122–6.

[54] Bird, P.A., A.G. Hill, and N. Houssami, *Poor hormone receptor expression in East African breast cancer: evidence of a biologically different disease?* Ann Surg Oncol, 2008. **15**(7): 1983–8.

[55] Raina, V., et al., *Clinical features and prognostic factors of early breast cancer at a major cancer center in North India. 2005;42.* Indian J Cancer, 2005. **42**: 40–45.

[56] Albain, K.S., D.C. Allred, and G.M. Clark, *Breast cancer outcome and predictors of outcome: are there age differentials?* J Natl Cancer Inst Monogr, 1994(16): 35–42.

[57] Kroman N1, J.M., Wohlfahrt J, Mouridsen HT, Andersen PK, Melbye M., *Factors influencing the effect of age on prognosis in breast cancer: population based study.* BMJ, 2000. **320**(7233): 474–479.

[58] Eng, A., V. McCormack, and I. dos-Santos-Silva, *Receptor-defined subtypes of breast cancer in indigenous populations in Africa: a systematic review and meta-analysis.* PLoS Med, 2014. **11**(9): e1001720.

[59] Mohammed, S.I. and J.B. Harford, *Sorting reality from what we think we know about breast cancer in Africa.* PLoS Med, 2014. **11**(9): e1001721.

[60] Awadelkarim, K.D., et al., *Ki-67 labeling index in primary invasive breast cancer from Sudanese patients: a pilot study.* ISRN Pathol, 2012. **2012 (Article ID: 232171)**: 1–6.

[61] Elhaj, A., A.I. Ismaeel, and K.D. Awadelkarim, *Male breast cancer patients: a retrospective study of patients characteristics and treatment outcome at the National Cancer Institute (NCI-UG)—Central Sudan.* Pan Arab J Oncol, 2012. **5**(1): 18–22.

[62] Pant, K. and U. Dutta, *Understanding and management of male breast cancer: a critical review.* Med Oncol, 2008. **25**(3): 294–8.

[63] Niewoehner, C.B. and A.E. Schorer, *Gynaecomastia and breast cancer in men.* BMJ, 2008. **336**(7646): 709–13.

[64] Awadelkarim, K.D., et al., *BRCA1 and BRCA2 status in a Central Sudanese series of breast cancer patients: interactions with genetic, ethnic and reproductive factors.* Breast Cancer Res Treat, 2007. **102**(2): 189–99.

[65] Fackenthal, J.D. and O.I. Olopade, *Breast cancer risk associated with BRCA1 and BRCA2 in diverse populations.* Nat Rev Cancer, 2007. **7**(12): 937–48.

[66] Oluwagbemiga, L.A., A. Oluwole, and A.A. Kayode, *Seventeen years after BRCA1: What is the BRCA mutation status of the breast cancer patients in Africa?—a systematic review.* Springerplus, 2013. **1**(1): 83.

[67] Masri, M.A., et al., *Minor role for BRCA2 (exon11) and p53 (exon 5-9) among Sudanese breast cancer patients.* Breast Cancer Res Treat, 2002. **71**(2): 145–7.

[68] Khairy, G.A., et al., *Bilateral breast cancer. Incidence, diagnosis and histological patterns.* Saudi Med J, 2005. **26**(4): 612–5.

[69] Siddig, A., et al., *Estrogen receptor alpha gene polymorphism and breast cancer.* Ann N Y Acad Sci, 2008. **1138**: 95–107.

[70] Siddig, A., et al., *HER-2/neu Ile655Val polymorphism and the risk of breast cancer.* Ann N Y Acad Sci, 2008. **1138**: 84–94.

[71] Yahia, Z.A., et al., *Epstein Barr virus: a prime candidate of breast cancer aetiology in Sudanese patients.* Infect Agent Cancer, 2014. **9**(1): 9.

[72] Fletcher, S.W. and J.G. Elmore, *Clinical practice. Mammographic screening for breast cancer.* N Engl J Med, 2003. **348**(17): 1672–80.

[73] Galukande, M. and E. Kiguli-Malwadde, *Rethinking breast cancer screening strategies in resource-limited settings.* Afr Health Sci, 2010. **10**(1): 89–92.

[74] Harford, J.B., *Breast-cancer early detection in low-income and middle-income countries: do what you can versus one size fits all.* Lancet Oncol, 2011. **12**(3): 306–12.

[75] Yip, C.H., et al., *Guideline implementation for breast healthcare in low- and middle-income countries: early detection resource allocation.* Cancer, 2008. **113**(8 Suppl): 2244–56.

[76] WHO Position Paper on Mammography Screening, in *WHO Guidelines Approved by the Guidelines Review Committee*. 2014: Geneva.

[77] AbdElrahman, S.H. and M.A.A. Yousif, *Self examination of the breast for early detection of breast cancer: the role of medical students in the faculty of medicine – University of Gezira – Sudan*. Sudanese J Publ Health, 2006. **1**(1): 36–42.

[78] AbdElrahman, S.H., I.M. Elbashir, and A.A. Mohamadani, *The prevention of cancer through community-based interventionS (CBIS) in low-resource populations in Gezira state, Central Sudan*, in *27th Annual Meeting of the Internal Association of Cancer Registries*. 2005: Entebbe, Uganda.

[79] Abuidris, D.O., et al., *Breast-cancer screening with trained volunteers in a rural area of Sudan: a pilot study*. Lancet Oncol, 2013. **14**(4): 363–70.

[80] Elhaj, A.M., A.A. Elshaikh, and A.A. Mohammadani, *National guidelines for management of breast cancer: for enforcement or persuasion?* Sudan Med J, 2012. **48**(3): 213–218.

[81] Awadelkarim, K.D., et al., *Tissue microarray (TMA) versus whole section immunohistochemistry in the assessment of ER/PR and Her-2/neu status in a breast cancer series from Sudan*. Breast J, 2013.

[82] Fisher, B., et al., *Twenty-year follow-up of a randomized trial comparing total mastectomy, lumpectomy, and lumpectomy plus irradiation for the treatment of invasive breast cancer*. N Engl J Med, 2002. **347**(16): 1233–41.

[83] van Dongen, J.A., et al., *Long-term results of a randomized trial comparing breast-conserving therapy with mastectomy: European Organization for Research and Treatment of Cancer 10801 trial*. J Natl Cancer Inst, 2000. **92**(14): 1143–50.

[84] Veronesi, U., et al., *Twenty-year follow-up of a randomized study comparing breast-conserving surgery with radical mastectomy for early breast cancer*. N Engl J Med, 2002. **347**(16): 1227–32.

[85] Preker, A., et al., *Scaling up health professional education: opportunities and challenges for Africa*, in *Force for Scaling Up Education and Training for Health Workers, Global Health Workforce Alliance, World Bank*, 2008: Washington, D.C.

[86] Deantonio, L., et al., *Hypofractionated radiation therapy for breast cancer: Long-term results in a series of 85 patients*. Tumori, 2016: 0.

[87] Whelan, T.J., et al., *Long-term results of hypofractionated radiation therapy for breast cancer*. N Engl J Med, 2010. **362**(6): 513–20.

[88] Wolff, A.C., et al., *American Society of Clinical Oncology/College of American Pathologists guideline recommendations for human epidermal growth factor receptor 2 testing in breast cancer*. Arch Pathol Lab Med, 2007. **131**(1): 18–43.

[89] Parkin, D.M., et al., *Changing cancer incidence in Kampala, Uganda, 1991-2006*. Int J Cancer. **126**(5): 1187–95.

[90] Nyagol, J., et al., *Routine assessment of hormonal receptor and her-2/neu status underscores the need for more therapeutic targets in Kenyan women with breast cancer.* Anal Quant Cytol Histol, 2006. **28**(2): 97–103.

[91] Oluwatosin, O.A., *Rural women's perception of breast cancer and its early-detection measures in Ibadan, Nigeria.* Cancer Nurs, 2006. **29**(6): 461–6.

[92] Dye, T.D., et al., *Complex care systems in developing countries: breast cancer patient navigation in Ethiopia.* Cancer. **116**(3): 577–85.

[93] Awadelkarim, K.D., *Research infrastructure: use foreign aid to help African science.* Nature, 2013. **495**(7440): 174.

Chapter 2

Histopathological Characteristics: Clinical Course of Breast Cancer Subtypes Depending on the ER(+) (–)/ PR(+) (–) Receptor Status

Nilufer Bulut

Additional information is available at the end of the chapter

http://dx.doi.org/10.5772/66176

Abstract

Breast cancer patients were divided into separate groups, which were the estrogen receptor (ER)+/progesterone receptor (PR)+ HER2–, the ER or PR+ HER2–, the ER+/ PR+ HER2+, the ER or PR+ HER2+, the ER–/PR– HER2–, and the ER–/PR– HER2+ groups. Patients with the ER/PR(+)/HER2– subtype breast cancers show better clinical prognosis compared to the hormone-negative, triple-negative (TN), and HER2+ subtypes. TN, HER2+ tumors in postmenopausal women were of higher grade, showing lymph node and lymphovascular invasion with poor prognosis in all case series. However, the ER+/PR–/HER2+ subgroup had the lowest survival rates in 2- and 5-year follow-ups. Comparison between the ER+PR+HER2+ and ER+PR–HER2– subgroups showed that HER2– status is an indicator of improved prognosis in long-term follow-up. Single hormone receptor (HR)(+) status, particularly HER2(–) cases, was in between the favorable and poor survival subgroups. The ER–, PR–, and HER2+ properties were found to be risk factors for frequent recurrences. In this chapter, breast cancer subtypes are compared with each other. Results from different studies highlight the importance of ER/PR/HER2 receptor variations in the choice of treatment and prognosis of breast cancer

Keywords: breast cancer subtype, estrogen/progesterone receptor, survival, treatment

1. Introduction

Breast cancer is common among women between the ages of 50 and 60 years and is one of the leading causes of disease-related deaths [1]. There is no single marker that determines the clinical properties and treatment of breast cancer. The main factors affecting the choice of treatment, prognosis of the disease, and the predictability of the tumor include size, invasion into the lymph nodes, lymphovascular invasion (LVI), grade, age at diagnosis, menopausal status, surgical margins, estrogen and progesterone receptors (ER/PR), and HER2 oncogene [2–7].

About 70% of all breast cancers are hormone receptor (HR)-positive [4]. PR is the gene which regulates estrogen, and single hormone receptor positivity increases aggressiveness compared to ER+PR+ tumors, and is an indicator of poor prognosis [4]. Receptor positivity is often inversely related to the presence of HER2 oncogene [6]. ER/PR-negative HER2+ tumors, high grade, large tumor volume, and invasion into the lymph nodes indicate the need for an aggressive course of treatment [6]. Hormone receptor positivity is responsive to hormonal treatment, while HER2 positivity is responsive to trastuzumab treatment, and this helps guide clinicians in the optimal choice of treatment. Recently developed diagnostic methods, the definition of subtypes, goal-directed therapy, intensive chemotherapy, and hormonal therapies have increased the survival rates in breast cancers.

The biological properties of breast cancers tend to vary depending on ER, PR, and HER2 expression [5]. Breast cancers are divided into four subgroups based on ER and PR gene heterogeneity: luminal A (ER or PR+, HER2-negative), luminal B (ER- or PR-positive, HER2-positive), ER-PR-HER2-positive, and triple-negative (ER-PR-HER2−) types [8].

Adjuvant endocrine therapy and/or chemotherapy are given in luminal A (HR+/HER2−) cancers depending on tumor volume, lymph node status, and 21-gene recurrence score [9]. On the other hand, luminal B (HR+/HER2+) tumors are more aggressive, and anthracycline- and trastuzumab-based multichemotherapeutic agents are preferred in their treatment [9]. In luminal cancers, short-term prognosis and response to hormonal therapy are better compared to the other subgroups [9].

Luminal A tumors show the best progression, while TN tumors have the worst [10]. Luminal B type exhibits poor ER expression compared to luminal A tumors. The possibility of early relapse is also higher than with luminal A tumor [8]. With luminal B tumors, insensitivity to endocrine treatment is also higher than with HR+/HER2−, while chemotherapy resistance is more frequent than with TN and HER2+ tumors [8]. Invasion into the lymph nodes is also more common in luminal B tumors compared to that in luminal A [11, 12].

Triple negative and HER2 (+) breast cancers also exhibit poor clinical features and prognosis [13]. Recurrence and metastasis rates in TN breast cancers are particularly higher than in other subgroups due to their high grade and proliferative properties [13].

The aim of this section is to divide breast cancers into subgroups based on their receptor status, to compare ER (+) breast cancers with other subgroups (ER-PR+/− HER2+/−, ER-PR− HER2−, and ER-PR-HER2+), to determine the risk factors affecting the prognosis of the disease, and to compare the overall survival (OS) periods. Aside from the aforementioned risk factors, the study also aimed to evaluate the effects of the ER and PR status on tumor characteristics, as well as their impact on prognosis during long-term follow-up. Furthermore, the study emphasized that multiple chemotherapy combined with hormonal treatment cannot ensure the expected survival rates in the HR+ patients.

2. Clinical features and differences of tumor subgroups

The clinical, histopathological, and genetic subtypes of patients with breast cancer are important in the prognosis of the disease and in the choice of chemotherapy. Breast cancers have a considerably heterogeneous structure, and they are divided into at least four subtypes. Among these, luminal A cancers have the best prognosis, whereas TN and ER-PR-HER2+ subgroups possess the poorest prognosis. The prognosis of ER or PR (+) HER2 (+) luminal B subtype falls somewhat in between these subgroups. ER+PR-HER2− tumors, in particular, are associated with aggressive biology, hormonal treatment unresponsiveness resulting from PR gene loss, and resistance to chemotherapy [8]. PR negativity is related to a high relapse rate despite chemotherapy and endocrine treatment. However, in a meta-analysis performed by Early Breast Cancer Trialists' Collaborative Group (EGCTCG), hormonal treatment administration in ER(+) tumors regardless of the PR status was shown to improve the disease-free survival (DFS) [8].

ER positivity is a good predictive factor for the effectiveness of hormonal treatment, and 5-year hormonal therapy decreases the mortality rate by 5.6% [7]. In a previous study, prognosis in the first 3 years of ER(+) tumors was shown to be good, although survival in the longer term was fairly poor. Gradually, endocrine therapy resistance is the main factor that blocks the success of hormonal treatment [14].

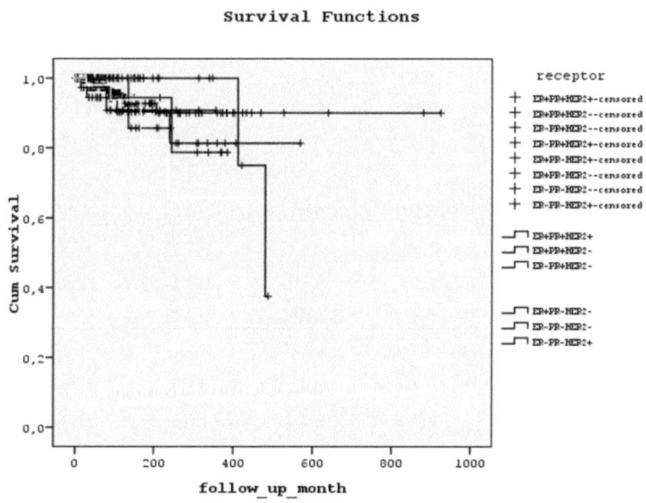

Figure 1. Analysis of overall survival of breast cancer subtypes by log-rank test [15].

Chemotherapy in HR-negative patients is known to improve DFS and OS [7]. In one study where HR+ patients with early-stage breast cancer received chemotherapy followed by subsequent 5-year hormonal treatment, the best survival rates were observed in the ER+/PR +HER2− and ER+/PR-HER2− subgroups (2-, 5-, and 10-year survival rates for these two groups were 96%, 83%, 68% and 87%, 81%, 81%, respectively). The shortest survival was observed in the ER+PR− and HER2+ cases (2-, 5-, and 10-year survival: 66, 33, and 0%, respectively), followed by TN (2-, 5-, and 10-year survival: 71, 64, and 64%, respectively) and HER2+ (2-, 5-, and 10-year survival: 82, 71, and 0%, respectively) cases. ER+PR+HER2− cases exhibited the longest survival (2-, 5-, and 10-year survival: 96, 83, and 68%, respectively). Meanwhile, single HR+/HER2+ cases (2-, 5-, and 10-year survival: 90, 90, and 0%, respectively) and HER2− cases (2-, 5-, and 10-year survival: 92, 92, and 46%, respectively) were found to have survival rates in between those of other subgroups [15] (**Figure 1** and **Table 1**). However, Bae et al. [4] surprisingly demonstrated that PR(+) tumors have poor prognosis compared to PR(−) tumors.

	ER+PR+ HER2− *N* = 1360 (47.7%)	**ER-PR+ HER2− *N* = 76 (2.7%)**	**ER+PR− HER2− *N* = 150 (5.3%)**	**ER+PR+ HER2+ *N* = 221 (7.8%)**	**ER-PR+ HER2+ *N* = 44 (1.5%)**	**ER+PR− HER2+ *N* = 59 (2.1%)**	**ER-PR− HER2− *N* = 311 (10.9%)**	**ER-PR− HER2+ *N* = 220 (7.7%)**	***p*-Value**
Age									
≤40	4.0%	0.3%	0.5%	1.1%	0.1%	0.2%	1.3%	0.8%	0.001
41-59	26.8%	1.7%	2.1%	4.8%	0.9%	1.0%	5.9%	3.7%	
≥60	17%	0.7%	2.7%	1.9%	0.5%	0.8%	3.7%	3.2%	
Menopause									
Pre	23.9%	1.4%	1.4%	4.3%	0.7%	0.8%	5.4%	3.5%	0.001
Peri	2.9%	0.2%	0.3%	0.6%	0.1%	0.2%	0.7%	0.6%	
Post	20.7%	1.0%	3.5%	2.8%	0.7%	1.1%	4.9%	3.7%	
Stage									
I	12%	0.4%	1.0%	1.2%	0.1%	0.3%	1.9%	0.9%	0.001
II	19.1%	1.1%	1.7%	2.8%	0.4%	0.7%	4.9%	2.1%	
III	10%	0.6%	1.5%	2.4%	0.5%	0.8%	2.1%	2.7%	
IV	7.1%	0.5%	1.2%	1.5%	0.5%	0.3%	2.2%	2.0%	
Lymph node									
N0	23.1%	1.2%	2.1%	3.1%	0.2%	0.8%	5.4%	2.2%	0.001
N1	14.4%	0.8%	1.9%	2.1%	0.6%	0.5%	3.3%	2.1%	
N2	6.6%	0.6%	0.8%	1.3%	0.3%	0.4%	1.5%	1.5%	
N3	4.4%	0.2%	0.6%	1.6%	0.4%	0.4%	1.2%	2.0%	
Grade									
I	8.8%	0.2%	0.6%	0.3%	0%	0.1%	0.2%	0.2%	0.001
II	27.5%	0.7%	2.9%	3.2%	0.4%	1.0%	2.4%	2.6%	
III	17.3%	1.8%	2.1%	4.7%	1.2%	1.1%	8.8%	5.4%	
Lymphovascular invasion (LVI)									
Yes	30.4%	1.9%	3.4%	7.1%	1.3%	1.9%	7.1%	7.6%	0.001
No	17.7%	0.8%	2.4%	3.3%	0.9%	0.4%	4.2%	2.1%	
Survival									
2 y	96%	92%	87%	97%	90%	66%	71%	82%	0.001
5 y	83%	92%	81%	86%	90%	33%	64%	71%	
10 y	68%	46%	81%	46%	0%	0%	64%	0%	

Table 1. Subtype features and clinical course of breast cancer [15].

In a previous study, it was determined that 1974 patients (69.3%), including those with lymph node invasion or who underwent breast-protective surgery, were treated with radiotherapy [15], while a total of 2797 patients received chemotherapy and/or hormonal therapy. Hormonal therapy included tamoxifen and aromatase inhibitors or switch combinations. Patients received chemotherapy regimens combined with endoxan, anthracycline, fluorouracil, taxane, trastuzumab, platine, cyclophosphamide, and methotrexate [15]. In another study, it was determined that, compared to the HR+ subtype, the HR− subtype is less commonly treatable by surgery, and more often treated through radiotherapy [16]. Nowadays, the main treatment for HR− tumors is surgery, radiotherapy, and chemotherapy [16]. The different treatment options that are available, as well as racial reasons and tumor subgroups, help explain the observed differences in survival rates [16].

2.1. Demographic and ethnic characteristics

Luminal A (ER-PR+)-type tumors are large volume and advanced stage tumors that are more common among young women of nonhispanic, black, and hispanic races [9]. Luminal B (ER+/PR+ or PR−) tumors, on the other hand, are high-incidence tumors that are observed among young people of nonhispanic, Asian, and hispanic races [9]. When the ER+PR− and ER+PR+ subgroups are compared independently of the HER2 status, it can be seen that ER-PR+ tumors are generally observed among women less than 50 years old, and that these tumors are generally advanced stage upon diagnosis. However, these tumors also have a low incidence among women of nonhispanic, white race. ER-PR+ subtype occurrence is higher among nonhispanic black women. Compared with nonhispanic white women, ER-PR+ subtype among nonhispanic black women also exhibits poorer prognosis [9]. Thus, the heterogeneity in genes also affects prognosis.

The location of the tumor, as well as tumor stage, and the presence of axillary lymph node involvement are all closely interrelated with breast cancer subtypes [17]. Luminal A tumors show the highest axillaries lymph involvement [17]. Late identification of tumor hypothetically explains the high mortality rate [17]. In one study, a relationship between the location and type of tumor was identified, and luminal A tumors were found to frequently occur in the upper outer quadrant of the breast [17]. Again, oral contraceptive use was found to be meaningfully associated with breast cancer subtype. Oral contraceptive use was observed more frequently in the luminal A group compared with the luminal B, basal, and HER2(+) groups [17]. While ovarian hormones and reproductive pattern appear in many studies to play a significant role in breast cancer growth, another study performed on 1326 Mexican women described that the number of pregnancies, gestational age, and menopause status were not risk factors for breast cancer [17].

Luminal A tumors are commonly observed among high-income, nonhispanic black race women living in cities. Compared with the ER+PR+ subtype, the incidence of the ER-PR+ is 1.7 times higher among individuals under the age of 50 [9]. The clinic and demographic characteristics of luminal A and B subtypes are different [9]. These differences are due to the effects of estrogen and progesterone in tumor progression [9]. Estrogen suppresses progression, while progesterone causes tumors to progress aggressively. In ER(−) tumors, high progesterone levels cannot be balanced by the estrogen levels, and this leads to the progression of the tumor [9].

A limited number of studies have researched the relationship between subtype of breast cancer and the socioeconomic and health-care conditions of the patients [16]. The study determined that good health care is closely associated with higher socioeconomic conditions, and that living in larger cities it facilitates patients' access to and compliance with treatment [16].

2.2. Prognosis, survival, and risk factors that affect them

In one study population, ER-PR+HER2 (+)/(−) patients showed poorer survival compared to the ER+PR+HER2 (+)/(−) group [15]. Similarly, other studies showed PR-HER2+ tumors to have high recurrence scores [18]. Recurrence risk (RR) in the ER-PR+ and ER+PR− tumors was determined as 2.1 and 1.4%, respectively [19]. Single hormone receptor positivity results in a poor prognosis and affects treatment response [20]. Additionally, lymph node invasion is seen more frequently in luminal B tumors compared to luminal A tumors, and is associated with poor prognosis [11]. A high Ki-67 index is characterized by lower patient age, larger tumor volume, positive lymph nodes, ER/PR negativity, and HER2 positivity [11, 13, 20, 21].

In most studies, TN and HER2+ tumors showed the poorest survival rates [22, 23]. In a study by You et al. [1], early-stage tumors without lymph node invasion and with improved histological appearance resulted in better survivals in all molecular subtypes. High-stage disease and HR negativity were associated with poor survival rates. As HR (−) subtypes develop and advance more rapidly than HR (+) tumors, they are usually detected in advanced stages [16]. Breast cancer mortality in HR (−) subtypes is two times more than HR (+) subtypes (HR: 1.91; 95% confidence interval (CI): 1.88–1.94) [16]. TN cases have the lowest survival rates, with 5- and 10-year survival being 63 and 44%, respectively [20].

In one study, both ER+PR-HER2+ and ER-PR-HER2+ subgroups received combined regimens such as trastuzumab and anthracycline/or taxane, carboplatine chemotherapies. However, the study found that ER+PR− leads to poorer prognosis with these treatment regimens. This result may have been due to the following factors: choice of treatment not being specific enough for the group, or not applied in sufficient or equal numbers, unresponsiveness to hormonal maintenance treatment due to ER positivity, small number of patients, and response to chemotherapy that varies according to the intrinsic profile of the tumor and HER2 positivity [5, 12, 15, 24].

The longer survival rate of ER+PR+/HER2 (+)(−) tumors compared to HER2+ and TN− tumors is due to their early-stage detection, absence of lymph node invasion, and the ability to administer hormonal treatment for at least 5 years (aromatase inhibitor following 2- or 3-year tamoxifen therapy) in addition to a combined chemotherapy regimen, no matter what the intrinsic profile of the tumor is.

In some studies, HR+HER2− tumors were found to have shorter OS and DFS periods, while their overall recurrence was more frequent than the single HR+HER2+ luminal B tumors [12]. Ki-67 indices of these tumors were high due to their high-grade property and lymph node invasion. Although HER2 positivity is a criterion of poor prognosis, anti-HER2 treatments may decrease the negative effects of this factor. Thus, high Ki-67 index in ER+ tumors is an important criterion which determines prognosis [12]. Additionally, 25–50% of ER+PR+ tumors are resistant to hormonal treatment. Genetic and non-genetic interferences between the ER and growth factors may lead to hormone resistance [14], but the exact mechanism that is implicated has not yet been understood. Genetic testing is not commonly performed to determine tumor subtypes or select treatment, and treatment alternatives are usually applied based on the receptor and clinicopathological data. However, genetic variations and ethnic differences may alter the prognosis of the disease [25]. Consequently, different response rates have been observed in many of the studies. These findings suggest that oncogenes in different pathways should be investigated to further improve treatment alternatives.

One study evaluated ER+, ER-PR+, TN, and HER2+ patients who were mostly premenopausal. As such, 54.1% of the patients in the study were premenopausal, while 45.1% were postmenopausal. In other studies, triple-negative breast cancer (TNBC) or PR− subtypes were found to be more frequent in postmenopausal women [2, 15, 26]. PR-negative breast cancers are frequently observed during the postmenopausal period. Some studies have shown that, due to the higher level of progesterone in premenopausal women, the incidence of ER-PR+ subtypes is considerably higher among individuals under the age of 50 [9]. The high levels of progesterone increase the invasiveness of breast cancer cells, and hence the risk of metastasis in premenopausal patients [9].

The initial metastatic site was bone in the HR+ (56.5%) patients, followed by liver, lung, and multiple organ invasions. In TN (12.9%) and HER2+ patients (11.5%), the disease progressed into multiple organ metastases. Recurrences were observed at the following rates in different tumor subtypes: in 215 (44.9%) of the patients with luminal A tumors, in 56 (11.6%) of the patients with luminal B tumors, in 61 (12.9%) of the patients with TN tumors, and in 54 (11.5%) of the patients with HER2+ tumors [15]. When HR+/HER2(+)(−) patients were compared to ER-PR-HER2− and ER-PR-HER2+ patients, the TN and HER2+ patients were found to be mostly postmenopausal, N+, high-stage and high-grade ($p = 0.001$) (**Table 2**) [15]. Each increase of age by a decade also raised the risk of recurrence (RR = 0.4, 95% CI, 0.3–0.6, $p = 0.001$) (**Table 2**). High-stage, high-grade tumors with node positivity and LVI showed higher recurrence risk. ER negativity led to a 1.5-fold increase in recurrence risk (RR = 1.5, 95% CI, 1.3–1.9, $p = 0.001$), while PR negativity led to a 1.4 fold increase (RR = 1.4, 95% CI, 1.2–1.8, $p = 0.001$) (**Table 2**). HER2 positivity (RR = 0.7, 95% CI, 0.6–0.9, $p = 0.025$) was also associated with a higher recurrence risk.

However, the Carolina Breast Cancer Study Group did not identify any differences in menopausal status between the molecular subtypes [2]. Devi et al. [26] reported high frequency of TNBC among postmenopausal women, which may have been due to ethnic differences and gene heterogeneity. Jenkins et al. [3] also reported increased luminal A and B tumors and decreased basal-like tumors with increasing age. TN and the basal-like subtype are particularly more common in the young population, whereas the HR+/HER2+ luminal B subtype is more frequent in patients above 60 years of age [3].

	RR	95% CI	*p*-Value
Age			
41–59/<40	0.6	0.4–0.8	**0.003**
>60/<40	0.4	0.3–0.6	**0.001**
Stage (2,3,4)/1			
3/1	2.1	0.3–15	**0.027**
2/1	0.4	0.2–0.9	**0.040**
Grade (III/II)/I			
III/I	1.7	1.1–2.6	**0.014**
II/I	1.2	0.8–1.9	0.311
LVI (yes/no)	0.6	0.5–0.8	**0.003**
Node (3,2,1/0)			
3/0	1.8	1.4	**0.001**
2/0	1.6	1.2–2.1	**0.001**
1/0	1.1	0.8–1.4	0.386
ER negative	1.5	1.3–1.9	**0.001**
PR negative	1.4	1.2–1.8	**0.001**
HER2 positive	0.7	0.6–0.9	**0.025**

Table 2. Univariate Cox-regression analysis of factors associated with recurrence in patients with subgroups [15].

Furthermore, PR negativity is not related with age and menopausal status; however, it is associated with high grade and proliferation index [8]. Ki-67 index is described as being more than 30% in ER+PR-HER2− tumors ($p = 0.006$) [8]. Epidermal growth factor (EGFR) expression is higher in PR− tumors [4]. PR negativity in our patients resulted in different survival rates depending on the HER2+/− status (2-, 5-, and 10-year survival being 66%, 33%, 0% and 87%, 81%, 81%, respectively) [15]. In addition, ER-PR+ tumors had poorer prognosis compared to ER+PR+ tumors. ER-PR+ tumor incidence has been reported as 1.5–3.4% [4]. In addition, ER-PR+ and ER+PR− tumor incidences were reported to be 4.2 and 7.4%, respectively. Altogether, ER+PR+HER2− tumors were the most frequent in younger women below 40 years of age, and in older women above 60 years of age (4.0 and 17.0%, respectively).

HR+ tumors have often lower grade compared to TN and HER2+ subgroups, showing a slow progression in the long term [27]. Recurrence in these slowly enlarging tumors after a 10-year follow-up appears to be associated with the 5–10-year hormonal treatments that continue after chemotherapy. In ER+HER2− tumors, the mortality rate increases in the 10–15-year follow-ups [27].

In one study, HER2 positivity was found to be 7.8% in ER+PR+ patients and 3.6% in patients with single HR positivity. This ratio was found to vary from 10 to 20% in other studies [15, 21, 28]. In agreement with the findings of other studies, we observed similar survival rates in ER +HER2+ and ER+HER2− groups, despite HER2 positivity [29]. When luminal A (mean survival: 5030 day) and luminal B (mean survival:4718 day) patients were compared, HER2+ (mean survival:3149 day) patients were found to have lower survival rates (**Figure 2** and **Table 3**).

The California Breast Cancer Study Group also reported the highest mortality rates for ER-HER2+ tumors in the 10-year or longer follow-up [29].

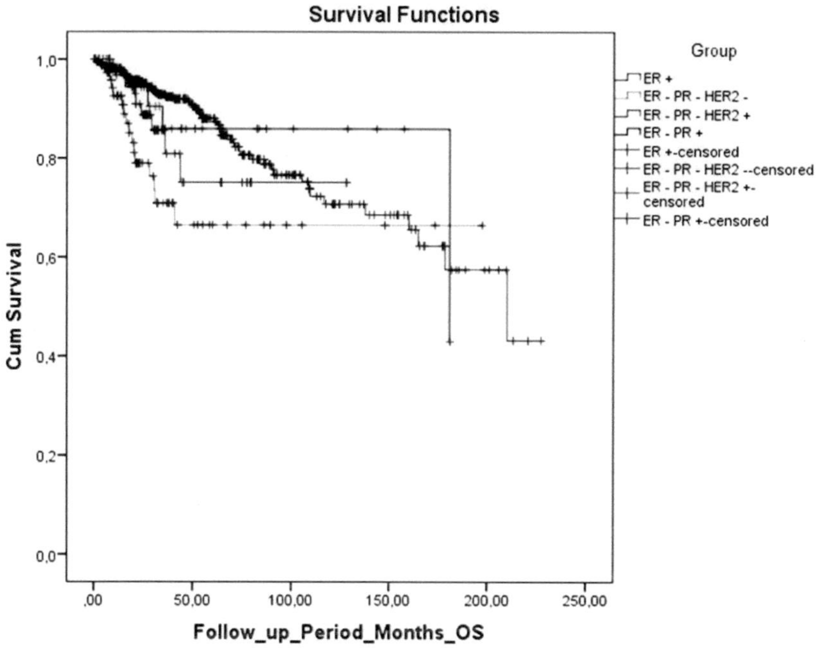

Figure 2. Analysis of overall survival of breast cancer subtypes by Kaplan-Meier. ER+ cases were determined to have longer survival rates when compared to non-luminal HER2+, HR-HER2–, and luminal B tumors. HER2+, HR-HER2–, and luminal B tumors [15].

	Number of patients	Number of case observed	Percent of case observed	Mean survival (day)	*P*-value
ER+	396	57	85.6	5030.747	**0.010***
ER-PR+	78	5	86.5	4718.160	
HER2+	37	9	87.0	3149.519	
TN	69	16	79.5	4150.100	
Total	**580**	**87**	**85%**	**4940.640**	

* HER2+ patients were found to have lower survival rates than others $p<0.05$

Table 3. Survival analysis of tumor subgroups [15].

3. Conclusion

HR+ tumors are the most frequently observed breast cancer subtype. ER+PR– and ER-PR+ tumors have a particularly poorer prognosis compared to the ER+PR+ subtypes. In addition to the poor prognosis factor (i.e., due to HER2 positivity), being ER− or PR− may further reduce the tumor's treatment responsiveness and survival, while increasing the risk of recurrence. In the clinical practice, the receptor status of the tumor should be determined to elucidate the intrinsic gene profile of the tumor, as this will assist and provide guidance in choosing the appropriate treatment.

Abbreviations

EGFR	epidermal growth factor
EGCTCG	early breast cancer trialists
ER	estrogen receptor
DFS	disease-free survival
HR	hormone receptor
LVI	lymphovascular invasion
OS	overall survival
PR	progesterone receptor
RR	recurrence risk
TNBC	triple-negative breast cancer

Author details

Nilufer Bulut

Address all correspondence to: ferlut@hotmail.com

Kanuni Sultan Suleyman Education and Search Hospital, Istanbul, Turkey

References

[1] You JM., Kim YG., Moon HG., Nam SJ., Lee JW., Lim W., et al. Survival improvement in Korean breast cancer patients due to increases in early-stage cancers and hormone receptor positive/HER2 negative subtypes: A nationwide registry-based study. J Breast Cancer 2015; 18(1): 8–15.

[2] Song Q., Huang R., Li J., Fan J., Zheng S., Zhang B, et al. The diverse distribution of risk factors between breast cancer subtypes of ER, PR and HER2: A 10-year retrospective multi-center study in China. PLoS One 2013;8:1–7.

[3] Jenkins EO., Deal AM., Anders CK., Prat A., Perou CM., Carey LA., et al. Age-specific changes in intrinsic breast cancer subtypes: A focus on older women. Oncologist 2014; 19:1076–83.

[4] Bae SY., Kim S., Lee JH., Lee H., Lee SK., Kil WH., et al. Poor prognosis of single hormone receptor-positive breast cancer: similar outcome as triple-negative breast cancer. BMC Cancer 2015; 15(138): 1–9.

[5] Yang XR., Claude CJ., Goode EL., Couch FJ., Nevanlinna H., Milne RL., et al. Associations of breast cancer risk factors with tumor subtypes: A pooled analysis from the breast cancer association consortium studies. J Natl Cancer Inst 2011; 103(3):250–63.

[6] Mahmood H., Faheem M., Mahmood S., Sadiq M., Irfan J. Impact of age, tumor size, lymph node metastasis, stage, receptor status and menopausal status on overall survival of breast cancer patients in Pakistan. Asian Pac J Cancer Prev 2015;16: 1019–24.

[7] He J., Wang H., Ma F., Feng F., Lin C., Qian H. Prognosis of lymph node-negative breast cancer: Association with clinicopathological factors and tumor associated gene expression. Oncol Lett 2014; 8:1717–24.

[8] Zong Y., Zhu L., Wu J., Chen X., Huang O., Fei X., et al. Progesterone receptor status and Ki-67 index may predict early relapse in luminal B/HER2 negative breast cancer patients: A retrospective study. PLoS One 2014;9:1–8.

[9] Andreana NH., Julie JR., Manohar R., David HG., Michele LC. HER2 status and disparities in luminal breast cancers. Cancer Med 2016; 1–7.

[10] Andrade ACM., Ferreira JCA., Guimaraes BD., Barros AWP., Almeida GS., Weller M. Molecular breast cancer subtypes and therapies in a public hospital of Northeastern Brazil. BMC Women's Health. 2014; 14(110): 1–9.

[11] Inic Z., Zegarac M., Inic M., Marcovic I., Kozomara Z., Djurisic I., et al. Difference between luminal A and luminal B subtypes according to Ki-67, tumor size, and progesterone receptor negativity providing prognostic information. Clin Med Insights Oncol 2014; 8: 107–11.

[12] Yan J., Liu XL., Han LZ., Xiao G., Li NL., Deng YN., et al. Relation between Ki-67, ER, PR, Her2/neu, p21, EGFR, and TOPII-α expression in invasive ductal breast cancer patients and correlations with prognosis. Asian Pas J Cancer Prev 2015; 16: 823–29.

[13] Galukande M., Wabinga H., Mirembe F., Karamagi C., Asea A. Molecular breast cancer subtypes prevalence in an indigenous Sub Saharan African population. Pan Afr Med J 2014; 17: 1–7.

[14] Jamshed A., Shah MA., Murtaza G., Mehmood T., Chaudry SJ., Loya A., Hameed S. Clinical outcome of primary non-metastatic breast cancer: A single institution experience. Indian J Cancer 2016; 52: 191–25.

[15] Nilufer B., Kadri A. Does estrogen receptor determination affect prognosis in early stage breast cancers? Int J Clin Exp Med 2015; 8(11): 21454–9.

[16] Tomi A., Justin XM., Akinyemi IO., John WW., Sean FA. Racial disparities in individual breast cancer outcomes by hormone-receptor subtype, area-level socio-economic status and healthcare resources. Breast Cancer Res Treat 2016; 157(3): 575–86.

[17] Gabriel PR., Catalina AM., Ivonne MOC., Jose RGS. The association of subtypes of breast cancer with tumour characteristic and reproductive factors in 1326 Mexican women. Contemp Oncol(pozn) 2015; 19(6): 462–6.

[18] Bharti JN., Rani P., Kamal V., Agarwal N. Angiogenesis in breast cancer and its correlation with estrogen, progesterone receptors and other prognostic factors. J of Clin Diagn Res 2015;9(1): 5–7.

[19] Dunnwald LK., Rossing MA., Li CI. Hormone receptor status, tumor characteristics and prognosis: a prospective cohort of breast cancer patients. Breast Can Res 2007; 9: 1–10.

[20] Dong G., Wang D., Liang X., Gao H., Wang L., Yu X., et al. Factors related to survival rates for breast cancer patients. Int J Clin Exp Med 2014; 7(10): 3719–24.

[21] Mahyari HM., Khosravi A., Monfared ZE. Human epidermal growth factor receptor 2 and estrogen receptor status in respect to tumor characteristics in non-metastatic breast cancer. Tanaffos 2014; 13(1): 26–34.

[22] Onitilo AA., Engel JM., Greenlee RT., Mukesh BN. Breast cancer subtypes based on ER/PR and HER2 expression: comparison of clinicopathologic features and survival. Clin Med Res 2009; 7: 1–13.

[23] Pal S., Lüchtenborg M., Davies EA., Jack RH. The treatment and survival of patients with triple negative breast cancer in a London population. Springerplus 2014; 3(553): 1–5.

[24] Prat A., Carey LA., Adamo B., Vidal M., Tabernero J., Cortes J., et al. Molecular features and survival outcomes of the intrinsic subtypes within HER2-positive breast cancer. J Natl Cancer Inst 2014; 106(8): 1–8.

[25] Song N., Choi JY., Sung H., Jeon S., Chung S., Park SK., et al. Prediction of breast cancer survival using clinical and genetic markers by tumor subtypes. PLoS One 2015; 13: 1–15.

[26] Devi CR., Tang TS., Corbex M. Incidence and risk factors for breast cancer subtypes in three distinct South-East Asian ethnic groups: Chinese, Malay and natives of Sarawak, Malaysia. Int J Cancer 2012; 131: 2869–77.

[27] Kontani K., Hashimoto S., Murazawa C., Norimura S., Tanaka H., Ohtani M., et al. Factors responsible for long term survival in metastatic breast cancer. World J Surg Oncol 2014; 12(344): 1–9.

http://dx.doi.org/10.5772/66176

[28] Yan M., Schwaederle M., Arguello D., Millis SZ., Gatalica Z., Kurzrock R. HER2 expression status in diverse cancers: review of results from 37,992 patients. Cancer Metastasis Rev 2015; 34: 157–64.

[29] Keegan THM., Press DJ., Tao L., DeRouen C., Kurian AW., Clarke CA., et al. Impact of breast cancer subtypes on 3-year survival among adolescent and young adult women. Breast Cancer Res 2013;15: 1–12.

Chapter 3

Breast Cancer as an Epstein-Barr Virus (EBV)-Associated Malignancy

Ghimja Fessahaye and Muntaser E. Ibrahim

Additional information is available at the end of the chapter

http://dx.doi.org/10.5772/66988

Abstract

The Epstein Barr Virus is among the very first oncogenic viruses to be identified as culprits of human malignancies. Its role as an etiologic agent of breast cancer however remains debated despite mounting molecular evidence. In this chapter we address the challenge of multiple molecular etiologies of breast cancer (BC) with emphasis on the Epstein Barr Virus (EBV) as a potential causative agent within a frame work of gene/environment interaction. We also hope to contribute to a critique of the a concept of universal single agent or gene in cancer etiology. In addition to reviewing further reasons of why EBV should be considered a tumor virus, coupling molecular targets at the initiation stage, we examine evidence for the culpability of EBV as oncogenic virus in relation to the genetic and epigenetic events that leads to carcinogenesis of cancer; and the subsequent downstream interaction including genetic and epigenetic modifiers of signaling and molecular function underlying the cancerous phenotype. The TNF family is taken as an example of how the epigenetic reprogramming process, impacts molecular targets and how these combined interplay of molecular events impinges on pathogenesis and malignancy of breast cancer in humans.

Keywords: Epstein-Barr virus, breast cancer, genetics, epigenetics, microRNA, tumor necrosis factor

1. Introduction

1.1. Breast cancer etiology

Although the prevalence of breast cancer (BC) is relatively lower in sub-Saharan Africa compared to that of the "western" countries, it is characterized by aggressive nature and target more women at a younger age [1]. BC etiology is not yet entirely understood, but its incidence is thought to be partially explained by environmental factors including viruses such as EBV [2]. Recently, a growing pile of evidence has accumulated with regard to the association of cancers and viruses. Viruses are believed to cause from 15 to 25% of all malignancies and this percentage will increase by more than 50% in 2030 in developing countries [3, 4]. As transforming agents, viruses, seem ideal culprit in causing cell transformation. More recently, the virus was reported as a main culprit of breast cancer in Sudan [5]. A putative role for viruses was speculated based on the limited contribution of mutational events within tumor suppressors such as BRCA1, BRCA2, and p53 to breast cancer etiology [6]. Epigenetic silencing was also envisaged as an obvious candidate to entertain. The fact that methylation lies prominently at the interface of genes and the environment, and the known link between selfish DNA (viruses) and methylation makes it particularly important in understanding both short- and long-term evolutionary effects in oncology. Interestingly, in the same subset of BC tissues where fragments of the virus DNA were detected by *in situ* hybridization in nearly all samples, significant epigenetic silencing of tumor suppressers was observed in a limited but key set of genes such as BRCA1, BRCA2, and p14 [5].

1.2. Genetic and epigenetic modifiers in breast cancer

A transcriptome study for virus-host interaction identified few of the main partners of EBV in the host cell [7] as of oncogenic potential. This is essential for a framework we are proposing in the current chapter. The framework (**Figure 1**) suggested by us and other authors [8, 9] entails the involvement of both genetic and epigenetic modifiers to converge on a cancer phenotype. However, we propose, in addition, an earlier role for the EBV virus in initiating that sequel of events through interaction of viral proteins and nucleic acid with key cellular components in the target cell (stem cell). Prominent among these cellular partners are RNA-binding proteins like ELAVL1/HuR, and editing genes like APOBEC/AID in the genomic side and DNMT, TET, and HDAC in the epigenetic side. One significant feature especially in the RNA-binding proteins is the plethora of potential targets and partners which could partly explain the wide spectrum of biological mechanisms involved and targeted by these events. Moreover, the virus molecular interaction could provide a plausible explanation to the features of organization described in previous publications [10] and increasingly ascribed to DNA/RNA editing and RNA-binding proteins like ELAVL1/HuR in addition to miRNA regulation. ELAVL1 has been reported to show marked centrality in a colorectal cancer family in which EBV infection is speculated to have a role [10]. The protein turned to display similar centrality among differentially methylated genes in breast cancer cases that had strong EBV positivity by *in situ* hybridization (**Figure 2**). This does not preclude a role for individual proteins like C-Fos, an established EBV partner [7], which has also been identified as independent predictor of decreased survival in breast cancer.

We simply try to differentiate between major upstream effecter molecules and downstream by-products of interaction like c-Fos and several other molecules; and cancer as a system and polygenic complex phenomenon, versus the rarity of a cancers of Mendelian-like monogenic inheritance where one or few molecules are key in determining a tumor phenotype.

http://dx.doi.org/10.5772/66988

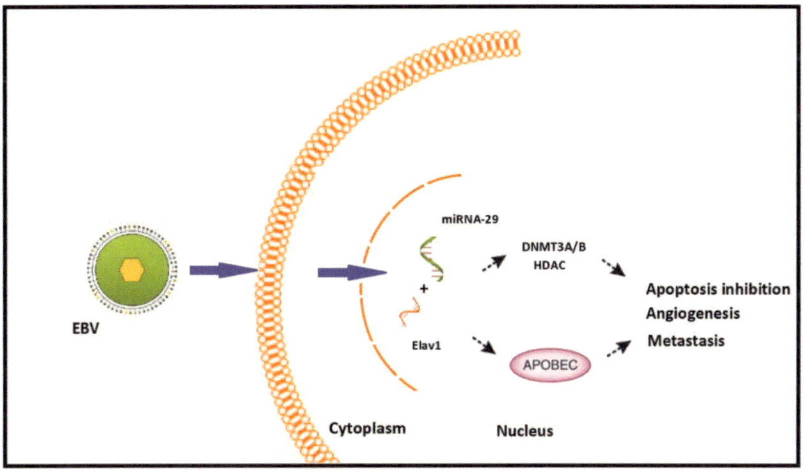

Figure 1. The oncogenic potential of EBV is outlined in the figure, where the interaction of viral proteins and nucleic acid (LNP, LNP2, BZLF, etc.) with key cellular components (ELAVL1/Hur, miRNA29) in the target cell (stem cell) dictates the consequent pathogenesis and carcinogenesis processes impinged by downstream molecules (e.g., APOBEC3) and involving both genetic and epigenetic modifiers.

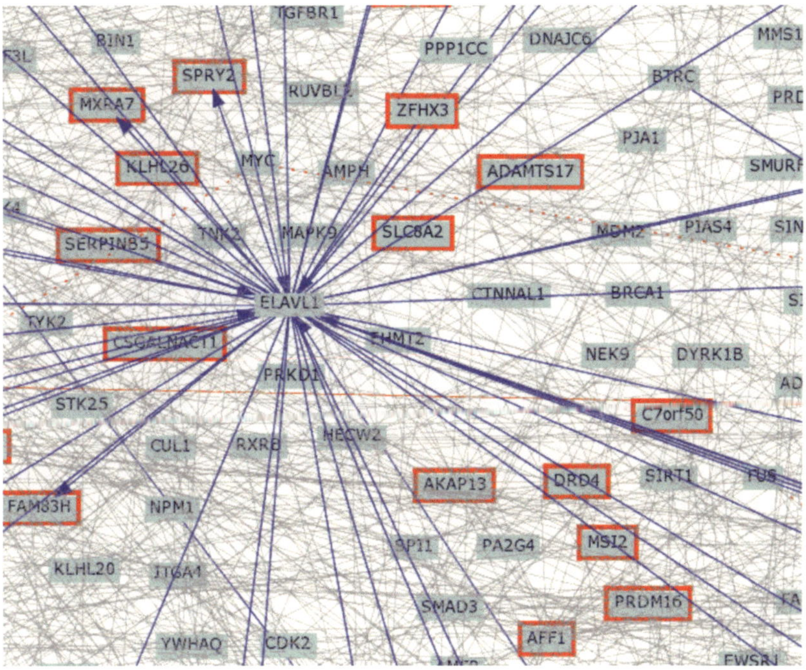

Figure 2. The centrality of ELAVL1/Hur is demonstrated through an interaction network of differentially methylated genes in breast cancer cases with strong EBV positivity using *in situ* hybridization from Sudan, using the program Cognosante.

2. Breast cancer and EBV

2.1. EBV infection molecular interaction and latency

EBV has been used routinely in laboratories to create cell lines for decades [11]. Furthermore, it has been found in breast tissue and is frequently found in breast secretions including breast milk [12]. EBV can infect mammary epithelial cells and its DNA fragment (p31) is capable of inducing immortalization in these cells [13]. This cosmopolitan γ-herpes virus infects usually at younger age. Its main target are B lymphocytes but it has a potential to infect epithelial cells as well and thus is associated with various lymphoid and epithelial malignancies and is incriminated as a carcinogenic agent by the World Health Organization [14].

EBV is closely associated with endemic Burkitt's lymphoma in sub-Saharan Africa [15] which earned the area the lymphoma belt due to such high frequency among children. The virus is associated with a horde of other malignancies in the tropics, such as nasopharyngeal carcinoma (NPC), gastric cancer, and breast cancer, although most studies regarding the controversial role of the virus as a cofactor in BC were done in countries outside of Africa. The variable prevalence of EBV in different regions is an indicator of the importance of the environmental and geographic cofactors in the development of such association and the diseases [16].

One key question to be entertained is why some oncogenic viruses like human papillomavirus (HPV) and EBV although common infections tend to develop cancer in some individuals whereas others remain asymptomatic? Should we speculate population-specific susceptibility factors that predispose to cancer in the human genome? Or whether some viral strains have more oncogenic potential as the case of HPV16, and 18 and EBV Type I, II and Type III? are there specific role and molecular basis of epigenetic silencing in inactivation of tumor suppressors, both of which environmental geographical cofactors play an important role in determining the strength of the association of malignancy with EBV [17] and hence variation in susceptibility may be influenced by factors such as geographical and immunological differences and ethnicity [18, 19].

The natural host of the virus is B-lymphocyte to which the virus gains entry through a type two complement receptor (CR2/CD21) [20]. Although breast cancer cells normally do not express the receptor CD21 [21], the range of viral tropism could be widened through the targeting of stem cells which are capable of expressing a wider range of receptor repertoires. EBV can infect primary mammary epithelial cells (MECs) that express CD21 and EBV infection leads to the expansion of early MEC progenitor cells with a stem cell phenotype, activates mesenchymal epithelial transition (MET) signaling and enforces a differentiation block. Hu et al. report that EBV can infect primary human mammary epithelial cells (MECs) but not tumor cells leading to phenotypic changes consistent with transformation [22]. Latent membrane protein-2A (LMP2A) may induce a stem cell state, evidenced by an enhanced self-renewal and transformational capacity, and also increases the number of tumor initiating cells *in vivo*, thus potentially rendering a B-lymphocyte into a cancer stem cell. This viral protein plays a key role not only in EBV latency and persistence but also in the progression of EBV-associated cancers such as NPC in which it was expressed in about half of the samples [23, 24]. It affects hedgehog signaling and induces stem cell behavior in epithelial cells [25].

When MECs were implanted as xenografts, EBV infection cooperated with activated Ras and accelerated the formation of breast cancer [22]. A human gene expression signature for MECs infected with EBV, termed EBVness, was associated with high grade, estrogen-receptor-negative status, p53 mutation, and poor survival. In 11/33 EBVness-positive tumors, EBV-DNA was detected by fluorescent *in situ* hybridization for the viral LMP1 and BXLF2 genes [22]. The observations that CD21 was absent on all of the tumor cell lines, none of which became infected, and that analysis of the TCGA breast cancer RNAseq data revealed no active transcription of EBV [26, 27] suggest that the EBV DNA detected in a subset of human breast cancers, is an inactive remnant of a previously active EBV infection that might have occurred in mammary epithelial cells years or even decades prior to cancer formation and which is no longer required once malignant transformation has occurred [22]. However, the strong EBV signals detected by the *in situ* hybridization in tumor tissues in the study by Yahia et al. [5] while being absent from the safety margin requires some explanation. The presence of EBV-DNA and an APOBEC mutational signature correlated with adverse clinicopathological features, however, the presence of the virus is not always a requirement for tumor growth, consistent with a "hit and-run" mechanism which would also explain why mining of the TCGA RNAseq data did not show active transcription of EBV [26, 27].

Following EBV infection, the host cell is affected through different mechanisms pertaining to the viral lytic and lysogenic survival strategies. The infection that usually occurs during childhood triggers the immune machinery which attempts to clear the virus, and this may probably be to its own advantage to control the development of another intruder, the tumor. The majority of the asymptomatic carriers harbor up to 50 EBV genomes per million B cells [28]. A virus may trick the host cellular machinery and enter into latency phase. Histone acetylation plays an important role in the switch between the lytic and lysogeny phases by regulating BZLF promoter known as Z. It has been suggested that the balance between recruitment of histone acetyltransferases versus histone deacetylases by transacting factors promotes and decides the switch between latency and lytic reactivation [29]. Viral latency may eventuate in carcinogenesis provided the presence of conducive host (susceptibility factors) and viral (oncogenic latency proteins) exists. During latency the virus successfully evade the host's immune system and persists within the B cells by decreasing its contents to few latent genes [30], six nuclear antigens, three latent membrane proteins and two abundant untranslated RNAs and can persist without being recognized by the immune system and with little interference with the health of the host. Functionally, the oncogenic potential of the virus is associated with its latency molecules such as latent membrane protein-1 (LMP1) [31], but some studies however, reported that this form of the virus (latency) to be associated with good prognosis, while on the other hand its lytic form to be a sign of worse outcome [32]. These, and the authors conclude that this might possibly occur through non-specific anti-tumoral immune response and they consider the virus as a 'double faceted' infectious agent at a time acting as a co-factor for the anti-tumoral immune response. However, this is contradicted by the fact that in patients with good prognosis high frequency of interferon (IFN)-γ and tumor necrosis factor (TNF)-α producing cells were observed, which indicates the existence of a Th1-type polarized immune response in the tumor [32]. Inflammation may also contribute to cancerous and precancerous conditions, mainly through signaling of the highly central and pivotal protein NFkB.

The mechanism which disturbs this perfect host-virus equilibrium which is indicated by the majority asymptomatic carriers is not known yet. It could be inherent in the host or in the virus or in both? EBV usually infects immunosuppressed/immunocompromised individuals [33]. Most of the post-transplant lymphoproliferative disorders (PTLD) which are more common in immunosuppressed transplant patients are EBV-associated [34]. The association with PTLD has been observed particularly following allogenic stem cell transplantation (SCT) [35], which brings the element of the stem cell factor in EBV-associated cancer [36] and may account for receptor promiscuity.

2.2. EBV and APOBEC3 as a genomic modifier

Of the several molecules that confer the spectacularly wide genotypic and phenotypic changes, characteristic of the cancer cell is the APOBEC/AID family of enzymes. Editing by apolipoprotein B editing catalytic subunits proteins 3 (APOBEC3s) is a strong and well-conserved system of the innate immunity that mutates and inactivates viral genomes [37, 38]. These proteins are involved in the system of innate defense against exogenous viruses and endogenous retroelements. EBV genomes in EBV-transformed oligoclonal B-cell lines can be edited by at least one APOBEC3 enzyme [39]. It is possible that APOBEC3 increases the chance of viral DNA integration in the host by inducing mutations and genome instability after viral infection [40].

In an analysis of the TCGA breast cancer data mentioned earlier, EBVness correlated with the presence of the APOBEC mutational signature. Recently, APOBEC3 proteins linked the viral infections to cancer development [41], and now recognized as key players in cancer-associated somatic mutation processes that seem to influence cancer development and progression [42, 43]. In breast cancer, APOBEC3B mRNA was found to be overexpressed in the normal breast epithelial cells transfected with HPV [44], indicating a possible role of APOBEC-mediated mutagenesis in HPV-driven tumor development [45]. APOBEC3G was found to be highly expressed in colorectal tumors and hepatic metastasis, and it has been proposed to promote colorectal cancer hepatic metastasis through miR29 downregulation and consequent derepression of MMP2, a known metastasis activator [46]. Also, it has been involved in microRNA regulation [47].

Both molecules, APOBEC3 [10] and miRNA [Yousif submitted], have been implicated in Sudanese multicase colorectal family, with the striking finding of identify by state of tumor tissues between distant relatives, in contrast to a limited similarity between relatives (identity by decent).

2.3. EBV as a potential epigenome modifier

The relationship between EBV and the epigenetic machinery particularly methylation of CpG moieties is too obvious to oversee. It is embedded in the distant evolutionary relationship of viruses and DNA modification systems of selfish DNA. Several tumors are associated with arthrobacter luteus (Alu) elements in which tumor suppressor genes are more enriched [48] and other markers of selfish DNA including the recently recognized N6-methyladenosine (m6A), the most common internal messenger RNA modification found in eukaryotes and also in RNA of

http://dx.doi.org/10.5772/66988

nuclear-replicating viruses [49]. This modification is catalyzed by an evolutionarily conserved, nuclear, multicomponent enzyme. One of whose subunits, methyltransferase-like 3(METTL3), has been identified and a METTL3 knockout model resulted in an apoptosis phenotype [50]. The infected and EBV transformed cancer cell employs a bundle of these tools including the above, HDAC, methylating enzymes like DNMTA/B to its advantage and survival. Methylome analysis may provide further clues to the contribution of epigenetics to the tumorigenesis process in dictating the function of key cancer genes and genomes.

DNA hypermethylation in cancer genomes usually occurs in the promoter regions of tumor suppressor genes, which can result in silencing of tumor suppressor [51]. In contrast, DNA hypomethylation often targets DNA repeats, which may induce genomic instability and mutation events in cancer genomes [52]. There is evidence that promoter hypomethylation of some genes may be associated with the tumor progression and metastasis of some cancers [53] as well as the initiation of inflammation and immunomodulation [54].The role of DNMT3B in the altered methylation and inactivation of genes in human tumor cells as well as its role in the maintenance of the transformed phenotype is well established. It has significant site selectivity that is distinct from DNMTA1, regulates aberrant gene silencing, and is essential for cancer cell survival [55]. DNMT3A and DNMT3B repress transcription independent of their methylating activities, and this repression is partially dependent upon histone deacetylase activity (HDAC) [56]. DNMT3B-mediated gene suppression may involve both methylation-dependent and methylation-independent HDAC-dependent mechanisms. Histone acetylation, a component of an epigenetic mechanism has a role in the initiation and progression of human cancer as a result of post transcriptional modification [57]. Aberration in HDACs leads to transcriptional repression in genes involved in proliferation, differentiation, invasion, and metastasis [58]. HDAC9 an important factor in mammary carcinogenesis [59] overexpression was associated with higher rates of gene transcription and increased epigenetic marks on the HDAC9 promoter. Methylome of BC is a foundation for metastatic risk "CpG island methylator phenotype (CIMP)" in breast cancer is not yet clearly defined as is in colon cancer, in which it is defined by promoter hypermethylation of at least three of five specific methylation markers [60]. In one study, lobular breast carcinoma was revealed with the highest number of differentially methylated CpG sites indicating its epigenetic unstableness [61]. EBV protein, LMP2A, can cause activation of (DNMT1), which in turn hypermethylate a tumor suppressor gene, PTEN in EBV-associated gastric cancer [62]. DNMT1 over expression mediated by EBV LMP1 and LMP2 and Oncogenic EBV gene, LMP1, can upregulate all of the DNA methyltransferases (DNMTs) [63]. DNMT3b overexpression contributes to a hypermethylator phenotype in human breast cancer cell lines [64], and LMP2a functions in the initiation and progression of cancer by inducing the cancer stem-like cells [24] as aforementioned.

Differential methylation analysis of whole methylome data of breast cancer cases from Sudan provided a possible link between these entities. The results reveal epigenetic dysregulation of major developmental pathways including hippo signaling pathway [Alsiddig, 2015, data online, pending submission], thus providing not only a clue to the stem cell dimension of the disease but also insights to subsequent pathognomonic features of cancer process. It also demonstrated the presence of significant enrichment of EBV-associated pathways with a significant score.

3. TNFα gene methylation

An insightful example of the contribution of the methylation phenotype to breast cancer through modulation of key cancer-related genes is the TNFα. Genetic as well as epigenetic aberrations at the promoter of TNF-α has been reported; its promoter can be methylated with functional modification, and eight DNA variants or "SNPs" have been described within the TNF promoter as reviewed by Bayley et al. [65].

Methylated TNFα promoter and TNFα exon1 were associated with significant suppression of TNF in colorectal tumors [66], although, this has to be reconciled with a contrasting report of TNF-α shown to be highly expressed in breast carcinomas [67]. TNF-α is a multifunctional cytokine that plays important roles in diverse cellular events such as cell survival, proliferation, differentiation, and death. However, when chronically produced and inflammation persists in the tumor microenvironment it may have a critical role in the promotion and progression of cancers by DNA damage, enhancing proangiogenic functions, increasing the expression of matrix metalloproteinases (MMP) and endothelial adhesion molecules and inducing growth-promoting hormones and chemokines that promote tumor development [68]. TNF-α can promote EMT of MCF-7 cells and activates cell migration [69]. This transition generates stem-cellness [70]. Activation of regulatory T cells (Tregs) can cause immunosuppression and has resulted from prolonged exposure to TNF-α [71], which could have a cancer-promoting effect. TNF is hence believed to be a double-edged sword that could be either pro- or antitumorigenic, this double standard phenomenon is also seen in severe infectious diseases such as malaria in which fatal cerebral malaria is associated with high circulating levels of this cytokine [72]. Environmental factors such as malaria exerts selective pressure on the TNF loci and is reflected on common polymorphisms in the human genome like the TNF (–308G/A) in the TNF promoter (–308G/A). This SNP which was found to be associated with protection from malaria [72] was found to be associated with susceptibilities to various types of cancer [73]. This influence on the susceptibility to cancer may be associated with altered TNF production or a neighboring gene in tight-linkage disequilibrium. These reports indirectly suggest that TNF has a tumor-promoting role and that TNF promoter SNPs could be a predictor for cancer risk.

The CD40 ligand (CD40L), a glycoprotein involved in B cell proliferation, antigen presenting cell activation, and member of the TNF receptor ligand family, was reported to confer protection from severe malaria has also significant functional homology with EBV LMP1. In the malaria endemic area of eastern Sudan, elevated levels of CD40L expression were observed in comparison to naive healthy controls from nonmalaria areas.

In an analysis of the methylome of subset of human triple-negative breast cancer the analysis identified significant enrichment in methylation phenotypes of the tumor necrosis factor (TNF) and TNF receptor family (**Table 1**). The attempts to dissect the functionality of the TNF promoter have all concentrated on the genetic aspects of TNF gene regulation, but now with the increasing interest in the epigenetic control of gene regulation and possible significance for disease, it is surprising that little attention has been paid to the possibility that aberrant methylation could play a role in TNF dysregulation.

TNF-α stimulates many signaling pathways by binding to two receptors, TNFR1 (p55) and TNFR2 (p75) [68, 74]. TNFR-1 is ubiquitously expressed, whereas TNFR-2 is mainly expressed in immune cells [75].

Gene symbol	Site of hypermethylation	Site of hypomethylation
TNF	TSS 1500, promoter	–
TNFRSF1A	Body	–
TNFAIP3	Body	–
TNFRSF1B	Body	–
TNFSF11	5′ UTR, promoter, exon	5′ UTR, promoter
TNFRSF10D	Exon, body, promoter	Body
TNFAIP8L1	TSS1500, promoter	–
TNFRSF19	5′ UTR, exon, body, promoter,	–
CIQTNF4	5′ UTR, body, promoter	Exon
C1QTNF5	5′ UTR, body, 3′ UTR, promoter	–
TNFRSF13C	TSS1500, promoter	–
C1QTNF9	TSS1500, promoter	–
TNFRSF13B	TSS1500, promoter	–
TNFRSF11A	TSS1500, promoter	Body
TNFRSF8	Promoter	–
C1QTNF7	Exon	–
TNFAIP8L3	Body	–
C1QTNF1	Body	–
TNFSF12-TNFSF13	Body	–
TNFSF8	–	Body
TNF18	–	Body
C1QTNF6	–	Body
C1QTNF8	–	3′ UTR

Table 1. Differentially methylated TNF and TNF receptor family genes at various CpG sites from Sudanese breast cancer samples, indicating the significant enrichment in methylation phenotypes in this important family of genes and being a target of epigenetic modification in a directed tumorigenesis process.

4. Gene chromosome location and breast cancer

Another key class of molecules identified through this approach is the hypomethylated olfactory receptor genes in Sudanese breast cancer samples. Significant enrichment of differentially hypomethylated olfactory receptor family members were mapped to chromosomes 1 specifically to chr1q44 (*P*-value, 6.867e-20) a cytoband known to be one of the viral integration sites [76]. Moreover, this location is also associated with autoimmune diseases [77] and chronic inflammatory responses induced by physical stimuli from the environment [78]. It seems that the virus selects this environmentally prone site.

According to various studies, chromosome 1 aberration is associated with different cancers, such as neuroblastoma [79], cervical [80], and colorectal [81]. In breast cancer, gains at 1q are found in over 50% of breast tumors [82]. It is reported that the long arm of chromosome1 to be usually associated with karyotypic changes seen in breast cancer and is believed that the development of breast cancer might be caused by inactivation of a gene (s) located on 1q23-32 [83].

5. miRNA as epigenetic actor in breast cancer

microRNA(miRNA) is naturally involved in the biological process across the carcinogenesis from initiation to metastasis and this occurs through the spectrum of genetic and epigenetic mechanisms of the cell. Several miRNA have been reported to be involved in the myriad of the biological processes, for example miR-22 (chromosome 17) can regulate breast cancer stemness and metastasis through a TET-dependent chromatin remodeling [84], and miR-373, miR-520 were found to promote migration and invasion of BC cells.

A differential analysis of the methylome dataset of a Sudanese breast cancer cases and controls identified hypomethylated sites for six different miRNAs, including miR-153-2, miR-2276, miR-30B, miR-1204, miR-141, and miR-300 [Alsiddig, 2015 data on line, pending submission]. Only miR-153-2, miR-2276, and miR30B had been previously associated with breast cancer [85–87]. miR153-2 was of particular interest, since numerous studies linked miR153 to a myriad of epithelial cancers. One study demonstrated that miR-153 upregulation promotes prostate cancer proliferation through downregulation of PTEN tumor suppressor gene [88].A test dataset The Cancer Genome Atlas (TCGA), contained methylation data for 90 samples of healthy individuals and 638 samples of primary tumor. The authors found miR153-2 promoter to be significantly hypomethylated at the exact same CpG sites. Interestingly, another epigenetic regulators, TET2, and TET3 are among the listed targets of miR153-2 as predicted by TargetScan algorithm.

RNA-binding protein sometimes have the same target sequence as miRNA and a notable example is miRNA 29 which competes with ELAVL1 on the same regulatory sites.miRNA29b Stops protein production from other genes that play vital role in metastasis and its isoform are shown to regulate various aspects of the carcinogenesis process in different tumors. However, its target site homology with a key RNA-binding protein like ELAV1/Hur suggest that this micro RNA may play a critical role in the early phase of viral pathogenesis and in coupling of downstream key players like TNFα as shown in **Figure 1**.

6. Conclusion

In this chapter, we review some examples pertinent to questions as of why EBV should be considered a tumor virus, examine molecular evidence for the culpability of EBV as oncogenic virus in relation to the established cases of EBV cancer oncogenesis; the cancer target cell and stem cell, which bring the element of development as an epigenetic reprogramming process, linking the breast cancer methylome differential methylation to developmental and EBV, dwelling on EBV molecular targets, and how the combined interplay of molecular events in human impinges on pathogenesis and malignancy of breast cancer.

Author details

Ghimja Fessahaye and Muntaser E. Ibrahim*

*Address all correspondence to: mibrahim@iend.org

Unit of Diseases and Diversity, Department of Molecular Biology, Institute of Endemic Diseases, University of Khartoum, Khartoum, Sudan

References

[1] Fregene, A. & Newman, L.A. (2005) Breast cancer in sub-Saharan Africa: how does it relate to breast cancer in African-American women? *Cancer* 103:1540–1550.

[2] Pogo, B.G. & Holland, J.F. (1997) Possibilities of a viral etiology for human breast cancer. A review. *Biol Trace Elem Res*. 56:131–142.

[3] Boccardo, E. & Villa, L.L. (2007) Viral origins of human cancer. *Curr Med Chem*. 14 (24): 2526–2539.

[4] Harford, J.B. (2012) Viral infections and human cancers: the legacy of Denis Burkitt. *Br J Haematol*. 156:709–718.

[5] Yahia, Z.A., Adam, A.A., Elgizouli, M., Hussein, A., Masri, M.A., Kamal, M., et al. (2014) Epstein-Barr virus: a prime candidate of breast cancer etiology in Sudanese patients. *Infect Agent Cancer*. 9(1): 9.

[6] Masri, M.A., Abdel Seed, N.M., Fahal, A.H., Romano. M., Baralle, F., El Hassan, A.M., et al. (2002) Minor role for BRCA2 (exon11) and p53 (Exon 5-9) among Sudanese breast cancer patients. *Breast Cancer Res Treat*. 71(2):145–147.

[7] Arvey, A., Tempera I., Tsai K., Chen, H., Tikhmyanova, N. &Klichinsky, M. Leslie C, Lieberman PM (2012) An atlas of the Epstein-Barr virus transcriptome and Epigenome reveals host-virus regulatory interaction. Cell Host Microbe 12 (2): 233-245.

[8] Chan, T.A., Glockner, S., Yi, J.M., Chen, W., VanNeste, L., Cope, L.et al. (2008) Convergence of mutation and epigenetic alterations identifies common genes in cancer that predict for poor prognosis. *PLoS Med*. 5:823–838.

[9] You, J.S. & Jones, P.A. (2012) Cancer genetics and epigenetics: Two sides of the same coin? *Cancer Cell*. 22(1): 9–20.

[10] Suleiman, S.H., Koko, M.E., Nasir, W. H., Elfateh, O., Elgizouli, U. K., Abdallah, M. O. E., et al. (2015) Exome sequencing of a colorectal cancer family reveals shared mutation pattern and predisposition circuitry along tumor pathways. *Front Genet*. 6: 288.

[11] Bass, H., Walters, R. & Darke, C. (2004) Provision of Epstein- Barr virus-transformed B-cell lines in a routine tissue typing laboratory: practicalities and applications. *Eur J Immuno Genet*.31: 87–92.

[12] Glenn, W.K., Whitaker, N.J. & Lawson, J.S. (2012) High risk human papillomavirus and Epstein-Barr virus in human breast milk. *BMC Res. Notes* 5: 477.

[13] Gao, Y., Lu, Y.J., Xue, S.A., Chen, H., Wedderburn, N. & Griffin, B.E. (2002) Hypothesis: a novel route for immortalization of epithelial cells by Epstein-Barr virus. *Oncogene*. 21: 825–835.

[14] IARC, (1997) Epstein-Barr virus and Kaposi's sarcoma herpesvirus/herpesvirus 8. IARC *Monog*r *Eval Carcinog Risks Hum*. 70: 1–492.

[15] Tang, W., Harmon, P., Gulley, M.L., Mwansambo, C., Kazembe, P.N., Martinson, F., et al. (2010) Viral response to chemotherapy in endemic burkitt lymphoma. *Clin Cancer Res. 16*(7): 2055–2064.

[16] Hsu, J.L. & Glaser, S.L. (2000) Epstein-Barr virus-associated malignancies: epidemiologic patterns and etiologic implications. *Crit. Rev Oncol Hematol*.34(1): 27–53.

[17] Lopategui, J.R., Gaffey, M.J. &Weiss, L.M. (1994) Detection of Epstein-Barr viral RNA in sinonasal undifferentiated carcinoma from Western and Asian patients. *Am J SurgPathol*.18: 391–398.

[18] Fina, F., Romain, S., Ouafik, L., Palmari, J., Ayed, F.B., Benharkat, S., et al. (2001) Frequency and genome load of Epstein-Barr virus in breast cancers from different geographical areas. *Br J Cancer. 84* (6): 783–790.

[19] Thompson, M.P. & Kurzrock, R.(*2004*) Epstein-Barr virus and cancer. *Clin Cancer Res*. 10: 803–821.

[20] Nemerow, G. R., Luxembourg, A. T. & Cooper, N. R. (1994) CD2I/ CR2, its role in EBV infection and immune function. *Epstein-Barr Reports*. 1: 59–64.

[21] Speck, P. & Longnecker, R. (2000) Infection of breast epithelial cells with Epstein-Barr virus via cell-to-cell contact. *J Natl Cancer Inst*.92: 1849–1851.

[22] Hu, H., Luo, M.L., Desmedt, C., Nabavi, S., Yadegarynia, S., Hong, A., et al. (2016) Epstein–Barr virus infection of mammary epithelial cells promotes malignant transformation. *EBioMedicine*.9: 148–160.

[23] Pegtel, D.M., Subramanian, A., Sheen, T.S., Tsai, C.H., Golub, T.R. & Thorley-Lawson, D.A. (2005) Epstein-Barr-virus-encoded LMP2A induces primary epithelial cell migration and invasion: possible role in nasopharyngeal carcinoma metastasis. *J Virol*. 79: 15430–15442.

[24] Kong, Q.L., Hu, L.J., Cao, J.Y., Huang, Y.J., Xu, L.H., Liang, Y., et al. (2010) Epstein-Barr virus-encoded LMP2A induces an epithelial–mesenchymal transition and increases the number of side population stem-like cancer cells in nasopharyngeal carcinoma. *PLoS Pathogens*. 6(6): e1000940.

[25] Port, R.J., Pinheiro-Maia, S., Hu, C., Arrand, J.R., Wei, W., Young, L.S., et al. (2013) Epstein-Barr virus induction of the Hedgehog signaling pathway imposes a stem cell phenotype on human epithelial cells. *J Pathol*. 231: 367–377.

[26] Khoury, J.D., Tannir, N.M., Williams, M.D., Chen, Y., Yao, H., Zhang, J., & Thompson (2013) Landscape of DNA virus associations across human malignant cancers: analysis of 3,775 cases using RNA-Seq. *J. Virol*. 87: 8916–8926.

[27] Tang, K.W., Alaei-Mahabadi B., Samuelsson T., Lindh M. & Larsson E. (2013) The landscape of viral expression and host gene fusion and adaptation in human cancer. *Nat Commun*. 4: 2513.

[28] Gulley, M.L. (*2001*) Molecular diagnosis of Epstein-Barr virus- related diseases. *J Mol Diagn*. 3:1–10.

[29] Homa, N.J., Salinas, R., Forte, E., Robinson, T.J., Garcia-Blanco, M.A. & Luftig, M.A. (2013) Epstein-Barr virus induces global changes in cellular mRNA isoform usage that are important for the maintenance of latency. *J Virol*. 87(22): 12291–12301.

[30] Thorley-Lawson, D.A. (2001) Epstein–Barr virus: exploiting the immune system. *Nat Rev Immunol*. 1: 75–82.

[31] Goormachtigh, G., Ouk, T.S., Mougel, A., Tranchand-Bunel, D., Masy, E., Le Clorennec, C., et al. (2006) Auto activation of the Epstein-Barr virus oncogenic protein LMP1 during Type II latency through opposite roles of the NF-κB and JNK signaling pathways. *J Virol*. 80(15): 7382–7393.

[32] Marrão, G., Habib, M., Paiva, A., Bicout, D., Fallecker, C., Franco, S., et al. (2014) Epstein-Barr virus infection and clinical outcome in breast cancer patients correlate with immune cell TNF-α/IFN-γ response. *BMC Cancer*. 14: 665.

[33] Raab-Traub, N. (1996) Pathogenesis of Epstein-Barr virus and its associated malignancies. *Semin Virol*. 7: 315–323.

[34] Niedobitek, G., Meru, N. & Delecluse, H.J. (2001) Epstein-Barr virus infection and human malignancies. *Int J Exp Pathol*. 82(3): 149–170.

[35] Sundin, M., Le Blanc, K., Ringden, O., Barkholt, L., Omazic, B., Lergin, C., et al. (2006) The role of HLA mismatch, splenectomy and recipient Epstein-Barr virus seronegativity as risk factors in post-Transplant-lymphoproliferative disorder following allogeneic hematopoietic stem cell transplantation. *Haematologica*. 91(8): 1059–1067.

[36] vanEsser, J.W., van der Holt, B., Meijer, E., Niesters, H.G., Trenschel, R., Thijsen, S.F., et al. (2001) Epstein-Barr virus (EBV) reactivation is a frequent event after allogeneic stem cell transplantation (SCT) and quantitatively predicts EBV-lymphoproliferative disease following T-cell–depleted SCT. *Blood*. 98(4): 972–978.

[37] Cullen, B.R. (2006) Role and mechanism of action of the APOBEC3 family of antiretroviral resistance factors. *J Virol.* 80(3): 1067–1076.

[38] Willems, L. & Gillet, N. A. (2015). APOBEC3 interference during replication of viral genomes. *Viruses.* 7(6): 2999–3018.

[39] Suspene, R., Aynaud, M.M., Koch, S., Pasdeloup, D., Labetoulle, M., Gaertner, B., et al. (2011) Genetic editing of herpes simplex virus 1 and Epstein-Barr herpesvirus genomes by human APOBEC3 cytidine deaminases in culture and in vivo. *J Virol.* 85(15): 7594–7602.

[40] Shi, Y., Peng, S.L., Yang, L.F., Chen, X., Tao, Y.G., & Cao, Y. (2016). Co-infection of Epstein-Barr virus and human papillomavirus in human tumorigenesis. *Chin J Cancer.*35:16.

[41] Downey, R.F., Sullivan, F.J., Wang-Johanning, F., Ambs, S., Giles, F.J. & Glynn, S.A. (2015) Human endogenous retrovirus K and cancer: innocent bystander or tumorigenic accomplice? *Int J Cancer.* 137: 1249–1257.

[42] de Bruin, E.C, McGranahan, N., Mitter, R., Salm, M.,Wedge, D.C., Yates, L. et al. (2014) Spatial and temporal diversity in genomic instability processes defines lung cancer evolution. *Science.* 346: 251–256.

[43] Rebhandl, S., Huemer, M., Greil, R. & Geisberger, R. (2015) AID/APOBEC deaminases and cancer. *Oncoscience.* 2(4): 320–333.

[44] Burns, M.B., Lackey, L., Carpenter, M.A., Rathore, A., Land, A.M., Leonard, B., et al. (2013) APOBEC3B is an enzymatic source of mutation in breast cancer. *Nature.* 494: 366–370.

[45] Henderson, S., Chakravarthy, A., Su, X., Boshoff, C. & Fenton, T.R. (2014) APOBEC-mediated cytosine deamination links PIK3CA helical domain mutations to human papillomavirus driven tumor development. *Cell Rep.* 7: 1833–1841.

[46] Ding, Q.Q., Chang, C.J., Xie, X.M., Xia, W.Y., Yang, J.Y., Wang, S.C., et al. (2011) APOBEC3G promotes liver metastasis in an orthotopic mouse model of colorectal cancer and predicts human hepatic metastasis. *J Clin Invest.* 121: 4526–4536.

[47] Liu, C., Zhang, X., Huang, F., Yang, B., Li, J., Liu, B., et al. (2012) APOBEC3G inhibits MicroRNA-mediated repression of translation by interfering with the interaction between Argonaute-2 and MOV10. *J Biol Chem.* 287(35): 29373–29383.

[48] Zhang, W., Edwards, A., Fan, W., Deininger, P & Zhang, K. (2011) Alu distribution and mutation types of cancer genes. *BMC Genomics.*12: 157.

[49] Luo, G.Z., MacQueen, A., Zheng, G., Duan, H., Dore, L. C., Lu, Z., Liu J, Chen K, Jia G, Bergelson J & He, C. (2014) Unique features of the m^6A methylome in *Arabidopsis thaliana. Nat. Commun.* 5: 5630.

[50] Liu, J., Yue, Y., Han, D., Wang, X., Fu, Y., Zhang, L., et al. (2014) A METTL3-METTL14 complex mediates mammalian nuclear RNA N6- adenosine methylation. *Nat Chem Biol.* 10: 93–95.

[51] Esteller, M. (2005) Aberrant DNA methylation as a cancer-inducing mechanism. *Annu Rev Pharmacol Toxicol.* 45: 629–656.

[52] Howard, G., Eiges, R., Gaudet, F., Jaenisch, R. & Eden, A.(2008) Activation and transposition of endogenous retroviral elements in hypomethylation induced tumors in mice. *Oncogene*. 27: 404–408.

[53] Ehrlich, M. (2009).DNA hypomethylation in cancer cells. *Epigenomics*. 1(2): 239–259.

[54] Shen, X., He, Z., Li, H., Yao, C., Zhang, Y., He, L., et al. (2012) Distinct functional patterns of gene promoter hypomethylation and hypermethylation in cancer genomes. *PLoS ONE*. 7(9): e44822.

[55] Beaulieu, N., Morin S., Chute I.C., Robert M.F., Nguyen H. & MacLeod, A.R. (2002) An essential role for DNA methyltransferase DNMT3B in cancer cell survival. *J Biol Chem*. 277: 28176–28181.

[56] Bachman, K.E., Rountree, M.R. & Baylin, S.B. (2001). Dnmt3a and Dnmt3b are transcriptional repressors that exhibit unique localization properties to heterochromatin. *J Biol Chem*. 276: 32282–32287.

[57] Shi, B. & Xu, W. (2013) The development and potential clinical utility of biomarkers for HDAC inhibitors. *Drug Discoveries & Therapeutics*. 7: 129– 136.

[58] Glozak, M. & Seto, E. (2007) Histone deacetylases and cancer. *Oncogene*. 26: 5420–5432.

[59] Lapierre, M., Linares, A., Dalvai, M., Duraffourd, C., Bonnet, S., Boulahtouf, A., et al. (2016) Histone deacetylase regulates breast cancer cell proliferation and the response to histone deacetylase inhibitors. *Oncotarget*. 7(15): 19693– 19708.

[60] Weisenberger, D.J., Siegmund, K.D., Campan, M., Young, J., Long, T.I., Faasse, M.A., et al. (2006) CpG island methylator phenotype underlies sporadic microsatellite instability and is tightly associated with BRAFmutation in colorectal cancer. *Nat Genet*. 38(7): 787–793.

[61] Roessler, J., Ammerpohl, O., Gutwein, J., Steinemann, D., Schlegelberger B., Weyer, V., et al. (2015) The CpG island methylator phenotype in breast cancer is associated with the lobular subtype. *Epigenomics*. 7(2):187–199.

[62] Hino, R., Uozaki, H., Murakami, N., Ushiku, T., Shinozaki, A., Ishikawa, S., et al. (2009) Activation of DNA methyltransferase 1 by EBV latent membrane protein 2A leads to promoter hypermethylation of PTEN gene in gastric carcinoma. *Cancer Res*. 69: 2766–2774.

[63] Tsai, C.N., Tsai, C.L., Tse, K.P., Chang, H.Y. & Chang, Y.S. (2002) The Epstein-Barr virus oncogene product, latent membrane protein 1, induces the downregulation of E-cadherin gene expression via activation of DNA methyltransferases. *Proc Natl Acad Sci USA*. 99(15): 10084–10089.

[64] Roll, J. D., Rivenbark, A. G., Jones, W. D. & Coleman, W. B. (2008). DNMT3b over expression contributes to a hypermethylator phenotype in human breast cancer cell lines. *Molecular Cancer*.7: 15.

[65] Bayley, J.P., Ottenhoff, T.H.M. & Verweij, C.L. (2004) Is there a future for TNF promoter polymorphisms? *Genes Immun*. 5: 315–329.

[66] Ganapathi, S.K., Beggs, A.D., Hodgson, S.V. & Kumar, D. (2014) Expression and DNA methylation of TNF, IFNG and FOXP3 in colorectal cancer and their prognostic significance. *Br J Cancer*. 111: 1581–1589.

[67] Soria, G., Ofri-Shahak, M., Haas, I., Yaal-Hahoshen, N., Leider-Trejo, L., Leibovich-Rivkin, T., et al. (2011) Inflammatory mediators in breast cancer: coordinated expression of TNFα & IL-1β with CCL2 & CCL5 and effects on epithelial-to-mesenchymal transition. *BMC Cancer*.11:130.

[68] Balkwill, F. (2006) TNF-alpha in promotion and progression of cancer. *Cancer Metastasis Rev*. 25: 409–416.

[69] Dong, R., Wang, Q., He, X.L., Chu, Y.K., Lu, J.G. & Ma, Q.J. (2007) Role of nuclear factor kappa B and reactive oxygen species in the tumor necrosis factor-a-induced epithelial-mesenchymal transition of MCF-7 cells. *Braz J Med Biol Res*. 40(8): 1071–1078.

[70] Mani, S.A., Guo, W., Liao, M.J., Eaton, E.N., Ayanan, A., Zhou, A.Y. et al. (2008) The epithelial-mesenchymal transition generates cells with properties of stem cells. *Cell*. 133: 704–771.

[71] Chen, X., Baumel, M., Mannel, D.N., Howard, O.M. & Oppenheim, J.J. (2007) Interaction of TNF with TNF receptor type 2 promotes expansion and function of mouse CD4+CD25+ T regulatory cells. *J Immunol*. 179: 154–161.

[72] McGuire, W., Hill, A. V. S., Allsopp, C. E. M., Greenwood, B. M. & Kwiatkowski, D. (1994) Variation in the TNF-a promoter region associated with the susceptibility to cerebral malaria. *Nature*. 371: 508–510.

[73] Wang, X., & Lin, Y. (2008). Tumor necrosis factor and cancer, buddies or foes? *Acta Pharmacol Sin*. 29(11): 1275–1288.

[74] Madhusudan, S., Foster, M., Muthuramalingam, S.R., Braybrooke, J.P., Wilner, S., Kaur, K., et al. (2004) A phase II study of Etanercept (Enbrel), a tumor necrosis factor inhibitor in patients with metastatic breast cancer. *Clin Cancer Res*. 10: 6528–6534.

[75] Aggarwal, B.B. (2003) Signalling pathways of the TNF superfamily: a double-edged sword. *Nat Rev Immunol*. 3: 745–756.

[76] Morissette, G. & Flamand, L. (2010) Herpesviruses and chromosomal integration. *J Virol*. 84: 12100–12109.

[77] Kenealy, S. J., Herrel, L. A., Bradford, Y., Schnetz-Boutaud, N., Oksenberg, J. R., Hauser, S. L., et al. (2006) Examination of seven candidate regions for multiple sclerosis: strong evidence of linkage to chromosome 1q44. *Genes and Immunity*.7(1): 73–76.

[78] Hoffman, H. M., Wright, F. A., Broide, D.H., Wanderer, A.A., Kolodner, R.D. (2000) Identification of a locus on chromosome 1q44 for familial cold urticaria. *Am J Hum Genet*. 66: 1693–1698.

[79] Christiansen, H. & Lampert, F. (1988) Tumour karyotype discriminates between good and bad prognostic outcome in neuroblastoma. *Br J Cancer*. 57: 121–126.

http://dx.doi.org/10.5772/66988

[80] Sreekantaiah, C., Bhargava, M.K. & Shetty, N.J. (1988) Chromosome 1 abnormalities in cervical carcinoma. *Cancer*. 62(7): 1317–1324.

[81] Couturier-Turpin, M.J., Esnous, C., Louvel, A., Poirier, Y. & Couturier, D. (1992) Chromosome 1 in human colorectal tumors. Cytogenetic research on structural changes and their significance. *Hum Genet*. 88: 431–438.

[82] Orsetti, B., Nugoli, M., Cervera, N., Lasorsa, L., Chuchana, P., Rougé, C., et al. (2006) Genetic profiling of chromosome 1 in breast cancer: mapping of regions of gains and losses and identification of candidate genes on 1q. *Br J Cancer*. 95(10): 1439–1447.

[83] Chen, L. C., Dollbaum, C. & Smith, H. S. (1989) Loss of heterozygosity on chromosome 1q in human breast cancer. *Proc. Natl. Acad. Sci. U.S.A.* 86(18), 7204–7207.

[84] Song, S.J., Poliseno, L., Song, M.S, Ala, U., Webster, K., Ng, C., et al. (2013) MicroRNA-antagonism regulates breast cancer stemness and metastasis via TET-family-dependent chromatin remodeling. *Cell*. 154: 311– 324.

[85] Anaya-Ruiz, M., Cebada, J., Delgado López-G, Sánchez-Vázquez, M.L., Pérez-Santos, J.L.(2013) miR-153 silencing induces apoptosis in the MDA-MB-231 breast cancer cell line. *Asian Pac J Cancer Prev*. 14(5): 2983–2986.

[86] Ouzounova, M., Vuong, T., Ancey P., Ferrand, M., Durand, G., Le-CalvezKelm, F., et al. (2013) "MicroRNA miR-30 family regulates non-attachment growth of breast cancer cells. *BMC Genomics*. 14: 139.

[87] Torkashvand S, Damavandi Z, Mirzaei B, Tavallaei M, Vasei M, Mowla SJ. (2016) Decreased expression of bioinformatically predicted piwil2-targeting microRNAs, miR-1267 and miR-2276 in breast cancer. *Arch Iran Med*.19(6): 420–425.

[88] Wu, Z., He, B., He, J. & Mao, X. (2013) Up regulation of miR-153 promotes cell proliferation via downregulation of the PTEN tumor suppressor gene in human prostate cancer. *Prostate*. 73 (6): 596–604.

Chapter 4

Early-Stage Progression of Breast Cancer

William Kietzman, Anna T. Riegel and Virginie Ory

Additional information is available at the end of the chapter

http://dx.doi.org/10.5772/65633

Abstract

Breast cancer can be defined as a group of diseases with heterogeneous origins, molecular profiles and behaviors characterized by uncontrolled proliferation of cells within the mammary tissue. Around one in eight women in the US will develop breast cancer in their lifetime, making it the second most frequently diagnosed cancer behind skin cancer [1]. In 2015, an estimated 231,840 cases of invasive carcinoma were diagnosed, and over 40,000 deaths were caused by breast cancer which accounts for almost 7% of all cancer mortality each year [1, 2]. In 2015, 60,290 cases of in situ breast cancer were diagnosed, representing over 14% of all new cancer cases among women and men [1]. The steep increase in diagnosis of early-stage breast cancer over the past 10 years is believed to be a result of more frequent mammography. However, since over half of these in situ lesions will not progress to invasive breast cancer, controversies have arisen about approaches to treatment and prevention of progression of early-stage in situ breast cancer. Understanding the mechanisms of transition of normal breast to in situ pre-neoplastic lesions and invasive breast cancer is currently a major focus of breast cancer research with implications for preventive and clinical management of breast cancer. In this review, we give an overview of current knowledge on the molecular and pathological changes that occur during early-stage progression of breast cancer and describe some of the current models that are used to study this process.

Keywords: ductal carcinoma in situ, molecular and cellular drivers of invasive progression, early-stage breast cancer models

1. Pathophysiology of breast cancer

1.1. Anatomy and histology of the normal mammary gland

Within each mammary gland, there are 15–20 lobes containing 20–40 smaller compartments called lobules. Each lobule is composed of 10–100 grapelike clusters of milk-secreting glands termed acini, which are connected to lactiferous ducts [3]. The epithelium throughout the acini and ducts consists of two layers: an inner layer of polarized and cuboidal luminal cells that encapsulate a central lumen, and a basal outer layer of myoepithelial cells with contractile properties conferring these cells an active role in the milk excretion during lactation [3, 4]. Myoepithelial cells also ensure the maintenance of the adjacent luminal epithelial cell polarity and the synthesis of a laminin-rich basement membrane (BM) that forms a structural barrier separating the glandular epithelium from the stroma [5]. In the normal mammary gland, luminal epithelial cells are characterized by the expression of the luminal cytokeratins CK7, CK8 and CK18, sialomucin, epithelial-specific antigen, occludin and integrin β4 [5, 6]. On the other hand, myoepithelial cells express the basal cytokeratins CK5, CK14 and CK17 along with CD10/CALLA, alpha-smooth actin and P63 [6, 7]. The stroma surrounding the mammary gland consists of an insoluble extracellular matrix (laminin, fibronectin, collagen, proteoglycans), mesenchymal cells (fibroblasts, adipocytes, endothelial cells and resident immune cells), and various growth factors and cytokines [8]. Aberrant interactions between mammary epithelial cells and the stroma may lead to structural and functional alterations of the mammary gland biology and ultimately promote breast malignancy [8].

1.2. Hyperplasia/atypical hyperplasia and "in situ" carcinoma histopathology

Many suspicious mammograms or palpable findings turn out to be benign lesions following breast biopsy [9]. However, based on the histopathological report and family history, about 3–10% of these benign lesions are considered to be at high risk of later breast cancer and are referred to as atypical hyperplasia [10, 11]. Atypical hyperplasia is a premalignant lesion diagnosed based on the architectural pattern, cytology and the disease extent and is traditionally classified into two subtypes: atypical ductal hyperplasia (ADH) and atypical lobular hyperplasia (ALH) [12]. The absolute risk of developing breast cancer has been estimated at about 30% for women diagnosed with atypical hyperplasia after 25 years of follow-up [13].

"In Situ" carcinoma, also known as stage 0 breast cancer, is defined by the clonal proliferation of neoplastic epithelial cells within the ducts (e.g., ductal carcinoma in situ) or the lobules (e.g., lobular carcinoma In Situ) of the mammary gland. "In Situ" means that cancer epithelial cells remain confined inside the mammary ducts or lobules with no evidence of cancer cell invasion into the surrounding stroma [1]. Ductal carcinoma in situ (DCIS) incidence has risen, and it accounts for 15–20% of the breast cancer currently diagnosed as a result of increased screening mammography in the past 30 years [14, 15].

Even if DCIS is not immediately life-threatening, 14–53% of untreated DCIS lesions will progress to invasive ductal carcinoma (IDC) with considerable inconsistency in the timing and nature of this transition [16–20]. The most widely accepted model of breast carcinogenesis is the model of "linear" progression that hypothesizes that DCIS is an obligate precursor of IDC evolving through sequential stages, dependent upon early genetic and/or epigenetic changes [21–26].

1.3. DCIS: treatment perspectives

Generally, surgery alone will reduce the risk of mortality following DCIS to less than 5% for lumpectomy and 1% for mastectomy [27]. Surgery followed by radiation and/or hormonal therapy may not alter overall survival dramatically but tends to reduce recurrence, and in the case of hormonal therapy, contralateral breast cancers [28–30]. Decisions regarding therapy are made on a case-by-case basis in function of the clinical presentation and patient choice. Though controversy remains surrounding treatment strategies, generally an argument with concerns of overtreatment voiced against fears of under-treatment; it seems unlikely that current paradigms will change without further research and understanding into the natural history of DCIS progression and identification of clinically actionable markers of risk.

1.4. Profiling of DCIS

Using molecular profiling, Perou et al. first described the subtypes of human breast cancer generating four intrinsic subtypes: luminal A, luminal B (that are frequently ER (estrogen receptor) and PR (progesterone receptor) positive); HER2+ (human epidermal growth factor receptor); and basal-like (frequently HER2-,ER-, PR- also known as triple negative) [31]. These subtypes are utilized currently to subcategorize breast cancer and have demonstrated clinical applicability as individual subtypes display differences in biology and behavior that inform prognosis and course of treatment [31–33].

In 2008, Tamimi et al. performed tissue microarrays for demonstrably reliable [34–37] surrogates for the intrinsic subtypes identified by Perou et al. in 2000 in order to evaluate the prevalence of these phenotypes among DCIS cases. A large cohort of both DCIS and IDC samples were analyzed by immunohistochemistry for ER, PR, HER2, cytokeratin 5/6 and epidermal growth factor receptor (EGFR) and were classified based on expression of these markers. It was discovered that though all of the subtypes are represented in DCIS, the relative frequency differs significantly between DCIS and IDC. HER2 and luminal B subtypes were significantly enriched in the DCIS samples (13.2 and 13.6%, respectively) relative to invasive lesions (5.2 and 5.7%, respectively). In contrast, it was observed that the luminal A subtype was significantly more frequent in invasive carcinoma (73.4%) than in DCIS (62.5%). The triple negative/basal-like category was somewhat more prevalent in invasive carcinoma (10.9%) than in DCIS (7.7%). These discrepancies have been recapitulated by several other studies utilizing genetic means that corroborate this and other histological studies [38–42].

2. Drivers of malignant progression of early-stage breast cancer

Two types of mechanisms drive the invasive progression of DCIS: genetic and/or epigenetic modifications occurring in tumor epithelial cells, or nongenetic aberrations as a result of the bidirectional interactions between cancer epithelial cells and their microenvironment. No molecular markers have been convincingly validated to predict which subsets of DCIS are expected to progress to IDC. Nevertheless, a plethora of studies have demonstrated that the most significant changes in gene expression profiles are observed during the transition from normal tissue to DCIS [43] and revealed that the genetic patterns observed in IDC are already present in DCIS, suggesting a probable common origin [24, 44].

2.1. Genomic changes during progression

In addition to HER2, ER and PR status, similarities between DCIS and IDC begin broadly with chromosomal aberrations that are present in both invasive and in situ stages of disease [45–48]. Several studies have demonstrated that the majority of DCIS cases harbor large copy number alterations that appear to have origins in the transition from normal mammary epithelium to ADH, indicative of a role in early tumorigenesis [40, 48, 49]. The general profile and distribution of DCIS copy number variation have proven to very nearly match that which was previously established for invasive breast cancer with 63% of the peak regions overlapping and 21% within 10 Mb of peak regions established in IDC [46, 48, 50, 51]. Many of the most frequently observed and well-characterized alterations in invasive cancer, including gains on 1q, 5p, 8q, 12q, 16p, 20q and Xq along with losses on 8p, 9p, 11q, 13q, 14q, 16q, 17p and Xp, were similar among ADH, DCIS and IDC [45, 52]. It has been demonstrated that, on average, 83% (range 59–100%) of matched DCIS and IDC genome sample displays the exact same copy number status [48, 53]. A large body of work has failed to find significant, nonrandom discrepancies in the quantity or quality of DCIS copy number aberrations relative to invasive carcinoma [24, 25, 44, 52, 54–60]. These data support the notion of clonal disease origins and add evidence to the case that DCIS is a precursor lesion to invasive stages. Some studies have shown these genetic alterations to increase in frequency during progression from ADH through DCIS to IDC [24, 45, 49]. This suggests that at least some of the genomic alterations may be required for progression though they could be indicative of global genomic instability resulting in the accumulation of chromosomal gains and losses over time. Some studies utilizing matched synchronous ipsilateral DCIS and IDC have identified potential copy number variations that may be related to progression including amplification of genes mediating proliferative, invasive and migratory function such as the growth factor receptor, fibroblast growth factor receptor 1 [61], V-myc avian myelocytomatosis viral oncogene homolog (MYC) [62] and cyclin D1 [63] in invasive disease relative to in situ lesions. Despite these findings, it appears that these changes alone are not necessary or sufficient to drive the acquisition of an invasive phenotype and tend to be inconsistent across individual studies [45–47].

2.2. Transcriptomic and proteomic changes during progressions

In a 2015 study by Abba et al., the full exome, transcriptome and methylome of 30 pure high-grade DCIS cases were examined. 100% of DCIS cases displayed numerous somatic mutations, 62% harboring mutations in known and potential cancer driver genes; though moderately lower than invasive disease, overall the mutational profile of DCIS is remarkably similar to later stages [40]. Not all DCIS cases with chromosomal copy number variation also exhibit mutations in driver genes, which could suggest that chromosomal alteration proceeds some mutation and is a very early event in the natural history of breast cancer [25, 40]. In fact, only 10% of cases in this study displayed unaltered chromosomal copy number and cancer driver genes. They report evidence of P53 pathway inactivation in every lesion analyzed; regardless of its mutation status or intrinsic subtype, a provocative finding as P53 inactivation is not commonplace in all varieties of invasive disease [64, 65]. Other studies have found P53 mutation in anywhere from 15 to 22% of cases [66–69]. A higher frequency was observed in high-grade lesions, a trend that is reflected in invasive breast cancer [66, 67]. Overall, this study concluded that on a whole, the molecular profiles they identified in DCIS were indistinguishable from invasive cancer suggesting that the known major genomic anomalies present in later stages of disease are present in their in situ origins. The results of this study corroborate earlier studies comparing the molecular profiles of ADH, DCIS and IDC, all of which find that the stages of breast cancer progression are extremely similar to one another, providing evidence in support of the now widely held notion that the gene and protein expression changes present in IDC proceed the transition from in situ [39, 40, 43, 70–75].

A recent study by Lesurf et al. compared DCIS and IDC after stratifying by intrinsic subtype and was able to identify differential and highly specific gene sets that distinguish IDC from DCIS [38]. The gene sets are remarkably distinct with no single gene present in every subtype's "invasion signature." It is thus possible that previous studies lack of stratification by subtype could have generated systematic errors in attempts to identify genetic predictors of progression. Strengthening this case, when genetic analysis is performed without intrinsic subtype stratification, it generates relatively inconclusive differentially expressed gene lists with significant overlap relative to previous lists generated without stratification [39, 43, 70, 74, 76, 77]. These previously generated gene lists have not be overwhelmingly useful as predictive tools for progression of DCIS, making Lesurf's findings of invasive signatures valuable. Further work needs to be done to validate these signatures before anyone can comfortably rely on them for consideration in therapy.

DCIS has also been analyzed at the proteomic level, and compared to normal ductal and lobular units, this has revealed that alterations in protein expression occur during carcinogenesis [72]. Proteins that have been identified to be significantly differentially expressed between normal structures and in situ carcinoma have functions ranging from control of cytoskeletal architecture, intracellular trafficking, apoptosis, chaperone functions to regulation of genomic stability [72]. Differential expression of actin-binding proteins was considered to be an unusual finding as remodeling of the actin cytoskeleton tends to be related to lamellar protrusions utilized in invasion and motility, and DCIS is defined as a pre-invasive lesion [72]. It seems that, in a manner similar to the genomic and transcriptomic variation observed in breast cancer progression, proteomic alterations are an early event in the natural history of tumor progression and do not display extensive changes in the transition from in situ.

2.3. Epigenomic changes during progression

Based on the overall lack of differences observed at both the global genomic and transcriptomic levels, some have postulated that epigenetic alterations, inheritable changes that do not modify DNA sequences, may be involved in the transition from in situ to IDC. DNA methylation is a common mechanism of gene promoter silencing [78–80] and has been demonstrated to increase in breast tumorigenesis [81–83]. In comparing normal breast epithelium, ADH, DCIS and IDC, Park et al. noted an increase in methylation status of interrogated breast cancer-specific CpG islands in the transition from normal to ADH and again when comparing

DCIS to ADH though DCIS and IDC did not differ in methylation levels or frequencies. Even the earliest morphologically identifiable stages of breast disease, columnar cell lesions, display an increase in the number of methylated genes, with a similar profile to DCIS and IDC [84]. This suggests that changes in methylation frequency and patterning are an early event in the natural history of breast cancer and may not significantly contribute to the transition between disease stages.

Outside of methylation status, chromatin remodeling via modification of histone residues results in differential gene transcription and has been linked to carcinogenesis [85–87]. Hints at the importance of chromatin remodeling in DCIS formation and progression have been demonstrated with over expression of chromatin remodeling proteins associated with transformation of premalignant lesions and poor prognosis in invasive disease [88, 89]. One study has even demonstrated that overexpression of the chromatin remodeling protein EZH2 is able to drive the acquisition of malignant phenotypes in immortalized mammary epithelial cells [88]. Chromatin remodeling also appears to be involved in the epithelial to mesenchymal transition, a process reported to be important in the DCIS transition to IDC [76, 90].

Another mechanism of epigenetic gene regulation is the expression of microRNAs (miRNAs) which are short noncoding sequences that are able to bind and repress translation of messenger RNAs [91, 92]. When compared to normal breast epithelium, DCIS miRNA profiles do display differences such as increased miR-21 and decreased miR-98 and let-7, though these changes are consistent between DCIS and IDC [93]. Some studies have identified potential miRNA invasive signatures highlighting differential expression of a subset of miRNAs in the transition from DCIS to IDC while others have found essentially no difference between the two [38, 40, 94]. Further studies will need to be done to validate the potential pro-invasive effect of miRNAs that could be involved in the transition to invasive carcinoma.

A more recently recognized mechanism of epigenetic regulation is the alternative splicing of mRNA transcripts, allowing for the generation of multiple unique proteins from the same message, which may have differential and even opposing functions [95, 96]. For example, our lab has studied the role of the nuclear co-activator and oncogene, amplified in breast cancer 1 (AIB1), and we have identified an alternatively processed transcript of the mRNA which generates a shorter form of the protein named AIB1-Δ4 [97]. We have demonstrated an upregulation of this variant in breast cancer and have associated the alternative processing with loss of a regulatory domain, potentiating the oncogenic function of AIB1 [97]. Our lab has also shown that AIB1 is upregulated in the transition from normal breast to DCIS and maintained in the transition to invasive carcinoma [98]. It is possible that given the enhanced oncogenic activity of Δ4 and correlation of this variant with metastatic capability that alternative splicing of this oncogene could play a role in progression from DCIS to invasive disease. Future investigation into alternative splicing in the acquisition of invasive capacity could yield fruitful results in understanding, predicting and potentially preventing progression.

Overall the epigenetic changes interrogated as a potential drivers of tumor progression have returned similar results to genetic and proteomic investigations—differences between invasive and in situ disease are minimal suggesting that epigenetic alterations seen in advanced disease are present from an early stage in the natural progression of breast cancer [81, 84, 99].

2.4. Tumor microenvironment components driving invasive progression

Breast cancer cells are integrated within a complex microenvironment that has been increasingly recognized to influence tumor initiation and invasiveness [100, 101]. The tumor microenvironment (TME) is composed of multiple stromal cells (e.g., myoepithelial cells, fibroblasts, immune cells and adipocytes), insoluble extracellular matrix (ECM), newly formed vasculature, as well as growth factors and cytokines [101].

2.4.1. Myoepithelial cells

The disruption of the myoepithelial cell layer that separates in situ lesions from the surrounding breast stroma is considered to be the initial step required for DCIS to progress to IDC [102–106]. Normal myoepithelial cells secrete proteinase inhibitors along with factors like thrombospondin, laminin and the oxytocin receptor that ensure the maintenance of BM integrity and suppress epithelial cell proliferation and invasion [104, 105]. By contrast, cancer-associated myoepithelial cells (CAMs) aid in BM destruction through proteinase production [5, 107]. Though they appear genomically normal, CAMs are significantly different from those associated with normal ductal structures in terms of gene expression and tumor-suppressive function [73, 102, 106, 108] and engage in paracrine signaling with adjacent cancer cells [109, 110]. One such signaling axis is the upregulation of the chemokine CXCL14 which has been demonstrated to positively influence proliferation, migration and invasion of cancer epithelial cells [73]. Loss of tumor-suppressive signaling and the loss of this physical cell barrier along with associated ECM signaling unleash progressive potential [5, 102, 106, 111, 112].

2.4.2. Immune cells

In response to impairment of the BM, tumor cells express chemokines (e.g., colony-stimulating factor 1 receptor) that attract macrophages within the TME [113, 114]. Tumor-associated macrophages (TAMs), mainly of M2 phenotype, can constitute up to 50% of the breast tumor mass [115], and increased TAMs density has been shown to relate poor prognosis in most human tumors [114, 116]. M2-type TAMs are critical modulators that potentiate the invasion of tumor cells through various mechanisms: secretion of chemotactic factors (e.g., EGF) [117], pro-angiogenic molecules (e.g., vascular endothelial growth factor) [118] and anti-inflammatory cytokines (such as interleukin-10) [119, 120], as well as remodeling of the ECM [121]. Tumor infiltrating lymphocytes (TILs) have also been identified as a prognostic factor in breast cancer, generally associated with improved survival, decreased distant recurrence and increased metastatic latency predicting a better response to therapeutic interventions and overall survival [122–126]. Though there have been many studies on the importance of immune presence and regulation in advanced breast cancers, the immune infiltrate in DCIS specifically is less well characterized and has only recently started to be evaluated. A novel 2016 study by Thompson et al. investigated the immune microenvironment of 27 DCIS cases of known intrinsic subtype [127, 128]. CD3+ T cells were the predominate lymphocyte subtype across all DCIS cases with CD4+ T-helper cells making up a slightly larger proportion compared to CD8+ effector T cells. Also present, though at a lower frequency were CD20+ B cells and FoxP3+ T regulatory cells. Interestingly, it was noted that the DCIS cases included that had concurrent invasive disease tended to have more CD20+ B cell and CD8+ T cell infiltrate. Additionally, the DCIS cases known to recur later had greater CD8+ T cells than other subsets of DCIS cases and also displayed an increased relative presence of regulatory T cells than those that did not [127]. These findings suggest that an active adaptive immune response is mounted early in the natural history of breast cancer and that suppression of the host immune system constitutes another crucial step in the malignant progression through the inhibition of immune effector cells (e.g., myeloid-derived suppressor cells) and the stimulation of immunosuppressive cells (e.g., regulatory T cells) [129].

2.4.3. *Fibroblasts*

Cancer-associated fibroblasts (CAFs) are predominant components of the TME that enhance tumor growth and invasiveness by conferring a mesenchymal-like phenotype in premalignant mammary epithelial cells [130]. CAFs create a pro-tumorigenic environment through high deposition, cross-linking and remodeling of the ECM [131], and by regulating the immune polarization [52]. In breast cancer carcinoma, transforming growth factor beta (TGF-β), stromal cell-derived factor-1, platelet-derived growth factor α/β and interleukin 6 are the major tumor-derived factors that have been described to induce CAFs activation [132–134]. Reciprocally, CAFs secrete tumor-promoting factors, such as hepatocyte growth factor, that stimulate the invasive behavior of DCIS cells [135]. Co-implantation of CAFs with DCIS cells has been shown to increase the invasive capacity of the in situ lesions [136, 137]. For instance, the presence of CAFs resulted in activation of cyclooxygenase-2 (COX-2) in the epithelial component, driving cancer progression [136]. It should be noted that COX-2 expression was demonstrated to be one of three markers, along with P16 and Ki-67 that were found to be associated with significantly increased risk of invasive recurrence within 8 years of initial diagnosis and treatment of DCIS [138].

2.4.4. *Extracellular matrix*

Factors that mediate ECM remodeling and degradation have been of interest in studying the transition of DCIS to invasive disease as destruction of the BM is a hallmark of progression. Several studies have shown matrix metalloproteinases (MMPs) such as MMP1, 2 11, 12 and 13 as well as other proteases and protease inhibitors such as cathepsins, PLAU, SERPINS and metallopeptidase inhibitors to be regulated, up and down respectively, in both DCIS and invasive cancer-associated stromal cells [73, 74, 139]. These expression changes are further linked to poor prognosis and likely related to the acquisition of invasive capacity [73, 74, 139]. Lyons et al. suggested that mammary gland involution, which is a natural driving force of ECM remodeling following pregnancy [140–142], may recapitulate alterations that occur in the initiation of tumor progression [143]. They demonstrated in a mouse model of involution that xenografted MCF10DCIS.com cells grown in this environment formed larger more invasive lesions marked by increased fibrillar collagen deposition and COX-2 expression and that anti-inflammatory treatments with NSAIDs were able to at least partially prevent this progression [143].

http://dx.doi.org/10.5772/65633

2.4.5. *Neovasculature*

In order to sustain their expanding neoplastic growth and eventually disseminate to distant sites, tumors are capable of stimulating the formation of new blood vessels, a process referred to as angiogenesis [144]. Strikingly, the tumor-associated neovasculature is observed early during carcinogenesis in both murine and human premalignant, noninvasive lesions [145, 146]. The transition from dormant nonvascularized hyperplasia to vascularized proliferative tumor requires the cooperation of various TME cell types (e.g., endothelial and pericytes) and is regulated by counteracting molecules, of which the main pro- and anti-angiogenic factors are vascular endothelial growth factor-A and thrombospondin-1, respectively [147].

2.4.6. *Adipocytes*

Lastly, at earlier stages, the level of invasiveness of breast tumor ductal epithelial cells is increased as a result of the secretion and processing of ECM molecules by the mammary adipocytes, especially type VI collagen [148, 149].

3. Experimental models of early-stage breast cancer

Our understanding of the natural history of early-stage breast cancer remains challenging due to the tumor heterogeneity and requires the implementation of experimental models that are capable of mimicking all aspects of the disease. Cell lines and mouse models are valuable tools routinely used to investigate the mechanisms underlying the initiation and progression of breast cancer and will be reviewed in this section.

3.1. In vitro models

3.1.1. *Normal breast epithelial cell lines*

Most in vitro studies aiming to model early-stage breast cancer are based on the utilization of immortalized mammary epithelial cells

3.1.1.1. *MCF10A cell line*

MCF10A cell line is the most commonly used breast epithelial cell line to model normal breast epithelium. This immortal cell line was generated from the fibrocystic breast tissue of a 36-year-old patient and emerged spontaneously as a result of continuous trypsin-versene passages [150]. These cells are considered as "normal" breast epithelial cells based on various characteristics commonly found in the normal glandular epithelium, including lack of tumorigenicity, anchorage-dependent growth, as well as hormonal and growth factor-dependent proliferation in vitro. MCF10A cells are ER negative and express wild-type P53 [151] along with markers of basal-like cells, such as P63 [152, 153]. Although MCF10A cells are non-transformed and exhibit near diploidy, cytogenetic analyses revealed that these cells are karyotypically abnormal following immortalization. Their genetic abnormalities include amplification of the oncogene MYC and the deletion of the chromosomal locus containing genes regulating the cellular senescence, especially P14ARF and P16 [150]. These latter molecular characteristics render MCF10A cell line particularly adapted for oncogenic transformations. Cui et colleagues recently reported that MCF10A cells do not fully recapitulate in vitro the architectural features of normal human breast tissue most likely due to epigenetic derivations driven by the immortalization process and a continuous culture [154].

3.1.1.2. Primary mammary epithelial cell lines

In vitro systems using primary human mammary epithelial cells (HMEC) are believed to be a more reliable model of normal breast epithelial cells. Usually easily isolated from reduction mammoplasty tissues, the life span and propagation of HMEC in vitro remain challenging as they stop doubling and undergo cellular senescence after several passages [155]. In addition, these cells tend to lose their lineage commitment as well as their capacity to grow and normally differentiate when cultured ex vivo. To overcome the senescence block, primary human epithelial cells have been immortalized using exogenous expression of viral oncogenes [156] and the telomerase reverse transcriptase [157]. None of these strategies is capable of maintaining these cells in culture without permanently altering their normal phenotype and genetic background. Schlegel and colleagues in collaboration with our laboratory recently established a novel method that can be used to indefinitely propagate a wide range of normal primary epithelial cells, including breast cells [158, 159]. This technique is based on the coculture of primary epithelial cells in presence of irradiated fibroblasts and requires the utilization of a specialized medium containing a Rho-kinase inhibitor. The resultant cells, also referred to as conditionally reprogrammed cells (CRCs), although highly proliferative, remain karyotypically normal, non-tumorigenic [158] and exhibit hallmarks of adult stem cells [159, 160]. Because human breast CRCs can be genetically modified in culture and implanted into mouse models as discussed below, the CRC system appears as an in vitro method of choice to study the phenotypic and molecular alterations underlying the benign to malignant transition in breast cancer.

3.1.2. Early-stage breast cancer cell lines

To explore the mechanisms promoting the invasive progression of DCIS, the scientific community has at its disposal few cellular models, although no single cell line is capable of fully recapitulating the different subtypes of DCIS tumors.

3.1.2.1. MCF10DCIS.com cell line

The majority of research studies focused on early-stage breast cancer utilized the premalignant MCF10A series established by Miller and Colleagues [161, 162]. One of these variants, termed MCF10DCIS.com, was isolated upon successive passages in culture of lesions obtained from xenografted MCF10AT cells [162]. At the molecular level, MCF10DCIS.com is a ER-negative basal-like cell line that expresses high levels of signaling proteins well-known to play a crucial role in malignant progression, including CD44v, HER2, COX-2, Smad4, Stat3, Pak4 and the phosphorylated forms of ERK and AKT [163]. Similarly, a gain of function mutation conferring an increased oncogenic potential to the phosphatidylinositol 3-kinase has also been found in MCF10DCIS.com cells [164]. Of note, although MCF10DCIS.com cells are considered as a model of early-stage disease, these cells secrete a significant amount of the metastatic galectin-3-binding protein [165], which suggests that they also contain precursors with metastatic capacities. The essential advantage of using MCF10DCIS.com cells relies on their ability to give rise to fast-growing and comedo-like DCIS tumors when injected into xenograft mouse model [162, 166]. The particular features of the tumors derived from MCF10DCIS.com xenograft will be described in the next section.

3.1.2.2. SUM cell lines

Eleven breast cancer cell lines, referred to as SUM, have been generated by Forozan et al. from different subtypes of primary breast tumors [167]. Two of them, called SUM-102 and SUM-225 cells, were immortalized from human DCIS tumors containing microinvasive lesions or from recurrent lesions formed in the chest wall of a patient with DCIS history that did not receive chemotherapy treatment, respectively. SUM-102 cells express CK19 and are considered as basal B-type breast cancer cells [167, 168]. These cells also overexpress Cyclin D1 while they possess mutations in PIK3CA, P16 [169] and checkpoint kinase 2 genes [170]. On the other hand, SUM-225 cells are ER and PR negative, whereas they are amplified for HER2 and are thus classified as luminal epithelial cells [167, 171]. Of note, a P53 missense mutation frequently observed in breast cancer within the sequence encoding the DNA-binding region has also been found in SUM-225 cells [171]. Like MCF10DCIS.com cells, SUM-225 cells generate tumors resembling human DCIS lesions when injected into immuno-compromised mice [166].

3.1.2.3. 21T cell lines

Band and colleagues developed another series, named 21T, including four cell lines established from the tumor tissues of a 36-year-old woman that was first diagnosed with stage 3 intraductal carcinoma, then developed lung metastases 1 year later [172]. 21PT and 21NT cells were both isolated and immortalized from the primary breast tumor and were found to resemble ADH and DCIS, respectively. Phenotypically, 21PT cells are normal spindle epithelial cells, whereas 21NT cells are polygonal-shaped tumor cells of different sizes. At the molecular level, these two cell lines are aneuploid, HER2-amplified and are believed to not express ER and PR, reflecting the original patient biopsy. The most striking difference between 21PT and 21NT cells relies on their ability to form tumors when grown into immunodeficient mice, and this tumorigenic property was shown to be restricted to 21NT cells [172, 173].

3.1.2.4. Other immortalized cell lines

To date, two additional early-stage breast cancer cell lines have been reported: h.DCIS.01 cells established from columnar cell hyperplastic lesions [77] and FSK-H7 cells isolated from human DCIS tumors positive for HER2 [166]. Similar to the previous cell lines, h.DCIS.01 and FSK-H7 cells are capable of producing xenograft tumors in vivo as reviewed previously [77, 166]. In addition to these established cell lines, various technologies have been developed to generate primary breast cancer cell lines representing the full spectrum of human breast cancer subtypes, such as the mammary-optimized EpiCult-B technology and the CRC system (described above) [158, 159, 174]. The CRC system is particularly advantageous as it allows for isolation and rapid expansion of tumor cells from a core needle biopsy of human or murine breast cancer [158, 174]. Notably, primary murine CRCs are able to form tumors recapitulating the original carcinoma when implanted orthotopically into syngeneic mice [159].

As previously discussed in this chapter, signals from the breast microenvironment play a key role in the differentiation and maintenance of normal breast epithelial cells [8], as well as during breast cancer initiation and progression [101]. For these reasons, homotypic culture of breast cancer cell lines does not provide the optimal system for studying the multicellular complexity of breast carcinogenesis. This latter limitation emphasizes the importance of developing in vitro culture systems that allow investigations of the cross talk between breast cancer epithelial cells and the surrounding stroma.

3.2. In vitro models for tumor-stromal interactions

Breast cancer cells cultured ex vivo in three-dimensional and heterotypic systems represent advanced and effective tools for elucidating the morphological and molecular changes governing the epithelial-stromal interactions during breast cancer invasive progression. Besides recapitulating the breast cellular complexity, organotypic 3D cultures are also practicable systems for experimental research and manipulations of cell lines.

3.2.1. Three-dimensional culture systems

Morphogenesis and homeostasis of the normal breast epithelium depend on the balanced relationship between ductal epithelial cells and the ECM [175]. Conversely, the altered communication between epithelial cells and ECM results in the loss of polarity together with the invasion of epithelial cells through the ECM and ultimately contributes to cancer initiation and progression. Breast epithelial cells grown in three-dimensional (3D) systems can recapitulate the architectural and functional features of the glandular epithelium in vivo in response to molecular signals provided by the ECM substratum [176, 177]. The development of biologically relevant 3D models relies on matching specific matrices and culture media with specific cell types. Particularly, mammary epithelial cells are capable of forming differentiated and functional organoids that resemble normal mammary acini when grown within substrata rich in collagen I [178] or laminin [179], and under culture conditions allowing their survival and proliferation [180, 181]. The vast majority of the 3D cultures of breast epithelial cells imply the utilization of an ECM secreted by the Englebreth-Holm-Swarm mouse tumor cells and commercially available as Matrigel™ [179]. Matrigel™ is composed of laminin, collagen IV, entactin and proteoglycans and is supposed to mimic the ductal BM. Monotypic and Matrigel™-based 3D culture assays recapitulating the breast epithelial signaling have been originally developed by Brugge, Bissell and colleagues in order to unravel the morphogenetic processes supporting the normal mammary gland development and its tumorigenesis [180–182]. Notably, Petersen et al. reported that normal breast cells seeded singly within Matrigel™ are capable of forming spherical, polarized and growth-arrested acini-like structures with a central hollow lumen and deposition of BM rich in laminin V and collagen IV [176, 180]. By contrast, breast tumor cells failed to adopt acini-like phenotypes and instead evolved into poorly differentiated, non-polarized and highly disordered aggregates when grown in Matrigel™ [176].

3D culture systems offer the opportunity to investigate a large spectrum of phenotypic effects mediated by oncogenes and tumor suppressors on the architecture of breast epithelia by using two main strategies. The first strategy intends to reconstruct the tumorigenic phenotypes as a result of targeted genetic modifications in normal epithelial cells. For example, Muthuswamy et al. demonstrated that MCF10A cells genetically engineered to overexpress the oncogene HER2 can give rise to hyperproliferative multi-acinar structures showing filled lumina and loss of the apicobasal polarization when cultured in homotypic 3D assays [183]. These disorganized structures are characterized by the absence of invasive properties and thus mirror the histopathological hallmarks of precancerous epithelial cells, especially human DCIS. The second strategy aims to genetically manipulate breast cancer cells to possibly restore the organized and polarized phenotype observed in the normal breast duct. Recently, our laboratory followed this strategy to delineate the functional role of the oncogene AIB1 during DCIS progression [98]. We demonstrated that small hairpin RNA (shRNA)-mediated knockdown of AIB1 in MCF10DCIS.com cells generates more normal acini-like spheroids with deposition of laminin V to the periphery when these knockdown cells are grown in Matrigel™, overall suggesting that AIB1 plays a key role in the maintenance of the DCIS-like structure in 3D culture.

Besides alterations of the normal breast acinar architecture, the invasion of malignant epithelial cells into the surrounding stroma relies on their migratory properties and implies the protease-mediated disruption of the BM barrier [73]. 3D culture techniques can be applied to assess the migratory behavior of breast cancer cells through specific 3D matrices in response to particular cytokines [184]. As an illustration, Zaman and colleagues revealed that the co-overexpression of the oncogenes HER2 and 14-3-3ζ in MCF10A cells significantly induces their motility within 3D type I collagen matrices in a stiffness-dependent manner [185].

Homotypic organoid models involving a single cell type grown within reconstituted BM matrices remain the most simplistic approach used to appreciate the epithelial-stromal interactions. Significant technological progresses had been made in the past decade to provide the cancer cell scientists with a variety of evolved 3D coculture systems reflecting more faithfully the breast cellular complexity in vivo.

3.2.2. Heterotypic 3D culture systems

Multiple organotypic coculture systems have been elaborated to selectively investigate the cross talk between preneoplastic breast epithelial cells and particular stromal cells, such as myoepithelial cells, fibroblasts and macrophages.

3.2.2.1. Myoepithelial cells

As previously discussed, myoepithelial cells play an essential role in preventing breast cancer dissemination by expressing genes specifically responsible of maintaining a polarized bilayered acinar organization [186]. To decipher the molecular mechanisms underlying the tumor-suppressive role of myoepithelial cells, Petersen and colleagues recently developed 3D cocultures of human primary luminal and myoepithelial cells isolated from either normal breast reduction mammoplasty or breast tumor tissues [5]. They confirmed that luminal epithelial cells embedded in type I collagen matrices required the presence of normal myoepithelial cells to form polarized acini-like structures. By contrast, 3D collagen cocultures of luminal epithelial cells with tumor-derived myoepithelial cells fail to generate properly polarized organoids as a consequence of decreased synthesis of functional laminin I by tumor myoepithelial cells.

3.2.2.2. Fibroblasts

In addition to being the most abundant cancer-associated stromal cells present in the TME, CAFs have been largely shown to modulate the invasive transition of breast cancer [130]. To better comprehend the influence of the cross talk fibroblasts-epithelial cells during early-stage breast cancer, Sadlonova et al. grew premalignant breast MCF10AT cells on top of Matrigel™ in the presence of primary fibroblasts [187]. Only fibroblasts purified from normal breast reduction mammoplasty were able to notably suppress MCF10AT cell growth in 3D culture, whereas breast cancer-derived fibroblasts reduced the proliferation of these transformed cells to a lesser extent. Those results further indicate that upon their malignant conversion, breast cancer epithelial cells become insensitive to the tumor growth inhibitors synthesized by stromal fibroblasts, which underlines the importance of establishing new treatment paradigms for early-stage breast cancer based on recovering the tumor-suppressive function of fibroblasts.

3.2.2.3. Macrophages

Similar heterotypic 3D coculture strategies have been applied to elucidate the molecular mechanisms by which macrophages modulate the behavior of tumor cells during breast carcinogenesis [188, 189]. As an example, Balkwill and colleagues plated MCF-7 cells or human mammary epithelial cells genetically immortalized with hTERT, on top of Matrigel™ [188]. Then, they tested the invasive phenotype of these two breast cancer cells along with the level of expression of 22 inflammatory-related genes in the presence of macrophages, previously isolated from human bone marrow and seeded into a modified Boyden chamber to avoid direct cell-to-cell contact. This method permitted them to prove that the cancer cell ability to invade through Matrigel™ is induced when cocultured with macrophages. This invasive phenotype was further correlated to increased activation of JNK and NF-Kappa B pathways. Linde et al. investigated the macrophage-mediated invasive properties of tumor cells using an approach that integrates macrophages into cocultures of tumor cells with fibroblasts [189]. They plated tumor cells on top of collagen I-rich dermal equivalents containing macrophages derived from bone marrow alone or together with primary dermal fibroblasts. Using this tri-culture model, they concluded that activation of macrophages toward M2 phenotype promotes cancer cell invasion through the proteolytic degradation of the BM likely due to increased levels of MMP-2 and MMP-9 [189]. Although this model was developed using tumor cells derived from squamous cell carcinoma, it was successfully generated in both a murine and human background, and its applicability can presumably be extended to study the interactions between early-stage breast tumor cells and TAMs.

The establishment of a wide collection of heterotypic 3D models and their interchangeable utilization have allowed the extensive study of the molecular roles of each cellular component within the breast TME during carcinogenesis. In addition, these models are easily reproducible and particularly handy for the development of targeted therapies. However, even if organotypic 3D cultures are preferred to in vitro models for the identification of new stromal targets for breast cancer progression, only in vivo models have yet been able to thoroughly recapitulate the complexity of the tumor-stromal interactions that govern breast tumor initiation and invasiveness.

3.3. Mouse models

3.3.1. Xenograft mouse models

Xenografts of human breast cancer cell lines or tissues implanted into immuno-compromised recipient mice represent powerful tools for understanding the multiple aspects of the human disease within an in vivo context. Athymic nude, severe combined immune deficient (SCID), NOD/SCID IL2Rgamma^{null} (NGS) and "humanized" NSG mice are the most commonly utilized immunodeficient animals [190]. Two types of xenograft mouse models of breast cancer are usually established: through subcutaneous injection [162], or after orthotopic transplantation of cancer cells or tissues into the mammary fat pad or the duct [166, 173, 191]. Breast cancer cell lines can be genetically manipulated prior to being grafted into mice, which allows to study the tumorigenic properties of specific factors on the tumor take, growth and dissemination in vivo [98]. On the other hand, the actual human cancer tissue can be used to rapidly generate xenograft tumors recapitulating the cellular and molecular heterogeneity inherent to a particular cancer [191]. As a result, xenograft mouse models are frequently employed to predict the tumor response to clinically relevant drugs as well as their possible adverse effects and thus have served as preclinical models for multiple clinical trials [190]. In order to identify the possible factors driving the invasive transition of DCIS, various xenograft models of human DCIS have also been developed based on the utilization of the DCIS cell lines reviewed above, especially MCF10ADCIS.com [162, 166, 192], 21NTci [173] and SUM-225 cells [166].

3.3.1.1. MCF10ADCIS.com xenograft models

As previously discussed, MCF10ADCIS.com cells are capable of engendering tumors containing comedo-like DCIS lesions that resemble human high-grade DCIS and that spontaneously evolve to IDC in a time-dependent manner when implanted into immunodeficient mice [162, 192]. Polyak and colleagues extensively studied this animal model and revealed that MCF10DCIS.com cells are unique bipotent progenitors capable of differentiating into both luminal and myoepithelial cells following subcutaneous injection into female nude mice [192]. MCF10ADCIS.com xenograft tumors displayed DCIS-like lesions filled with luminal epithelial cells expressing ESA, CD44, CK17, cadherin 1 and vimentin, surrounded by an outer layer of myoepithelial cells positive for P63, CD10 and α-smooth muscle actin, and by a BM rich in laminin V. In addition, they demonstrated that luminal and myoepithelial cells, purified from MCF10ADCIS.com tumors, differentially expressed factors that belong to signaling pathways known to modulate their functional phenotype, especially TGF-β, hedgehog, cell adhesion and P63 signal transduction pathways. Interestingly, these gene expression patterns were similar to those observed in primary DCIS tissues. As mentioned above, the tumorigenic properties of factors possibly involved in breast cancer progression can be investigated using xenograft animal models upon implantation of genetically engineered breast cancer cells. Our laboratory recently used this approach to elucidate the pro-oncogenic function of AIB1 in early-stage breast cancer using the MCF10ADCIS.com xenograft model [98]. Because high levels of AIB1 were found in MCF10ADCIS.com cell line, we transduced these cells with shRNAs directed against AIB1 prior to injection into nude mice. Decreased expression of AIB1 in MCF10ADCIS.com cells resulted in reduced tumor growth and development in vivo. Additionally, MCF10ADCIS.com xenograft tumors deficient in AIB1 exhibited smaller DCIS lesions containing fewer tumor-initiating cells (TIC) and myoepithelial progenitor cells, and those cellular alterations were correlated with downregulation of NOTCH, HER2 and HER3 signaling pathways. Overall, our data indicated for the first time that AIB1 is required for the initiation and preservation of DCIS lesions in part through maintenance of the TICs subpopulation, thus suggesting that AIB1 may serve as a novel therapeutic target for early-stage breast cancer.

3.3.1.2. 21T xenograft model

As detailed previously, 21PT and NT cell lines are primary tumor-derived cells believed to mimic early-stage breast cancer when implanted into the mammary fat pad of female nude mice at 8–9 weeks of age [173]. Souter et al. reported that 21PT cells were not tumorigenic or metastatic in vivo and instead formed xenograft structures that shared features of ADH. Furthermore, atypical/neoplastic and normal/benign epithelial cells were shown to coexist within 21PT xenograft tissues. Conversely, 21NT cells were able to give rise to malignant lesions in about 20% of the mice, and the resultant tumors displayed intermediate to high-grade DCIS lesions, with no evidence of invasive progression. Interestingly, 21NT-derived lesions exhibited phenotypic traits identical to the ones obtained in MCF10ADCIS.com xenograft mouse model, although in contrast to 21NT tumors, MCF10ADCIS.com tumors ultimately progress to IDC as a result of RAS-induced transformation.

3.3.1.3. Mouse intraductal models

Most of the xenograft models are obtained upon subcutaneous injection of cancer cells and thus fail to replicate the early steps of breast carcinogenesis that occur inside the mammary duct. In order to better recreate the natural progression of DCIS within conditions mimicking the stromal microenvironment, Medina and colleagues developed a novel method based on the intraductal transplantation of human breast cancer cells into immunodeficient female mice [166]. To generate this unique mouse intraductal model, they injected the previously described DCIS cell lines, MCF10ADCIS.com, SUM-225 and FSK-H7 cells, through the nipple directly into the mammary ducts of 6- to 10-week-old SCID-beige mice. Following intraductal transplantation, all three cells lines were able to form DCIS-like lesions that slowly evolved into IDC in 90% of the mice. Unlike subcutaneous injection, the intraductal transplantation of MCF10ADCIS.com cells into immuno-compromised mice gave rise to cribriform DCIS, whereas SUM-225 and FSK-H7 cells displayed comedo and apocrine-like DCIS lesions, respectively. Using immunostaining analyses, Behdoh et al. further reported that SUM-225 and FSK-H7 xenograft samples are characterized by the overexpression of HER2 along with moderate expression of CK8 and 19. MCF10ADCIS.com-derived tumors were also positively stained for CK8 although they contained lesions classified as basal-like as they express CK5. More recently, Behbod et colleagues extended the intraductal mouse model to primary human DCIS [191]. They successfully xenotransplanted DCIS cell lines, derived from eight different patient samples, within the mammary duct of 8- to 10-week-old virgin NSG mice. At 8 weeks, the tissues collected from the xenografted tumors exhibited noninvasive lesions that closely resemble human DCIS and that retain the histopathological and molecular hallmarks of the patient's original biopsy. Strikingly, the engraftment of primary DCIS cells obtained from human tumors was only permitted using mice depleted in both mature T and B cells, suggesting that T and B cells both regulate the tumor growth of primary cells into in vivo models. Altogether, the mammary intraductal mouse model thus appears as the most suitable xenograft model of DCIS to deciphering the cellular and molecular processes that underline the epithelial-stromal cell cross talk during the initiation and invasive transition of DCIS.

As the fundamental role exerted by the tumor microenvironment during early-stage breast cancer is increasingly recognized, the subcutaneous implantation of cancer cells into mouse models deficient in T and B lymphocytes remains problematic and may result in decreased tumor take and abnormal cancer progression. To overcome this critical limitation, "humanized" mouse models have been generated based on the engraftment of human $CD34^+$ hematopoietic stem cells onto irradiated NOD/SCID mice [193] and the orthotopic implantation into cleared mammary fat pads humanized using stromal cells of human origin [194]. Humanized mice represent very promising models for better defining the tumorigenic properties of tumor-associated stromal cells during breast cancer development. This strategy can further be used to create a wide range of analogous models reflecting the various subtypes of DCIS.

3.3.2. *Genetically engineered mouse models*

Genetically engineered mouse models (GEMM) constitute invaluable resources for experimentally examining the in vivo function of specific oncogenes or tumor suppressor genes within immunocompetent animals. The primary benefit of employing GEMM as model of human cancer is that this approach allows modulation of the expression of particular genes in a tissue and time-specific fashion. Many GEMM models of breast cancer are currently available and are of two kinds: transgenic models in which specific oncogenes are overexpressed, and knockout models created upon targeted deletion of tumor suppressors [195]. In the following section, we will focus on GEMM that were found to develop tumors containing early-stage breast cancer lesions, especially DCIS.

3.3.2.1. Transgenic mouse models

In transgenic mouse models, the transcription of particular oncogene is induced throughout the mammary luminal epithelium under the control of strong mammary-specific epithelial promoters, of which the mouse mammary tumor virus (MMTV) and the whey acidic protein (WAP) are the most frequently utilized [195]. Transgenic mammary carcinoma models usually give rise to highly penetrant tumors after short latency. To date, few transgenic mouse models of human breast cancer have been shown to develop premalignant and DCIS-like lesions. They are discussed below.

3.3.2.1.1. MMTV-neu mouse model

Given the undeniable association of *neu* (e.g., HER2) amplification with DCIS [196], two mouse models expressing high levels of *neu* driven by the MMTV promoter have been created. Jolicoeur and colleagues established a model by genetically modifying mice to strongly express the activated form of *neu* [197]. As expected, multifocal mammary adenocarcinomas were observed in 5- to 10-month-old transgenic females. The *c-neu* overexpressing tumors displayed undifferentiated lesions resembling human comedo-type DCIS mixed with cytologically normal epithelium. Interestingly, the majority of the primary tumors had the potential to metastasize to the lung. Muller and colleagues developed a transgenic model bearing the unactivated form of *neu* fused to MMTV promoter [198]. The latter transgenic animals gave rise to focal mammary tumors highly metastatic and histologically identical to those induced by the activated *neu*, although after a longer latency period. Using this model, our laboratory demonstrated that the development of early-stage lesions and invasive mammary cancer depends upon the oncogene AIB1 [199].

3.3.2.1.2. MMTV-PyV-mT mouse model

MMTV-PyV-mT mouse model is another frequently used mouse model of premalignant mammary cancer in which the MMTV promoter has been manipulated to target the expression of the polyomavirus middle T antigen (PyV-mT) [198]. The resultant transgenic mice rapidly developed multifocal tumors in all mammary glands associated with secondary lung metastases. Maglione et al. characterized this transgenic model and reported that 5-week-old MMTV-PyV-mT mice carry tumors which contain high-grade, poorly differentiated, ADH-like lesions [200]. Furthermore, those lesions were ER positive and exhibited aberrant vasculature and myoepithelium.

3.3.2.1.3. WAP-T mouse model

The WAP promoter sequence has also been employed to induce mammary intraepithelial neoplasia in mice. Tzen et al. initially applied this strategy to drive the murine mammary epithelial cell transformation through WAP-mediated increased transcription of the SV40 large T antigen (SV40 TAg) [201]. SV40 TAg possesses the unique properties to physically interact with both P53 [202] and the retinoblastoma protein [203] and abrogate their tumor-suppressive function, leading to cellular hyperproliferation. Deppert and colleagues recently expanded the histological analysis of the WAP-T transgenic mouse model and reported that these animals carried multifocal DCIS-like carcinomas progressing to IDC after a short latency period [204]. Notably, the resultant in situ carcinoma was composed of differentiated lesions showing tubular and papillary architecture comparable to those diagnosed in human DCIS.

3.3.2.1.4. C3(1)-SV40 TAg mouse model

Because MMTV and WAP were shown to be regulated by hormones [205, 206], Dr. Green's laboratory engineered a novel transgenic model by transcriptionally overexpressing the SV40 TAg in the mammary and prostate glands under the hormone-independent control of the C3(1) component of the prostate steroid-binding protein (PSBP) 5′ flanking sequence [207]. All C3(1)-SV40 TAg female mice bore mammary tumors that were found to share similar histologic and molecular hallmarks of human infiltrating ductal carcinoma in a predictable time-dependent manner. Eight-week-old transgenic mice, in fact, did exhibit ADH-like lesions that evolve into DCIS at about 12 weeks, invasive carcinoma at 16 weeks of age and ultimately metastasized into the lung with a 15% incidence. In addition, well-known chromosomal and molecular aberrations driving mammary carcinogenesis were also observed in C3(1)-SV40 TAg mice, thus suggesting that this transgenic model provides the unique opportunity to assess the antitumor potential of targeted therapies.

3.3.2.1.5. MMTV-tTA/tetop-SV40 TAg/tetop ERα mouse model

Increased levels of ERα in mammary epithelial cells are believed to be correlated to initiation and progression of premalignant breast cancer [208]. In order to corroborate this hypothesis, our collaborator Dr. Furth established a unique mouse model with dominant gain of ERα by breeding together three types of transgenic animals expressing: (i) the tetracycline-responsive transactivator tTA under control of MMTV promoter (MMTV-tTA); (ii) SV40 TAg under control of the tetracycline-responsive promoter (tetop); (iii) FLAG-tagged ERα under control of tetop [209, 210]. Strikingly, 4-month-old triple transgenic mice (MMTV-tTA/tetop-SV40 TAg/tetop-ERα) gave rise to ERα positive and estrogen-sensitive mammary tumors that contained preneoplastic lesions identical to those found in human ADH and DCIS. Using the double transgenic mice MMTV-tTA/tetop ERα, Frech et al. further reported that the rate of mammary epithelial cell proliferation was higher in ADH and DCIS lesions and was accompanied by increased expression of cyclin D1 in the nuclear compartment of these cells [210]. Altogether, this work reported for the first time that high ERα expression can promote the benign to cancerous transformation of mammary epithelial cells in vivo and provided unique mouse models to unravel the neoplastic events regulated by ERα signalings.

3.3.2.1.6. GEMM-based syngeneic transplantation models

Due to the time-consuming nature of using GEMM and their costs, various methods have recently emerged based on the establishment of stable mammary intraepithelial neoplasia outgrowth (MIN-O) lines derived from tumors carried by GEMM, such as MMTV-PyV-mT [211], P53 knockout [212] and MMTV-*Neu* mice [159]. The orthotopic serial transplantation of these MIN-O cell lines into immunocompetent syngeneic mice has been proven to faithfully mimic the human disease and offered the opportunity to well-characterize the molecular mechanisms underlying breast cancer progression. As an illustration, Gregg and colleagues obtained MIN-O lines from MMTV-PyV-mT premalignant lesions and serial transplanted these lines into the cleared mammary fat pads of FVB females [211]. Those PyV-mT lines formed DCIS-like lesions that were able to progress to IDC in a predictable manner and that were undistinguishable from the parental tumors with respect to their histology and molecular profiles. MIN-O lines purified from mice depleted in the suppressor gene P53 [213] and implanted into the cleared fat pads of P53 wild-type BALB/c mice developed DCIS-like and invasive lesions [212]. Similarly to the PyV-mT-derived MIN-O cells, the resultant ductal-like outgrowths were capable of recapitulating the different stages of DCIS progression from ADH to IDC. Our laboratory recently extended this approach to MIN-O lines isolated from MMTV-*Neu* tumors using the CRC technology described previously [159]. The main advantage of this strategy is to allow the indefinite propagation of those lines ex vivo without the need for serial transplantation. Remarkably, MMTV-*Neu* MIN-O cells orthotopically transplanted into syngeneic females gave rise to lesions that retained the histopathological features of the original mammary tumors, underscoring the unique potential of using this approach to generate a wide range of GEMM-based preclinical models.

4. Conclusion

In summary, the molecular and cellular profiling of early-stage breast cancer using in vitro and in vivo models that reflect the heterogeneity of the disease have drastically allowed for improved understanding of the mechanisms underlying invasive progression of DCIS. As no individual model is capable of recapitulating the complexity of the human tumors, efforts should be made in the future to develop integrated strategies for better defining the drivers of early-stage progression of breast cancer and thus open new avenues for targeted therapy.

Acknowledgements

This work was funded in part by RO1CA205632 (ATR) and the Nina Hyde Center Breast Cancer Fund (ATR).

Author details

William Kietzman, Anna T. Riegel and Virginie Ory*

*Address all correspondence to: vo24@georgetown.edu

Department of Oncology, Lombardi Comprehensive Cancer Center, Georgetown University, Washington, DC, USA

References

[1] American Cancer Society. Breast Cancer Facts & Figures 2013-2014. Atlanta: American Cancer Society, Inc. 2013.

[2] Research Data (1973–2013) [Internet]. 2016:1–1. Retrieved from: www.seer.cancer.gov.

[3] Hassiotou F, Geddes D. Anatomy of the human mammary gland: Current status of knowledge. Clin Anat 2013;26:29–48.

[4] Schmeichel KL, Bissell MJ. Modeling tissue-specific signaling and organ function in three dimensions. J Cell Sci 2003;116:2377–88.

[5] Gudjonsson T, Rønnov-Jessen L, Villadsen R, Rank F, Bissell MJ, Petersen OW. Normal and tumor-derived myoepithelial cells differ in their ability to interact with luminal breast epithelial cells for polarity and basement membrane deposition. J Cell Sci 2002;115:39–50.

[6] Yaziji H, Gown AM, Sneige N. Detection of stromal invasion in breast cancer: the myoepithelial markers. Adv Anat Pathol 2000;7:100–9.

[7] Barbareschi M, Pecciarini L, Cangi MG, Macrì E, Rizzo A, Viale G, et al. P63, a p53 homologue, is a selective nuclear marker of myoepithelial cells of the human breast. Am J Surg Pathol 2001;25:1054–60.

[8] Polyak K, Kalluri R. The role of the microenvironment in mammary gland development and cancer. Cold Spring Harb Perspect Biol 2010;2:a003244–4.

[9] Gutwein LG, Ang DN, Liu H, Marshall JK, Hochwald SN, Copeland EM, et al. Utilization of minimally invasive breast biopsy for the evaluation of suspicious breast lesions. Am J Surg 2011;202:127–32.

[10] Simpson JF. Update on atypical epithelial hyperplasia and ductal carcinoma in situ. Pathology 2009;41:36–9.

[11] Hartmann LC, Sellers TA, Frost MH, Lingle WL, Degnim AC, Ghosh K, et al. Benign breast disease and the risk of breast cancer. N Engl J Med 2005;353:229–37.

[12] Ellis IO. Intraductal proliferative lesions of the breast: morphology, associated risk and molecular biology. Mod Pathol 2010;23(Suppl 2):S1–7.

[13] Page DL, Schuyler PA, Dupont WD, Jensen RA, Plummer WD, Simpson JF. Atypical lobular hyperplasia as a unilateral predictor of breast cancer risk: a retrospective cohort study. Lancet 2003;361:125–9.

[14] Ernster VL, Ballard-Barbash R, Barlow WE, Zheng Y, Weaver DL, Cutter G, et al. Detection of ductal carcinoma in situ in women undergoing screening mammography. J Natl Cancer Inst 2002;94:1546–54.

[15] van Dongen JA, Holland R, Peterse JL, Fentiman IS, Lagios MD, Millis RR, et al. Ductal carcinoma in-situ of the breast; second EORTC consensus meeting. Eur J Cancer 1992;28:626–9.

[16] Rosen PP, Braun DW, Kinne DE. The clinical significance of pre-invasive breast carcinoma. Cancer 1980;46:919–25.

[17] Eusebi V, Feudale E, Foschini MP, Micheli A, Conti A, Riva C, et al. Long-term follow-up of in situ carcinoma of the breast. Semin Diagn Pathol 1994;11:223–35.

[18] Page DL, Dupont WD, Rogers LW, Jensen RA, Schuyler PA. Continued local recurrence of carcinoma 15–25 years after a diagnosis of low grade ductal carcinoma in situ of the breast treated only by biopsy. Cancer 1995;76:1197–200.

[19] Collins LC, Tamimi RM, Baer HJ, Connolly JL, Colditz GA, Schnitt SJ. Outcome of patients with ductal carcinoma in situ untreated after diagnostic biopsy: results from the Nurses' Health Study. Cancer 2005;103:1778–84.

[20] Erbas B, Provenzano E, Armes J, Gertig D. The natural history of ductal carcinoma in situ of the breast: a review. Breast Cancer Res Treat 2006;97:135–44.

[21] Wellings SR, Jensen HM. On the origin and progression of ductal carcinoma in the human breast. J Natl Cancer Inst 1973;50:1111–8.

[22] Carter CL, Corle DK, Micozzi MS, Schatzkin A, Taylor PR. A Prospective-Study of the Development of Breast-Cancer in 16,692 Women with Benign Breast Disease. Am J Epidemiol 1988;128:467–77.

[23] Kuerer HM, Albarracin CT, Yang WT, Cardiff RD, Brewster AM, Symmans WF, et al. Ductal carcinoma in situ: state of the science and roadmap to advance the field. J Clin Oncol 2009;27:279–88.

[24] O'Connell P, Pekkel V, Fuqua SA, Osborne CK, Clark GM, Allred DC. Analysis of loss of heterozygosity in 399 premalignant breast lesions at 15 genetic loci. J Natl Cancer Inst 1998;90:697–703.

[25] Hwang ES, DeVries S, Chew KL, Moore DH, Kerlikowske K, Thor A, et al. Patterns of chromosomal alterations in breast ductal carcinoma in situ. Clin Cancer Res 2004;10:5160–7.

[26] Buerger H, Simon R, Schäfer KL, Diallo R, Littmann R, Poremba C, et al. Genetic relation of lobular carcinoma in situ, ductal carcinoma in situ, and associated invasive carcinoma of the breast. MP, Mol Pathol 2000;53:118–21.

[27] Morrow M. Refining the use of endocrine therapy for ductal carcinoma in situ. J Clin Oncol 2012;30:1249–51.

[28] Fisher B, Dignam J, Wolmark N, Wickerham DL, Fisher ER, Mamounas E, et al. Tamoxifen in treatment of intraductal breast cancer: National Surgical Adjuvant Breast and Bowel Project B-24 randomised controlled trial. Lancet 1999;353:1993–2000.

[29] Allred DC, Anderson SJ, Paik S, Wickerham DL, Nagtegaal ID, Swain SM, et al. Adjuvant tamoxifen reduces subsequent breast cancer in women with estrogen receptor-positive ductal carcinoma in situ: a study based on NSABP protocol B-24. J Clin Oncol 2012;30:1268–73.

[30] Margolese RG, et al. Anastrozole versus tamoxifen in postmenopausal women with ductal carcinoma in situ undergoing lumpectomy plus radiotherapy (NSABP B-35): a randomised, double-blind, phase 3 clinical trial. Lancet 2016;387:849–56.

[31] Perou CM, Sørlie T, Eisen MB, van de Rijn M, Jeffrey SS, Rees CA, et al. Molecular portraits of human breast tumours. Nature 2000;406:747–52.

[32] Dai X, Li T, Bai Z, Yang Y, Liu X, Zhan J, et al. Breast cancer intrinsic subtype classification, clinical use and future trends. Am J Cancer Res 2015;5:2929–43.

[33] Parker JS, Mullins M, Cheang MCU, Leung S, Voduc D, Vickery T, et al. Supervised risk predictor of breast cancer based on intrinsic subtypes. J Clin Oncol 2009;27:1160–7.

[34] Cheang MCU, Voduc D, Bajdik C, Leung S, McKinney S, Chia SK, et al. Basal-like breast cancer defined by five biomarkers has superior prognostic value than triple-negative phenotype. Clin Cancer Res 2008;14:1368–76.

[35] Abd El-Rehim DM, Pinder SE, Paish CE, Bell J, Blamey RW, Robertson JFR, et al. Expression of luminal and basal cytokeratins in human breast carcinoma. J Pathol 2004;203:661–71.

[36] Abd El-Rehim DM, Ball G, Pinder SE, Rakha E, Paish C, Robertson JFR, et al. High-throughput protein expression analysis using tissue microarray technology of a large well-characterised series identifies biologically distinct classes of breast cancer confirming recent cDNA expression analyses. Int J Cancer 2005;116:340–50.

[37] van de Rijn M, Perou CM, Tibshirani R, Haas P, Kallioniemi O, Kononen J, et al. Expression of cytokeratins 17 and 5 identifies a group of breast carcinomas with poor clinical outcome. Am J Pathol 2002;161:1991–6.

[38] Lesurf R, Aure MR, Mørk HH, Vitelli V, Oslo Breast Cancer Research Consortium (OSBREAC), Lundgren S, et al. Molecular features of subtype-specific progression from ductal carcinoma in situ to invasive breast cancer. Cell Rep 2016;16:1166–79.

[39] Hannemann J, Velds A, Halfwerk JBG, Kreike B, Peterse JL, van de Vijver MJ. Classification of ductal carcinoma in situ by gene expression profiling. Breast Cancer Res 2006;8:R61.

[40] Abba MC, Gong T, Lu Y, Lee J, Zhong Y, Lacunza E, et al. A molecular portrait of high-grade ductal carcinoma in situ. Cancer Res 2015;75:3980–90.

[41] Meijnen P, Oldenburg HSA, Loo CE, Nieweg OE, Peterse JL, Rutgers EJT. Risk of invasion and axillary lymph node metastasis in ductal carcinomain situ diagnosed by core-needle biopsy. Br J Surg 2007;94:952–6.

[42] Clark SE, Warwick J, Carpenter R, Bowen RL, Duffy SW, Jones JL. Molecular subtyping of DCIS: heterogeneity of breast cancer reflected in pre-invasive disease. Br J Cancer 2011;104:120–7.

[43] Porter D, Lahti-Domenici J, Keshaviah A, Bae YK, Argani P, Marks J, et al. Molecular markers in ductal carcinoma in situ of the breast. Mol Cancer Res 2003;1:362–75.

[44] Buerger H, Otterbach F, Simon R, Poremba C, Diallo R, Decker T, et al. Comparative genomic hybridization of ductal carcinoma in situ of the breast—evidence of multiple genetic pathways. J Pathol 1999;187:396–402.

[45] Gao Y, Niu Y, Wang X, Wei L, Lu S. Genetic changes at specific stages of breast cancer progression detected by comparative genomic hybridization. J Mol Med 2009;87:145–52.

[46] Liao S, Desouki MM, Gaile DP, Shepherd L, Nowak NJ, Conroy J, et al. Differential copy number aberrations in novel candidate genes associated with progression from in situ to invasive ductal carcinoma of the breast. Genes Chromosom Cancer 2012;51:1067–78.

[47] Yao J, Weremowicz S, Feng B, Gentleman RC, Marks JR, Gelman R, et al. Combined cDNA array comparative genomic hybridization and serial analysis of gene expression analysis of breast tumor progression. Cancer Res 2006;66:4065–78.

[48] Johnson CE, Gorringe KL, Thompson ER, Opeskin K, Boyle SE, Wang Y, et al. Identification of copy number alterations associated with the progression of DCIS to invasive ductal carcinoma. Breast Cancer Res Treat 2012;133:889–98.

[49] Xu S, Wei B, Zhang H, Qing M, Bu H. Evidence of chromosomal alterations in pure usual ductal hyperplasia as a breast carcinoma precursor. Oncol Rep 2008;19:1469–75.

[50] Chin K, DeVries S, Fridlyand J, Spellman PT, Roydasgupta R, Kuo W-L, et al. Genomic and transcriptional aberrations linked to breast cancer pathophysiologies. Cancer Cell 2006;10:529–41.

[51] Haverty PM, Fridlyand J, Li L, Getz G, Beroukhim R, Lohr S, et al. High-resolution genomic and expression analyses of copy number alterations in breast tumors. Genes Chromosom Cancer 2008;47:530–42.

[52] Liao D, Luo Y, Markowitz D, Xiang R, Reisfeld RA. Cancer associated fibroblasts promote tumor growth and metastasis by modulating the tumor immune microenvironment in a 4T1 murine breast cancer model. PLoS One 2009;4:e7965.

[53] Vincent-Salomon A, Lucchesi C, Gruel N, Raynal V, Pierron G, Goudefroye R, et al. Integrated genomic and transcriptomic analysis of ductal carcinoma in situ of the breast. Clin Cancer Res 2008;14:1956–65.

[54] Aubele M, Mattis A, Zitzelsberger H, Walch A, Kremer M, Welzl G, et al. Extensive ductal carcinoma In situ with small foci of invasive ductal carcinoma: evidence of genetic resemblance by CGH. Int J Cancer 2000;85:82–6.

[55] Leong AS, Sormunen RT, Vinyuvat S, Hamdani RW, Suthipintawong C. Biologic markers in ductal carcinoma in situ and concurrent infiltrating carcinoma. A comparison of eight contemporary grading systems. Am J Clin Pathol 2001;115:709–18.

[56] Farabegoli F, Champeme M-H, Bieche I, Santini D, Ceccarelli C, Derenzini M, et al. Genetic pathways in the evolution of breast ductal carcinoma in situ. J Pathol 2002;196:280–6.

[57] Burstein HJ, Polyak K, Wong JS, Lester SC, Kaelin CM. Ductal carcinoma in situ of the breast. N Engl J Med 2004;350:1430–41.

[58] Simpson PT, Reis-Filho JS, Gale T, Lakhani SR. Molecular evolution of breast cancer. J Pathol 2005;205:248–54.

[59] Castro NP, Osório CABT, Torres C, Bastos EP, Mourão-Neto M, Soares FA, et al. Evidence that molecular changes in cells occur before morphological alterations during the progression of breast ductal carcinoma. Breast Cancer Res 2008;10:R87.

[60] Iakovlev VV, Arneson NCR, Wong V, Wang C, Leung S, Iakovleva G, et al. Genomic differences between pure ductal carcinoma in situ of the breast and that associated with invasive disease: a calibrated aCGH study. Clin Cancer Res 2008;14:4446–54.

[61] Jang MH, Kim EJ, Choi Y, Lee HE, Kim YJ, Kim JH, et al. FGFR1 is amplified during the progression of in situ to invasive breast carcinoma. Breast Cancer Res 2012;14:R115.

[62] Robanus-Maandag EC, Bosch CAJ, Kristel PM, Hart AAM, Faneyte IF, Nederlof PM, et al. Association of C-MYC amplification with progression from the in situ to the invasive stage in C-MYC-amplified breast carcinomas. J Pathol 2003;201:75–82.

[63] Burkhardt L, Grob TJ, Hermann I, Burandt E, Choschzick M, Jänicke F, et al. Gene amplification in ductal carcinoma in situ of the breast. Breast Cancer Res Treat 2010;123:757–65.

[64] Gasco M, Shami S, Crook T. The p53 pathway in breast cancer. Breast Cancer Res 2002;4:70–6.

[65] Pharoah PD, Day NE, Caldas C. Somatic mutations in the p53 gene and prognosis in breast cancer: a meta-analysis. Br J Cancer 1999;80:1968–73.

[66] Done SJ, Eskandarian S, Bull S, Redston M, Andrulis IL. p53 missense mutations in microdissected high-grade ductal carcinoma in situ of the breast. J Natl Cancer Inst 2001;93:700–4.

[67] O'Malley FP, Vnencakjones CL, Dupont WD, Parl F, Manning S, Page DL. P53 mutations are confined to the comedo type ductal carcinoma in-situ of the breast—immunohistochemical and sequencing data. Lab Invest 1994;71:67–72.

[68] Lukas J, Niu N, Press MF. p53 mutations and expression in breast carcinoma in situ. Am J Pathol 2000;156:183–91.

[69] Polyak K. Molecular alterations in ductal carcinoma in situ of the breast. Curr Opin Oncol 2002;14:92–6.

[70] Ma X-J, Salunga R, Tuggle JT, Gaudet J, Enright E, McQuary P, et al. Gene expression profiles of human breast cancer progression. Proc Natl Acad Sci USA 2003;100:5974–9.

[71] Nagaraja GM, Othman M, Fox BP, Alsaber R, Pellegrino CM, Zeng Y, et al. Gene expression signatures and biomarkers of noninvasive and invasive breast cancer cells: comprehensive profiles by representational difference analysis, microarrays and proteomics. Oncogene 2006;25:2328–38.

[72] Wulfkuhle JD, Sgroi DC, Krutzsch H, McLean K, McGarvey K, Knowlton M, et al. Proteomics of human breast ductal carcinoma in situ. Cancer Res 2002;62:6740–9.

[73] Allinen M, Beroukhim R, Cai L, Brennan C, Lahti-Domenici J, Huang H, et al. Molecular characterization of the tumor microenvironment in breast cancer. Cancer Cell 2004;6:17–32.

[74] Schuetz CS, Bonin M, Clare SE, Nieselt K, Sotlar K, Walter M, et al. Progression-specific genes identified by expression profiling of matched ductal carcinomas in situ and invasive breast tumors, combining laser capture microdissection and oligonucleotide microarray analysis. Cancer Res 2006;66:5278–86.

[75] Seth A, Kitching R, Landberg G, Xu J, Zubovits J, Burger AM. Gene expression profiling of ductal carcinomas in situ and invasive breast tumors. Anticancer Res 2003;23:2043–51.

[76] Knudsen ES, Ertel A, Davicioni E, Kline J, Schwartz GF, Witkiewicz AK. Progression of ductal carcinoma in situ to invasive breast cancer is associated with gene expression programs of EMT and myoepithelia. Breast Cancer Res Treat 2012;133:1009–24.

[77] Lee S, Stewart S, Nagtegaal I, Luo J, Wu Y, Colditz G, et al. Differentially expressed genes regulating the progression of ductal carcinoma in situ to invasive breast cancer. Cancer Res 2012;72:4574–86.

[78] Jones PA, Laird PW. Cancer epigenetics comes of age. Nat Genet 1999;21:163–7.

[79] Baylin SB, Chen WY. Aberrant gene silencing in tumor progression: implications for control of cancer. Cold Spring Harb Symp Quant Biol 2005;70:427–33.

[80] Newell-Price J, Clark A, King P. DNA methylation and silencing of gene expression. Trends Endocrinol Metab 2000;11:142–8.

[81] Park SY, Kwon HJ, Lee HE, Ryu HS, Kim S-W, Kim JH, et al. Promoter CpG island hypermethylation during breast cancer progression. Virchows Arch 2011;458:73–84.

[82] Widschwendter M, Jones PA. DNA methylation and breast carcinogenesis. Oncogene 2002;21:5462–82.

[83] Sproul D, Nestor C, Culley J, Dickson JH, Dixon JM, Harrison DJ, et al. Transcriptionally repressed genes become aberrantly methylated and distinguish tumors of different lineages in breast cancer. Proc Natl Acad Sci USA 2011;108:4364–9.

[84] Verschuur-Maes AHJ, de Bruin PC, van Diest PJ. Epigenetic progression of columnar cell lesions of the breast to invasive breast cancer. Breast Cancer Res Treat 2012;136:705–15.

[85] Jones PA, Baylin SB. The epigenomics of cancer. Cell 2007;128:683–92.

[86] Shain AH, Giacomini CP, Matsukuma K, Karikari CA, Bashyam MD, Hidalgo M, et al. Convergent structural alterations define SWItch/Sucrose NonFermentable (SWI/SNF) chromatin remodeler as a central tumor suppressive complex in pancreatic cancer. Proc Natl Acad Sci USA 2012;109:E252–9.

[87] Nair SS, Kumar R. Chromatin remodeling in cancer: a gateway to regulate gene transcription. Mol Oncol 2012;6:611–9.

[88] Kleer CG, Cao Q, Varambally S, Shen R, Ota I, Tomlins SA, et al. EZH2 is a marker of aggressive breast cancer and promotes neoplastic transformation of breast epithelial cells. Proc Natl Acad Sci USA 2003;100:11606–11.

[89] Ding L, Erdmann C, Chinnaiyan AM, Merajver SD, Kleer CG. Identification of EZH2 as a molecular marker for a precancerous state in morphologically normal breast tissues. Cancer Res 2006;66:4095–9.

[90] McDonald OG, Wu H, Timp W, Doi A, Feinberg AP. Genome-scale epigenetic reprogramming during epithelial-to-mesenchymal transition. Nat Struct Mol Biol 2011;18:867–74.

[91] Hannon GJ, Rossi JJ. Unlocking the potential of the human genome with RNA interference. Nature 2004;431:371–8.

[92] Sætrom P, Snøve O, Rossi JJ. Epigenetics and microRNAs. Pediatr Res 2007;61:17R–23R.

[93] Farazi TA, Horlings HM, Hoeve Ten JJ, Mihailovic A, Halfwerk H, Morozov P, et al. MicroRNA sequence and expression analysis in breast tumors by deep sequencing. Cancer Res 2011;71:4443–53.

[94] Volinia S, Galasso M, Sana ME, Wise TF, Palatini J, Huebner K, et al. Breast cancer signatures for invasiveness and prognosis defined by deep sequencing of microRNA. Proc Natl Acad Sci USA 2012;109:3024–9.

[95] Black DL. Mechanisms of alternative pre-messenger RNA splicing. Annu Rev Biochem 2003;72:291–336.

[96] Matlin AJ, Clark F, Smith CWJ. Understanding alternative splicing: towards a cellular code. Nat Rev Mol Cell Biol 2005;6:386–98.

[97] Chien CD, Kirilyuk A, Li JV, Zhang W, Lahusen T, Schmidt MO, et al. Role of the nuclear receptor coactivator AIB1-Delta4 splice variant in the control of gene transcription. J Biol Chem 2011;286:26813–27.

[98] Ory V, Tassi E, Cavalli LR, Sharif GM, Saenz F, Baker T, et al. The nuclear coactivator amplified in breast cancer 1 maintains tumor-initiating cells during development of ductal carcinoma in situ. Oncogene 2014;33:3033–42.

[99] Moelans CB, Verschuur-Maes AHJ, van Diest PJ. Frequent promoter hypermethylation of BRCA2, CDH13, MSH6, PAX5, PAX6 and WT1 in ductal carcinoma in situ and invasive breast cancer. J Pathol 2011;225:222–31.

[100] Bissell MJ, Radisky D. Putting tumours in context. Nat Rev Cancer 2001;1:46–54.

[101] Quail DF, Joyce JA. Microenvironmental regulation of tumor progression and metastasis. Nat Med 2013;19:1423–37.

[102] Polyak K, Hu M. Do myoepithelial cells hold the key for breast tumor progression? J Mammary Gland Biol Neoplasia 2005;10:231–47.

[103] Cichon MA, Degnim AC, Visscher DW, Radisky DC. Microenvironmental influences that drive progression from benign breast disease to invasive breast cancer. J Mammary Gland Biol Neoplasia 2010;15:389–97.

[104] Adriance MC, Inman JL, Petersen OW, Bissell MJ. Myoepithelial cells: good fences make good neighbors. Breast Cancer Res 2005;7:190–7.

[105] Sternlicht MD, Kedeshian P, Shao ZM, Safarians S, Barsky SH. The human myoepithelial cell is a natural tumor suppressor. Clin Cancer Res 1997;3:1949–58.

[106] Sternlicht MD, Barsky SH. The myoepithelial defense: A host defense against cancer. Med Hypotheses 1997;48:37–46.

[107] Kleer CG, Bloushtain-Qimron N, Chen Y-H, Carrasco D, Hu M, Yao J, et al. Epithelial and stromal cathepsin K and CXCL14 expression in breast tumor progression. Clin Cancer Res 2008;14:5357–67.

[108] Hilson JB, Schnitt SJ, Collins LC. Phenotypic alterations in ductal carcinoma in situ-associated myoepithelial cells: biologic and diagnostic implications. Am J Surg Pathol 2009;33:227–32.

[109] Moinfar F, Man YG, Arnould L, Bratthauer GL, Ratschek M, Tavassoli FA. Concurrent and independent genetic alterations in the stromal and epithelial cells of mammary carcinoma: Implications for tumorigenesis. Cancer Res 2000;60:2562–6.

[110] Kurose K, Hoshaw-Woodard S, Adeyinka A, Lemeshow S, Watson PH, Eng C. Genetic model of multi-step breast carcinogenesis involving the epithelium and stroma: clues to tumour-microenvironment interactions. Hum Mol Genet 2001;10:1907–13.

[111] Place AE, Jin Huh S, Polyak K. The microenvironment in breast cancer progression: biology and implications for treatment. Breast Cancer Res 2011;13:227.

[112] Barsky SH, Karlin NJ. Myoepithelial cells: autocrine and paracrine suppressors of breast cancer progression. J Mammary Gland Biol Neoplasia 2005;10:249–60.

[113] Scholl SM, Pallud C, Beuvon F, Hacene K, Stanley ER, Rohrschneider L, et al. Anti-colony-stimulating factor-1 antibody staining in primary breast adenocarcinomas correlates with marked inflammatory cell infiltrates and prognosis. J Natl Cancer Inst 1994;86:120–6.

[114] Lin EY, Gouon-Evans V, Nguyen AV, Pollard JW. The macrophage growth factor CSF-1 in mammary gland development and tumor progression. J Mammary Gland Biol Neoplasia 2002;7:147–62.

[115] Lewis CE, Pollard JW. Distinct role of macrophages in different tumor microenvironments. Cancer Res 2006;66:605–12.

[116] Bingle L, Brown NJ, Lewis CE. The role of tumour-associated macrophages in tumour progression: implications for new anticancer therapies. J Pathol 2002;196:254–65.

[117] Wyckoff J, Wang W, Lin EY, Wang Y, Pixley F, Stanley ER, et al. A paracrine loop between tumor cells and macrophages is required for tumor cell migration in mammary tumors. Cancer Res 2004;64:7022–9.

[118] Giraudo E, Inoue M, Hanahan D. An amino-bisphosphonate targets MMP-9-expressing macrophages and angiogenesis to impair cervical carcinogenesis. J Clin Invest 2004;114:623–33.

[119] Coussens LM, Werb Z. Inflammation and cancer. Nature 2002;420:860–7.

[120] Biswas SK, Mantovani A. Macrophage plasticity and interaction with lymphocyte subsets: cancer as a paradigm. Nat Immunol 2010;11:889–96.

[121] Yamaguchi H, Pixley F, Condeelis J. Invadopodia and podosomes in tumor invasion. Eur J Cell Biol 2006;85:213–8.

[122] Emens LA. Breast cancer immunobiology driving immunotherapy: vaccines and immune checkpoint blockade. Exp Rev Anticancer Ther 2012;12:1597–611.

[123] Cimino-Mathews A, Ye X, Meeker A, Argani P, Emens LA. Metastatic triple-negative breast cancers at first relapse have fewer tumor-infiltrating lymphocytes than their matched primary breast tumors: a pilot study. Hum Pathol 2013;44:2055–63.

[124] Loi S, Sirtaine N, Piette F, Salgado R, Viale G, Van Eenoo F, et al. Prognostic and predictive value of tumor-infiltrating lymphocytes in a phase III randomized adjuvant breast cancer trial in node-positive breast cancer comparing the addition of docetaxel to doxorubicin with doxorubicin-based chemotherapy: BIG 02-98. J Clin Oncol 2013;31:860–7.

[125] Adams S, Gray RJ, Demaria S, Goldstein L, Perez EA, Shulman LN, et al. Prognostic value of tumor-infiltrating lymphocytes in triple-negative breast cancers from two phase III randomized adjuvant breast cancer trials: ECOG 2197 and ECOG 1199. J Clin Oncol 2014;32:2959–66.

[126] Loi S, Michiels S, Salgado R, Sirtaine N, Jose V, Fumagalli D, et al. Tumor infiltrating lymphocytes are prognostic in triple negative breast cancer and predictive for trastuzumab benefit in early breast cancer: results from the FinHER trial. Ann Oncol 2014;25:1544–50.

[127] Thompson E, Taube JM, Elwood H, Sharma R, Meeker A, Warzecha HN, et al. The immune microenvironment of breast ductal carcinoma in situ. Mod Pathol 2016;29:249–58.

[128] Schalper KA, Velcheti V, Carvajal D, Wimberly H, Brown J, Pusztai L, et al. In situ tumor PD-L1 mRNA expression is associated with increased TILs and better outcome in breast carcinomas. Clin Cancer Res 2014;20:2773–82.

[129] Lindau D, Gielen P, Kroesen M, Wesseling P, Adema GJ. The immunosuppressive tumour network: myeloid-derived suppressor cells, regulatory T cells and natural killer T cells. Immunology 2013;138:105–15.

[130] Dumont N, Liu B, DeFilippis RA, Chang H, Rabban JT, Karnezis AN, et al. Breast fibroblasts modulate early dissemination, tumorigenesis, and metastasis through alteration of extracellular matrix characteristics. Neoplasia 2013;15:249–62.

[131] Bhowmick NA, Neilson EG, Moses HL. Stromal fibroblasts in cancer initiation and progression. Nature 2004;432:332–7.

[132] Kojima Y, Acar A, Eaton EN, Mellody KT, Scheel C, Ben-Porath I, et al. Autocrine TGF-beta and stromal cell-derived factor-1 (SDF-1) signaling drives the evolution of tumor-promoting mammary stromal myofibroblasts. Proc Natl Acad Sci USA 2010;107:20009–14.

[133] Bronzert DA, Pantazis P, Antoniades HN, Kasid A, Davidson N, Dickson RB, et al. Synthesis and secretion of platelet-derived growth-factor by human-breast cancer cell-lines. Proc Natl Acad Sci USA 1987;84:5763–7.

[134] Hugo HJ, Lebret S, Tomaskovic-Crook E, Ahmed N, Blick T, Newgreen DF, et al. Contribution of fibroblast and mast cell (Afferent) and tumor (Efferent) IL-6 effects within the tumor microenvironment. Cancer Microenviron 2012;5:83–93.

[135] Jedeszko C, Victor BC, Podgorski I, Sloane BF. Fibroblast hepatocyte growth factor promotes invasion of human mammary ductal carcinoma in situ. Cancer Res 2009;69:9148–55.

[136] Hu M, Peluffo G, Chen H, Gelman R, Schnitt S, Polyak K. Role of COX-2 in epithelial-stromal cell interactions and progression of ductal carcinoma in situ of the breast. Proc Natl Acad Sci USA 2009;106:3372–7.

[137] Orimo A, Gupta PB, Sgroi DC, Arenzana-Seisdedos F, Delaunay T, Naeem R, et al. Stromal fibroblasts present in invasive human breast carcinomas promote tumor growth and angiogenesis through elevated SDF-1/CXCL12 secretion. Cell 2005;121:335–48.

[138] Kerlikowske K, Molinaro AM, Gauthier ML, Berman HK, Waldman F, Bennington J, et al. Biomarker expression and risk of subsequent tumors after initial ductal carcinoma in situ diagnosis. J Natl Cancer Inst 2010;102:627–37.

[139] Finak G, Bertos N, Pepin F, Sadekova S, Souleimanova M, Zhao H, et al. Stromal gene expression predicts clinical outcome in breast cancer. Nat Med 2008;14:518–27.

[140] Strange R, Li F, Saurer S, Burkhardt A, Friis RR. Apoptotic cell-death and tissue remodeling during mouse mammary-gland involution. Development 1992;115:49–58.

[141] Lund LR, Rømer J, Thomasset N, Solberg H, Pyke C, Bissell MJ, et al. Two distinct phases of apoptosis in mammary gland involution: Proteinase-independent and -dependent pathways. Development 1996;122:181–93.

[142] O'Brien J, Lyons T, Monks J, Lucia MS, Wilson RS, Hines L, et al. Alternatively activated macrophages and collagen remodeling characterize the postpartum involuting mammary gland across species. Am J Pathol 2010;176:1241–55.

[143] Lyons TR, O'Brien J, Borges VF, Conklin MW, Keely PJ, Eliceiri KW, et al. Postpartum mammary gland involution drives progression of ductal carcinoma in situ through collagen and COX-2. Nat Med 2011;17:1109–15.

[144] Folkman J. Tumor angiogenesis: therapeutic implications. N Engl J Med 1971;285:1182–6.

[145] Raica M, Cimpean AM, Ribatti D. Angiogenesis in pre-malignant conditions. Eur J Cancer 2009;45:1924–34.

[146] Hanahan D, Folkman J. Patterns and emerging mechanisms of the angiogenic switch during tumorigenesis. Cell 1996;86:353–64.

[147] Bergers G, Benjamin LE. Tumorigenesis and the angiogenic switch. Nat Rev Cancer 2003;3:401–10.

[148] Iyengar P, Combs TP, Shah SJ, Gouon-Evans V, Pollard JW, Albanese C, et al. Adipocyte-secreted factors synergistically promote mammary tumorigenesis through induction of anti-apoptotic transcriptional programs and proto-oncogene stabilization. Oncogene 2003;22:6408–23.

[149] Iyengar P, Espina V, Williams TW, Lin Y, Berry D, Jelicks LA, et al. Adipocyte-derived collagen VI affects early mammary tumor progression in vivo, demonstrating a critical interaction in the tumor/stroma microenvironment. J Clin Invest 2005;115:1163–76.

[150] Soule HD, Maloney TM, Wolman SR, Peterson WD, Brenz R, McGrath CM, et al. Isolation and characterization of a spontaneously immortalized human breast epithelial-cell line, Mcf-10. Cancer Res 1990;50:6075–86.

[151] Merlo GR, Basolo F, Fiore L, Duboc L, Hynes NE. P53-dependent and P53-independent activation of apoptosis in mammary epithelial-cells reveals a survival function of Egf and insulin. J Cell Biol 1995;128:1185–96.

[152] Neve RM, Chin K, Fridlyand J, Yeh J, Baehner FL, Fevr T, et al. A collection of breast cancer cell lines for the study of functionally distinct cancer subtypes. Cancer Cell 2006;10:515–27.

[153] DiRenzo J, Signoretti S, Nakamura N, Rivera-Gonzalez R, Sellers W, Loda M, et al. Growth factor requirements and basal phenotype of an immortalized mammary epithelial cell line. Cancer Res 2002;62:89–98.

[154] Qu Y, Han B, Yu Y, Yao W, Bose S, Karlan BY, et al. Evaluation of MCF10A as a reliable model for normal human mammary epithelial cells. PLoS One 2015;10:e0131285.

[155] Kuilman T, Michaloglou C, Mooi WJ, Peeper DS. The essence of senescence. Genes Dev 2010;24:2463–79.

[156] Van der Haegen BA, Shay JW. Immortalization of human mammary epithelial cells by SV40 large T-antigen involves a two step mechanism. In Vitro Cell Dev Biol 1993;29A:180–2.

[157] Roig AI, Eskiocak U, Hight SK, Kim SB, Delgado O, Souza RF, et al. Immortalized epithelial cells derived from human colon biopsies express stem cell markers and differentiate in vitro. Gastroenterology 2010;138:1012–5.

[158] Liu X, Ory V, Chapman S, Yuan H, Albanese C, Kallakury B, et al. ROCK inhibitor and feeder cells induce the conditional reprogramming of epithelial cells. Am J Pathol 2012;180:599–607.

[159] Saenz FR, Ory V, AlOtaiby M, Rosenfield S, Furlong M, Cavalli LR, et al. Conditionally reprogrammed normal and transformed mouse mammary epithelial cells display a progenitor-cell-like phenotype. PLoS One 2014;9:e97666.

[160] Suprynowicz FA, Upadhyay G, Krawczyk E, Kramer SC, Hebert JD, Liu X, et al. Conditionally reprogrammed cells represent a stem-like state of adult epithelial cells. Proc Natl Acad Sci USA 2012;109:20035–40.

[161] Dawson PJ, Wolman SR, Tait L, Heppner GH, Miller FR. MCF10AT: A model for the evolution of cancer from proliferative breast disease. Am J Pathol 1996;148:313–9.

[162] Miller FR, Santner SJ, Tait L, Dawson PJ. MCF10DCIS.com xenograft model of human comedo ductal carcinoma in situ. J Natl Cancer Inst 2000;92:1185–6.

[163] So JY, Lee HJ, Kramata P, Minden A, Suh N. Differential expression of key signaling proteins in MCF10 cell lines, a human breast cancer progression model. Mol Cell Pharmacol 2012;4:31–40.

[164] Chakrabarty A, Rexer BN, Wang SE, Cook RS, Engelman JA, Arteaga CL. H1047R phosphatidylinositol 3-kinase mutant enhances HER2-mediated transformation by heregulin production and activation of HER3. Oncogene 2010;29:5193–203.

[165] Mbeunkui F, Metge BJ, Shevde LA, Pannell LK. Identification of differentially secreted biomarkers using LC-MS/MS in isogenic cell lines representing a progression of breast cancer. J Proteome Res 2007;6:2993–3002.

[166] Behbod F, Kittrell FS, LaMarca H, Edwards D, Kerbawy S, Heestand JC, et al. An intraductal human-in-mouse transplantation model mimics the subtypes of ductal carcinoma in situ. Breast Cancer Res 2009;11:R66.

[167] Forozan F, Veldman R, Ammerman CA, Parsa NZ, Kallioniemi A, Kallioniemi OP, et al. Molecular cytogenetic analysis of 11 new breast cancer cell lines. Br J Cancer 1999;81:1328–34.

[168] Ethier SP, Mahacek ML, Gullick WJ, Frank TS, Weber BL. Differential isolation of normal luminal mammary epithelial-cells and breast-cancer cells from primary and metastatic sites using selective media. Cancer Res 1993;53:627–35.

[169] Hollestelle A, Elstrodt F, Nagel JHA, Kallemeijn WW, Schutte M. Phosphatidylinositol-3-OH kinase or RAS pathway mutations in human breast cancer cell lines. Mol Cancer Res 2007;5:195–201.

[170] Wasielewski M, Hanifi-Moghaddam P, Hollestelle A, Merajver SD, van den Ouweland A, Klijn JGM, et al. Deleterious CHEK2 1100delC and L303X mutants identified among 38 human breast cancer cell lines. Breast Cancer Res Treat 2009;113:285–91.

[171] Barnabas N, Cohen D. Phenotypic and molecular characterization of MCF10DCIS and SUM breast cancer cell lines. Int J Breast Cancer 2013;2013:872743–16.

[172] Band V, Zajchowski D, Swisshelm K, Trask D, Kulesa V, Cohen C, et al. Tumor progression in four mammary epithelial cell lines derived from the same patient. Cancer Res 1990;50:7351–7.

[173] Souter LH, Andrews JD, Zhang G, Cook AC, Postenka CO, Al-Katib W, et al. Human 21T breast epithelial cell lines mimic breast cancer progression in vivo and in vitro and show stage-specific gene expression patterns. Lab Invest 2010;90:1247–58.

[174] Alamri AM, Kang K, Groeneveld S, Wang W, Zhong X, Kallakury B, et al. Primary cancer cell culture: mammary-optimized vs conditional reprogramming. Endocr Relat Cancer 2016;23:535–54.

[175] Rizki A, Bissell MJ. Homeostasis in the breast it takes a village. Cancer Cell 2004;6:1–2.

[176] Petersen OW, Ronnovjessen L, Howlett AR, Bissell MJ. Interaction with basement-membrane serves to rapidly distinguish growth and differentiation pattern of normal and malignant human breast epithelial-cells. Proc Natl Acad Sci USA 1992;89:9064–8.

[177] Barcelloshoff MH, Aggeler J, Ram TG, Bissell MJ. Functional-differentiation and alveolar morphogenesis of primary mammary cultures on reconstituted basement-membrane. Development 1989;105:223.

[178] Emerman JT, Enami J, Pitelka DR, Nandi S. Hormonal effects on intracellular and secreted casein in cultures of mouse mammary epithelial-cells on floating collagen membranes. Proc Natl Acad Sci USA 1977;74:4466–70.

[179] Li ML, Aggeler J, Farson DA, Hatier C, Hassell J, Bissell MJ. Influence of a reconstituted basement-membrane and its components on casein gene-expression and secretion in mouse mammary epithelial-cells. Proc Natl Acad Sci USA 1987;84:136–40.

[180] Debnath J, Muthuswamy SK, Brugge JS. Morphogenesis and oncogenesis of MCF-10A mammary epithelial acini grown in three-dimensional basement membrane cultures. Methods 2003;30:256–68.

[181] Lee GY, Kenny PA, Lee EH, Bissell MJ. Three-dimensional culture models of normal and malignant breast epithelial cells. Nat Meth 2007;4:359–65.

[182] Debnath J, Brugge JS. Modelling glandular epithelial cancers in three-dimensional cultures. Nat Rev Cancer 2005;5:675–88.

[183] Muthuswamy SK, Li D, Lelievre S, Bissell MJ, Brugge JS. ErbB2, but not ErbB1, reinitiates proliferation and induces luminal repopulation in epithelial acini. Nat Cell Biol 2001;3:785–92.

[184] Friedl P, Wolf K. Tumour-cell invasion and migration: diversity and escape mechanisms. Nat Rev Cancer 2003;3:362–74.

[185] Baker EL, Srivastava J, Yu D, Bonnecaze RT, Zaman MH. Cancer cell migration: integrated roles of matrix mechanics and transforming potential. PLoS One 2011;6:e20355.

[186] Barsky SH. Myoepithelial mRNA expression profiling reveals a common tumor-suppressor phenotype. Exp Mol Pathol 2003;74:113–22.

[187] Sadlonova A, Novak Z, Johnson MR, Bowe DB, Gault SR, Page GP, et al. Breast fibroblasts modulate epithelial cell proliferation in three-dimensional in vitro co-culture. Breast Cancer Res 2005;7:R46–59.

[188] Hagemann T, Wilson J, Kulbe H, Li N, Leinster DA, Charles K, et al. Macrophages induce invasiveness of epithelial cancer cells via NF-kappa B and JNK. J Immunol 2005;175:1197–205.

[189] Linde N, Gutschalk CM, Hoffmann C, Yilmaz D, Mueller MM. Integrating macrophages into organotypic co-cultures: a 3D in vitro model to study tumor-associated macrophages. PLoS One 2012;7:e40058.

[190] Richmond A, Su Y. Mouse xenograft models vs GEM models for human cancer therapeutics. Dis Model Mech 2008;1:78–82.

[191] Valdez KE, Fan F, Smith W, Allred DC, Medina D, Behbod F. Human primary ductal carcinoma in situ (DCIS) subtype-specific pathology is preserved in a mouse intraductal (MIND) xenograft model. J Pathol 2011;225:565–73.

[192] Hu M, Yao J, Carroll DK, Weremowicz S, Chen H, Carrasco D, et al. Regulation of in situ to invasive breast carcinoma transition. Cancer Cell 2008;13:394–406.

[193] Bernard D, Peakman M, Hayday AC. Establishing humanized mice using stem cells: maximizing the potential. Clin Exp Immunol 2008;152:406–14.

[194] Kuperwasser C, Chavarria T, Wu M, Magrane G, Gray JW, Carey L, et al. Reconstruction of functionally normal and malignant human breast tissues in mice. Proc Natl Acad Sci USA 2004;101:4966–71.

[195] Borowsky AD. Choosing a mouse model: experimental biology in context--the utility and limitations of mouse models of breast cancer. Cold Spring Harb Perspect Biol 2011;3:a009670–0.

[196] van de Vijver MJ, Peterse JL, Mooi WJ, Wisman P, Lomans J, Dalesio O, et al. Neuprotein overexpression in breast cancer. Association with comedo-type ductal carcinoma in situ and limited prognostic value in stage II breast cancer. N Engl J Med 1988;319:1239–45.

[197] Bouchard L, Lamarre L, Tremblay PJ, Jolicoeur P. Stochastic appearance of mammary-tumors in transgenic mice carrying the Mmtv/C-Neu oncogene. Cell 1989;57:931–6.

[198] Guy CT, Webster MA, Schaller M, Parsons TJ, Cardiff RD, Muller WJ. Expression of the Neu Protooncogene in the mammary epithelium of transgenic mice induces metastatic disease. Proc Natl Acad Sci USA 1992;89:10578–82.

[199] Fereshteh MP, Tilli MT, Kim SE, Xu J, O'Malley BW, Wellstein A, et al. The nuclear receptor coactivator amplified in breast cancer-1 is required for Neu (ErbB2/HER2) activation, signaling, and mammary tumorigenesis in mice. Cancer Res 2008;68:3697–706.

[200] Maglione JE, Moghanaki D, Young L, Manner CK, Ellies LG, Joseph SO, et al. Transgenic Polyoma middle-T mice model premalignant mammary disease. Cancer Res 2001;61:8298–305.

[201] Tzeng YJ, Guhl E, Graessmann M, Graessmann A. Breast-cancer formation in transgenic animals induced by the whey acidic protein Sv40 T-antigen (Wap-Sv-T) hybrid gene. Oncogene 1993;8:1965–71.

[202] Mietz JA, Unger T, Huibregtse JM, Howley PM. The transcriptional transactivation function of wild-type-P53 is inhibited by Sv40 large T-antigen and by Hpv-16 E6-oncoprotein. EMBO J 1992;11:5013–20.

[203] Dyson N, Buchkovich K, Whyte P, Harlow E. The cellular 107K protein that binds to adenovirus E1A also associates with the large T antigens of SV40 and JC virus. Cell 1989;58:249–55.

[204] Schulze-Garg C, Löhler J, Gocht A, Deppert W. A transgenic mouse model for the ductal carcinoma in situ (DCIS) of the mammary gland. Oncogene 2000;19:1028–37.

[205] Pittius CW, Sankaran L, Topper YJ, Hennighausen L. Comparison of the regulation of the whey acidic protein gene with that of a hybrid gene containing the whey acidic protein gene promoter in transgenic mice. Mol Endocrinol 1988;2:1027–32.

[206] Cato AC, Weinmann J, Mink S, Ponta H, Henderson D, Sonnenberg A. The regulation of expression of mouse mammary tumor virus DNA by steroid hormones and growth factors. J Steroid Biochem 1989;34:139–43.

[207] Green JE, Shibata MA, Yoshidome K, Liu ML, Jorcyk C, Anver MR, et al. The C3(1)/SV40 T-antigen transgenic mouse model of mammary cancer: ductal epithelial cell targeting with multistage progression to carcinoma. Oncogene 2000;19:1020–7.

[208] Shoker BS, Jarvis C, Sibson DR, Walker C, Sloane JP. Oestrogen receptor expression in the normal and pre-cancerous breast. J Pathol 1999;188:237–44.

[209] Tilli MT, Frech MS, Steed ME, Hruska KS, Johnson MD, Flaws JA, et al. Introduction of estrogen receptor-alpha into the tTA/TAg conditional mouse model precipitates the development of estrogen-responsive mammary adenocarcinoma. Am J Pathol 2003;163:1713–9.

[210] Frech MS, Halama ED, Tilli MT, Singh B, Gunther EJ, Chodosh LA, et al. Deregulated estrogen receptor alpha expression in mammary epithelial cells of transgenic mice results in the development of ductal carcinoma in situ. Cancer Res 2005;65:681–5.

[211] Namba R, Maglione JE, Young L, Borowsky AD, Cardiff RD, MacLeod CL, et al. Molecular characterization of the transition to malignancy in a genetically engineered mouse-based model of ductal carcinoma in situ. Mol Cancer Res 2004;2:453–63.

[212] Medina D, Kittrell FS, Shepard A, Stephens LC, Jiang C, Lu J, et al. Biological and genetic properties of the p53 null preneoplastic mammary epithelium. FASEB J 2002;16:881–3.

[213] Kuperwasser C, Hurlbut GD, Kittrell FS, Dickinson ES, Laucirica R, Medina D, et al. Development of spontaneous mammary tumors in BALB/c p53 heterozygous mice—a model for Li-Fraumeni syndrome. Am J Pathol 2000;157:2151–9.

Section 2

Cell and Molecular Biology of Breast Cancer

Chapter 5

GWAS in Breast Cancer

Paulo C.M. Lyra-Junior, Nayara G. Tessarollo,
Isabella S. Guimarães, Taciane B. Henriques,
Diandra Z. dos Santos, Marcele L.M. de Souza,
Victor Hugo M. Marques, Laura F.R.L. de Oliveira,
Krislayne V. Siqueira, Ian V. Silva,
Leticia B.A. Rangel and Alan T. Branco

Additional information is available at the end of the chapter

http://dx.doi.org/10.5772/67223

Abstract

Breast cancer is the most diagnosed cancer in women, and the second cause of cancer-related deaths among women worldwide. It is expected that more than 240,000 new cases and 40,450 deaths related to the disease will occur in 2016. It is well known that inherited genetic variants are drivers for breast cancer development. There are many mechanisms through which germline genetic variation affects prognosis, such as BRCA1 and BRCA2 genes, which account for approximately 20% of the increased hereditary risks. Therefore, it is evident that the genetic pathways that underlie cancer development are complex in which networks of multiple alleles confer disease susceptibility and risks. Global analyses through genome-wide association studies (GWAS) have revealed several *loci* across the genome are associated with the breast cancer. This chapter compiles all breast GWAS released since 2007, year of the first article published in this area, and discuss the future directions of this field. Currently, hundreds of genetic markers are linked to breast cancer, and understanding the underlying mechanisms of these variants might lead to the discover of biomarkers and targets for therapy in patients.

Keywords: breast cancer, genome-wide association studies (GWAS), susceptibility, *Loci*, SNPs

1. Introduction

One of the main goals of human genetics is to understand genetic pathways underlying traits. It has been highly successful the gene mapping of disorders with a Mendelian pattern of inheritance using the tendency of genes and other genetic markers to be inherited together. It is well known that genetic variants underlying these single-gene Mendelian disorders are rare in the population and tend to be highly penetrant, which means that a high percentage of carriers of the genotype will manifest the phenotype. On the other hand, mapping of non-Mendelian (or complex) traits, cases in which variants in multiple genes contribute to the phenotype, was only possible after sequencing and study of the human genome. Inherited variants underlying complex diseases, opposing the Mendelian disorders, have modest penetrance but higher frequency in the population [1–4] (**Figure 1**). Thus, efforts have been made to identify genes and pathways that control human traits, and, in the future, predict illness and establish more appropriated methods of treatment.

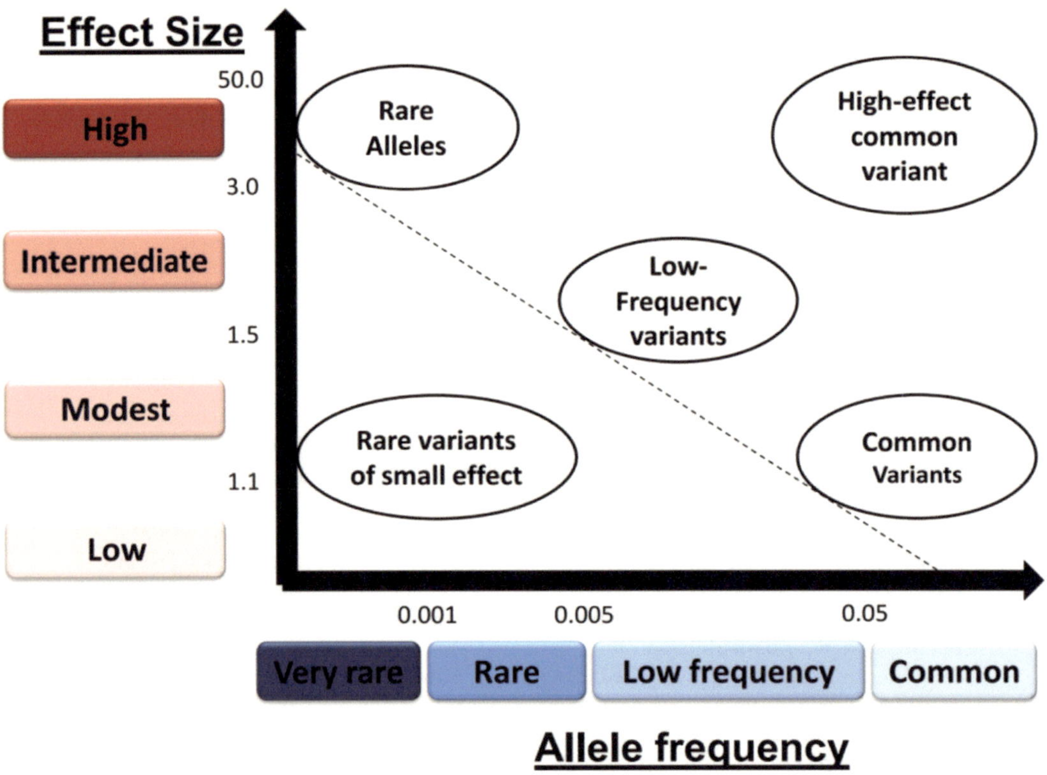

Figure 1. Features of genetic variants and correlation with disease severity. The panel shows the correlation between the frequency of alleles and the severity of the disease (odds ratio). Accordingly, Mendelian diseases (top left circle) have high effect on the individual, but the frequency of such mutations in the population is very rare. On the other hand, very rare variants with small effect (bottom left circle) are also found in the population, these features restrain the establishment of a reliable correlation between phenotype and genotype. GWAS have focused on identifying a massive number of genetic variants, which can be separated as (i) common variants associated with high effect size (top right circle) and (ii) abundant common alleles with apparent very low impact on human health (bottom right circle). Adapted from Manolio et al. [95].

http://dx.doi.org/10.5772/67223

A reflection of the urgency to unveil this research field is notable when looking through breast cancer numbers. Worldwide, the scenario is dramatic, with more than one million new cases of breast cancer diagnosed yearly (cancer genome atlas network 2012), and the fifth cause of death from cancer overall. In developing countries, breast cancer is the second cause of death from cancer and accounts for 15.4% of overall cancer-related deaths in women [5]. Moreover, it corresponds to the most common cancer-related death in women in the less developed regions (14.3%). In the United States, breast cancer is the second cause of cancer-related deaths among women, and it is estimated that one of eight American women will develop invasive breast cancer over the course of her lifetime. Accordingly, in the year of 2016, only in the United States, more than 240,000 new cases of the disease and 40,450 related deaths are expected [6].

Breast cancer comprises multiple diseases harbouring different genetic alterations; each subtype responds differently to treatments, and this feature leads to distinct clinical outcomes [7, 8]. Based on tumour histological biomarkers, breast cancer can be separated into three basic clinical types, such as HR positive (estrogen receptor and progesterone receptor), HER2+ (human epidermal growth factor receptor 2 positive), and triple-negative breast cancer, which are an essential part of the diagnostic workup of all breast cancer patients [9]. Approximately, 85% of all breast cancers are HR positive, about 20% are HER2+ and nearly 15% are triple-negative.

It is well understood that breast cancer is a complex and heterogeneous disease with a multifactorial etiology involving genetic, dietary, hormonal and reproductive factors. Among these, genetic is of particular importance. Epidemiological studies estimate that women with history of breast cancer in a first-degree relative show nearly twofold higher risk to develop breast cancer than women without a family history, indicating that the genetic factors are important determinants of disease risk [10]. At least 10–15% of all breast cancer cases may be due to the inheritance of a single gene mutation or multiple genetic variants [10, 11]. In the 1990s, two major susceptibility genes for breast cancer, breast cancer 1 (BRCA1) and breast cancer 2 (BRCA2), were the first ones to be identified on the long arm of chromosome 17 and the short arm of chromosome 13, respectively [12–14]. These genes are responsible for 20–30% of hereditary breast cancer cases worldwide. BRCA1 and BRCA2 are important on the maintenance of genome stability by playing a critical role in the regulation of different cellular processes, such as transcription, cell cycle, DNA repair, cell proliferation and differentiation, in response to DNA damage [15]. Indeed, woman carrying such pathogenic variants have an increased risk of 60–80% of breast cancer [16, 17]. Moreover, inherited BRCA1/2 gene mutations are associated with a 39–80% lifetime risk of female breast cancer [18–21]. It is also well established that BRCA1/2 carriers with breast cancer have a strong lifetime risk of developing contralateral breast cancer range from 10 to 40% and are 2–6 times higher than the risk for non-carriers [22–27].

The identification of mutations in BRCA, considered as a critical factor for the development of breast cancer in some women, has boosted the interest of scientists to discover more mutations that drive tumour development. In this context, advances in DNA sequencing technologies empowered massive parallel sequencing, and, as a consequence, it has led to a fantastic discovery and assignment of other hereditary pre-disposition genes to high (TP53, PALB2, PTEN), moderated (CHEK2, ATM, NF1, NBN) and elevated, but imprecise, breast cancer risk (CDH1, STK11) [28–34]. Altogether, high and moderate penetrance breast cancer susceptibility mutations in these genes account for just over 30% of familial breast cancer cases, because linkage studies are not amenable to the identification of common alleles with small effects.

However, the major advance over the several years has led by genome-wide association studies (GWAS). This approach is based on genome-wide genotyping for thousands to millions of single-nucleotide polymorphisms (SNPs) in a large number of individuals and contrast between the groups with and without a specific phenotype. Therefore, this approach has successfully identified thousands of *loci* associated with hundreds of traits (National Human Genome Research Institute GWAS catalogue) [35]. Hence, this recent technology opens a new way to understand the underlying genetic causes of common diseases [1].

2. Genome-wide association studies

In the past, studying polymorphisms were limited by the technologies that only permitted analysis of one or a few *loci* at time, hence limiting the aims to particular genes or pathways. The selection for candidate genes or pathways to be studied were based on the potential relation with carcinogenesis, metabolism, cell cycle control and hormone synthesis. Therefore, the initial studies focused on single nucleotide polymorphisms which were associated with a crucial role in the cell functionality. With the advancement of techniques, sets of tagged SNPs included 'known common variants' across a gene. However, even though the number of candidates being analysed have increased, the number of well-validated association in those studies did not increase as expected. Association studies, involving direct testing of genetic polymorphisms in large series of cases versus controls, provide a powerful approach to identify lower penetrance alleles that cannot be detected by genetic linkage studies [36, 37]. However, additional susceptibility genes in which rare coding variants are associated with a moderate cancer risk have emerged through candidate gene re-sequencing [38].

GWAS have emerged as a powerful new approach that has the capacity of analysing the whole human genome in order to identify common variations in the population possibly associated with genetic factors of a specific disease. In other words, the intent of GWAS is to predict who is at the risk and develop new strategies for prevention and treatments of genetic diseases [39]. One of the initial successes of GWAS was the identification of the *complement factor* H gene as a major risk factor for age-related macular degeneration [40–42].

The GWAS technology is based on genotyping platforms (chip-based microarray technology) that can evaluate hundreds to thousands of SNPs simultaneously. The two primary platforms that have been used for most GWAS were developed by Illumina (San Diego, CA) and Affymetrix (Santa Clara, CA). These two competing technologies use different approaches to detect SNP variation. Accordingly, the Affymetrix platform prints short DNA sequences on a chip that recognizes a specific SNP allele. Alleles (i.e. nucleotides) are detected by a differential

DNA hybridization between the samples. Illumina, on the other hand, uses a bead-based technology with slightly longer DNA sequences to detect alleles. The Illumina technology is more expensive, but provides better specificity. Hence, it is possible to conduct association studies using sets of SNPs that tag most known common variants in the genome, and therefore, scan for the associations without prior knowledge of function or position [39, 43].

GWAS arrays have identified SNPs that are associated with many complex diseases or traits [44]; although they do not contain all mapped SNPs, rather they contain only index SNPs that represent SNPs in the same linkage disequilibrium (LD) block. The SNPs identified by GWAS are significantly correlated with a disease (or case) and are called as risk-associated SNPs, and the genomic regions containing the SNPs are called as risk *loci* for that particular disease [45, 46]. One common trend of the SNPs associated with the trait is that they are not frequently found in coding regions of the genome. Instead, most of them are located in non-coding regions of the genome and are equally distributed between intronic and intergenic compartments [47, 48]. This might initially reduce the potential of the index, SNPs being the causal, but it is important to keep in mind that all the SNPs in the same haplotype block with the index SNP could possibly play the role of a causal SNP. A commonly used approach to investigate SNPs other than the index SNPs present on the standard GWAS array has been to use an LD calculation [49–51] together with the 1000 Genomes Project reference panels from different populations [52, 53].

To move from the index SNP to a more refined list of putative causal SNPs located within the identified region, another approach called fine-mapping has also been used. Fine-mapping studies employ dense genotyping arrays that contain all common SNPs within the previously identified risk *loci*, which together with imputation [49–51] allow investigators to perform a more complete analysis of the risk regions. The most fine-mapping analyses have been done by international consortia with the shared interests for specific diseases or traits; examples include: the immunochip [54], the metabochip [55], the iCOGs array [56] and the Oncoarray [57].

3. GWAS in breast cancer

Over the past years, the results from GWAS have been published for breast cancer reporting well-validated novel associations. In total, these scans have identified approximately 100 common genetic susceptibility *loci* for breast cancer risk, and as additional scans are ongoing at some point, the number of cancer susceptibility *loci* is likely to change rapidly over the next years. This is only possible because there are many worldwide consortium groups, for example Asia Breast Cancer Consortium (ABCC) and Breast Cancer Association Consortium (BCAC), and it is through them that has been possible identifying the susceptibility of SNPs in large-scale and different populations.

The first GWAS for breast cancer was published in 2007 and identified novel susceptibility *loci* associated with this illness. Accordingly, as in reference [58], they studied 4398 breast cancer cases and 4316 controls, followed by a third stage in which 30 SNPs were tested for confirmation in 21860 cases and 22578 controls from 22 studies. In total 227876 SNPs were analyzed, which represented a coverage of approximately 77% of known common SNPs in Europeans at $r^2 > 0.5$. As a result, they found five novel independent *loci* associated with the breast cancer ($P < 10^{-7}$ using a stratified Cochran-Armitage trend test). The genes found around four *loci* are plausible causative genes (FGFR2, TNRC9, MP3K1 and LSP1). The most strongly associated SNP was in the intron 2 of the FGFR2 gene, a receptor tyrosine kinase that is amplified and overexpressed in 5–10% of breast tumours [59]. The 16q *locus* contains the candidate genes *TNRC9* and *LOC643714*. The function of *TNRC9* genes is currently unknown; however, the presence of the HMG box motif suggests that it possibly acts as a transcription factor [60]. MAP3K1, located at the 5q *locus*, is a gene involved in signal transduction and has not been previously reported to be involved with cancer. LSP1 is located at 11p *locus* and is an F-actin bundling cytoskeletal protein expressed in hematopoietic and endothelial cells. Other evidence of association pointed to a SNP around the H19 gene, a maternally imprinted gene that encodes an untranslated mRNA closely involved in regulation of IGF2. The fifth *locus* is an interval of 110 kb lacking known genes and located in the genomic region 8q24. Despite the absence of genes in the segment of 110 kb, the region 8q24 contains *loci* associated with prostate and colorectal cancers. The second stage of this study identified 1792 SNPs with *P*-value < 0.05, while the estimated by chance would be 1343. These observations have indicated that many additional common susceptibility alleles might be identifiable by this approach, but the detection of further susceptibility *loci* is associated with the increased coverage and use of larger number of cases and controls [58].

In the following years, nine articles using GWAS to identify genetic factors linked with breast cancer were published [61–69]. These works have not only increased the number of new markers associated with the illness, but also validated the genetic factors that were previously identified. Furthermore, the cancer genetic markers of susceptibility (CGEMS) group detected the association of FGFR2 in a second genome scan, genotyping 528,173 SNPs in 1145 cases of invasive breast cancer among postmenopausal white women and 1142 controls they detected a set of four SNPs in intron 2 of FGFR2 [62]. All the variants are related with FGFR2 expression in normal breast tissue, and interesting two of them are likely related to biological mechanism for interrupting active transcription factor-binding sites [70]. The deCODE group later on, using approximately 1000 unselected breast cancer cases and illumina 317k panel, found two additional *loci* at 2q and 5p [61, 63]. A further *locus* on 6q was identified by Gold et al. [64] studying 249 familial Ashkenazi Jewish breast cancer cases. This region contains two potential candidate genes, ECHDC1 and RNF146. The CGEMS group again added two novel *loci* with genome-wide significance: (i) one SNP, on the genomic region 1p11.2 neighbouring NOTCH2 and FCGR1B, is predominantly associated with estrogen receptor-positive breast cancer; (ii) the second SNP is located on chromosome 14q24.1, localizes to RAD51L1, a prior candidate pathway for breast cancer susceptibility [67]. Additional *loci* associated with the breast cancer were found with a more refined analysis of the first GWAS. Accordingly, Ahmed et al. [66] tested over 800 promising associations in the two stages involving 37,012 cases and 40,069 controls from 33 studies in the CGEMS and BCAC, finding strong evidence for additional susceptibility *loci* on 3p24 and 17q23.2; the causative genes include SLC4A7 and NEK10 on 3p and COX11 on 17q. Finally, Zheng et al. [65] conducted a GWAS among Chinese women and studied 607,728 SNPs in 1505 cases and 1522 controls; this analysis revealed 29 promising SNPs. The SNP at 6q25.1, located upstream of the estrogen receptor 1 gene (ESR1), exhibited consistent association with breast cancer across all the three stages performed, providing strong evidence of a susceptibility *locus* for breast cancer.

In 2010, a group conducted a new GWAS in which 582,886 SNPs were genotyped in 3659 cases with a family history of the disease and 4897 controls. They identified five new susceptibility *loci* on the chromosomes 9, 10 and 11, and found three SNPs in the 6q25.1, 8q24 and 11p15 regions with a higher correlation risk to develop cancer than the ones reported previously [69]. In the same year, other group, based on the fact that the germline BRCA1 mutations predispose to breast cancer, aimed to identify genetic modifiers of this risk in 1193 individuals with BRCA1 mutations who were diagnosed with invasive breast cancer under the age 40. This group was contrasted with 1190 BRCA1 carriers without breast cancer diagnosis over age 35. The first stage of this study had led to the identification of 96 SNPs; after the further stages of analysis, five SNPs on 19p13 were highly associated with breast cancer risk and also associated with triple-negative breast cancer in a separate study of 2301 triple-negative cases and 3949 controls [68].

Three studies were published in 2011 revealing new *loci* associated with the breast cancer. Haiman et al. [71] searching for common risk alleles for ER-negative breast cancer, combined GWAS data from women of African ancestry (1004 ER-negative cases and 2745 controls) and European ancestry (1718 ER-negative cases and 3670 controls). This study was further replicated with an additional 2292 ER-negative cases and 16,901 controls of European ancestry. Their conclusion pinpointed a common risk variant for ER-negative breast cancer at the TERT-CLPT1L *locus* on chromosome 5p15 in multiple populations. Furthermore, the same variant was also significantly associated with the triple-negative breast cancer, particularly in younger women (<50 years old). Cai et al. [72] published a four-stage GWAS including 17,153 cases and 16,943 controls among East-Asian women, after analysing 684,457 SNPs. The final result revealed one SNP at 10q21.2 (ZNF365) strongly implicated as a genetic risk variant for breast cancer among East-Asian women. Fletcher et al. [73] compared 296,114 tagging SNPs in 1694 cases of breast cancer and 2365 controls, with validation in three independent series totalling 11,880 cases and 12,487 controls, identifying a novel *locus* risk for breast cancer at 9q31.2 (the nearest genes around the SNP found are KLF4, RAD23B and ACTL7A), as well two variants mapping to 6q25.1, a *locus* previously reported. Although approximately 25 common genetic susceptibility *loci* have been identified to be independently associated with breast cancer risk, the genetic risk variants reported only explain a small fraction of the heritability of breast cancer.

Long et al. [74] aimed to discover novel genetic susceptibility *loci* for breast cancer, therefore they conducted a four-stage GWAS in 19,091 cases and 20,606 controls of East-Asian descent (Chinese, Korean and Japanese women were included). It was analysed 690,947 SNPs, from this group the final stage showed an SNP in chromosome 6q25.1, near to TGF-β activated kinase (TAB2), with consistent association with breast cancer risk across all four stages, reaching a *P*-value of 3.8×10^{-12} when the analysis was done with all samples combined. In addition, they identified two possible susceptibility SNPs, one located in the intron 5 of the ESR1 gene and the other at 11q24.3, with consistent association in each of the four stages. Kim et al. [75] conducted a GWAS to evaluate previously identified *loci* in Korean woman and to identify additional novel breast cancer susceptibility variants. Accordingly, they conducted a three-stage GWAS that included 6322 cases and 5897 controls. The results revealed one SNP in the epidermal growth factor receptor (ERB4) gene, located at chromosome 2q34, and showed that seven breast cancer susceptibility *loci* that were previously identified in European and/or Chinese population could be directly replicated in Korean women. Another GWAS study was conducted in Japanese patients with hormone receptor-positive, invasive breast cancer receiving adjuvant tamoxifen therapy. This study detected significant associations with recurrence-free survival of15 SNPs on nine chromosomal *loci* 1p31, 1q41, 5q33, 7p11, 10q22, 12q13, 13q22, 18q12 and 19p13. Among them, the one in the C10orf11 gene in 10q22 was significantly associated with recurrence-free survival in breast cancer patients treated with tamoxifen [76]. Besides these articles, two more were published in the same year. Ghoussaini et al. [77] reported a follow up of 72 promising associations from two independent GWAS using approximately 70,000 cases and 68,000 controls from 41 case-control studies and nine breast cancer GWAS. Through this study, three new breast cancer risk *loci* on 12p11 (PTHLH gene), 12q24 and 21q21 (NRIP1 gene) were identified. An interesting fact was that two SNPs were associated only with ER-positive disease, whereas the SNP on 12p11 was associated with similar relative risks for both ER-negative and ER-positive breast cancer. Because the GWAS of breast cancer separated by immunohistochemical have revealed *loci* contributing to the susceptibility of ER-negative subtypes. Siddiq et al. [78] conducted a large meta-analysis of ER-negative disease, comprising 4754 ER-negative cases and 31,663 controls from three GWAS, to identify additional genetic variants for ER-negative breast cancer. They performed an *in silico* replication with 86 SNPs using a *P*-value $\leq 10^{-5}$ in an additional population of 11,209 cases of breast cancer, where 946 were with ER-negative disease, and 16,057 controls of Japanese, Latino and European ancestry. As result two novel *loci* were identified, one at 6q14 and other at 20q11. At the *locus* 6q14 the SNP was associated with breast cancer and both ER-positive and ER-negative disease. In contrast, the SNP at 20q11 was associated with ER-negative breast cancer, but showed weaker association with overall breast cancer and no association with ER-positive disease. This work also confirmed three known *loci* associated with both ER-negative and ER-positive breast cancer. These findings highlight the relevance of large-scale collaborative studies to identify novel breast cancer risk *loci*.

In order to obtain a more comprehensive knowledge on the genetic factors controlling breast cancer development, the project collaborative oncological gene-environment study (COGS) was created through collaboration among four consortia [56]. The project consisted of a meta-analysis of nine GWAS, involving 10,052 breast cancer cases and 12,575 controls of European ancestry. 29,807 SNPs were selected for further genotyping. The selected SNPs were genotyped in 41 studies in BCAC, using 45,290 cases and 41,880 controls in European ancestry population. Another important point of the study was the custom Illumina iSelect genotyping array (iCOGS) utilized that comprises more than 200,000 SNPs. The combined efforts identified SNPs at 41 new breast cancer susceptibility *loci* at genome-wide significance ($P < 5 \times 10^{-8}$). Two other studies were published in 2013. One aimed to identify further cancer risk-modifying *loci* using multi-stage GWAS of 11,705 BRCA1 carriers (5920 diagnosed with breast cancer and 1839 diagnosed with ovarian cancer); further replication was done with an additional sample of 2646 BRCA1 carriers. Looking specifically at breast cancer factors they identified a novel risk modifier *locus* at 1q32 for BRCA1 carriers [79]. The other study was focused on identification of susceptibility *loci* specific to ER-negative disease, using a meta-analysis of 3 GWAS with 4193 ER-negative breast cancer cases and 35,194 controls with a series of 40 follow-up studies and also used the iCOGS to genotype. Their conclusion reported SNPs at four *loci*, 1q32.1 (MDM4 and LGR6), 2p24.1 and 16q12.2 associated with ER-negative but not ER-positive breast cancer. Once again providing further evidence for distinct etiological pathways associated with invasive ER-positive and ER-negative breast cancer [80].

GWAS have also been proven to be a powerful strategy to identify genetic factors associated with adverse reactions caused by drugs. The first GWAS for chemotherapy-induced alopecia was conducted in Japanese breast cancer patients, and identified SNPs significantly associated with drug-induced grade 2 alopecia. For instance, the rs3820706 (calcium channel voltage-dependent subunit beta) on 2q23 and its nearby SNP rs16830728 could be associated with significant molecular alterations in genes such as ion channel-related genes and genes related to the β-catenin signalling pathway [81].

The lack of concordance among some studies for breast cancer led a group to study 41 common non-synonymous SNP (nsSNP) for which evidence of association with breast cancer risk had been previously reported. This work combined 38 studies of white European women (46,450 cases and 42,600 controls), and showed strong association for one previously reported, 7q21; one novel susceptibility *locus*, 3p21 and the third *locus* is located in an established breast cancer susceptibility region, 3p24 [82]. Another study with 22,780 cases and 24,181 controls provided additional insights into the genetics and biology of breast cancer in East Asian women. It was identified that three genetic *loci* located at 1q32.1, 5q14.3 and 15q26.1 were recently associated with breast cancer risk [83]. Purrington et al. [84], interested on identify *loci* that influence triple-negative breast cancer risk, conducted a two-stage GWAS of triple-negative breast cancer with 1529 cases and 3399 controls in the first stage and 2148 cases and 1309 controls in the second. Variants at 19p13.1 and PTHLH *loci* showed significant association in both stages. Moreover, 25 SNPs already known as breast cancer susceptibility were associated with risk of triple-negative breast cancer ($P < 0.05$).

One particular article published in 2014 called attention for running a meta-analysis of GWAS of three mammographic density phenotype: dense area, non-dense and percent density in up to 7916 women in stage 1 and 10,379 women in the second stage. The results showed *loci* that reached genome-wide significance for all three phenotypes, for dense area (AREG, ESR1, ZNF365, LSP1, IGF1, TMEM184B and SGSM3), non-dense area (8p11.23) and percent density (PRDM6, 8p11.23 and TMEM184B). Interestingly, some regions are known as breast cancer susceptibility *loci* and the others regions were found, after a large meta-analysis, to be associated with breast cancer ($P < 0.05$). Based on the ability to identify known as well as putative novel breast cancer *loci* by studying mammographic density phenotypes, the authors demonstrated the power of using quantitative intermediate phenotypes to discover new disease *loci* [85].

In 2015, there were more than 90 established breast cancer risk *loci*, with 57 new ones, revealed through GWAS during 2013 and 2014. Nevertheless, new studies were published identifying new susceptibility *loci*. A group performed a meta-analysis restricted to women of European ancestry. They worked with 11 GWAS comprising of 15,748 breast cancer cases and 18,084 controls, and 46,785 cases and 42,892 controls from 41 studies genotyped on iCOGS, and used imputation to estimate genotypes for more than 11 million SNPs, identifying 15 novel *loci* associated with breast cancer at $P < 5x10^{-8}$ [85]. Palomba et al. [86], also following the assumption that analyses in genetically-homogeneous population could represent an additional approach to detect low penetrance alleles, conducted a GWAS study comparing 1431 Sardinian patients with non-familial, BRCA1/2-mutation-negative breast cancer to 2171 healthy Sardinian blood donors, where 2,067,645 SNPs were analysed. The study concludes the role of TOX3 and FGRF2 as breast cancer susceptibility genes in BRCA1/2-wild-type breast cancer patients from Sardinian population.

In 2016, three GWAS were three GWAS were published describing novel genetic susceptibility *loci*. It was a study including 14,224 cases and 14,829 controls of East Asian women, where two SNPs in two *loci* were found to be associated with breast cancer risk at the genome-wide significance level, one at 1p22.3 and other at 21q22.12 [87]. The identification of four previously unidentified *loci* including the ones at 13q22 (KLF5), 2p23.2 (WDR43) and 2q33 (PPIL3) with genome-wide significant association with ER-negative breast cancer, performing a meta-analysis of 11 GWAS consisting of 4939 ER-negative cases and 14,352 controls, combined with 7333 ER-negative cases and 42,468 controls and 15,252 BRCA1 mutation carriers genotyped on the iCOGS array [88]. GWAS also can be useful to identify SNPs associated with response to anthracycline-based neoadjuvant chemotherapy in breast cancer patients. A group identified two SNPs that were significantly associated with pathologic complete response after neoadjuvant chemotherapy. After the validation using 401 patients who received anthracycline-based neoadjuvant regimens the authors found that only one SNP, located in the WT1 gene, was associated with the pathologic complete response after anthracycline-based neoadjuvant therapy, suggesting that WT1 may be a potential target of anthracycline-based neoadjuvant therapy for breast cancer [89].

4. Conclusion

GWAS have been successful in identifying many genetic variants that are significantly associated with human diseases. However, a gap has emerged between the ability to detect these associations and the ability to meaningfully interpret their biological significance [90]. Currently, the challenges facing GWAS include the translation of associated *loci* into suitable biological hypotheses, missing heritability [91], and the understanding of how multiple modestly associated *loci* within genes interact to influence a phenotype [92]. Thus, the new trend for susceptibility *loci* identification has moved forward to describe precisely the functional weffects and target genes. The post-GWAS include detailed genetic and epidemiological dissection, bioinformatics prediction of functionality and *in vitro* and *in vivo* experimental verification of the molecular mechanisms for the causal variants and their target genes [93, 94]. Although identification of common risk variants is an emerging field, it will create a routine screening method for earlier diagnosis and direct breast cancer treatment strategies.

http://dx.doi.org/10.5772/67223

Abbreviations

GWAS	Genome-wide association studies
BRCA 1	Breast cancer 1 gene
BRCA 2	Breast cancer 2 gene
SNP	Single-nucleotide polymorphisms
HER 2+	Human epidermal growth factor receptor 2 positive
HR	Progesterone receptor
LOD	Logarithm of odds
LD	Linkage disequilibrium
TP53	Tumour protein p53
PALB2	Partner and localizer of BRCA2
PTEN	Phosphatase and tensin homolog
CHEK2	Checkpoint kinase 2
ATM	Serine/threonine kinase
NF1	Nuclear factor 1
NBN	Nibrin
CDH1	Cadherin-1
STK11	Serine/threonine kinase 11
FGFR2	Fibroblast growth factor receptor 2
TNRC9	Trinucleotide-repeat-containing 9
LSP1	Lymphocyte-specific protein 1
IGF2	Insulin-like growth factor 2
CGEMS	Cancer genetic markers of susceptibility
RNF146	RING finger protein 146
RAD51L1	DNA repair protein RAD51 homolog 2
NOTCH2	Neurogenic *locus* notch homolog protein 2
FCGR1B	Cluster of differentiation 64
BCAC	Breast Cancer Association Consortium
SLC4A7	Solute carrier family 4, sodium bicarbonate cotransporter, member 7
NEK10	NIMA-related kinase 10
COX11	Cytochrome C oxidase copper chaperone

ER	Estrogen receptor
KLF4	Kruppel-like factor 4
RAD23B	UV excision repair protein RAD23 homolog B
ACTL7A	Actin-like protein 7A
ESR1	Estrogen receptor 1
ERB4	Epidermal growth factor receptor
PTHLH	Parathyroid hormone-related protein
NRIP1	Nuclear receptor-interacting protein 1
COGS	Collaborative oncological gene-environment study
LGR6	Leucine-rich repeat-containing G-protein coupled receptor 6
AREG	Amphiregulin
ZNF365	Zinc finger protein 365
IGF1	Insulin-like growth factor 1
TMEM184B	Transmembrane protein 184B
SGSM3	Small G protein signaling modulator 3
KLF5	Krueppel-like factor 5
WDR43	WD repeat domain 43
PPIL3	Peptidyl-prolyl cis-trans isomerase-like 3
WT1	Wilms tumour protein

Author details

Paulo C.M. Lyra-Junior[1], Nayara G. Tessarollo, Isabella S. Guimarães[1], Taciane B. Henriques[1], Diandra Z. dos Santos[1], Marcele L.M. de Souza[1], Hugo M. Victor Marques[2], Laura F.R.L. de Oliveira[2], Krislayne V. Siqueira[2], Ian V. Silva[3], Leticia B.A. Rangel[1*] and Alan T. Branco[2]

*Address all correspondence to: lbarangel@yahoo.com

1 Laboratory of Cellular and Molecular Biology of Human Cancer, Department of Pharmaceutical Sciences and Biotechnology Program, Federal University of Espirito Santo State, Vitória, Brazil

2 Laboratory of Cellular and Molecular Biology of Human Cancer, Department of Pharmaceutical Sciences, Vitória, Brazil

3 Department of Morphology, Health Sciences Center, Federal University of Espirito Santo State, Vitória, Brazil

References

[1] Monteiro ANA, Freedman ML. Lessons from postgenome-wide association studies: functional analysis of cancer predisposition loci. Journal International Medicine. 2013; **274**: 414–424. DOI: 10.1111/joim.12085

[2] Venter JC, et al. The sequence of the human genome. Science. 2001; **291**: 1304–1351. DOI:10.1126/science.1058040

[3] Lander ES, et al. Initial sequencing and analysis of the human genome. Nature. 2001; **409**: 860–921. DOI: 10.1038/35057062

[4] Altshuler D, et al. Haplotype map of the human genome. Nature. 2005; **437**: 1299–1320. DOI: 10.1038/nature04226

[5] Ferlay J, et al. Cancer incidence and mortality worldwide: sources, methods and major patterns in GLOBOCAN 2012. International Journal Cancer. 2015; **136**: 359–386. DOI: 10.1002/ijc.29210. Epub 2014 Oct 9.

[6] American Cancer Society. Cancer Facts & Figures 2016. Atlanta: American Cancer Society; 2016.

[7] Perou CM, et al. Molecular portraits of human breast tumours. Nature. 2000; **406**: 747–752. DOI: 10.1038/35021093

[8] Sorlie T, et al. Gene expression patterns of breast carcinomas distinguish tumor subclasses with clinical implications. Proceedings of the National Academy of Sciences of the United States of America. 2001; **98**: 10869–10874. DOI: 10.1073/pnas.191367098

[9] Rakha EA, Chan S. Metastatic triple-negative breast cancer. Clinical Oncology. 2011; **23**: 587–600. DOI: 10.1016/j.clon.2011.03.013

[10] Collaborative Group on Hormonal Factors in Breast Cancer. Familial breast cancer: collaborative reanalysis of individual data from 52 epidemiological studies including 58,209 women with breast cancer and 101,986 women without the disease. The Lancet. 2001; **358**: 1389–1399. DOI: 10.1016/S0140-6736(01)06524-2

[11] Pharoah PD, et al. Polygenic susceptibility to breast cancer and implications for prevention. Nature Genetics. 2002; **31**: 33–36. DOI: 10.1038/ng853

[12] Miki Y, et al. A strong candidate for the breast and ovarian-cancer susceptibility gene BRCA1. Science. 1994; **266**: 66–71. DOI: 10.1126/science.7545954

[13] Friedman LS, et al. Confirmation of BRCA1 by analysis of germline mutations linked to breast and ovarian cancer in ten families. Nature Genetics. 1994; **8**: 399–404. DOI: 10.1038/ng1294-399.

[14] Wooster R, et al. Identification of the breast cancer susceptibility gene BRCA2. Nature. 1995; **378**: 789–792. DOI: 10.1038/378789a0

[15] Gudmundsdottir K, Ashworth A. The roles of BRCA1 and BRCA2 and associated proteins in the maintenance of genomic stability. Oncogene. 2006; **25**: 5864–5874. DOI: 10.1038/sj.onc.1209874

[16] Lakhani SR, et al. Prediction of BRCA1 status in patients with breast cancer using estrogen receptor and basal phenotype. Clinical Cancer Research. 2005; **11**: 5175–5180. DOI: 10.1158/1078-0432

[17] Foulkes WD, Shuen AY. In brief: BRCA1 and BRCA2. The Journal of pathology. 2013; **230**: 347–349. DOI: 10.1002/path.4205

[18] King M.C, Marks J.H, Mandell J.B. Breast and ovarian cancer risks due to inherited mutations in BRCA1 and BRCA2. Science. 2003; **302**: 643–646. DOI: 10.1126/science.1088759

[19] Chen S, Parmigiani G. Meta-analysis of BRCA1 and BRCA2 penetrance. Journal of Clinical Oncology. 2007; **25**: 1329–1333. DOI: 10.1200/JCO.2006.09.1066

[20] Mavaddat N, et al. Cancer risks for BRCA1 and BRCA2 mutation carriers: Results from prospective analysis of EMBRACE. Journal of the National Cancer Institute. 2013; **105**: 812–822. DOI: 10.1093/jnci/djt095

[21] Gabai-Kapara E, et al. Population-based screening for breast and ovarian cancer risk due to BRCA1 and BRCA2. Proceedings of the National Academy of Sciences of the United States of America. 2014; **111**: 14205–14210. DOI: 10.1073/pnas.1415979111

[22] Brekelmans CT, et al. Survival and prognostic factors in BRCA1-associated breast cancer. Annals of Oncology. 2006; **17**: 391–400. DOI: 10.1093/annonc/mdj095

[23] Graeser MK, et al. Contralateral breast cancer risk in BRCA1 and BRCA2 mutation carriers. Journal of Clinical Oncology. 2009; **27**: 5887–5892. DOI:10.1200/JCO.2008.19.9430

[24] Van Der Kolk DM, et al. Penetrance of breast cancer, ovarian cancer and contralateral breast cancer in BRCA1 and BRCA2 families: high cancer incidence at older age. Breast Cancer Research and Treatment. 2010; **124**: 643–651. DOI: 10.1007/s10549-010-0805-3

[25] Bernstein JL, et al. Contralateral breast cancer after radiotherapy among BRCA1 and BRCA2 mutation carriers: A WECARE study report. European Journal of Cancer. 2013; **49**: 2979–2985. DOI: 10.1016/j.ejca.2013.04.028

[26] Evans DG, et al. Contralateral mastectomy improves survival in women with BRCA1/2-associated breast cancer. Breast Cancer Research and Treatment. 2013; **140**: 135–142.DOI: 10.1007/s10549-013-2583-1

[27] Van den Broek AJ, et al. Impact of age at primary breast cancer on contralateral breast cancer risk in BRCA1/2 mutation carriers. Journal of Clinical Oncology. 2015; **34**: 409–418. DOI: 10.1200/JCO.2015.62.3942

[28] Giardiello FM, et al. Very high risk of cancer in familial Peutz-Jehgers syndrome. Gastroenterology. 2000; **119**: 1447–1453. DOI: 10.1053/gast.2000.20228

[29] Antoniou A, et al. Average risks of breast and ovarian cancer associated with BRCA1 or BRCA2 mutations detected in case series unselected for family history: a combined analysis of 22 studies. The American Society of Human Genetics. 2003; **72**: 1117–1130. DOI: 10.1086/375033

[30] The CHEK2 Breast Cancer Case-Control Consortium. CHEK2*1100delC and susceptibility to breast cancer: A collaborative analysis involving 10,860 breast cancer cases and 9,065 controls from ten studies. The American Society of Human Genetics. 2004; **74**: 1175–1182. DOI: 10.1086/421251

[31] Thompson D, et al. Cancer risks and mortality in heterozygous ATM mutation carriers. Journal of the National Cancer Institute. 2005; **97:** 813–822. DOI: 10.1093/jnci/dji141

[32] Rahman N, et al. PALB2, which encodes a BRCA2-interacting protein, is a breast cancer susceptibility gene. Nature Genetics. 2006; **39**: 165–167. DOI: 10.1038/ng1959

[33] Robson M. CHEK2, breast cancer, and the understanding of clinical utility. Clinical Genetics. 2010; **78**: 8–10. DOI: 10.1111/j.1399-0004.2010.01444.x

[34] Meindl A, et al. Germline mutations in breast and ovarian cancer pedigrees establish RAD51C as a human cancer susceptibility gene. Nature Genetics. 2010; **42**: 410–414. DOI: 10.1038/ng.569

[35] Manolio TA. Genomewide association studies and assessment of the risk of disease. The New England Journal of Medicine. 2010; **363**: 166–176. DOI: 10.1056/NEJMra0905980

[36] García-Closas M, Malats N, Silverman D, et al. NAT2 slow acetylation, GSTM1 null genotype, and risk of bladder cancer: results from the Spanish Bladder Cancer Study and meta-analyses. The Lancet. 2005; **366**: 649–59. DOI: 10.1016/S0140-6736(05)67137-1

[37] Cox A, et al. A common coding variant in CASP8 is associated with breast cancer risk. Nature Genetics. 2007; **39**: 352–358. DOI: 10.1038/ng1981

[38] Easton DF, Eeles RA. Genome-wide association studies in cancer. Human Molecular Genetics. 2008; **17**: R109–R115. DOI: 10.1093/hmg/ddn287

[39] Bush WS, Moore JH. Chapter 11: Genome-Wide Association Studies. PLoS Computation Biology. 2012; **8**: e1002822. DOI:10.1371/journal.pcbi.1002822

[40] Haines JL, et al. Complement factor H variant increases the risk of age-related macular degeneration. Science. 2005; **308**: 419–421. DOI: 10.1126/science.1110359

[41] Edwards AO, et al. Complement factor H polymorphism and age-related macular degeneration. Science. 2005; **308**: 421–424. DOI: 10.1126/science.1110189

[42] Klein RJ, Zeiss C, Chew EY, et al. Complement factor H polymorphism in age-related macular degeneration. Science. 2005; **308**: 385–389. DOI: 10.1126/science.1109557

[43] The Wellcome Trust Case Control Consortium. Genome-wide association study of 14,000 cases of seven common diseases and 3,000 shared controls. Nature. 2007; **447**: 661–678. DOI: 10.1038/nature05911

[44] Welter D, et al. The NHGRI GWAS catalog, a curated resource of SNP-trait associations. Nucleic Acids Research. 2014; **42**: 1001–1006. DOI: 10.1093/nar/gkt1229

[45] Li Y, et al. Genotype imputation. Annual Review Genomics Human Genetics. 2009; **10**: 387–406. DOI: 10.1146/annurev.genom.9.081307.164242

[46] Kichaev G, Pasaniuc B. Leveraging functional-annotation data in transethnic fine-mapping studies. American Journal Human Genetics. 2015; **97**: 260–271. DOI: 10.1016/j.ajhg.2015.06.007

[47] Freedman ML, Monteiro AN, Gayther SA et al. Principles for the post-GWAS functional characterization of cancer risk loci. Nature Genetics. 2011; **43**: 513–8. DOI:10.1038/ng.840.

[48] Blattler A, et al. Global loss of DNA methylation uncovers intronic enhancers in genes showing expression changes. Genome Biology. 2014; **15**: 469. DOI: 10.1186/s 13059-014-0469-0

[49] Howie BN, Donnelly P, Marchini JA. Flexible and accurate genotype imputation method for the next generation of genome-wide association studies. PLoS Genetics. 2009; **5**: e1000529. DOI: 10.1371/journal.pgen.1000529

[50] Li Y, et al. Mach: using sequence and genotype data to estimate haplotypes and unobserved genotypes. Genetic Epidemiology. 2010; **34**: 816–834. DOI: 10.1002/gepi.20533

[51] Browning SR, Browning BL. Rapid and accurate haplotype phasing and missing-data inference for whole-genome association studies by use of localized haplotype clustering. American Journal of Human Genetics. 2007; **81**: 1084–1097. DOI: 10.1086/521987

[52] Genomes Project C, et al. A global reference for human genetic variation. Nature. 2015; **526**: 68–74. DOI: 10.1038/nature15393

[53] 1000 Genomes Project Consortium, et al. An integrated map of genetic variation from 1092 human genomes. Nature. 2012; **491**: 56–65. DOI: .1038/nature11632

[54] Trynka G, Hunt KA, Bockett NA et al. Dense genotyping identifies and localizes multiple common and rare variant association signals in celiac disease. Nature Genetics. 2011; **43**: 1193–201. DOI: 10.1038/ng.998

[55] Voight BF, et al. The metabochip, a custom genotyping array for genetic studies of metabolic, cardiovascular, and anthropometric traits. PLoS Genetics. 2012; **8**: e1002793. DOI: 10.1371/journal.pgen.1002793

[56] Michailidou K, et al. Large-scale genotyping identifies 41 new loci associated with breast cancer risk. Nature Genetics. 2013; **45**: 353–361. DOI: 10.1038/ng.2563

[57] Available from: http://epi.grants.cancer/gov/oncoarray/ [Accessed: 2016-07-14].

[58] Easton DF, et al. Genome-wide association study identifies novel breast cancer susceptibility loci. Nature. 2007; **447**; 1087–1093. DOI: 10.1038/nature05887.

[59] Adnane J, et al. BEK and FLG, two receptors to members of the FGF family, are amplified in subsets of human breast cancers. Oncogene. 1991; **6**: 659–663.

[60] Brantjes H, et al. All Tcf HMG box transcription factors interact with Groucho-related co-repressors. Nucleic Acids Research. 2001; **29**: 1410–1419. DOI: 10.1093/nar/29.7.1410

[61] Stacey SN, et al. Common variants on chromosomes 2q35 and 16q12 confer susceptibility to estrogen receptor-positive breast cancer. Nature Genetics. 2007; **39**: 865–869. DOI: 10.1038/ng2064

[62] Hunter DJ, et al. A genome-wide association study identifies alleles in FGFR2 associated with risk of sporadic postmenopausal breast cancer. Nature Genetics. 2007; **39**: 870–874. DOI: 10.1038/ng2075

[63] Stacey SN, et al. Common variants on chromosome 5p12 confer susceptibility to estrogen receptor-positive breast cancer. Nature Genetics. 2008; **40**; 703–706. DOI: 10.1038/ng.131

[64] Gold B, et al. Genome-wide association study provides evidence for a breast cancer risk locus at 6q22.33. Proceedings of the National Academy of Sciences of the United States of America. 2008; **105**: 4340–4345. DOI: 10.1073/pnas.0800441105

[65] Zheng W, et al. Genome-wide association study identifies a new breast cancer susceptibility locus at 6q25.1. Nature Genetics. 2009; **41**: 324–328. DOI: 10.1038/ng.318

[66] Ahmed S, et al. Newly discovered breast cancer susceptibility loci on 3p24 and 17q23.2. Nature Genetics. 2009; **41**: 585–590. DOI: 10.1038/ng.354

[67] Thomas G, et al. A multistage genome-wide association study in breast cancer identifies two new risk alleles at 1p11.2 and 14q24.1 (RAD51L1). Nature Genetics. 2009; **41**: 579–584. DOI: 10.1038/ng.353

[68] Antoniou AC, et al. A locus on 19p13 modifies risk of breast cancer in BRCA1 mutation carriers and is associated with hormone receptor-negative breast cancer in the general population. Nature Genetics. 2010; **42**: 885–892. DOI:10.1038/ng.669

[69] Turnbull C, et al. Genome-wide association study identifies five new breast cancer susceptibility loci. Nature Genetics. 2010; **42**: 504–507. DOI: 10.1038/ng.586

[70] Meyer KB, et al. Allele-specific up-regulation of FGFR2 increases susceptibility to breast cancer. PLoS Biology. 2008; **6**: e108. DOI: 10.1371/journal.pbio.0060108

[71] Haiman CA, et al. A common variant at the TERT-CLPTM1L locus is associated with estrogen receptor-negative breast cancer. Nature Genetics. 2011; **43**: 1210–1214. DOI: 10.1038/ng.985

[72] Cai Q, et al. Genome-wide association study identifies breast cancer risk variant at 10q21.2: results from the Asia Breast Cancer Consortium. Human Molecular Genetics. 2011; **20**: 4991–4999. DOI: 10.1093/hmg/ddr405

[73] Fletcher O, et al. Novel breast cancer susceptibility locus at 9q31.2: results of a genome-wide association study. Journal of the National Cancer Institute. 2011; **103**: 425–435. DOI: 10.1093/jnci/djq563

[74] Long J, et al. Genome-wide association study in East Asians identifies novel susceptibility loci for breast cancer. PLoS Genetics. 2012; **8**: e1002532. DOI: 10.1371/journal.pgen.1002532

[75] Kim HC, et al. A genome-wide association study identifies a breast cancer risk variant in ERBB4 at 2q34: results from the Seoul Breast Cancer Study. Breast Cancer Research. 2012; **14**: R56. DOI: 10.1186/bcr3158

[76] Kiyotani K, et al. A genome-wide association study identifies locus at 10q22 associated with clinical outcomes of adjuvant tamoxifen therapy for breast cancer patients in Japanese. Human Molecular Genetics. 2012; **21**: 1665–1672. DOI: 10.1093/hmg/ddr597

[77] Ghoussaini M, et al. Genome-wide association analysis identifies three new breast cancer susceptibility loci. Nature Genetics. 2012: **44**: 312–318. DOI: 10.1038/ng.1049

[78] Siddiq A, et al. A meta-analysis of genome-wide association studies of breast cancer identifies two novel susceptibility loci at 6q14 and 20q11. Human Molecular Genetics. 2012; **21**: 5373–5384. DOI: 10.1093/hmg/dds381

[79] Couch FJ, et al. Genome-wide association study in BRCA1 mutation carriers identifies novel loci associated with breast and ovarian cancer risk. PLoS Genetics. 2013; **9**: e1003212. DOI: 10.1371/journal.pgen.1003212

[80] Garcia-Closas M, et al. Genome-wide association studies identify four ER negative-specific breast cancer risk loci. Nature Genetics. 2013; **45**: 392–398. DOI: 10.1038/ng.2561

[81] Chung R, et al. Roles of Wnt/β-catenin signalling pathway in the bony repair of injured growth plate cartilage in young rats. Bone. 2013; **52**: 651–658. DOI: 10.1016/j.bone.2012.10.035

[82] Milne RL, et al. Common non-synonymous SNPs associated with breast cancer susceptibility: findings from the Breast Cancer Association Consortium. Human Molecular Genetics. 2014; **23**: 6096–6111. DOI: 10.1093/hmg/ddu311

[83] Cai Q, et al. Genome-wide association analysis in East Asians identifies breast cancer susceptibility loci at 1q32.1, 5q14.3 and 15q26.1. Nature Genetics. 2014; **46**: 886–890. DOI: 10.1038/ng.3041

[84] Purrington KS, et al. Genome-wide association study identifies 25 known breast cancer susceptibility loci as risk factors for triple-negative breast cancer. Carcinogenesis. 2014; **35**: 1012–1019 DOI: 10.1093/carcin/bgt404

[85] Michailidou K, et al. Genome-wide association analysis of more than 120,000 individuals identifies 15 new susceptibility loci for breast cancer. Nature Genetics. 2015; **47**: 373–380. DOI: 10.1038/ng.3242

[86] Palomba G, et al. Genome-wide association study of susceptibility loci for breast cancer in Sardinian population. BMC cancer. 2015; **15**: 383. DOI: 10.1186/s12885-015-1392-9

[87] Han MR, et al. Genome-wide association study in East Asians identifies two novel breast cancer susceptibility loci. Human Molecular Genetics. 2016; **0**: 1–11. DOI: 10.1093/hmg/ddw164

[88] Couch FJ, et al. Identification of four novel susceptibility loci for oestrogen receptor negative breast cancer. Nature Communication. 2016; **7**: 11375. DOI: 10.1038/ncomms11375

[89] Wu L, et al. A genome-wide association study identifies WT1 variant with better response to 5-fluorouracil, pirarubicin and cyclophosphamide neoadjuvant chemotherapy in breast cancer patients. Oncotarget. 2016; **7**: 5042–5052. DOI: 10.18632/oncotarget.5837

[90] Qian DC, et al. Identification of shared and unique susceptibility pathways among cancers of the lung, breast, and prostate from genome-wide association studies and tissue-specific protein interactions. Human Molecular Genetics. 2015; **24**: 7406–7420. DOI: 10.1093/hmg/ddv440

[91] Cantor RM, Lange K, Sinsheimer JS. Prioritizing GWAS results: A review of statistical methods and recommendations for their application. American Journal of Human Genetics. 2010; **86**: 6–22. DOI: 10.1016/j.ajhg.2009.11.017

[92] Peng G, et al. Gene and pathway-based second-wave analysis of genome-wide association studies. European Journal of Human Genetics. 2010; **8**: 111–117. DOI: 10.1038/ejhg.2009.115

[93] Edwards SL, et al. Beyond GWASs: illuminating the dark road from association to function. American Journal of Human Genetics. 2013; **93**: 779–797. DOI: 10.1016/j.ajhg.2013.10.012

[94] Fachal L. Dunning AM. From candidate gene studies to GWAS and post-GWAS analyses in breast cancer. Current Opinion in Genetics & Development. 2015; **30**: 32–41. DOI: 10.1016/j.gde.2015.01.004

[95] Manolio TA, et al. Finding the missing heritability of complex diseases. Nature. 2009; **461**: 747–53. DOI: 10.1038/nature08494

Chapter 6

Circulating Tumor Cells in Breast Cancer: A Potential Liquid Biopsy

Mohamed Kamal, Wajeeha Razaq, Macall Leslie,
Smita Adhikari and Takemi Tanaka

Additional information is available at the end of the chapter

http://dx.doi.org/10.5772/66439

Abstract

Circulating tumor cells (CTCs) have emerged as a new generation of liquid biomarker that allows for noninvasive longitudinal disease monitoring. CTCs represent a rare cell population in the blood, surrounded by billions of hematopoietic cells. Due to the rarity of CTCs in the blood, the isolation of pure CTCs' populations has proven to be challenging. However, a number of new technologies have emerged using CTCs cytometric/immunological and physical characteristics. Currently, patients with greater than 5 CTCs have a shorter progression-free survival, as compared with those with less than 5 CTCs per 7.5 ml of whole blood. Although the CTC count itself is an independent prognostic marker, the field is shifting toward understanding metastasis-relevant marker expression on CTCs for the improvement of the prognostic significance of CTCs. This chapter first introduces the principles of CTC isolation and detection methods, then the clinical utility of CTCs for prediction of prognosis and therapy response. Lastly, the heterogeneity of CTCs will be discussed.

Keywords: circulating tumor cell (CTC), breast cancer, liquid biomarker, metastasis

1. Introduction

Breast cancer is the most commonly diagnosed malignancy as well as one of the leading causes of cancer deaths. Treatment strategies in early-stage breast cancer are directed toward radical cure and prevention of recurrence or the development of metastatic diseases. However, once metastatic disease has been detected, alleviation of symptoms or palliative care becomes the focus, with the aim of extending overall and disease-free survival (DFS). Current methods of disease monitoring are limited to radio-imaging of detectable metastatic lesions and/or elevation of tumor markers in the serum. Due to a lack of sensitive and specificity, accurate disease monitoring remains a challenge. Recently, however, circulating tumor cells (CTCs) have received significant attention as a new class of "liquid biopsy" that would enable longitudinal and noninvasive disease monitoring in order to capture an overall snapshot of individual disease.

The presence of cancer cells in the circulation was recognized as early as the nineteenth century, when the Australian physician Thomas Ashworth detected the presence of cells in the blood that were similar to those from the primary tumor of a woman with metastatic breast cancer (MBC) [1]. The early 1900s yielded few descriptions of the isolation of tumor cells from the blood [2, 3]. In 1960, Alexander and Spriggs undertook cytopathologic analysis for the presence of CTCs in the blood of 140 cancer patients of various sites [4]. Although CTCs were detected in only seven of these cases, each of those patients had a markedly short survival of only several months, reinforcing the rarity as well as the potential clinical significance of CTCs. In addition to these early clinical investigations, parallel efforts using animal models to elucidate the process of cancer cell dissemination have further highlighted the clinical relevance of CTCs [5, 6]. Despite growing awareness throughout the twentieth century of CTCs' potential impact, their clinical implication was not robustly examined until the early 2000s. In 2002, Fehm et al. conducted cytogenetic analyses of cells obtained from the blood of cancer patients of several types, including breast, and compared chromosome profiles to those from their primary tumors, finding similar malignant features and chromosomal abnormalities between the two. The first large, multi-institutional clinical study evaluating the prognostic value of CTCs in patients with MBC was conducted in 2004 by Cristofanilli et al. Their study concluded that patients with 5 or more CTCs found in 7.5 ml of pretreatment blood have shorter progression-free survival (PFS) compared to those with less than 5 CTCs [7]. Since then, multiple studies have followed investigating the clinical validity of CTCs in the prediction of prognosis and therapy response.

These initial findings not only revealed that cancer cells in the circulation originate from the solid primary tumor but also provided new insight into the hematogenous metastasis pathway. Since the majority of breast cancer-related deaths are caused by distant organ metastasis rather than primary tumor burden, understanding this pathway is of great consequence to clinicians and researchers working to reduce breast cancer mortality. The completion of metastasis requires a sequential multistep process, the first step of which is local invasion. Increased motility facilitates the entry of cancer cells from the primary tumor into the blood stream. Vascular circulation is the interface between the primary tumor and the target organ for metastasis, making cancer cells disseminated in the blood a critical driver of metastasis. Although the drastic environmental change from a static solid tumor to dynamic blood flow eliminates many of the intravasated tumor cells, those that survive and adhere firmly to the vessel surface of a distant organ complete the next step in the metastasis pathway. The firm adhesion of CTCs to the endothelium under dynamic blood flow triggers permeabilization of endothelial tight junctions, subsequently allowing transendothelial migration of CTCs and eventual growth at distant organs [8]. Each of these steps is rate-limiting, and failure of even one inhibits metastasis. Thus, only a small fraction of the cancer cells disseminated from the primary tumor into circulation eventually give rise to overt organ metastasis.

In this chapter, we discuss the different platforms used to isolate CTCs from the blood as well as their clinical relevance in predicting prognosis and treatment response. The cytological features and heterogeneity among CTCs will also be examined. Finally, throughout the chapter, we will explore new avenues of research on CTCs and their implications in establishing CTCs as the new "liquid biopsy."

2. Isolation and enumeration of CTCs

CTCs represent a rare cell population in the blood; therefore, they must be well distinguished from blood and other noncancerous cells (such as epithelial, fibroblast, and endothelial cells) present in the circulation [9–11]. Successful detection of CTCs is comprised of two consecutive steps: (1) enrichment, the separation of CTCs from blood cells and (2) confirmation, the identification of CTCs based on their unique biological characteristics. Currently, the main principles guiding CTC enrichment are based on the unique biological, morphological, and physiochemical characteristics that distinguish CTCs from other cells in circulation [12, 13]. However, each method faces its own difficulties. For example, CTC collection based on biological properties using surface markers will automatically eliminate CTCs without the marker expression. By contrast, enrichment by density, charge, or size collects any circulating cell with those prerequisite properties. A combinatorial approach may overcome current technology limitations. Additionally, a better understanding of the properties of CTCs may lead to the development of new enrichment criteria. Since strategies for CTC enrichment and identification vary in their respective strengths and weaknesses, the method of enrichment should be determined by the end point of individual studies. This section introduces commonly used CTC enumeration and identification methodologies and further discusses the advantages and potential pitfalls of each enrichment principle.

2.1. Isolation based on biological characteristics of CTCs

Breast cancer originates from epithelial cells in the mammary duct; thus, CTCs with positive expression of epithelial surface markers (cytokeratins and/or EpCAM) have traditionally been the focus of enrichment methodologies. CTCs are enriched by their affinity to bind antibodies against epithelial surface markers and excluded by the presence of the common leukocyte marker (CD45) as well as cytologic criteria [14]. This principle is the most widely adopted basis for enrichment techniques, and automated devices have been developed and commercialized for this application. While high reproducibility, specificity, and automation are major strengths, CTCs without epithelial marker expression likely escape inclusion by this method. Given the importance of epithelial mesenchymal transition (EMT) in invasion and metastasis, the potential exclusion of CTCs with weak or no epithelial marker expression should be considered [15, 16].

2.1.1. CellSearch® system (Veridex, LLC)

The CellSearch® system is a Food and Drug Administration (FDA)-approved CTC isolation device that is widely utilized for CTC enumeration in clinical studies. CellSearch's enrichment method relies on affinity binding of CTCs to magnetic ferrofluids attached to anti-EpCAM antibodies. EpCAM positive pools are then further used for enumeration by positive expression of cytokeratins $8^+/18^+$ and/or 19^+ that collocate with DAPI and the absence of CD45 [17]. Whole blood is processed using an automated blood cell diluting apparatus (CellPrep and Immunicon) and then immunomagnetically labeled $EpCAM^+$ cells are concentrated using an external magnetic field. Finally, the immunomagnetically labeled cells are analyzed using either the CellSpotter Analyzer or the CellTracks Analyser II which examine cell morphology and staining patterns for CTC confirmation [17, 18]. The CTC criteria used in these methods are (1) an intact cell with a round to oval morphology and at least 4 μm in size; (2) positive for DAPI with a nucleus inside the cytoplasm (of at least >50%) and a nucleus area smaller than the cytoplasm, and (3) positive for cytokeratins and negative for CD45 [19]. One advantage of the CellSearch® System is that blood is collected in a CellSave tube which contains a mixed fixative. CTCs remain stable for 96 hours and can be transported at room temperature for later analysis. Since the CellSearch® system is semiautomated, the reproducibility of this study is high with minimal inter- or intrareader variability.

Using CellSearch®, Cristofanilli et al. were the first to report that circulating epithelial cells are rare in healthy women and those with benign tumors (0.1 ± 0.2 per 7.5 ml blood). Additionally, they found 5 CTCs per 7.5 ml blood to be a reliable cutoff for the prediction of patient survival among women with malignant breast tumors. A study of 517 breast cancer patients showed that patients at or above this cutoff had a shorter median PFS (2.7 months vs. 7.0 months; $p < 0.001$) and shorter overall survival (OS) (10.1 months vs. >18.0 months; $p < 0.001$) when compared to those with fewer than 5 CTCs. These data demonstrate that the number of CTCs prior to treatment is an independent predictor of PFS and OS in patients with MBC [7].

2.1.2. *Adnatest (AdnaGen AG)*

Adnatest is an immunomolecular assay that combines immunomagnetic-based enrichment with multiplex reverse transcription polymerase chain reaction (RT-PCR). In the initial isolation step, $EpCAM^+$/$MUC1^+$ CTCs are enriched using magnetized antibodies and further identified by tumor-associated gene expression [20–22]. Since phenotypic changes occur in cancer cells throughout the disease course and in response to therapies, cancer cells in the primary tumor as well as in the circulation are diverse in their gene expression. Considering the heterogeneity of cancer cells, the most prominent advantage of Adnatest is that it allows use of a variety of antibody-based selection markers, thereby minimizing false negative and false positive results. Bredemeier et al. enriched CTCs in 62 MBC patients using immunomagnetic beads that target EpCAM, epithelial growth factor receptor (EGFR), and HER2. The enriched CTCs were then characterized by their expression of tumor-related genes using a multiplex qPCR assay (AdnaTest EMT-2/StemCellDetect™). Using this approach, authors of the study established a panel of nine genes able to identify differential expression of each phenotype— epithelial (*EpCAM*), EMT (*PIK3CA, AKT2*), stem cell (*ALDH1*), drug resistant (*ERCC1, AURKA*), receptor positive (*ERBB2, ERBB3,* and *EGFR*), and leukocyte control (*CD45*) [23]. Adnatest is capable of detecting as few as 2 CTCs in 5 ml of blood [20, 22] and in a comparative study showed greater sensitivity than the CellSearch® system in detecting CTCs (53 vs. 47% CTC positive, respectively, in a sample of 55 MBC patients) [24].

2.1.3. *CTC-Chip*

A surface coating of anti-EpCAM antibody enables the microfluidic CTC-Chip to capture $EpCAM^+$ cells in its channel while eliminating those that are negative under precisely controlled laminar flow conditions. Etched in silicon and no larger than a standard microscope slide [25], the CTC-Chip contains an array of microposts functionalized with anti-EpCAM antibodies and a pneumatic pump to establish flow, all enclosed by a manifold. Once a blood sample has been pumped through, the microchip is gradually flushed with PBS to remove any nonspecifically bound cells. To identify CTCs, the microchip is then stained with DAPI, pan-cytokeratins (1, 4, 5, 6, 8, 10, 13, 18, and 19), and CD45 using immunocytochemistry. Cells meeting the morphological characteristics of malignant tumor cells (such as cell size, shape, and nuclear size) and positive for cytokeratins are considered CTCs. Assessment of cell membrane integrity following this method showed substantial viability (98.5 ± 2.3%). Additionally, the CTC-Chip captures cells with low EpCAM expression as efficiently as cells with high expression. The CTC-Chip successfully identified CTCs in the peripheral blood of patients with metastatic disease in 115 of 116 (99%) samples, with a range of 5–1281 CTCs per ml [26].

2.1.4. *MagSweeper*

The MagSweeper is another EpCAM-based immunomagnetic cell separator. It uses a round-bottom, magnetic rod covered with an ultrathin (25 μm) nonadherent plastic sheath. This assembly is robotically swept through a well containing a blood sample labeled with anti-EpCAM functionalized paramagnetic beads (CELLection Epithelial Enrich Dynabeads: Invitrogen). The $EpCAM^+$ cells captured on the covered magnetic rod (MagSweeper) are transferred to and washed in a well containing PBS, then released into another well of PBS by removing the magnetic rod from its sheath. Finally, $EpCAM^+$ cells are further confirmed by morphology and gene expression profiles [27, 28]. The gene expression profiles of MCF7 cells incubated with anti-EpCAM magnetic beads before and after MagSweeper isolation were analyzed using microarray analysis and compared with a similar number of MCF7 cells grown in culture media. Statistical analysis indicated that the MagSweeper isolation process does not induce any significant perturbation in the gene expression profile of cells. Additionally, the use of 4.5-μm magnetic beads permits isolation of target $EpCAM^+$ cells, even with single-bead attachment, making the procedure suitable for isolation of CTCs with moderate-to-low EpCAM expression. However, the attachment of large magnetic beads to the cell surface may interfere with certain applications. An additional drawback is that normal $EpCAM^+$ cells present in the circulation are also potentially selected and need to be distinguished from CTCs at a microscopic level. MagSweeper technology succeeded in isolating CTCs from all MBC patients ($n = 47$) at an average of 12 ± 23 CTCs per 9 ml of blood, while no CTCs were found in samples derived from healthy donors [28].

2.1.5. *Vita-Assay™ (Vitatex Inc.)*

The Vita-Assay™ is a functional assay-based CTC enrichment method that takes advantage of invasive CTCs preferential adhesion to the cell adhesion matrix (CAM). Viable, invasive CTCs are captured on a plate coated with CAM-mimic, then further identified based on their proclivity to degrade and ingest the extracellular matrix. CTCs adhered to the Vita-Assay™ plate are released by the addition of an enzyme that dissolves the CAM coating, and then concentrated by centrifugation for cytologic analysis. This application's criteria for CTCs include positive CAM uptake (CAM^+) and negative hematopoietic lineage (HL) marker expression. Enumeration of CTCs by flow cytometry may be further validated by microscopic comparison of CTC and immune cell morphology. The Vita-Assay™ CTC-enrichment platform is capable of enriching rare and invasive CTCs and is not biased by surface markers, morphology, or size. Rather, since it focuses on the adhesive properties of CTCs, it offers a potentially robust capture method for invasive CTCs. Additionally, Vita-Assay™ allows for sensitive multiplex flow cytometric and microscopic detection of CTCs. Vita-Assay™ successfully detected CTCs in all blood samples from MBC patients (n = 10) with a range of 18–256 CTCs per ml. Moreover, CTCs were detected in blood samples of 28 of 54 (52%) stage I–III breast cancer patients with a mean count of 61 CTCs per ml [29].

2.2. Isolation based on physicochemical properties of CTCs

Several isolation methods take advantage of differences between the physicochemical properties of CTCs and other circulating cells. Enrichment methods have been developed for properties including size, density, and surface charge [30]. For example, the well-documented fact that carcinoma cells have larger overall size and denser nuclei than normal epithelial and immune cells has been adopted for CTC isolation [31, 32]. Similarly, nuclear condensation of carcinoma cells has led to the development of density-based CTC enrichment [33]. Lastly, differential surface charges between carcinoma and normal epithelial or immune cells are also a strategy used for CTC enrichment [34]. Enrichment strategies based on physiochemical properties have emerged in order to minimize bias (i.e., exclusion of non-EpCAM$^+$ cells); thus, the sensitivity of CTC isolation using these methods is high. However, their specificity is not always high due to the difficulty of completely eliminating potential leukocyte contamination during the enrichment step. Most of these methods rely on manual cytopathologic identification of CTCs, a highly laborious process with varied reproducibility depending on the pathologist. Despite this, the potential for versatile applications as well as live CTC collection remains major strengths of this method class.

2.2.1. Size and density

Since CTCs are larger in size than immune or red blood cells, two commercially available methods have used this principle to enrich CTCs. Using negative pressure or gravity, cells with diameter greater than the 6.5–8.0-μm pores are captured on porous membranes. This results in the acquisition of multiple types of cells, including CTCs, leukocytes, fibroblasts, normal epithelial, and endothelial cells. CTCs are then distinguished from immune cells by immunostaining and morphology. Although, different types of staining methods have been explored for reproducibility, no standard staining method for CTCs has been established thus far.

2.2.1.1. RareCells® system (Rarecells)

The RareCells® system allows performance of the Isolation by Size of Epithelial Tumor Cells test (ISET® test). The ISET® test enriches CTCs according to their size and subsequently identifies them based on their cytopathologic features. The RareCells® system is a negative depression-based filtration device. It consists of a 10-well filtration module that captures CTCs on a polycarbonate Track-Etch-type porous membrane [35–37]. Following red blood cell rupture and mild fixation, circulating cells smaller than 8 μm are filtered through the porous membrane, while those of a greater diameter are enriched on the membrane. The membranes may subsequently be stained for the detection of CTCs or stored for future analysis. The RareCells® system allows

http://dx.doi.org/10.5772/66439

for versatile applications, including both fixed and live CTC collection. Using ISET method, Hofman et al. conducted a blinded, multicenter study to assess the feasibility of CTC identification using cytopathologic criteria. CTCs were defined as circulating nonhematologic cells exhibiting at least 4 of the following criteria: irregular nuclei, anisonucleosis (ratio >0.5), high nuclear/cytoplasmic ratio, nuclei larger than 24 μm, or the presence of tridimensional sheets. Based on these criteria, CTCs were only detected in the blood of patients with malignant disease and were absent in healthy subjects [38]. The RareCells® system has shown successful detection of CTCs in breast cancer, melanoma, and nonsmall cell lung cancer cases [37, 39–41]. In a comparison between the RareCells® system and CellSearch®, the RareCells® system displayed greater sensitivity of detection (93% vs. 40%, respectively) and yielded higher median CTC counts [42].

2.2.1.2. OncoQuick® tube (Greiner Bio-One)

This separation device is composed of a centrifugation tube containing a liquid density separation medium and porous barrier membrane optimized for the enrichment of CTCs from blood. During the enrichment step, blood is layered on top of the gradient and then centrifuged. CTCs are enriched in the fluid above the porous barrier and collected in a tube by centrifugation. Following immunocytochemistry, CTCs are identified as cytokeratin-positive (7, 8, and 18) and CD45 negative with intact nuclei and an increased nuclear-cytoplasmic ratio [43, 44]. The purity and efficacy of CTC enrichment using OncoQuick® are higher than that with Ficoll, which traps up to 25 times more blood mononuclear cells [45]. However, detection sensitivity using OncoQuick® was found to be lower than CellSearch® (23% vs. 54%; $p < 0.001$) [43].

2.2.2. Electrical properties

CTCs have a unique surface charge that distinguishes them from other cells. Thus, a dielectrophoretic flow field can be used to fractionate CTCs from blood cells based on their differential electrical properties [34].

2.2.2.1. DEPArray™ technology (Silicon Biosystems)

Utilizing this principle, DEPArray™ is an automated instrument that can identify, quantify, and recover individual rare cells. It is used as a second purification step after initial EpCAM-based CTC enrichment methods. The individually isolated CTCs using DEPArray™ are then identified based on their morphological and immunocytochemical features. The system includes the DEPArray™ cartridge and DEPArray™ analysis platform. The single-use, microfluidic cartridge contains an array of individually controllable electrodes, each with embedded sensors. This circuitry enables the creation of dielectrophoretic cages around cells. After imaging, individual CTCs are gently moved into the holding chamber for isolation and recovery. The DEPArray™ analysis platform utilizes image-based selection to allow identification and isolation of CTCs on the DEPArray™ cartridge. The system uses a six-channel fluorescent microscope and a CCD camera to capture images and identify cells demonstrating the desired fluorescence labeling and morphological characteristics. The main advantage of DEPArray™ is its ability to eliminate mononuclear cell cross contamination from the preenriched CTC pool. Image-based selection enables the isolation of specific rare cells from other cell types. Moreover, the DEPArray™ system yields high-quality nucleic acids for molecular investigations, since the

Detection strategy		Detection method	Advantages	Disadvantages
Biological	EpCAM expression	CellSearch® System [17]	Semiautomated system FDA approved Quantification of CTCs	Only epithelial CTCs are captured and mesenchymal cells are discarded
		CTC-chip [25]	Captured cells are suitable for molecular analyses High detection rate Quantification of CTCs	
		IsoFlux	NSG applicable Custom design for CTC isolation Semiautomated system	
		Herringbone-Chip (HB-Chip) [98]	Enhanced platform for CTC isolation Allows detection of microclusters of CTCs	
		MagSweeper [27, 28]	Automated immunomagnetic isolation Allows for gene expression profiling analysis	
	EpCAM and MUC1 expression	AdnaTest [20–22]	High sensitivity Multiplex PCR assays	CTCs cannot be morphologically characterized
	EpCAM expression and microfluidic	SIM-Chip [99]	Single-cell isolation High purity and recovery without cell damage	Possible cell damage
Physicochemical	Size	RareCells® system [35–37]	Single CTC morphological, immunocytological, and genetic analyses High sensitivity and specificity	Cross contamination with other rare blood cells such as megakaryocytes and large monocytes
		ScreenCell® [100]	Isolation of live cells and allows for tissue culture experiments	
		Celsee PREP™ slide	Highly efficient CTC detection with high sensitivity and specificity Immunohistochemistry, DNA, and mRNA analyses Single cell analyses Automatic imaging system	
	Surface charge	DEPArray™ [46]	Single cell isolation High quality nucleic acids for molecular investigations (elimination of blood cells cross contamination)	

Detection strategy		Detection method	Advantages	Disadvantages
Functional	Secretion	EPISPOT [101]	Detects viable cells	Detects only Epithelial CTCs
	Matrix adhesion	Vita-Assay™ [29]	Enriches viable CTCs from blood up to one-million fold	Limited only to invasive CTCs which are able to ingest cell matrix

Table 1. Summary of approaches used for CTC isolation and their relevant devices.

cells receive minimal disturbance during capture or transport. Additionally, the DEPArray™ system allows for the isolation of single cells, making it a promising contributor to the understanding of CTC heterogeneity [46].

A summary for the CTC methods discussed in this chapter along with other methods is described in **Table 1**.

3. Clinical utility of CTCs as a biomarker

Liquid biopsy is a clinically amenable method to enable real-time and longitudinal disease monitoring. Currently, available serum markers lack the specificity and sensitivity needed for clinical management of breast tumors. Since the detection of CTCs became feasible, a number of clinical studies have undertaken exploration of whether CTCs could provide a new minimally invasive, longitudinal disease monitoring strategy in breast cancer [7, 47]. The ability of CTCs to predict disease progression in both early and MBC as well as in different tumor subtypes is currently under investigation. Moreover, several clinical trials have investigated the use of CTCs as an early therapy response marker. This section discusses the potential use of CTCs as a biomarker for prognosis and therapy response in breast cancer.

3.1. Prediction of prognosis of metastatic breast cancer by CTC

In a landmark study, Cristofanilli et al. conducted the first large, multi-institutional clinical study to evaluate the utility of CTCs as a predictive biomarker for disease progression in patients with MBC. Using the CellSearch® system, CTCs were enumerated from 177 patients with measurable MBC from 20 clinical centers across the United States. Of these, 49% had ≥5 CTCs per 7.5 ml of blood at baseline prior to treatment. When compared to patients with fewer than 5 CTCs at baseline, these patients had shorter median PFS (2.7 months vs. 7.0 months; $p < 0.001$) and OS (10.1 months vs. >18 months; $p < 0.001$). After 4 months, 10 of the 177 patients had died, each showing an average of 3000 CTCs per 7.5 ml of blood at baseline [7]. This data clearly indicated that the presence of CTCs is strongly associated with poor outcomes in MBC patients. When another study, conducted by Nakamura et al., examined the correlation between CTC count and OS, increased risk was found for patients with higher pretreatment counts Hazard Ratio (HR): 2.4 for patients with 5–10 CTCs; (95% CI, 0.72–8.24, $p = 0.1481$); HR: 13.95 for patients with 21–100 CTCs; (95% CI, 4.57–42.55, $p < 0.0001$). Furthermore, when the OS of patients with ≥5 CTCs was compared to those with <5 CTCs, the HR was 3.1 times higher (95% CI, 1.49–6.29, $p = 0.002$) [47]. This relationship has been further confirmed by both meta- and pooled analyses [48–50]. Comprehensive meta-analysis of 49 studies, including a total of 6825 patients (Early stage [M0, $n = 2993$], metastatic [M1, $n = 3069$], and pooled patients with I–IV stages [$n = 763$]) found that CTC count was significantly associated with shorter PFS and OS in both early stage and MBC patients (HR: 1.78; 95% CI, 1.52–2.09, $p < 0.001$ for PFS; HR: 2.33; 95% CI, 2.09–2.60, $p < 0.001$ for OS in MBC patients) [48]. Additionally, pooled analysis of 20 studies from 17 European breast cancer centers found similar trends. In this cohort of 1944 MBC patients, 46.9% had a CTC count of ≥5 CTCs per 7.5 ml at baseline, which was associated with both decreased PFS (HR: 1.92; 95% CI, 1.73–2.14, $p < 0.0001$) and OS (HR: 2.78; 95%CI, 2.42–3.19, $p < 0.0001$) compared to those with <5 CTCs [49]. In another recent meta-analysis of 24 studies including 3701 MBC patients, in 1 and 2 years PFS and OS rates (respectively), higher CTC counts correlated with shorter PFS [50].

Since the studies included in these analyses varied in CTC detection method and time point of blood draw, Zhang et al. evaluated whether these differences affect the prognostic value of CTC counts. Using a subgroup analysis stratified by detection method and time point of blood sampling, their meta-analysis found that the prognostic value of CTCs in PFS was significant in studies using RT-PCR (HR: 2.58; 95% CI, 1.99–3.35) or CellSearch® methodologies (HR: 1.85; 95% CI, 1.53–2.25). This demonstrated that CTCs are a reliable prognostic marker from pre-dose/preoperative blood in patients with MBC, regardless of other differences in study design [51]. Similarly, CTC counts have also been shown to be a prognostic marker in the postdose blood of MBC patients receiving their first cycle of first-line treatment [7, 52].

Together, these studies lay the foundation for CTCs as a valid and reliable prognostic indicator both before and after breast cancer treatment. Given their promising clinical application, the question of whether CTCs are superior to other prognostic factors has also been addressed. A multivariate, Cox proportional hazards regression analysis showed that CTC count at baseline was the most significant predictor of both PFS and OS, regardless of histology grade, recurrence, de novo stage IV breast cancer, or hormone and HER2 receptor status. Moreover, in a retrospective analysis of MBC patients, comparison of the prognostic significance of CTCs with tumor burden, therapy type, and receptor subtype showed that CTCs were an independent predictor of prognosis [7, 53].

3.2. Prediction of prognosis of nonmetastatic breast cancer by CTCs

As mediators of metastasis, CTCs' presence and role in advanced breast cancer cases have received much attention. However, their implications in nonmetastatic cases have been a focus of investigation as well. Using mRNA expression of cytokeratin 19 (CK19) to identify CTCs, Stathopoulou et al. detected CTCs in the blood of 148 patients with operable breast cancer prior to initiation of adjuvant therapy. For stage I and II breast cancer, the presence of $CK19^+$, CTCs was an independent prognostic factor associated with early relapse ($p < 0.001$) and disease-related death ($p = 0.01$) during a median follow-up of 28 months [54]. Using the same approach, Xenedis et al. analyzed 167 node-negative breast cancer patients before the initiation of therapy and found 21.6% of the patients had $CK19^+$ CTCs, which were associated with early relapse ($p < 0.001$) and disease-related death ($p < 0.008$). Multivariate analysis further confirmed the detection of $CK19^+$ CTCs in the blood of node-negative patients is an independent prognostic factor [55].

The largest study on CTCs conducted in an adjuvant setting was the SUCCESS study, which included 2026 patients (median follow-up of 35 months) and collected CTCs after surgery and chemotherapy. The presence of even one CTC before adjuvant systemic treatment was associated with poor disease-free survival and OS. Additionally, node-positive patients were found to have CTCs more frequently than node-negative patients. In a subgroup analysis, the presence of CTCs was not significantly associated with DFS in node-negative patients; however, in node-positive patients, CTC was proportionally associated with number of node involvement and poor prognosis (positive node number of 1–3; $p = 0.008$), 4–9; $p < 0.001$; ≥10; $p = 0.001$). Patients who had CTCs present both before and after systemic chemotherapy had the worst 3 years DFS of any group in this study. Multivariate analysis further confirmed that detection of CTCs prior to chemotherapy was an independent prognostic factor for DFS (HR: 2.11; 95% CI,1.49–2.99, $p < 0.0001$) and OS (HR: 2.18; 95% CI,1.32–3.59, $p = 0.002$) in early breast cancer patients [56]. Although the study provided valuable prognostic data, its clinical significance remains uncertain since it only provided a short follow-up time. Two separate studies have found the presence of one or more CTCs to be of prognostic significance in nonmetastatic, chemotherapy-naïve (HR: 4.62 for PFS; 95% CI, 1.79–11.9, p = 0.005; HR: 4.04 for OS; 95% CI, 1.28–12.8, $p = 0.011$; [57]) and surgery-naïve patients (HR: 2.72 for relapse-free survival (RFS); 95% CI,1.57–4.72, $p < 0.001$; HR: 2.29 for OS; 95% CI, 1.12–4.67, p = 0.02;[58]). Moreover, a meta-analysis of 49 studies ($n = 6825$ of both early breast cancer and MBC patients) showed that in early breast cancer patients, CTC count correlated with both shorter DFS (HR: 2.86; 95% CI, 2.19–3.75, $p < 0.001$) and OS (HR: 2.78; 95% CI, 2.22–3.48, $p < 0.001$) [51]. Similar to MBC patients, posttherapy CTC count was shown to be an independent prognostic factor in non-MBC patients. In a study of stage I–III node-negative breast cancer patients ($n = 175$) who had completed adjuvant chemotherapy, Ignatiadis et al. detected CTCs using a panel of three biomarkers (CK19, mammaglobin (MGB1), and HER2) using RT-PCR. The detection of all three markers was associated with shorter DFS (for $CK19^+$; HR: 2.967; 95% CI, 1.64–5.34, $p < 0.001$, for MGB1+; HR: 3.275; 95% CI, 1.58–6.76, $p = 0.001$, and for HER2+; HR: 2.869; 95% CI,1.63–5.02, $p < 0.001$) in univariate analysis [59]. While these studies suggest the independent prognostic significance of CTCs in non-MBC patients both before and after adjuvant chemotherapy, the data remains somewhat controversial.

Kuniyoshi et al. reported no correlation between PFS and the presence of CK19 or HER2 CTCs in non-MBC patients ($n = 167$) at baseline or the first two subsequent follow-ups during chemotherapy [60]. This data was further supported by the recently published results from the SUCCESS-A trial, a randomized, multicenter trial (EudraCT2005000490-21) that evaluated the prognostic value of CTCs in 1221 early-stage (94% of patients were stages I and II) breast cancer patients prior to adjuvant chemotherapy. Using a density gradient followed by labeling with the anticytokeratin antibody, the SUCCESS-A trial detected CTCs in only 20.6% of all patients, and univariate analyses demonstrated that the presence of one or more CTCs had no significant impact on DFS or OS over a median follow-up of 64 months [61]. The inconsistent results regarding the prognostic utility of CTC counts in non-MBC patients may be partially attributable to the use of different CTC detection methods. While studies using the

CellSearch® system have consistently reported CTCs as a significant independent prognostic marker in non-MBC patients, those using other methods (such as mRNA or cytokeratin-protein expression) yielded data to the contrary. These conflicting reports underscore the need for standardization of CTC-detection methodologies.

3.3. Subtype-dependent prognostic significance of CTCs

Breast cancer is a heterogeneous disease, and large-scale gene expression analysis of primary tumors has made it possible to stratify clinical cases into four intrinsic subtypes based on receptor expression—Luminal A, Luminal B, HER2+, and triple negative (TN). These subtypes are significantly associated with differences in clinical outcomes and define a patient's course of therapy. In a large retrospective study using CellSearch®, Giordano et al. addressed subtype-specific differences among CTCs in 517 MBC patients prior to first course of therapy. CTC counts were predictive of prognosis in Luminal and TN breast cancer subtypes but were less so in the HER2-positive subtype. In Luminal A patients, the median OS and PFS of those with ≥5 CTCs ($n = 292$) were significantly shorter than those with <5 CTCs (OS, 18.8 vs. 48.7 months; $p < 0.001$; and PFS, 5.9 vs. 7.1; $p = 0.004$). Within the TN subtype, patients with >5 CTCs ($n = 124$) had a median OS significantly shorter than patients with <5 CTCs (10.4 vs. 17.8 months respectively; $p = 0.001$); however, there was little difference in median PFS for these patients (PFS, 5.1 vs. 4.8, respectively; $p = 0.274$). By contrast, among HER2$^+$ patients, there was no significant association between CTC count and OS or PFS (median OS, 27.2 vs. 21.4 months; $p = 0.991$; median PFS 7.6 vs. 8.6; $p = 0.458$) [62]. Likewise, another retrospective study using CellSearch® found similar trends in the relationship between CTCs and subtype among MBC patients. Patients were stratified into groups based on their CTC count at baseline (0, 1–4, or ≥ 5 CTCs) and subtype. Similar to Giordano's findings, CTCs were predominately found in patients with Luminal-A/Luminal-B/HER2-negative subtypes. Moreover, patients of all subtypes, except HER2$^+$, with no CTCs detected in the blood had a better prognosis compared with those with 1–4 or >5 CTCs [63]. However, a large, multicenter study conducted in Germany found that CTC count at baseline was positively associated with shorter OS in all tumor subtypes, including HER2$^+$ patients [64]. Additionally, two recent reports have investigated the prognostic role of CTCs, specifically in TN subtype. A meta-analyses including 10 studies with a total of 642 metastatic and nonmetastatic TN breast cancer patients found the presence of CTCs, predicted aggressive disease progression (HR: 2.18; 95% CI, 1.59–2.99, $p = 0.010$) and reduced OS (HR: 2.02; 95% CI, 1.59–2.57, $p = 0.169$) [65]. Additionally, Karhade et al. evaluated CTCs at baseline in 113 stage I–III nonmetastatic TN patients and found that presence of ≥2 CTCs predicted shorter PFS (HR: 8.30; 95% CI, 2.61–26.37, $p < 0.001$) and OS (HR: 7.19; 95% CI, 1.98–26.06, $p < 0.0004$) [66].

In summary, the prevalence and clinical relevance of CTCs vary by breast cancer subtype. Currently, data indicates that the prevalence of CTCs is high among metastatic Luminal A as well as both metastatic and nonmetastatic TN breast cancers. However, data regarding the prognostic significance in HER2+ tumors remains inconclusive.

3.4. Prediction of therapy response by CTCs

Neoadjuvant therapy is increasingly popular among patients (e.g., TN, HER2+, or large tumor burden, etc) who would qualify for adjuvant chemotherapy. Several studies have explored

http://dx.doi.org/10.5772/66439

the clinical validity of CTCs in this setting, specifically the REMAGUS02, GeparQuattro, and BEVERLY-2 trials. Each of these studies enumerated CTCs before and after neoadjuvant therapy, yet produced contradictory findings. The REMAGUS02 trial found no correlation between the presence of CTCs and pathological complete response, tumor size, grade, or lymph node status. However, multivariate analysis revealed that patients without CTCs before and after neoadjuvant therapy had better distant metastasis-free survival (DMFS) (before; Relative Risk (RR): 2.4; 95% CI,0.9–6, $p = 0.06$), although no difference was noted in DMFS or OS after a median follow-up of 70 months [67]. On the other hand, the GeparQuattro trial failed to show any correlation between the presence of CTCs and, worse, DFS or OS [68]. The BEVERLY-2 study, however, showed that the presence of CTCs at baseline was an independent prognostic factor for poor DFS (HR: 4.75; 95% CI,1.56–14.50, $p = 0.006$) at 3 years of follow-up [69]. Another study compared CTC enumeration with CT scan results in MBC patients following therapy. CTCs were measured at baseline and 4 weeks following therapy, and CT scans were obtained at 9–12-week intervals to assess response to therapy using RECIST criteria. CTC counts were reviewed by a local and central laboratory, while two central radiologists reviewed the CT scans. Superior interreader agreement for CTCs was observed at 0.7% variability, and radiological responses showed 15.2% variability. Patients with <5 CTCs following 4 weeks of therapy who had stable or partial response on the CT scans demonstrated the best median OS of 26.9 months. After these results, however, it is still unclear whether the change in therapy course can be based on CTC detection following chemotherapy in MBC patients [70]. In 2014, the first interventional study based on postchemotherapy CTC detection was launched by the SWOG trial. The main goal of the S0500 SWOG study was to demonstrate an OS benefit in CTC-positive patients who were nonresponsive to therapy by switching them from first to second-line therapy. Patients who had >5 CTCs after 3 weeks of therapy were randomized to ARM 1 (continuation of same therapy) or to ARM 2 (switch to second-line therapy). Disappointingly, no difference in OS or DFS was observed in either arm. There are several ongoing interventional clinical trials that stratify patients based on CTC count for either aggressive chemotherapy or hormonal therapy [52]. Another trial is investigating the change of therapy based on CTC number at the third or subsequent lines of therapy for MBC [71]. In conclusion, the present data is insufficient to recommend the use of CTC enumeration for risk stratification and treatment response. Also, early changes in therapy based on CTC enumeration in MBC patients are not recommended at this time, although ongoing studies may yield more definitive results.

4. CTC heterogeneity

A number of studies have addressed the heterogeneous nature of CTCs with the ultimate goal of understanding what molecular signature is required for successful metastasis. The two main phenomena that orchestrate tumor heterogeneity and metastases are cancer stem cells (CSC) and EMT. CSCs are pluripotent, highly resistant to conventional chemotherapy [72–74] and contribute to the heterogeneous nature of the tumor as well as its ability for self-renewal and metastasis [75]. Notably, not all tumor cells are capable of distant organ metastasis; CSCs seem to have such metastatic potential [76]. Likewise, the process of EMT plays an essential role in invasion and metastasis. At the primary tumor site, a subpopulation of cells loses their epithelial characteristics (such as cell polarity or adhesion to the matrix and other cells) and acquires mesenchymal features (including the ability to invade the basement membrane and surrounding tissues), which in turn supports eventual intravasation into the circulation, the first step in the metastatic cascade [77]. These two processes are interconnected, adding further complexity to our understanding of metastasis. Recent studies have shown a direct link between EMT and CSCs in breast cancer, suggesting that EMT generates cancer cells with stem cell-like traits. Mani et al. showed that the induction of EMT in immortalized human mammary epithelial cells results in *de novo* expression of stem cell markers and the acquisition of functional stem cell properties, including the ability to form mammospheres [78–80]. Both CSC and EMT markers have been identified in CTCs, and while a CTC count itself is an independent prognostic marker, the addition of functional marker expression among CTCs will likely strengthen their prognostic value. This section specifically focuses on CTC heterogeneity of CSC and EMT nature.

4.1. Stem-like CTCs

CSCs are derived both intrinsically and extrinsically [72–74]; although the mechanism for extrinsic acquisition of CSC properties is not clearly understood, several lines of evidence suggest a close link to EMT [81–84]. CSCs are pluripotent and highly resistant to conventional chemotherapy [72–74]. Currently, there is no therapeutics effective in eradicating CSCs [85]; therefore, CTCs with CSC properties are postulated to be an important subset. In 2010, Theodoropoulos et al. investigated whether bulk CTCs contain a subset of cells with CSC characteristics. The protein expression of CSC markers CD44, CD24, and ALDH1 was assessed in cytokeratin+ CTCs isolated from MBC patients using immunofluorescence microscopy. In approximately 1500 CTCs identified from 20 MBC patients, 35.2% had the stem-like phenotype ($CD44^{+}/CD24^{-/low}$), whereas 17.7% of the CTCs were $ALDH1^{-high}/CD24^{-/low}$ [86]. This is in concordance with another study that found 19% of $EpCAM^{+}/Cytokeratin^{+}$ CTCs are also $CD44^{+}/CD24^{-/low}$ cells [87]. Further support came from an experimental model that demonstrated a stem-like $CD44^{+}$ CTC subset isolated from MBC patient blood having metastatic potential. Interestingly, the six recipient NSG, immunocompromised mice in this study developed multiple bone, lung, and liver metastases within 6–12 months following injection of bulk CTCs into their bone marrow, confirming the existence of metastatic-initiating cells (MICs) among CTCs. To determine the phenotype of the MIC-CTC subpopulation, flow cytometry analyses showed that all analyzed CTCs expressed CD44 and CD47. CD47 has been implicated in facilitating cancer cell evasion of the innate immune system through its inhibitory role in phagocytosis. Around 33% of $CD44^{+}/CD47^{+}$ CTCs express the hepatocyte growth factor (HGF) receptor MET, a tyrosine kinase involved in the activation of the migration and putative invasion program in several cancers. To functionally assess the presence of MICs in this cell population, $CD44^{+}/CD47^{+}/MET^{+/-}$ CTCs were isolated by FACS and directly transplanted into the femoral medullar cavity of an NSG recipient mouse. After 8 months, bone metastasis developed in the mouse, demonstrating that $CD44^{+}CD47^{+}MET^{+/-}$ CTCs contain functional MICs. These markers were further examined in four patients before and after disease progression. An increased frequency of CTCs with $CD44^{+}/CD47^{+}/MET^{+}$ was detected after disease progression (fold increase of 1.78; $p = 0.019$). Additionally, in a total of eight patients, those with >12 $CD44^+/CD47^+/MET^+$ (triple positive) CTCs per 7.5 ml of blood had significantly more metastasis sites than those with <12 triple positive CTCs (mean: 3.25 sites vs. 2.25 sites; $p = 0.03$), and the presence of $CD44^+/CD47^+/MET^+$ CTCs was associated with shorter OS (HR: 7.4; $p = 0.0246$) [88]. The association of CSC-CTCs with advanced disease was further supported by the work of Papadaki *et al.* who found that MBC patients have a higher percentage of $ALDH1^+$ CTCs than those with early breast cancer. $ALDH1^+$ CTCs were observed in 38.7% of CTCs from early-breast cancer patients compared to 83.5% from MBC patients [89]. Together, these data suggest that CTCs with CSC characteristics have more biological relevance for disease development, progression, and outcomes than bulk CTC data. However, the value of CSC-like CTCs in prognosis and therapy-response prediction requires further confirmation in a large prospective clinical study.

4.2. Mesenchymal CTCs

EMT contributes to the acquisition of invasiveness in cancer cells, and therefore it is believed that CTCs with mesenchymal features may contribute to metastasis. However, this question has not been extensively addressed due to the use of affinity-based CTC enrichment methods that rely on EpCAM and/or Cytokeratin markers, lacking mesenchymal cell surface marker selection. EMT is a gradual process that yields epithelial cells which have not gone through EMT, intermediate mesenchymal (cells that have partially completed EMT), and exclusively mesenchymal cells (ones that have completed EMT). Yu et al. characterized the EMT status of CTCs captured on the microfluidic herringbone chip with an antibody cocktail directed against EpCAM, EGFR, and HER2. These researchers established a quantifiable, dual-colorimetric RNA-in situ hybridization (ISH) assay to examine tumor cells for expression of seven pooled epithelial transcripts (Cytokeratin 5, 7, 8, 18, and 19, EpCAM, and Cadherin 1) and three mesenchymal transcripts (Fibronectin 1, Cadherin 2, and Serpin peptidase inhibitor/clade E [SERPINE1/PAI1]). Five categories of cells ranging from exclusively epithelial, intermediate (more epithelial, equal, and more mesenchymal), and exclusively mesenchymal were determined [90]. Similarly, a study by Polioudaki et al. used the ratio of Cytokeratin to Vimentin protein expression (measured by immunofluorescence) to study on a single cell basis the EMT status of 110 CTCs detected in 5 MBC patients. This study identified that 46% of CTCs were "epithelial," 5.4% were "mesenchymal," and 48.2% were "intermediate" [91]. The existence of CTCs across the EMT spectrum was further confirmed by another single cell level study. Using DEPArray to select viable CTCs from 56 MBC patients, Bulfoni et al. determined the EMT status of single CTCs by staining with an antibody cocktail that recognized both epithelial (EpCAM, E-Cad) and mesenchymal (CD44, CD146, and N-Cadherin) markers. This study also reported the presence of diverse CTC phenotypes based on their EMT statuses [92]. CTC heterogeneity was further investigated on a genetic level using single CTCs. Powell et al. were the first to perform microfluidic-based single cell transcriptional profiling of 87 cancer-associated and reference genes in CTCs. Their study found that CTCs are heterogeneous and can be separated into two major subgroups based on 31 highly expressed genes including mesenchymal and metastatic associated genes (*VIMENTIN, TGFß1, ZEB2, FOXC1, CXCR4, NPTN, S100A4, and S100A9*) [93].

Several studies have investigated the clinical relevance of CTCs based on their EMT status. Yu et al. reported the CTCs isolated from ER^+/PR^+ breast cancer patients were predominantly epithelial, whereas those from the TN and $HER2^+$ subtypes were predominantly mesenchymal in a sample of 41 MBC patients [90]. Similarly, Polioudaki et al. retrospectively analyzed 1000 CTCs isolated from 61 MBC patients at baseline using CellSearch® and investigated the correlation between the level of cytokeratin expression and tumor subtype. Interestingly, CTCs from TN patients showed a lower average cytokeratin expression level compared to those from the remaining patients (122 vs. 175; $p < 0.001$) [91]. Moreover, Kallergi et al. found that the proportion of CTCs coexpressing cytokeratins 7, 8, or 18 together with the mesenchymal marker Twist (measured by Immunofluorescence) is lower in patients with non-MBC than in patients with MBC (53% vs. 97%, respectively; $p < 0.001$). Similarly, the proportion of CTCs coexpressing cytokeratins and Vimentin was lower in patients with non-MBC than in those with MBC (56% vs. 74%; $p = 0.005$) [94]. Likewise, Papadaki et al. found that nuclear Twist localization was detected in the CTCs of 70.3% of MBC patients, whereas it was detected in only 32.3% of CTCs from early breast cancer patients [89]. Moreover, Markiewicz et al. found that CTCs isolated from lymph node-positive breast cancer patients are more frequently Vimentin and Snail mRNA expression positive compared to those from lymph node-negative patients [95]. Polioudaki et al. reported that 1-year OS of patients with high cytokeratin$^+$ CTCs was 73.3%, whereas 1-year OS declined by 46.2% in patients with low cytokeratin$^+$ CTCs ($p = 0.038$) [91].

4.3. CTC with CSC and EMT characteristics

Given the implications of both CSCs and EMT in metastasis, the existence of CTCs displaying both traits has been investigated. Aktas et al. tested the mRNA expression of three EMT markers (Twist1, Akt2, PI3Kα) and the CSC marker ALDH1 in CTCs from 39 MBC patients and found CTCs expressing at least one EMT marker, ALDH1, or both in 21 patients (81% of CTC-positive patients) [96]. The presence of CTCs coexpressing one of the EMT markers and ALDH1 was further confirmed by Raimondi et al. The mRNA expression of ALDH1 in bulk CTCs is correlated with the mRNA expression of Vimentin and Fibronectin ($p < 0.001$) [97]. Papadaki et al. further investigated the coexpression of ALDH1 and Twist in individual CTCs from both early and MBC patients and found that the prevalence of an $ALDH1^+/Twist^+$ subpopulation was significantly higher in MBC patients compared to those with early disease (76% vs. 15.4%, $p = 0.001$) [89]. Overall, these results indicate that the identification of a subpopulation of CTCs bearing mesenchymal properties, cancer stem cell characteristics, or both may help in discerning which patients are at higher risk for disease progression.

5. Summary

CTCs have received significant attention as a liquid biopsy to facilitate longitudinal disease monitoring. The current consensus based on large clinical studies is that CTC count is an independent prognostic marker in MBC, yet it is still controversial whether CTC count is predictive

http://dx.doi.org/10.5772/66439

of prognosis in non-MBC or could be used for monitoring of therapy response. Several clinical trials are currently ongoing to determine the utility of CTCs in making an early decision to change the course of therapy and spare toxicity. The isolation of CTCs has been a challenging task due to their rarity in the blood; however, a number of new isolation and detection strategies have emerged in the past 10 years, making CTC detection in relatively small amounts of blood feasible. The current challenge in this era is tackling the heterogeneous nature of CTCs and understanding which subpopulations drive metastasis. The count of CTCs with mesenchymal features was shown to be more sensitive in the prediction of prognosis than the number of bulk CTCs. Similarly, CTCs with both stem-like and mesenchymal features sensitively predicted prognosis. Currently, the detection of mesenchymal CTCs that have lost their epithelial markers requires laborious work necessitating either the detection of intracellular markers or mRNA expression. Therefore, discovery of a new CTC-specific functional surface marker that is relevant to metastasis would greatly advance the realistic clinical utility of CTCs. Additionally, in-depth understanding of CTC's heterogeneity utilizing single cell level analysis will improve our knowledge of hematogenous metastasis.

Abbreviations

AKT2	RAC-beta serine/threonine-protein kinase
ALDH1	Aldehyde dehydrogenase 1 family
AURKA	Aurora kinase A
BEVERLY-2	Single-arm phase II trial assessed the efficacy and safety of combining neoadjuvant chemotherapy with bevacizumab and trastuzumab for the treatment of HER2-positive breast cancer
CAM	Cell Adhesion Matrix
CCD	Charge-Coupled Devices
CD24	Signal transducer CD24 (Modulates B-cell activation responses)
CD44	CD44 antigen (receptor for hyaluronic acid)
CD45	Receptor-type tyrosine-protein phosphatase C
CD47	Leukocyte surface antigen CD47
CK19	Cytokeratin 19
CSC	Cancer Stem Cells
CT	Computerized tomography
CTCs	Circulating Tumor Cells
CXCR4	C-X-C chemokine receptor type 4

DAPI	4′,6-Diamidino-2-phenylindole
DEP	DielEctroPhoretic
DFS	Disease-Free Survival
DNA	Deoxyribonucleic acid
EGFR	Epithelial Growth Factor Receptor
EMT	Epithelial Mesenchymal Transition
EpCAM	Epithelial cell adhesion molecule
EPISPOT	EPithelial ImmunoSPOT
ER	Estrogen receptor
ERBB2	Receptor tyrosine-protein kinase erbB-2 (Gene)
ERBB3	Receptor tyrosine-protein kinase erbB-3 (Gene)
ERCC1	DNA excision repair protein ERCC-1
FDA	Food and Drug Administration
FOXC1	Forkhead box protein C1
HB	Heringbone
HER2	Receptor tyrosine-protein kinase erbB-2 (protein)
HGF	Hepatocyte growth factor
HL	Hematopoietic lineage
HR	Hazard ratio
ISET	Isolation by size of epithelial tumor cells test
ISH	In situ hybridization
MBC	Metastatic breast cancer
MET	The hepatocyte growth factor receptor
MGB1	Mammaglobin
MICs	Metastatic-initiating cells
mRNA	Messenger ribonucleic acid
MUC1	Mucin-1
NPTN	Neuroplastin
NSG	NOD Scid Gamma
OS	Overall Survival

PBS	Phosphate-Buffered Saline
PFS	Progression-Free Survival
PIK3CA	Phosphatidylinositol 4,5-bisphosphate 3-kinase catalytic subunit alpha isoform
PR	Progesterone receptor
REMAGUS02	Phase II clinical study: Standard Neoadjuvant Chemotherapy Versus Genomic Driven Chemotherapy in Patients With Breast Cancer
RNA	Ribonucleic acid
RR	Relative risk
RT-PCR	Reverse transcription polymerase chain reaction
S0500 SWOG	Treatment decision making based on blood levels of tumor cells in women with metastatic breast cancer receiving chemotherapy
S100A4	Gene encodes Protein S100-A4
S100A9	Gene encodes Protein S100-A9
SERPINE1/PAI1	Plasminogen activator inhibitor 1
SIM	Single-cell isolation microfluidic
SUCCESS	Simultaneous Study of Gemcitabine-Docetaxel Combination adjuvant treatment
TGFβ1	Transforming growth factor beta-1
TN	Triple negative
ZEB2	Zinc finger E-box-binding homeobox 2

Author details

Mohamed Kamal[1], Wajeeha Razaq[2], Macall Leslie[1], Smita Adhikari[1] and Takemi Tanaka[1,3*]

*Address all correspondence to: takemi-tanaka@ouhsc.edu

1 Stephenson Cancer Centre, Oklahoma University Health Science Center, OK, USA

2 Department of Hematology and Oncology, Stephenson Cancer Centre, School of Medicine, OK, USA

3 Department of Pathology, Stephenson Cancer Centre, School of Medicine, Oklahoma University Health Science Center, OK, USA

References

[1] Ashworth TR. A case of cancer in which cells similar to those in the tumors were seen in the blood after death. Medical Journal of Australia. 1869;14:146–9.

[2] Jonescu P. Über das Vorkommen von Geschwulstzellen im strömenden Blut von Tieren mit Impftumoren. Z Krebsforsch. 1931;33:264.

[3] Marcus H. Krebszellen im strömenden Blut. Z Krebsforsch. 1919;16.

[4] Alexander RF, Spriggs AI. The differential diagnosis of tumour cells in circulating blood. Journal of Clinical Pathology. 1960;13:414s24.

[5] Zeidman I. The fate of circulating tumor cells. I Passage of cells through capillaries. 1961;21(1):38–9.

[6] Romsdahl MD, Chu EW, Hume R, Smith RR. The time of metastasis and release of circulating tumor cells as determined in an experimental system. Cancer. 1961;14(4):883–8.

[7] Cristofanilli M, Budd GT, Ellis MJ, Stopeck A, Matera J, Miller MC. Circulating tumor cells, disease progression, and survival in metastatic breast cancer. The New England Journal of Medicine. 2004;351.

[8] Nguyen DX, Bos PD, Massague J. Metastasis: from dissemination to organ-specific colonization. Nature Reviews Cancer. 2009;9(4):274–84.

[9] Joosse SA, Gorges TM, Pantel K. Biology, detection, and clinical implications of circulating tumor cells. EMBO Molecular Medicine. 2015;7.

[10] Miller MC, Doyle GV, Terstappen LW. Significance of circulating tumor cells detected by the CellSearch system in patients with metastatic breast colorectal and prostate cancer. Journal of Oncology. 2010;2010:617421.

[11] Alix-Panabieres C, Schwarzenbach H, Pantel K. Circulating tumor cells and circulating tumor DNA. Annual Review of Medicine. 2012;63:199–215.

[12] Hu XC, Chow LW. Detection of circulating breast cancer cells with multiple-marker RT-PCR assay. Anticancer Research. 2001;21(1A):421–4.

[13] Hawes D, Neville AM, Cote RJ. Occult metastasis. Biomedicine & Pharmacotherapy = Biomedecine & Pharmacotherapie. 2001;55(4):229–42.

[14] Witzig TE, Bossy B, Kimlinger T, Roche PC, Ingle JN, Grant C, et al. Detection of circulating cytokeratin-positive cells in the blood of breast cancer patients using immunomagnetic enrichment and digital microscopy. Clinical Cancer Research. 2002;8(5):1085–91.

[15] Bednarz-Knoll N, Alix-Panabieres C, Pantel K. Plasticity of disseminating cancer cells in patients with epithelial malignancies. Cancer Metastasis Reviews. 2012;31(3–4):673–87.

[16] Mostert B, Kraan J, Sieuwerts AM, van der Spoel P, Bolt-de Vries J, Prager-van der Smissen WJ, et al. CD49f-based selection of circulating tumor cells (CTCs) improves detection across breast cancer subtypes. Cancer Letters. 2012;319(1):49–55.

[17] Kagan MH, Bendele MS, Mayes BS, Silvia BS, Repollet BS, Doyle DDS, Allard J, Tu N, Bui T, Russell T, Rao C, Hermann BS, Rutner MS, Terstappen LWMM. A sample preparation and analysis system for identification of circulating tumor cells. Journal of Clinical Ligand Assay. 2002;25:104 –10.

[18] Allard WJ, Matera J, Miller MC, Repollet M, Connelly MC, Rao C, et al. Tumor cells circulate in the peripheral blood of all major carcinomas but not in healthy subjects or patients with nonmalignant diseases. Clinical Cancer Research. 2004;10(20):6897–904.

[19] Farace F, Massard C, Vimond N, Drusch F, Jacques N, Billiot F, et al. A direct comparison of CellSearch and ISET for circulating tumour-cell detection in patients with metastatic carcinomas. British Journal of Cancer. 2011;105(6):847–53.

[20] Demel U, Tilz GP, Foeldes-Papp Z, Gutierrez B, Albert WH, Bocher O. Detection of tumour cells in the peripheral blood of patients with breast cancer. Development of a new sensitive and specific immunomolecular assay. Journal of Experimental & Clinical Cancer Research: CR. 2004;23(3):465–8.

[21] Zieglschmid V, Hollmann C, Gutierrez B, Albert W, Strothoff D, Gross E, et al. Combination of immunomagnetic enrichment with multiplex RT-PCR analysis for the detection of disseminated tumor cells. Anticancer Research. 2005;25(3A):1803–10.

[22] Lankiewicz S, Rivero BG, Bocher O. Quantitative real-time RT-PCR of disseminated tumor cells in combination with immunomagnetic cell enrichment. Molecular Biotechnology. 2006;34(1):15–27.

[23] Bredemeier M, Edimiris P, Tewes M, Mach P, Aktas B, Schellbach D, et al. Establishment of a multimarker qPCR panel for the molecular characterization of circulating tumor cells in blood samples of metastatic breast cancer patients during the course of palliative treatment. Oncotarget. 2016.

[24] Andreopoulou E, Yang LY, Rangel KM, Reuben JM, Hsu L, Krishnamurthy S, et al. Comparison of assay methods for detection of circulating tumor cells in metastatic breast cancer: AdnaGen AdnaTest BreastCancer Select/Detect versus Veridex CellSearch system. International Journal of Cancer. 2012;130(7):1590–7.

[25] Sequist LV, Nagrath S, Toner M, Haber DA, Lynch TJ. The CTC-Chip: an exciting new tool to detect circulating tumor cells in lung cancer patients. Journal of Thoracic Oncology. 2009;4(3):281–3.

[26] Nagrath S, Sequist LV, Maheswaran S, Bell DW, Irimia D, Ulkus L, et al. Isolation of rare circulating tumour cells in cancer patients by microchip technology. Nature. 2007;450(7173):1235–9.

[27] Ameri K, Luong R, Zhang H, Powell AA, Montgomery KD, Espinosa I, et al. Circulating tumour cells demonstrate an altered response to hypoxia and an aggressive phenotype. British Journal of Cancer. 2010;102(3):561–9.

[28] Talasaz AH, Powell AA, Huber DE, Berbee JG, Roh KH, Yu W, et al. Isolating highly enriched populations of circulating epithelial cells and other rare cells from blood using a magnetic sweeper device. Proceedings of the National Academy of Sciences of the United States of America. 2009;106(10):3970–5.

[29] Lu J, Fan T, Zhao Q, Zeng W, Zaslavsky E, Chen JJ, et al. Isolation of circulating epithelial and tumor progenitor cells with an invasive phenotype from breast cancer patients. International Journal of Cancer. 2010;126(3):669–83.

[30] den Toonder J. Circulating tumor cells: the Grand Challenge. Lab on a Chip. 2011;11(3):375–7.

[31] Kim MS, Sim TS, Kim YJ, Kim SS, Jeong H, Park J-M, et al. SSA-MOA: a novel CTC isolation platform using selective size amplification (SSA) and a multi-obstacle architecture (MOA) filter. Lab on a Chip. 2012;12(16):2874–80.

[32] Coumans FAW, van Dalum G, Beck M, Terstappen LWMM. Filter characteristics influencing circulating tumor cell enrichment from whole blood. PloS One. 2013;8(4):e61770.

[33] Paterlini-Brechot P, Benali NL. Circulating tumor cells (CTC) detection: Clinical impact and future directions. Cancer Letters. 2007;253(2):180–204.

[34] Moon H-S, Kwon K, Kim S-I, Han H, Sohn J, Lee S, et al. Continuous separation of breast cancer cells from blood samples using multi-orifice flow fractionation (MOFF) and dielectrophoresis (DEP). Lab on a Chip. 2011;11(6):1118–25.

[35] Rostagno P, Moll JL, Bisconte JC, Caldani C. Detection of rare circulating breast cancer cells by filtration cytometry and identification by DNA content: sensitivity in an experimental model. Anticancer Research. 1997;17(4A):2481–5.

[36] Vona G, Sabile A, Louha M, Sitruk V, Romana S, Schutze K, et al. Isolation by size of epithelial tumor cells : a new method for the immunomorphological and molecular characterization of circulatingtumor cells. The American Journal of Pathology. 2000;156(1):57–63.

[37] Dong X, Alpaugh KR, Cristofanilli M. Circulating tumor cells (CTCs) in breast cancer: a diagnostic tool for prognosis and molecular analysis. Chinese Journal of Cancer Research. 2012;24(4):388–98.

[38] Hofman VJ, Ilie MI, Bonnetaud C, Selva E, Long E, Molina T, et al. Cytopathologic detection of circulating tumor cells using the isolation by size of epithelial tumor cell method: promises and pitfalls. American Journal of Clinical Pathology. 2011;135(1):146–56.

[39] Pinzani P, Salvadori B, Simi L, Bianchi S, Distante V, Cataliotti L, et al. Isolation by size of epithelial tumor cells in peripheral blood of patients with breast cancer: correlation with real-time reverse transcriptase-polymerase chain reaction results and feasibility of molecular analysis by laser microdissection. Human Pathology. 2006;37(6):711–8.

[40] De Giorgi V, Pinzani P, Salvianti F, Panelos J, Paglierani M, Janowska A, et al. Application of a filtration- and isolation-by-size technique for the detection of circulating tumor cells in cutaneous melanoma. The Journal of Investigative Dermatology. 2010;130(10):2440–7.

[41] Hofman V, Ilie MI, Long E, Selva E, Bonnetaud C, Molina T, et al. Detection of circulating tumor cells as a prognostic factor in patients undergoing radical surgery for non-small-cell lung carcinoma: comparison of the efficacy of the CellSearch Assay and the isolation by size of epithelial tumor cell method. International Journal of Cancer. 2011;129(7):1651–60.

[42] Khoja L, Backen A, Sloane R, Menasce L, Ryder D, Krebs M, et al. A pilot study to explore circulating tumour cells in pancreatic cancer as a novel biomarker. British Journal of Cancer. 2012;106(3):508–16.

[43] Balic M, Dandachi N, Hofmann G, Samonigg H, Loibner H, Obwaller A, et al. Comparison of two methods for enumerating circulating tumor cells in carcinoma patients. Cytometry Part B, Clinical Cytometry. 2005;68(1):25–30.

[44] Konigsberg R, Obermayr E, Bises G, Pfeiler G, Gneist M, Wrba F. Detection of EpCAM positive and negative circulating tumor cells in metastatic breast cancer patients. Acta Oncologica. 2011;50.

[45] Gertler R, Rosenberg R, Fuehrer K, Dahm M, Nekarda H, Siewert JR. Detection of circulating tumor cells in blood using an optimized density gradient centrifugation. Recent Results in Cancer Research. 2003;162:149–55.

[46] The DEPArray™ System http://www.siliconbiosystems.com/deparray-system.

[47] Nakamura S, Yagata H, Ohno S, Yamaguchi H, Iwata H, Tsunoda N, et al. Multi-center study evaluating circulating tumor cells as a surrogate for response to treatment and overall survival in metastatic breast cancer. Breast Cancer. 2010;17(3):199–204.

[48] Zhang L, Riethdorf S, Wu G, Wang T, Yang K, Peng G. Meta-analysis of the prognostic value of circulating tumor cells in breast cancer. Clinical Cancer Research. 2012;18.

[49] Bidard FC, Peeters DJ, Fehm T, Nole F, Gisbert-Criado R, Mavroudis D. Clinical validity of circulating tumour cells in patients with metastatic breast cancer: a pooled analysis of individual patient data. Lancet Oncology. 2014;15.

[50] Lv Q, Gong L, Zhang T, Ye J, Chai L, Ni C, et al. Prognostic value of circulating tumor cells in metastatic breast cancer: a systemic review and meta-analysis. Clinical and Translational Oncology. 2015;18(3):322–30.

[51] Zhang L, Riethdorf S, Wu G, Wang T, Yang K, Peng G, et al. Meta-analysis of the prognostic value of circulating tumor cells in breast cancer. Clinical Cancer Research. 2012;18.

[52] Smerage JB, Barlow WE, Hortobagyi GN, Winer EP, Leyland-Jones B, Srkalovic G. Circulating tumor cells and response to chemotherapy in metastatic breast cancer: SWOG S0500. Journal of Clinical Oncology. 2014;32.

[53] Cristofanilli M, Broglio KR, Guarneri V, Jackson S, Fritsche HA, Islam R, et al. Circulating tumor cells in metastatic breast cancer: biologic staging beyond tumor burden. Clinical Breast Cancer. 2007;7(6):471–9.

[54] Stathopoulou A, Vlachonikolis I, Mavroudis D, Perraki M, Kouroussis C, Apostolaki S. Molecular detection of cytokeratin-19-positive cells in the peripheral blood of patients with operable breast cancer: evaluation of their prognostic significance. Journal of Clinical Oncology. 2002;20.

[55] Xenidis N, Perraki M, Kafousi M, Apostolaki S, Bolonaki I, Stathopoulou A, et al. Predictive and prognostic value of peripheral blood cytokeratin-19 mRNA-positive cells

detected by real-time polymerase chain reaction in node-negative breast cancer patients. Journal of Clinical Oncology. 2006;24(23):3756–62.

[56] Rack B, Schindlbeck C, Juckstock J, Andergassen U, Hepp P, Zwingers T, et al. Circulating tumor cells predict survival in early average-to-high risk breast cancer patients. Journal of the National Cancer Institute. 2014;106(5).

[57] Lucci A, Hall CS, Lodhi AK, Bhattacharyya A, Anderson AE, Xiao L, et al. Circulating tumour cells in non-metastatic breast cancer: a prospective study. Lancet Oncology. 2012;13.

[58] Hall C, Valad L, Lucci A. Circulating tumor cells in breast cancer patients. Critical Reviews in Oncogenesis. 2016;21(1-2):125–39.

[59] Ignatiadis M, Kallergi G, Ntoulia M, Perraki M, Apostolaki S, Kafousi M. Prognostic value of the molecular detection of circulating tumor cells using a multimarker reverse transcription-PCR assay for cytokeratin 19, mammaglobin A, and HER2 in early breast cancer. Clinical Cancer Research. 2008;14.

[60] Kuniyoshi RK, Gehrke Fde S, Alves BC, Vilas-Boas V, Colo AE, Sousa N, et al. Gene profiling and circulating tumor cells as biomarker to prognostic of patients with locoregional breast cancer. Tumour Biology. 2015;36(10):8075–83.

[61] Jueckstock J, Rack B, Friedl TW, Scholz C, Steidl J, Trapp E, et al. Detection of circulating tumor cells using manually performed immunocytochemistry (MICC) does not correlate with outcome in patients with early breast cancer—results of the German SUCCESS-A-trial. BMC Cancer. 2016;16:401.

[62] Giordano A, Giuliano M, Laurentiis M, Arpino G, Jackson S, Handy BC. Circulating tumor cells in immunohistochemical subtypes of metastatic breast cancer: lack of prediction in HER2-positive disease treated with targeted therapy. Annals of Oncology : Official Journal of the European Society for Medical Oncology/ESMO. 2012;23.

[63] Munzone E, Botteri E, Sandri MT, Esposito A, Adamoli L, Zorzino L, et al. Prognostic value of circulating tumor cells according to immunohistochemically defined molecular subtypes in advanced breast cancer. Clinical Breast Cancer. 2012;12(5):340–6.

[64] Wallwiener M, Hartkopf AD, Baccelli I, Riethdorf S, Schott S, Pantel K. The prognostic impact of circulating tumor cells in subtypes of metastatic breast cancer. Breast Cancer Research and Treatment. 2013;137.

[65] Lu YJ, Wang P, Wang X, Peng J, Zhu YW, Shen N. The significant prognostic value of circulating tumor cells in triple-negative breast cancer: a meta-analysis. Oncotarget. 2016; 7(24): 37361–9.

[66] Karhade M, Hall C, Mishra P, Anderson A, Kuerer H, Bedrosian I, et al. Circulating tumor cells in non-metastatic triple-negative breast cancer. Breast Cancer Research and Treatment. 2014;147(2):325–33.

[67] Bidard FC, Belin L, Delaloge S, Lerebours F, Ngo C, Reyal F, et al. Time-dependent prognostic impact of circulating tumor cells detection in non-metastatic breast cancer: 70-month analysis of the REMAGUS02 study. International Journal of Breast Cancer. 2013;2013:130470.

[68] Riethdorf S, Müller V, Zhang L, Rau T, Loibl S, Komor M, et al. Detection and HER2 expression of circulating tumor cells: prospective monitoring in breast cancer patients treated in the neoadjuvant GeparQuattro Trial. Clinical Cancer Research. 2010;16(9):2634–45.

[69] Pierga JY, Petit T, Levy C, Ferrero JM, Campone M, Gligorov J, et al. Pathological response and circulating tumor cell count identifies treated HER2+ inflammatory breast cancer patients with excellent prognosis: BEVERLY-2 survival data. Clinical Cancer Research. 2015;21(6):1298–304.

[70] Budd GT, Cristofanilli M, Ellis MJ, Stopeck A, Borden E, Miller MC, et al. Circulating tumor cells versus imaging—predicting overall survival in metastatic breast cancer. Clinical Cancer Research. 2006;12(21):6403–9.

[71] Bidard F-C, Asselain B, Baffert S, Brain E, Campone M, Delaloge S, et al. Abstract OT3-4-05: use of early CIRculating tumor CElls count changes to guide the use of chemotherapy in advanced metastatic breast cancer patients: the CirCe01 randomized trial. Cancer Research. 2012;72(24 Supplement):OT3-4-05-OT3-4-.

[72] Nguyen LV, Vanner R, Dirks P, Eaves CJ. Cancer stem cells: an evolving concept. Nature Reviews Cancer. 2012;12(2):133–43.

[73] Liu S, Cong Y, Wang D, Sun Y, Deng L, Liu Y, et al. Breast cancer stem cells transition between epithelial and mesenchymal states reflective of their normal counterparts. Stem Cell Reports. 2014;2(1):78–91.

[74] Dean M, Fojo T, Bates S. Tumour stem cells and drug resistance. Nature Reviews Cancer. 2005;5(4):275–84.

[75] Pece S, Tosoni D, Confalonieri S, Mazzarol G, Vecchi M, Ronzoni S, et al. Biological and molecular heterogeneity of breast cancers correlates with their cancer stem cell content. Cell. 2010;140(1):62–73.

[76] Idowu MO, Kmieciak M, Dumur C, Burton RS, Grimes MM, Powers CN, et al. CD44(+)/CD24(-/low) cancer stem/progenitor cells are more abundant in triple-negative invasive breast carcinoma phenotype and are associated with poor outcome. Human Pathology. 2012;43(3):364–73.

[77] Thiery JP. Epithelial-mesenchymal transitions in development and pathologies. Current Opinion in Cell Biology. 2003;15(6):740–6.

[78] Mani SA, Guo W, Liao MJ, Eaton EN, Ayyanan A, Zhou AY, et al. The epithelial-mesenchymal transition generates cells with properties of stem cells. Cell. 2008;133.

[79] Shipitsin M, Campbell LL, Argani P, Weremowicz S, Bloushtain-Qimron N, Yao J, et al. Molecular definition of breast tumor heterogeneity. Cancer Cell. 2007;11(3):259–73.

[80] Morel AP, Lievre M, Thomas C, Hinkal G, Ansieau S, Puisieux A. Generation of breast cancer stem cells through epithelial-mesenchymal transition. PLoS One. 2008;3(8):e2888.

[81] Yilmaz M, Christofori G. EMT, the cytoskeleton, and cancer cell invasion. Cancer Metastasis Reviews. 2009;28(1–2):15–33.

[82] Tsai JH, Yang J. Epithelial-mesenchymal plasticity in carcinoma metastasis. Genes & Development. 2013;27(20):2192–206.

[83] Puisieux A, Brabletz T, Caramel J. Oncogenic roles of EMT-inducing transcription factors. Nature Cell Biology. 2014;16(6):488–94.

[84] Kalluri R. EMT: when epithelial cells decide to become mesenchymal-like cells. Journal of Clinical Investigation. 2009;119(6):1417–9.

[85] Kano Y, Konno M, Kawamoto K, Tamari K, Hayashi K, Fukusumi T, et al. Novel drug discovery system for cancer stem cells in human squamous cell carcinoma of the esophagus. Oncology Reports. 2013.

[86] Theodoropoulos PA, Polioudaki H, Agelaki S, Kallergi G, Saridaki Z, Mavroudis D. Circulating tumor cells with a putative stem cell phenotype in peripheral blood of patients with breast cancer. Cancer Letters. 2010;288.

[87] Wang J, Cao MG, You CZ, Wang CL, Liu SL, Kai C, et al. A preliminary investigation of the relationship between circulating tumor cells and cancer stem cells in patients with breast cancer. Cellular and Molecular Biology. 2012;58 Suppl:OL1641–5.

[88] Baccelli I, Schneeweiss A, Riethdorf S, Stenzinger A, Schillert A, Vogel V. Identification of a population of blood circulating tumor cells from breast cancer patients that initiates metastasis in a xenograft assay. Nature Biotechnology. 2013;31.

[89] Papadaki MA, Kallergi G, Zafeiriou Z, Manouras L, Theodoropoulos PA, Mavroudis D, et al. Co-expression of putative stemness and epithelial-to-mesenchymal transition markers on single circulating tumour cells from patients with early and metastatic breast cancer. BMC Cancer. 2014;14:651.

[90] Yu M, Bardia A, Wittner BS, Stott SL, Smas ME, Ting DT. Circulating breast tumor cells exhibit dynamic changes in epithelial and mesenchymal composition. Science. 2013;339.

[91] Polioudaki H, Agelaki S, Chiotaki R, Politaki E, Mavroudis D, Matikas A, et al. Variable expression levels of keratin and vimentin reveal differential EMT status of circulating tumor cells and correlation with clinical characteristics and outcome of patients with metastatic breast cancer. BMC Cancer. 2015;15(1):1–10.

[92] Bulfoni M, Gerratana L, Del Ben F, Marzinotto S, Sorrentino M, Turetta M, et al. In patients with metastatic breast cancer the identification of circulating tumor cells in epithelial-to-mesenchymal transition is associated with a poor prognosis. Breast Cancer Research. 2016;18(1):1–15.

[93] Powell AA, Talasaz AH, Zhang H, Coram MA, Reddy A, Deng G, et al. Single cell profiling of circulating tumor cells: transcriptional heterogeneity and diversity from breast cancer cell lines. PLoS One. 2012;7(5):e33788.

[94] Kallergi G, Papadaki MA, Politaki E, Mavroudis D, Georgoulias V, Agelaki S. Epithelial to mesenchymal transition markers expressed in circulating tumour cells of early and metastatic breast cancer patients. Breast Cancer Research. 2011;13(3):R59.

[95] Markiewicz A, Ksiazkiewicz M, Welnicka-Jaskiewicz M, Seroczynska B, Skokowski J, Szade J, et al. Mesenchymal phenotype of CTC-enriched blood fraction and lymph node metastasis formation potential. PLoS One. 2014;9(4):e93901.

[96] Aktas B, Tewes M, Fehm T, Hauch S, Kimmig R, Kasimir-Bauer S. Stem cell and epithelial-mesenchymal transition markers are frequently overexpressed in circulating tumor cells of metastatic breast cancer patients. Breast Cancer Research. 2009;11.

[97] Raimondi C, Gradilone A, Naso G, Vincenzi B, Petracca A, Nicolazzo C. Epithelial-mesenchymal transition and stemness features in circulating tumor cells from breast cancer patients. Breast Cancer Research and Treatment. 2011;130.

[98] Stott SL, Hsu C-H, Tsukrov DI, Yu M, Miyamoto DT, Waltman BA, et al. Isolation of circulating tumor cells using a microvortex-generating herringbone-chip. Proceedings of the National Academy of Sciences. 2010;107(43):18392–7.

[99] Kim J, Cho H, Han SI, Han KH. Single-cell isolation of circulating tumor cells from whole blood by lateral magnetophoretic microseparation and microfluidic dispensing. Analytical Chemistry. 2016;88(9):4857–63.

[100] Desitter I, Guerrouahen BS, Benali-Furet N, Wechsler J, Janne PA, Kuang Y, et al. A new device for rapid isolation by size and characterization of rare circulating tumor cells. Anticancer Research. 2011;31(2):427–41.

[101] Alix-Panabieres C, Vendrell JP, Pelle O, Rebillard X, Riethdorf S, Muller V, et al. Detection and characterization of putative metastatic precursor cells in cancer patients. Clinical Chemistry. 2007;53(3):537–9.

Chapter 7

DNA Hypermethylation in Breast Cancer

Le Huyen Ai Thuy, Lao Duc Thuan and
Truong Kim Phuong

Additional information is available at the end of the chapter

http://dx.doi.org/10.5772/66900

Abstract

Cancer development is a complex process with multiple steps. Many factors, including radiation, chemicals, viruses, genetic and epigenetic changes, lead to abnormal proliferation of a single cell, which results in the outgrowth of a population of clonal-derived tumour cells. It has established that DNA hypermethylation, an epigenetic mechanism that occurred by the addition of a methyl group at 5′ position of the pyrimidine ring of cytosine residues at CpG islands through the action of DNA methyltransferase enzymes, has been considered as the cause of human tumorigenesis, including breast cancer development. Moreover, DNA hypermethylation holds a promising application as a potential biomarker for the early detection, prognosis and prediction of drug sensitivity in cancer. Therefore, this chapter focuses on the description and exemplification of the DNA hypermethylation changes, particularly, highlight the DNA hypermethylation as a potential biomarker applied in predictive, diagnostic, prognostic and therapeutic monitoring of breast cancer.

Keywords: breast cancer, epigenetics, hypermethylation, tumour suppressor gene

1. Introduction

Epigenetics, which was first coined by Waddington in 1942, literally means as 'outside conventional genetics', refers to the heritable, reversible changes in gene expression that occur without alteration DNA sequence [1]. Epigenetic modifications are natural processes and essential for mammalian development and cell proliferation. These epigenetic changes could also be affected by many random factors or environmental influences. Disruption of epigenetic modification resulting in regulating patterns of gene expression is the feature of a number of severe human diseases, including malignant cellular transformation [2–4]. Three main epigenetic modification systems, including DNA methylation, histone covalent modification, and non-coding RNA modification, leading to associated-gene silencing, have been observed [5, 6]. This chapter aims to introduce the reader to the concept of DNA methylation, especially DNA hypermethylation, with examples of its involvement in human breast cancer.

2. DNA hypermethylation: a kind of epigenetic modification that plays a key role in silencing tumour suppressor genes

DNA methylation is one of the epigenetic mechanisms that is closely associated with normal cell development and a number of key processes including imprinting, X-chromosome inactivation, repression of repetitive element transcription, chromatin organization, etc. [7–9]. Aberrant methylation patterns are known to be presented in the genomes of cancer cells. Two patterns of aberrant methylation have been observed, including global hypomethylation along the genome and hypermethylation at the specific sites, namely the CpG islands (CGIs) within the promoter regions, according to the decreased and increased the level of methyl group modification, respectively [4, 8, 10–12]. Disordered DNA methylation contributes to a number of human diseases, including breast cancer. Increased level of genome-wide hypomethylation results in increased chromosomal instability and activation of regulatory DNA sequences, including transcription of oncogenes, retrotransposons as well as genes encoding proteins involved in malignant cell development. DNA methylation refers to a covalent modification of cytosine ring at the 5′ position of a CpG dinucleotide by adding a methyl group in the 5th carbon of the ring using S-adenosyl methionine as a methyl donor (**Figure 1**) [8, 12].

This methylation process is catalysed by DNA (cytosine-5) methyltransferases (DNMTs). In mammalian, DNMTs are a highly conversed family protein encompassing DNMT1, DNMT2, DNMT3A, DNMT3B and DNMT3L, which could be distinguished by their function [13–15] (**Figure 2**). DNMT1 was the first methyltransferase to be discovered [1], then DNMT3 was discovered and characterized. Regarding to DNMTs function, DNMT3A and DNMT3B perform de novo methylation by adding the methyl groups to unmethylated CpG, which is responsible for the establishment of new methylation pattern in genomic DNA, whereas DNMT1, which has a high preference for hemi-methylated DNA, maintains the existence of methylation patterns following DNA replication on the newly synthesized strand [3, 4, 13, 14, 16, 17]. DNMT3L (DNA (cytosine-5-)-methyltransferase 3-Like) has no catalytic activity, DNMT3L has been shown to act as a general stimulatory factor for *de novo* methylation and facilitate methylation of DNMT3A and DNMT3B [2, 18].

The term CpG refers to the base cytosine (C) linked by a phosphate bond to the base Guanine (G) in the DNA nucleotide sequence, which usually cluster together in 'CpG islands (CGIs)' and typically locate at or near the promoters and transcription sites of genes. The molecular mechanisms underlying CpG island hypermethylation in many human cancers, including breast cancer, have been explored. The hypermethylation of CGIs located at tumour suppressor genes can result in transcriptional silencing of genes through a number of mechanisms, including (i) DNA hypermethylation directly affects the RNA polymerase II and DNA interactions by inhibiting the binding of transcriptional factors on specific sequences, such as AP-2, c-Myc/Myn, E2F, NF-κB, etc. and (ii) hypermethylated DNA recruits methyl-CpG binding proteins (MeCP1 and MeCP2), and methyl-CpG binding domain protein (MBD1, MBD2, MBD3 and MBD4) [4].

http://dx.doi.org/10.5772/66900

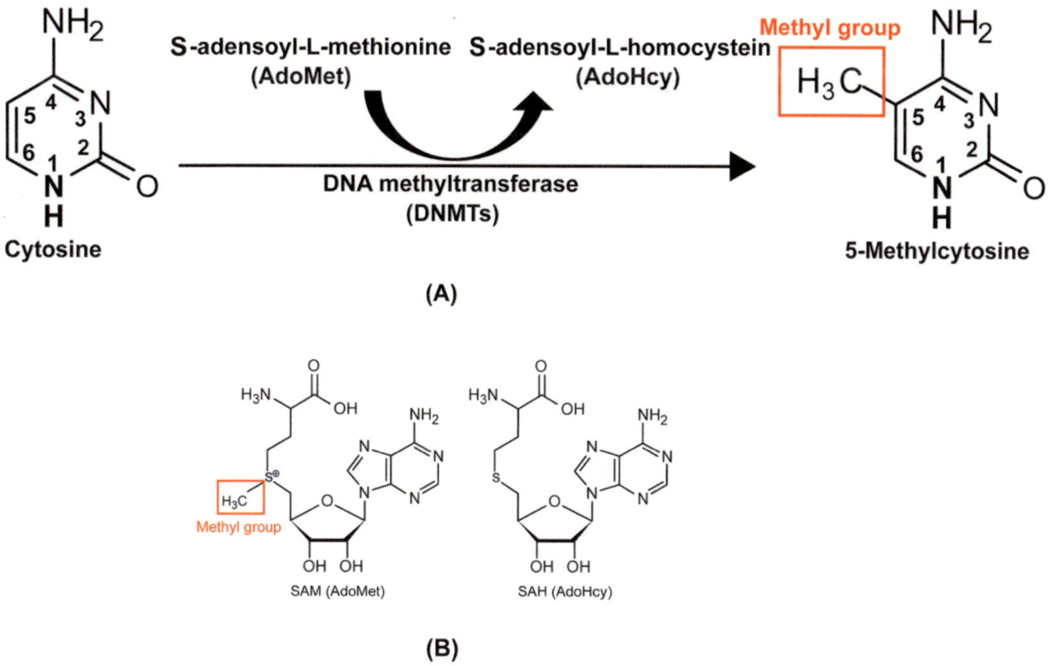

Figure 1. (A) The DNMTs catalyse the methyl cytosine modification. (B) The structure of SAM and SAH.

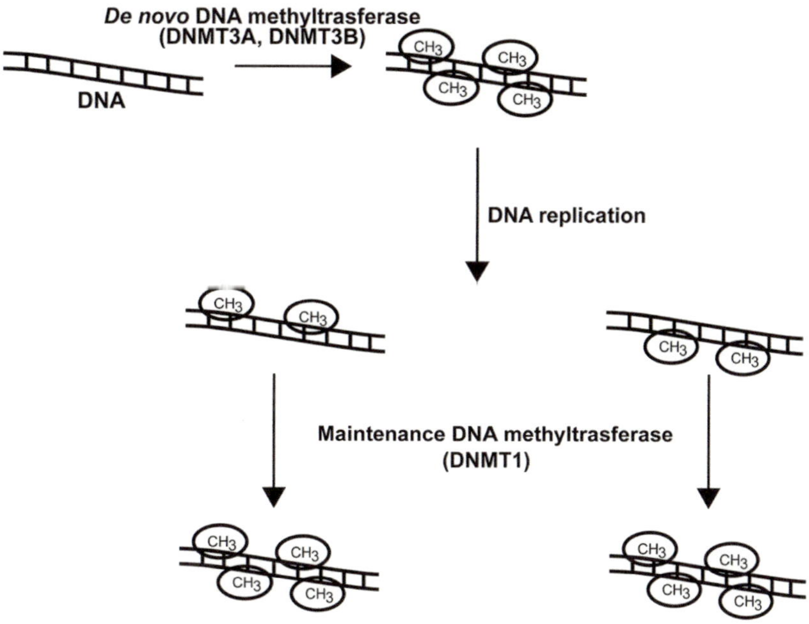

Figure 2. The roles of DNMTs.

Tumour suppressor genes (TSGs) normally suppress or negatively regulate cell proliferation by encoding proteins that block the action of growth-promoting proteins. A hallmark of cancer involves the loss of function of TSGs through the silencing genetic information. The silencing of TSGs by the high levels of 5-methylcytosine in their CpG island promoter regions, considered as the 'first and second hit', is equivalent to mutations and translocations, in Knudson's two-hit model of tumorigenesis [19, 20]. Here, the methyl groups become chemically bonded to the cytosine in CGIs, leading to disruption of the normally controlled cell proliferation and drive it to malignancy (**Figure 3**). Thus, the presence of m5CpG dinucleotide in tumour suppressor gene promoters is recognized as an important event in many human tumour types.

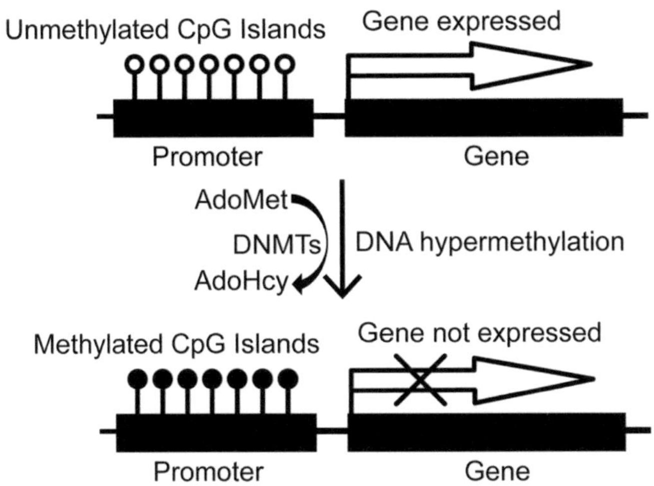

Figure 3. The typical CpG island of a tumour suppressor gene is represented in a normal and a tumour cell. White dots: unmethylated CpG; black dots: methylated CpG.

3. DNA methylation in circulation as a cancer biomarker

The high presence of cell-free circulating tumour DNA (ctDNA), which is derived from primary tumour cells, can be found in blood and non-invasive samples of patients with cancer, such as urine, brochoalveolar lavage, mammary aspiration fluids, saliva, sputum, etc. makes an ideal candidate biomarker for prognosis and early diagnosis of breast cancer. ctDNA can be distinguished from circulating DNA derived from healthy cells by the presence of genomic aberrant modifications. For example, upon the tumour development, ctDNA carries tumour specific epigenetic modifications, i.e. DNA hypermethylation, is released due to the lysis of circulating cancer cells or micro-metastases. Therefore, the detection of genetic and epigenetic alterations in ctDNA offers a potential source of development of prognostic and predictive biomarkers for cancer. Quantitative evaluation of ctDNA can reflect tumour burden relevant to provide information on genetic and epigenetic profiles associated with human cancer development. The concentration of methylated ctDNA is presented in an even smaller portion of this amount, thus, presenting a challenging substrate to work with. Fortunately, even in the low concentration, ongoing technical developments and much of the progress in molecular biological techniques have provided a chance that they can be directly applied in ctDNA collection and validation even smaller amounts of ctDNA [10, 21, 22].

4. Hypermethylation of TSGs in breast cancer: a prognostic and early diagnostic indicator

DNA aberrant methylation patterns, like hypermethylation of TSGs, global hypomethylation, etc. have been observed in human breast cancer. Silencing of TSGs expression by DNA hypermethylation provides a molecular mechanism by which DNA hypermethylation could trigger tumour development by interfering with the binding of transcription factors located at TSG gene's promoter. Thus, numerous studies have been attempted to focus on the role of hypermethylation of the TSG genes' promoter in breast cancer as well as the correlation between methylation of specific CGIs in TSGs and many breast cancer clinical states. **Table 1** shows the most relevant hypermethylated genes involve in various functions in breast cancer reported so far. Methylation of these TSG promoters is associated with the complete loss of TSG protein products in cancer cells and development of malignant phenotype.

TSGs	Function	Location
APC	Inhibitor of β-catenin, cell proliferation, migration and adhesion	5q21
BRCA1	DNA damage repair	17q21
Cyclin D2	Regulators of CDK kinases	12p13
GSTP1	Conjugation to Glutathione, prevention of oxidative DNA damage	11q13
$p16^{INK4a}$	Cyclin-dependent kinase inhibitor	9p21
PTEN	Negatively regulating AKT/PBK signalling pathway	10q23
RARβ	Retinoic acid receptor	3p24
RASSF1A	Ras effector homologue, cell cycle arrest	3p21
ZMYND10	Inhibitor of colony formation of cancer cells	3p21.3

Table 1. Examples of TSGs that undergo CpG island hypermethylation in breast cancer.

This DNA hypermethylation is a reversible signal, maybe due to the activity of Demethylase, which performs the reverse reaction to DNA methyltransferase and is an excellent candidate to be one of its important partners in shaping the methylation pattern of genomes [23, 24]. Thus, nowadays, many studies have been focused on an innovative approach in cancer treatments in which aimed to inhibit DNA hypermethylation and/or re-expression of silenced TSGs.

Therein, the hypermethylation of the CGIs promoter of *BRCA1* gene is now recognized as one of the most common molecular abnormalities associated with breast cancer development and is quoted as a significant example. *BRCA1* (Breast cancer 1) gene (HGNC: 1100; Entrez Gene: 672; OMIM: 113705; UniProtKB: P38398), which locates at 17q12-21, also known by many other names such as *IRIS*, *PSCP*, *BRCAI*, *BRCC1*, *RNF53*, *BROVCA1*, etc. is a tumour suppressor gene that conferred genetic pre-disposition to early onset of human breast and ovarian cancer [25–27]. This gene encodes a nuclear phosphoprotein that plays a role in maintaining genomic stability. The encoded protein combines with many other tumour suppressor, DNA damage sensors, and signal transducers to form a large multi-subunit protein complex that is called as BRCA1-associated genome surveillance complex (BASC). Therefore, the BRCA1 protein is involved in multifunction, such as repairing damaged DNA of double-stranded break, transcriptional regulation, ubiquitinylation, recombination and controlling the cell cycle check points as well as other functions. The hypermethylation of the *BRCA1* promoter has been considered as an inactivating mechanism of *BRCA1* expression, leading to breast tumourigenesis. In addition, some evidences have shown the significant association between the inactivation or low expression of BRCA1 protein expression and the aberrant methylation status of CGIs in the *BRCA1* promoter in breast cancer tumorigenesis.

It is well known that breast cancer constitutes a heterogeneous complex of diseases characterized by different distinct morphologies, biological behaviours and clinical outcomes. The classification and diagnosis of breast cancer have been based on the expression of different proteins, including estrogen receptor (ER), progesterone receptor (PR) and human epidermal growth factor receptor 2 (HER2) [28, 29]. An example of such a target molecular therapy is Trastuzumab (Herceptin®), which has been approved to directly against HER2-expressing tumours. Among the variety of breast cancer types, a subtype called triple-negative breast cancer (TNBC), which is clinically defined by the lack of expression of ER, PR and HER2, presents a challenge for effective clinical management [28]. Therefore, it is essential to find a reliable biomarker, which are not only useful for the screening, early diagnosis and prognosis prediction for breast cancer, but also provide insight into the mechanisms driving tumourigenesis as well as an innovative approach in breast cancer treatments.

Over the past few years, a considerable amount of studies has been conducted to evaluate the association between *BRCA1* promoter methylation and many clinicopathological characteristics of breast cancer. Therefore, tentatively, a meta-analysis was carried out, a total of 44 studies including 25 case-control studies and 19 cohort studies were eligible, enrolled into the meta-analysis research. According to our research, the prevalence of the hypermethylated *BRCA1* promoter has been reported to fall in the range from 9.1 to 59.2%, which was statistically significant higher in breast cancers than non-cancerous controls ($OR = 4.00$, 95% CI= 2.336–6.878, $P < 0.001$, **Figure 4**). Because of large heterogeneity ($P_H \leq <0.0001$, $I^2 = 73.82\%$), we continued to clarify the potential source of heterogeneity via stratified analysis based on sample materials, methods for identifying methylation and ethnicity; with the detailed results were summarized in **Table 2**.

As shown in **Table 2**, the pooled OR for *BRCA1* promoter hypermethylation in breast cancer tissues was 4.312 (95% CI = 2.395–7.765, $P < 0.001$) compared with normal or benign tissues, and was higher than the pooled OR in peripheral blood of breast cancer patients ($OR = 2.485$, 95% CI = 1.433–4.310, $P = 0.001$) compared with non-cancer controls. In addition, the pooled OR for *BRCA1* promoter hypermethylation detected by MSP was 5.059 (95% CI = 2.214–11.561, $P < 0.001$), significant higher than other methods ($OR = 2.506$; 95% CI = 1.409–4.457, $P = 0.002$). Meanwhile, the frequency of *BRCA1* promoter hypermethylation in Asians ($OR = 4.006$, 95% CI = 2.122–7.560; $P < 0.001$) was higher than in Caucasians ($OR = 2.291$, 95% CI = 1.147– 4.576, $P = 0.006$). Furthermore, our studies also demonstrated that the *BRCA1* promoter hypermethylation was significant correlated with the clinicopathological characteristics which included ages, meant that the prevalence of hypermethylation status was higher in the group of age under 55 (*OR* = 1.227, 95% CI = 1.604–1.414, *P* = 0.05) (**Figure 5**); histological grade, meant that the hypermethylated *BRCA1* in the case of histological grade 3 and 4 was higher than in the histological grade 1 and 2 (*OR* = 1.858, 95% CI = 1.499–2.301, *P* < 0.001) (**Figure 6**); disease stages, meant that the prevalence of the hypermethylation of *BRCA1* gene in the case of late stages was higher than in early stages (*OR* = 1.339, 95% CI = 1.023–1.752, *P* = 0.033) (**Figure 7**). Additionally, the hypermethylation status of *BRCA1* gene's promoter was correlated with the ER(−) (*OR*= 2.02, 95% CI = 1.525–2.675, *P* < 0.001), PR(−) (*OR* = 1.823, 95% CI = 1.374–2.41, *P* < 0.001) and especially with triple-negative phenotype (*OR* = 2.814, 95% CI = 1.811–4.371, *P* < 0.001) under fixed or random effect mode (**Figure 8**). Thus, those meta-analysis results confirmed that the *BRCA1* promoter hypermethylation was significant correlated with the increased risk of breast cancer, associated with several specific clinicopathological characteristics of breast cancer, which indicated that *BRCA1* promoter hypermethylation could be utilized as an effective biomarker in predictive and diagnostic breast cancer.

Study or Subgroup	Breast cancer		Non caner		Weight	Odds Ratio	Year
	Events	Totals	Events	Totals	(%)	M-H, Random, 95% CI	
Li 2015	24	49	11	49	6.87	3.316 (1.384-7.948)	2015
Al-Moghrabi 2014	22	155	13	143	7.28	1.654 (0.80-3.422)	2014
Gupta 2014	15	66	2	36	4.99	5 (1.07-23.275)	2014
Truong 2014	78	95	0	20	2.51	183.91 (10.608-3188.712)	2014
Hasan 2013	9	26	4	26	5.54	2.912 (0.765-11.888)	2013
Jung 2013	6	60	3	60	5.26	2.11 (0.503-8.866)	2013
Ben Gacem 2012	71	117	5	65	6.55	18.522 (6.918-49.591)	2012
Bosviel 2012	425	902	454	990	8.3	1.052 (0.878-1.260)	2012
Al-Moghrabi 2011	13	47	2	7	4.43	0.956 (9.164-5.556)	2011
Iwamoto 2011	31	162	27	200	7.68	1.516 (0.863-2.664)	2011
Wong 2011	28	255	0	3	2.35	0.877 (0.0442-17.416)	2011
Cho 2010	7	40	2	27	4.69	2.652 (0.507-13.878)	2010
Sharma 2010	25	100	0	30	2.54	20.603 (1.215-349.232)	2010
Buyru 2009	4	77	0	77	2.41	9.49 (0.502-179.359)	2009
Feng 2009	22	63	0	29	2.52	31.988 (1.865-548.572)	2009
Bagadi 2008	15	54	0	5	2.39	4.316 (0.225-82.810)	2008
Jing 2008	33	102	0	20	2.53	19.763 (1.160-336.76)	2008
Mirza 2007	13	50	0	5	2.38	3.96 (0.205-76.511)	2007
Wei 2005	39	131	0	3	2.35	2.989 (0.151-59.238)	2005
Parrella 2004	9	54	2	10	4.56	0.8 (0.145-4.409)	2004
Chen 2003	21	93	0	20	2.52	12.159 (0.706-209.450)	2003
Jerónimo 2003	11	27	0	12	2.42	17.424 (0.935-324.786)	2003
Esteller 2000	11	84	0	84	2.51	26.442 (1.532-456.524)	2000
Niwa 2000	10	32	0	32	2.47	30.333 (1.690-544.467)	2000
Dobrovic 1997	2	7	0	2	1.95	2.273 (0.0770-67.054)	1997
Total (95% CI)		**2848**		**1955**	**100**	**4.00 (2.336-6.878)**	
Total events	**944**		**525**				

Heterogeneity: Tai^2 =0.024, Chi^2=91.68, df=24 (P<0.0001),I^2 =73.82%
Test for overall effect: Z=5.04 (P<0.001)

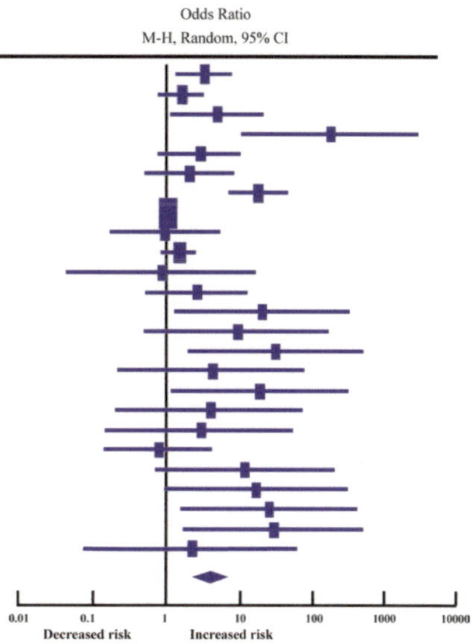

Figure 4. Forest plot for evaluating the association between *BRCA1* promoter methylation and breast cancer under fixed or random effect mode.

Up to now, a significant proportion of breast cancer patients who have poor prognosis will develop recurrence. This needs to find a more sensitive and specific biomarker, which can be a powerful prognostic indicator and help make therapeutic decisions to prolong the survival time of patients. Then, we included 10 articles provide disease-free survival (DFS) and/or overall survival (OS) to evaluate the role of the *BRCA1* promoter hypermethylation in the prognosis of breast cancer. Overall survival (OS), which was defined as the length of time from either the date of diagnosis or the start of treatment for breast cancer, that patients diagnosed with the disease are still alive, and disease-free survival (DFS), which was defined that the length of time after primary treatment for a cancer ends that the patient survives without any signs or symptoms of that cancer. In detail, in the Asian population, the OS and DFS were 2.163 (95% CI = 1.212–3.858, $P < 0.001$) and 2.47 (95% CI = 1.331–4.584, $P = 0.004$), respectively, using single variable analysis. In the case of using multiple variables analysis, the OS and DFS were 1.611 (95% CI = 1.116–2.324, $P = 0.011$), and 2.872 (95% CI = 1.389–5.937, $P = 0.004$), respectively. Those analytic results indicated that hypermethylated *BRCA1* gene's promoter was significant associated with OS, DFS, meant that it was poor prognosis to breast cancer patients, in both single and multiple variables analysis. Hence, *BRCA1* promoter hypermethylation is suggested to be a potential biomarker for prognostic assessment.

		Test of association			**Test of heterogeneity**		
Variables	*N*	**OR (95% CI)**	*Z*	*P*-**value**	**Model**	**Variables**	*N*
Total	25	4.00 (2.336–6.878)	5.04	<0.001	*R*	<0.0001	73.82%
Material							
Tissue	22	4.312 (2.395–7.765)	4.87	<0.001	*R*	0.0003	58.32%
Blood	10	2.485 (1.433–4.310)	3.24	0.001	*R*	0.0045	60.78%
Methods							
MSP	15	5.059 (2.214–11.561)	3.845	<0.001	*R*	0.0001	67.89%
Others	10	2.506 (1.409–4.457)	3.126	0.002	*R*	0.0049	61.97%
Ethnicity							
Caucasian	10	2.291 (1.147–4.576)	2.349	0.006	*R*	0.0375	49.25%
Asian	14	4.006 (2.122–7560)	4.282	<0.001	*R*	0.0060	55.60%
Africa	1	18.5217 (6.917–49.59)	5.809	<0,001	NA	NA	NA

Note: *N*: the total number of eligible studies; Caucasians included: American and Europeans, Australians. P_H: the *P*-value of *Q* test for heterogeneity among studies; F: fixed-effects model; R: random-effects model; NA: non-analysis.

Table 2. Overall and subgroups analyses of *BRCA1* methylation and breast cancer risk in 25 cases control studies.

Study or Subgroup	Early age Events	Early age Totals	Late age Events	Late age Totals	Weight (%)	Odds Ratio M-H, Random, 95% CI	Year
Li 2015	15	28	9	21	1.58	1.538 (0.492-4.808)	2015
Zhu 2015	69	117	68	122	7.79	1.142 (0.683-1.907)	2015
Hsu 2013	53	92	25	47	4.11	1.196 (0.590-2.424)	2013
Jacot 2013	12	80	6	75	1.91	2.029 (0.720-5.717)	2013
Xu 2013	159	597	135	566	29.18	1.159 (0.889-1.511)	2013
Bal 2012	6	18	5	27	1.08	2.2 (0.554-8.741)	012
Al-Moghrabi 2011	9	17	3	29	0.88	9.75 (2.115-44.945)	2011
Sharma 2010	12	41	15	59	2.58	1.214 (0.497-2.962)	2010
Chen 2009	71	273	68	263	13.74	1.008 (0.685-1.483)	2009
Xu 2009	259	434	245	417	27.42	1.039(0.790-1.366)	2009
Bagadi 2008	6	19	9	35	1.36	1.333 (0.390-4.557)	2008
Mirza 2007	8	22	5	28	1.21	2.629 (0.716-9.645)	2007
Birgisdottir 2006	9	66	4	77	1.36	2.882 (0.844-9.836)	2006
Wei 2005	23	68	15	67	3.38	2.278 (1.045-4.964)	2005
Chen 2003	9	33	12	60	2.08	1.5 (0.555-4.051)	2003
Miyamoto 2002	4	11	1	10	0.36	5.143 (0.465-56.899)	2002
Total (95% CI)		**1906**		**1903**		**1.227 (1.064-1.415)**	
Total events	**724**		**625**		**100**		

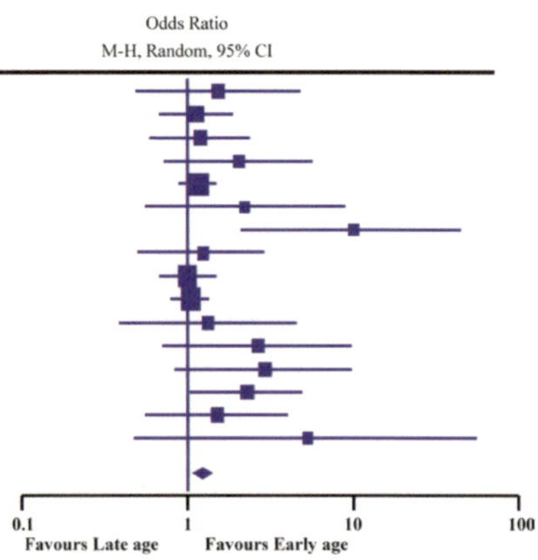

Heterogeneity: Chi^2 = 18.6297. df= 15 (P=0.2310); I^2 = 19.48%
Test for overall effect: Z = 2.82 (P= 0.005)

Figure 5. Forest plot for evaluating the association between *BRCA1* promoter methylation and ages under fixed or random effect mode.

Study or Subgroup	Early age		Late age		Weight	Odds Ratio	Year
	Events	Totals	Events	Totals	(%)	M-H, Random, 95% CI	
Zhu 2015	52	93	74	122	16.32	1216 (0.703-2.101)	2015
Otani 2014	7	20	7	9	1.48	6.5 (1.053-40.134)	2014
Hsu 2013	49	96	27	51	10.57	1.079 (0.547-2.130)	2013
Jacot 2013	2	52	16	103	2.14	4.598 (1.015-20.825)	2013
Jung 2013	1	40	5	20	0.98	13 (1.400-120.671)	2013
Xu 2013	229	898	42	139	31.83	1265 (0.855-1.872)	2013
Bal 2012	6	34	5	11	2.224	3.889 (0.887-17.059)	2012
Ben Gacem 2012	38	70	33	47	7.99	1.985 (0.908-4.340)	2012
Al-Moghrabi 2011	4	19	8	27	2.57	1.579 (0.398-6.264)	2011
Iwamoto 2011	22	133	7	21	4.74	2.523 (0.913-6.969)	2011
Sharma 2010	11	48	12	28	4.83	2.523 (0.922-6.903)	2010
Wei 2005	9	58	21	46	5.81	4.573 (1.827-11.447)	2005
Chen 2003	11	66	9	25	4.5	2.813 (0.992-7.974)	2003
Miyamoto 2002	0	7	5	14	0.53	8.684 (0.412-183.243)	2002
Niwa 2000	2	16	8	16	1.55	7 (1.185-41.360)	2000
Catteau 1999	2	38	9	50	1.92	3.951 (0.801-19.498)	1999
Total (95% CI)		1688		729	100	1.858 (1.499-2.301)	
Total events	445		288				

Heterogeneity: Chi² = 24.622. df= 15 (P=0.0553); I² = 39.08%
Test for overall effect: Z = 5.668 (P< 0.001)

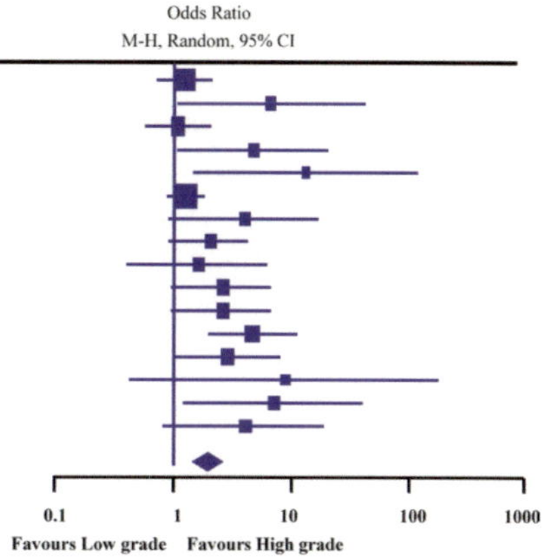

Figure 6. Forest plot for evaluating the association between *BRCA1* promoter methylation and histological tumour grades under fixed or random effect mode.

Study or Subgroup	Early Stage		Late Stage		Weight	Odds Ratio	Year
	Events	Totals	Events	Totals	(%)	M-H, Random, 95% CI	
Li 2015	18	31	6	18	5.21	0.361 (0.107-1.214)	2015
Saelee 2014	12	33	3	28	3.95	0.21 (0.0522-0.845)	2014
Jung 2013	5	53	1	7	1.43	1.6 (0.159-16.099)	2013
Sharma 2010	15	51	12	49	9.72	0.778 (0.159-16.099)	2010
Chen 2009	103	421	36	112	37.01	1.462 (0.928-2.304)	2009
Sharma 2009	9	59	18	42	8.72	4.167 (1.633-10.630)	2009
Bagadi 2008	7	27	8	27	5.37	1.203 (0.365-3.966)	2008
Mirza 2007	8	28	5	21	4.55	0.781 (0.214 to 2.856)	2007
Mirza 2007	8	28	5	21	4.55	0.781 (0.214-2.856)	2007
Wei 2005	17	85	12	27	8.91	3.2 (1.267-8.083)	2005
Chen 2003	12	67	9	26	7.33	2.426 (0.874 - 6.737)	2003
Catteau 1999	8	83	3	10	3.24	4.018 (0.864 - 18.676)	1999
Total (95% CI)		966		388	99.99	1.339 (1.023-1.752)	
Total events	222		118				

Heterogeneity: Chi² = 26.5643. df= 11 (P=0.0553); I² = 58.59%
Test for overall effect: Z = 2.127 (P< 0.033)

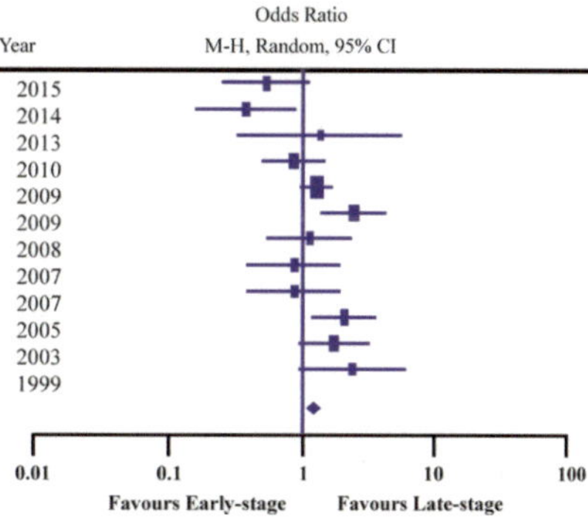

Figure 7. Forest plot for evaluating the association between *BRCA1* promoter methylation and disease stages under fixed or random effect mode.

Study or Subgroup	Triple negative		Triple positive		Weight	Odds Ratio	Year
	Events	Totals	Events	Totals	(%)	M-H, Random, 95% CI	
Saelee 2014	8	19	7	42	8.06	3.636 (1.074-12.315)	2014
Otani 2014	5	7	10	23	4.53	3.25 (0.519-20.370)	2014
Xu 2013	64	206	218	893	18.81	1.396 (1.001-1.946)	2013
Hsu 2013	16	21	61	117	9.42	2.938 (1.010-8.545)	2013
Jacot 2013	14	48	4	103	8.41	10.191 (3.139-33.084)	2013
Ben Gacem 2012	25	32	46	85	10.75	3.028 (1.182-7.755)	2012
Iwamoto 2011	7	11	24	142	7.4	8.604 (2.334-31.715)	2011
Sharma 2010	11	25	12	55	9.93	2.815 (1.019-7.780)	2010
Galizia 2010	14	44	14	68	11.63	1.8 (0.758-4274)	2010
Sharma 2009	15	40	12	49	11.06	1.85 (0.742-4.610)	2009
Total (95% CI)		**453**		**1577**	**100**	**2.814 (1.811-4.371)**	
Total events	**179**		**408**				

Heterogeneity: Tau² = 0.01, Chi² =19.6223, df= 9 (P=0.0204); I² = 54.13%
Test for overall effect: Z = 4.601 (P< 0.001)

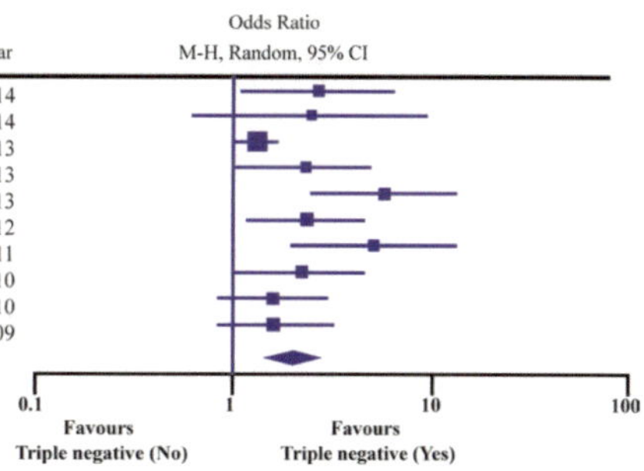

Figure 8. Forest plot for evaluating the association between *BRCA1* promoter methylation and triple negative phenotype under fixed or random effect mode.

5. DNA hypermethylation-targeted drug in cancer therapy

The process of DNA methylation is catalysed by DNMTs which typically occurs at CpG dinucleotides. As mentioned earlier, it is also a reversible process. Removal of a methyl group from DNA must involve a cleavage of a carbon-carbon bond, which is carried out by DNA demethylase (dMTase). In addition, the methylation reaction can be blocked by the inhibitors of DNA methylation drugs, such as 5-azacytidine, 5-aza-2′-deoxycytidine, etc. which contains a nitrogen in the place of carbon at 5′ position of cytosine ring (**Figure 9**) [30]. This drug is cooperated into DNA, then, replaces the natural base cytosine and acts as a potent inhibitor of the DNMTs, inducing the DNA demethylation [31]. Since DNA methylation is reversible, an aberrant hypermethylation of tumour suppression genes can be reverted. This consequently supports DNA methyltransferases (DNMTs) as attractive therapeutic targets. Indeed, epigenetic drugs (epi-drug)—methylation inhibitors through DNMT inactivation, used alone or in combination with other biomarkers, including by dietary agents, for targeted preventive and therapeutic interventions, have attracted attention recently.

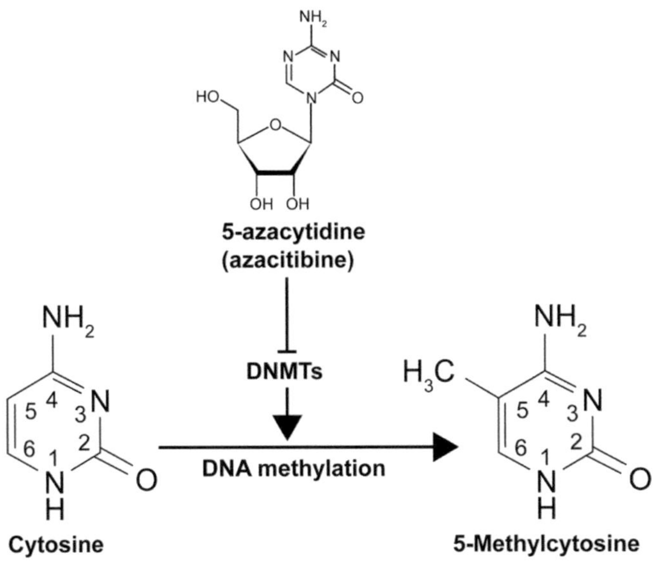

Figure 9. Inhibition of DNMTs by 5-azacytidine.

DNMT inhibitors (DNMTi), such as 5-azacytidine (azacitidine) and 5-aza-2′-deoxycytidine (decitabine) (**Figure 10**), are epi-drugs which are first announced and currently marketed as hypomethylation therapeutics. They are nucleoside analogues, derivatives of cytidine that work by incorporating into the DNA sequence at cytosine positions during DNA replication to be active and then form a suicidal covalent complex with the DNMTs. These drugs have been approved by Food and Drug Administration (FDA) for clinical tests on the myelodysplastic syndrome, malignant mesothelioma, pre-leukemic disease, breast cancer, nasopharyngeal carcinoma and some other diseases.

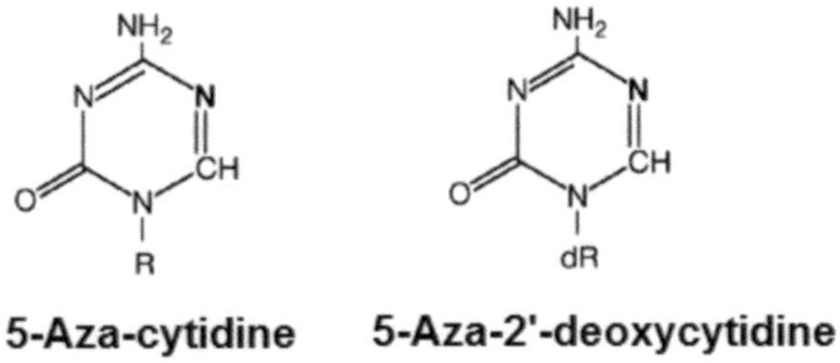

Figure 10. The structure of 5-azacytidine and 5-aza-2′-deoxycytidine.

Zebularine is another cytidine analog that has a mechanism similar to 5-azacytidine, integrating into DNA and forming a covalent bond with DNMT1, resulting in inhibition of methylation reaction. Moreover, Zebularine is reported that it is a DNMT1 inhibitor with low toxicity and has a high sensitivity in selective cancer cells. Particularly, this drug showed the reactivated functions on some important tumour suppressor genes that were disrupted in breast cancer cell lines, even at low concentrations. Although the drug is not yet FDA approved, a preclinical study on mouse models showed that Zebularine can inhibit DNA methylation and induce re-expression-silenced gene, even given orally.

Other trends related to DNA methylation including the inhibition of DNMTs through siRNA, ribozymes, antisense oligonucleotides have also been considered. Some drugs have proven effective impact on cell cultures, animal models and clinical trials as well such asMG98, a 20 bp anti-sense oligonucleotide that directly prevents the translation of DNMT1 or RG108—a new small molecule that can act on active site of DNMT1. Unlike the nucleoside analogs, RG108 did not demonstrate cytotoxic or genotoxic effects on cells even at high concentrations.

The combination of the histone deacetylase inhibitors (HDACi), such as Trichostatin A (TSA) and phenylbutyrate, with DNMTi is a new trend giving promising efficacy in the treatment of cancer. In breast cancer, triple negative metastatic patients that do not express estrogen receptor (ER), progesterone receptor (PR) and HER, do not respond to agents such as trastuzumab (Herceptin) and tamoxifen. Particularly, the loss of ER in some triple negative breast cancers is epigenetically silenced by abnormal methylation and histone modifications. Consequently, the patients express the resistance of anti-estrogen. Triple negative metastatic breast cancer patients were pre-treated with decitabine—a DNMTi and LBH 589—an HDACi, to restore the ER and then treated with tamoxifen. This combination can remove the epigenetic modifications including DNA methylation and histone deacetylation and reactivate ER. Thus, this reactivated ER cells become sensitive to agents like tamoxifen. Similarly, the combination of azacitidine with TSA also induces the re-expression of ER function to increase the sensitivity of breast cancer cell lines that previously show negative expression with ER in tamoxifen therapy or the combination of HDACi and trastuzumab has taken to effectively suppression of the development and apoptosis induction into breast cancer cells lines.

In addition, the combination of epi-drugs with chemotherapeutic agents or natural dietary ingredients also increases the effectiveness of treatment. A pre-clinical study has shown that the combination of decitabine and docetaxel (an anti-mitotic drug) can increase treatment outcomes against cancer cells in experiments conducted on breast cancer cell lines [32, 33]. Decitabine in combination with another substance, amsacrine or idarubicin, also shows therapeutic effect. Green tea polyphenol, (-)-epigallocatechin-3-gallate (EGCG), may cause re-modelling of chromatin structure and the ERα promoter by histone acetylation and DNA methylation mechanisms, and consequently reactivating ERα. The combination of TSA and EGCG leads to reactivation of numerous tumour suppressor genes by inhibiting directly or indirectly DNMTs. Dietary sulforaphane—an inhibitor of histone acetylation also shows very effective activity in the inhibition of proliferation and survival of breast cancer cells without affecting normal cells.

Therefore, methylation combined therapy is very promising in the treatment of breast cancer. Clinical trials in the combination of trastuzumab with HDACi for the treatment of breast cancer, and a phase II trial in breast cancer—valproic acid combined with FEC100 (5-fluorouracil, epirubicin and cyclophosphamide) also are being investigated. Up to date, several other classes of epi-drug have been studied, developed with new drugs, which based on the DNMT inhibitors, HDAC inhibitors, HMT inhibitors, etc. in early preclinical trial development.

6. Conclusion

DNA hypermethylation has become established in recent years as being one of the important causes of breast tumorigenesis and potential biomarkers in clinical applications, prognosis and early diagnosis of breast cancer. As the release of tumour-associated DNA into body fluids, thus the screening of plasma or serum DNA may provide information on epigenetic profiles which are tightly associated with breast cancer development, progression and response to therapies. This is the real advantage of an aberrant DNA methylation property as a great versatility, promising biomarker for the molecular monitoring of cancer patients, and applied in early detection, prognosis and predicting drug sensitivity in cancer.

Abbreviations

APC	Adenomatous Polyposis Coli
BASC	BRCA1-associated genome surveillance complex
BRCA1	Breast cancer 1
CGIs	CpG islands
CI	Confidence interval
ctDNA	Cell-free circulating tumour DNA
DFS	Disease free survival
DNMTi	DNA methyltransferase inhibitors

DNMTs	DNA methyltransferase
ER	Receptor
FDA	The Food and Drug Administration
GSTP1	*Glutathione S-transferase P1*
HDACi	Histone deacetylase inhibitors
HER2	Human epidermal growth factor receptor 2
m5CpG	Methyl-5-CpG
MBD	Methyl-CpG binding domain protein
OR	Risk ratio
OS	Overall survival
$p16^{INK4\alpha}$	CDK4 Inhibitor p16-INK4α
PR	Progesterone receptor
PTEN	Phosphatase and Tensin homolog
RARβ	Retinoic Acid Receptor Beta
RASSF1A	Ras Association domain Family 1 isoform A
TNBCs	Triple-negative breast cancer
TSA	Trichostatin A
TSG	Tumour suppressor gene
ZMYND10	Zinc Finger MYND-Type Containing 10

Author details

Le Huyen Ai Thuy*, Lao Duc Thuan and Truong Kim Phuong

*Address all correspondence to: thuy.lha@ou.edu.vn

Faculty of Biotechnology, Ho Chi Minh City Open University, Ho Chi Minh City, Viet Nam

References

[1] Waddington CH. The epigenotype. 1942. Int J Epidemiol. 2012;**41**(1):10–3. DOI: 10.1093/ije/dyr184.

[2] Jin B, Li Y, Robertson KD. DNA methylation: superior or subordinate in the epigenetic hierarchy?. Genes Cancer. 2011;**2**(6):607–17. DOI: 10.1177/1947601910393957.

[3] Kulis M, Esteller M. DNA methylation and cancer. Adv Genet. 2010;**70**:27–56. DOI: 10.1016/B978-0-12-380866-0.60002-2.

[4] Luczak MW, Jagodziński PP. The role of DNA methylation in cancer development. Folia Histochem Cytobiol. 2006;**44**(3):143–54.

[5] Chuang JC, Jones PA. Epigenetics and microRNAs. Pediatr Res. 2007;**61**(5 Pt 2):24R–29R. DOI: 10.1203/pdr.0b013e3180457684.

[6] Muntean AG, Hess JL. Epigenetic dysregulation in cancer. Am J Pathol. 2009;**175**(4):1353–61. DOI: 10.2353/ajpath.2009.081142.

[7] Jones M, Goodman SJ, Kobor MS. DNA methylation and healthy human aging. Aging Cell. 2015;**14**(6):924–32. DOI: 10.1111/acel.12349.

[8] Robertson KD. DNA methylation and human disease. Nat Rev Genet. 2005;**6**(8):297–610. DOI: 10.1038/nrg1655.

[9] Sadikovic B, Al-Romaih K, Squire JA, Zielenska M. Cause and consequences of genetic and epigenetic alterations in human cancer. Curr Genomics. 2008;**9**(6):394–408. DOI: 10.2174/138920208785699580.

[10] Diaz LA Jr, Bardelli A. Liquid biopsies: genotyping circulating tumor DNA. J Clin Oncol. 2014;**32**(6):579–86. DOI: 10.1200/JCO.2012.45.2011.

[11] Esteller M. CpG island hypermethylation and tumor suppressor genes: a booming present, a brighter future. Oncogene. 2002;**21**(35):5427–40. DOI: 10.1038/sj.onc.1205600.

[12] Yuanyuan D, Haiyang Z, Haiyan L, Xiaokun L, Shulin Y. DNA methylation as an early diagnostic marker of cancer (Review). Biomed Rep. 2014;**2**(3):326–30. DOI: 10.3892/br.2014.237.

[13] Bestor T, Laudano A, Mattaliano R, Ingram V. Cloning and sequencing of a cDNA encoding DNA methyltransferase of mouse cells. The carboxyl-terminal domain of the mammalian enzymes is related to bacterial restriction methyltransferases. J Mol Biol. 1988;**203**(4):971–83. DOI: 10.1016/0022-2836(88)90122-2.

[14] Kafri T, Ariel M, Brandeis M, Shemer R, Urven L, McCarrey J, et al. Developmental pattern of gene-specific DNA methylation in the mouse embryo and germ line. Genes Dev. 1992;**6**(5):705–14. DOI: 10.1101/gad.6.5.705.

[15] Zhang L, Long X. Association of BRCA1 promoter methylation with sporadic breast cancers: Evidence from 40 studies. Sci Rep. 2015;**5**:17869. DOI: 10.1038/srep17869.

[16] Bestor TH. The DNA methyltransferases of mammals. Hum Mol Genet. 2000;**9**(16):2395–402. DOI: 10.1093/hmg/9.16.2395.

[17] Okano M, Xie S, Li E. Cloning and characterization of a family of novel mammalian DNA (cytosine-5) methyltransferases. Nat Genet. 1998;**19**(3):219–20. DOI: 10.1038/890.

[18] Chen ZX, Mann JR, Hsieh CL, Riggs AD, Chédin F. Physical and functional interactions between the human DNMT3L protein and members of the de novo methyltransferase family. J Cell Biochem. 2005;9**5**(5):90–17. DOI: 10.1002/jcb.20447.

[19] Jones PA, Laird PW. Cancer epigenetics comes of age. Nat Genet. 1999;**21**(2):163–7. DOI: 10.1038/5947.

[20] Mossman D, Scott RJ. Epimutations, Inheritance and causes of aberrant DNA methylation in cancer. Hered Cancer Clin Pract. 2006;**4**(2):75–80. DOI: 10.1186/1897-4287-4-2-75.

[21] Schwarzenbach H, Pantel K. Circulating DNA as biomarker in breast cancer. Breast Cancer Res. 2015;**17**(1):136. DOI: 10.1186/s13058-015-0645-5.

[22] Warton K, Samimi G. Methylation of cell-free circulating DNA in the diagnosis of cancer. Front Mol Biosci. 2015;**2**:13. DOI: 10.3389/fmolb.2015.00013.

[23] Bhattacharya SK, Ramchandani S, Cervoni N, Szyf M. A mammalian protein with specific demethylase activity for mCpG DNA. Nature. 1999;**397**(6720):579–83. DOI: 10.1038/17533.

[24] Ramchandani S, Bhattacharya SK, Cervoni N, Szyf M. DNA methylation is a reversible biological signal. Proc Natl Acad Sci U S A. 1999;**96**(11):6107–12.

[25] Pang D, Zhao Y, Xue W, Shan M, Chen Y, Zhang Y, et al. Methylation profiles of the BRCA1 promoter in hereditary and sporadic breast cancer among Han Chinese. Med Oncol. 2012;**29**(3):1561–8. DOI: 10.1007/s12032-011-0100-0.

[26] Welcsh PL, King MC. BRCA1 and BRCA2 and the genetics of breast and ovarian cancer. Hum Mol Genet. 2001;**10**(7):705–13. DOI: 10.1093/hmg/10.7.705..

[27] Truong PK, Lao TD, Doan TP, Le TAH. BRCA1 promoter hypermethylation signature for early detection of breast cancer in the Vietnamese population. Asian Pac J Cancer Prev. 2014;**15**(22):9607–10.

[28] Perou CM. Molecular stratification of triple-negative breast cancers. Oncologist. 2010;**25**(Suppl 5):39–48. DOI: 10.1634/theoncologist.2010-S5-39.

[29] Subramaniam S, Bhoo-Pathy N, Taib NA, Tan GH, See MH, Jamaris S, et al. Breast cancer outcomes as defined by the estrogen receptor, progesterone receptor, and human growth factor receptor-2 in a multi-ethnic Asian Country. World J Surg. 2015;**39**(10):2450–8. DOI: 10.1007/s00268-015-3133-2.

[30] Herman JGT, Baylin SB. Gene silencing in cancer in association with promoter hypermethylation. N Engl J Med. 2003;**349**(21):2042–54. DOI: 10.1056/NEJMra02.

[31] Lo PK, Sukumar S. Epigenomics and breast cancer. Pharmacogenomics. 2008;**9**(12):1879–902. DOI: 10.2217/14622416.9.12.1879..

[32] Kastl L, Brown I, Schofield AC. Altered DNA methylation is associated with docetaxel resistance in human breast cancer cells. Int J Oncol. 2010;**36**(5):1235–41. DOI: 10.3892/ijo_00000607.

[33] Priya M, Amanda FC. Decitabine in the treatment of acute myeloid leukemia in elderly patients. Cancer Manag Res. 2014;**6**:53–61. DOI: 10.2147/CMAR.S40600.

Chapter 8

ErbB2 Receptor in Breast Cancer: Implications in Cancer Cell Migration, Invasion and Resistance to Targeted Therapy

Maria del Pilar Camacho-Leal,

Marianna Sciortino and Sara Cabodi

Additional information is available at the end of the chapter

http://dx.doi.org/10.5772/66902

Abstract

Overexpression of ErbB2 is found in several types of human carcinomas. In breast tumors, ErbB2 overexpression is detected in up to 20% of patients. Breast cancers in with amplification of ErbB2 are characterized by rapid tumor growth, lower survival rate and increased disease progression. The molecular mechanisms underlying the oncogenic action of ErbB2 involve a complex signaling network that tightly regulates malignant cell migration and invasion and hence metastatic potential. Recent efforts have been made to identify gene expression signatures of ErbB2-positive invasive breast cancers that may represent important mediators of ErbB2-induced tumorigenesis and metastatic progression.

In this chapter, we will discuss the canonical ErbB2 signaling pathways responsible for tumor growth and dissemination along with newly identified mediators such as adaptor protein p130Cas and miRNAs. From a therapeutic point of view, the treatment with anti-ErbB2 monoclonal antibody trastuzumab has greatly improved the outcomes of patients with ErbB2 aggressive cancer. Nevertheless, *de novo* and acquired resistance to trastuzumab therapy still represent a major clinical problem. In the second part of the chapter, we will provide an overview of the mechanisms so far implicated in the onset of resistance to targeted therapy and of the new strategies to overcome resistance.

Keywords: ErbB2, breast cancer, molecular mechanisms, treatment

1. Introduction

Breast cancer is the leading cause of cancer-related death in women worldwide [1]. Despite significant advances in breast cancer diagnosis and treatment, several major unresolved clinical and scientific problems still remain, such as the understanding of the causes of tumor progression and resistance and how to predict them.

ErbB2 is a well-known oncoprotein that belongs to the epidermal growth factor receptor epidermal growth factor receptor (EGFR) family. It is overexpressed approximately in 20% of invasive breast cancers [2]. In particular, overexpression of ErbB2 has been demonstrated to promote breast cancer invasion and metastasis and to correlate with poor patient survival [3–6]. ErbB2 is also overexpressed in noninvasive mammary ductal carcinomas *in situ* (DCIS) [7]. Indeed, ErbB2 amplification or overexpression seems to be crucial but not sufficient for the transition from *in situ* to invasive cancer and additional hits are required for the progression of ErbB2-positive tumors. Although the molecular and genetic events underlying ErbB2-positive tumor invasion and metastasis are still not fully understood, intense investigation has led to the notion that molecules involved in cell adhesion and migration are critical in this process [8].

The identification of the deregulated ErbB2 pathway in breast cancer pathogenesis has led to the development of ErbB2-targeted therapies. Although ErbB2 overexpression identifies patients who are likely to respond to therapy with trastuzumab, not all patients benefit from treatment. To date, approximately 15% of patients relapse after therapy due to *de novo* or acquired resistance, thus it is of extreme importance to better understand the factors that contribute to therapy resistance of ErbB2-positive breast cancer tumors in order to identify novel therapeutic strategies to overcome resistance [9–11].

2. Molecular mechanisms of ErbB2 activation

Downstream signaling pathways are activated upon ErbB2 receptor activation through either heterodimerization with ligand bound EGFR, ErbB3, or ErbB4 family receptors, or in presence of overexpression of ErbB2 due to gene amplification, by ligand independent homodimerization [12]. The homo/heterodimerization promotes the receptor activation that in turn leads to tyrosine phosphorylation of the C-terminal residues. Numerous phosphorylation sites exist within the cytoplasmic domain of ErbB2, these sites are essential for protein-protein interactions and induction of the signaling cascades downstream to ErbB2 receptor activation. To this regard, the activation of the phosphoinositide 3-kinase (PI3K) and Ras/RAF/MEK/ERK1/2 pathways are hallmarks of ErbB2 activation.

Besides the canonical interaction with the member of the ErbB family, it has been recently demonstrated that activation of ErbB2 can be induced through its interaction with additional transmembrane partners. Among them Mucin 1 that is overexpressed in breast cancer and has been shown to interact with EGFR and ErbB2 leading to activation of PI3K and MAPKs pathways [13]. In addition, it has been demonstrated that leptin receptor upon leptin binding can phos-

http://dx.doi.org/10.5772/66902

phorylate and activate ErbB2 contributing to activation of mitogen-activated protein kinase 1 (MAPK) activity [14]. It is worth noting that further amplification of the ErbB2 signaling may derive from its crosstalk with other signaling mediators. For instance, it has been demonstrated that ErbB2 can cross-talk with hormone receptors, insulin growth factor receptor (IGFR), protein phosphatases, transforming growth beta receptor (TGFR-beta) and ion channels resulting in a complex signaling network that contribute to tumor growth and progression [15].

2.1. Canonical ErbB2 signaling network

Several downstream signaling pathways are activated after ErbB2 receptor activation leading to the regulation of cell proliferation, growth and survival as well as invasion and angiogenesis [15]. Tyrosine residues phosphorylation resulting from receptor activation can recruit a variety of intracellular adaptor and scaffold proteins that in turn mediate the activation of downstream signaling pathways.

One of the most important pathways activated by ErbB2 signaling is the RAS-MAPK pathway [16]. The activation of the MAPK pathway controls cell proliferation, survival and migration and alteration of this pathway have been linked with many diseases including cancer.

Upon ErbB2 activation, the adaptor molecule growth factor receptor-bound protein 2 (GRB2) binds through its SH2 domain to the phosphorylated intracellular tail of ErbB2. GRB2 bound to the receptor recruits the adaptor protein son of sevenless (SOS) determining its activation. Active SOS can trigger the activation of RAS by inducing the transition the GDP-inactive to the GTP-active state. The activation of RAS promotes a cascade of downstream kinase activation that ultimately leads to the phosphorylation and activation of extracellular signal-regulated kinases 1 and 2 (ERK1, ERK2) [17, 18]. Activated ERK proteins phosphorylate a number of transcription factors such as Elk-1, c-Fos and c-Jun among others, that regulate the expression of genes implicated in cell growth, differentiation, proliferation, survival and migration [15, 19].

The PI3K/AKT is the second canonic pathway activated by ErbB2 and due to its relevance in cell proliferation, survival, protein synthesis, invasion and drug resistance has received much attention to develop anticancer targeted therapy [17, 18, 20]. Upon receptor activation, the p85 subunit of PI3K binds to tyrosine-phosphorylated residues of ErbB2. This recruitment determines the release of the 110 subunit of PI3K and allows the formation of PI3K heterodimers that can phosphorylate PIP2 substrate in PIP3 [21]. Ultimately PIP3 promotes the localization of AKT at cell membrane and its phosphorylation by PDK1 and mTOR complex 2. AKT represents the major effector of the PI3K/AKT signaling pathway leading to the regulation of many cell functions such as cell survival, cell growth and proliferation [21] (**Figure 1**).

2.2. ErbB2 signaling mediated by the adaptor proteins p130Cas

It is clear that activation of canonical ErbB2 signaling can be achieved through the recruitment of signaling proteins to the receptor. It is now emerging that p130Cas adaptor protein can mediate the activation of ErbB2 downstream signaling pathways. p130Cas/BCAR1 scaffold molecule is a signaling molecule involved in the linkage of actin cytoskeleton to the extracellular matrix during cell migration, cell invasion and cell transformation [22, 23] and it has

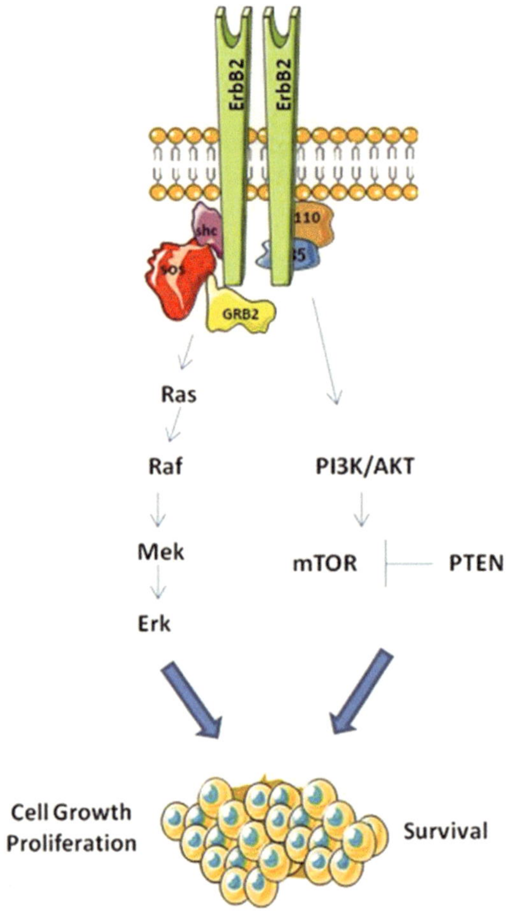

Figure 1. Canonical ErbB2 signaling network. ErbB2 activation leads to the activation of the phosphoinositide-3-kinase (PI3K)/AKT and the mitogen-activated protein kinase (RAS/RAF/MAPK) pathways that trigger cell proliferation, growth and survival.

been described as an essential transducer element in ErbB2 transformation and progression [24]. Due to its modular structure, p130Cas has been described to play a crucial role in signaling originating from many amplified or mutated oncogenes, by undergoing hyperphosphorylation and association with multiple signaling partners required for transformation [22].

It was recently demonstrated that overexpression of p130Cas in ErbB2 breast cancers correlates with poor survival and increased progression. In particular, p130Cas is required for ErbB2-dependent transformation and invasion both *in vitro* and *in vivo* models. Indeed, silencing of p130Cas is sufficient to inhibit ErbB2 orthotopic tumor growth in mice. The administration of p130Cas stabilized siRNAs by intranipple injection in the mammary glands of mice with spontaneous ErbB2 cancer lesions, significantly impaired lesions growth, indicating that p130Cas might be a potential therapeutic target [24]. It has also been reported that p130Cas binds to ErbB2 and its overexpression is sufficient to transactivate the ErbB2 receptor leading to the formation of a macromolecular signaling complex, in which Src and p125Fak kinases are present, that sustains ErbB2 downstream signaling pathways leading to activation of both MAPK and PI3K pathways regulating cell transformation, invasion and migration [24, 25]. Interestingly, concomitant p130Cas/ErbB2 overexpression accelerates the onset of mammary tumors, which are characterized at the molecular level by increased activation of c-Src and Akt [26]. Notably, a positive correlation between the expression of BCAR1/p130Cas and ErbB2 has been found in human breast cancers and the coexpression of these two genes is associated with shorter overall survival and a higher risk of developing distant metastasis [25, 26] (**Figure 2**).

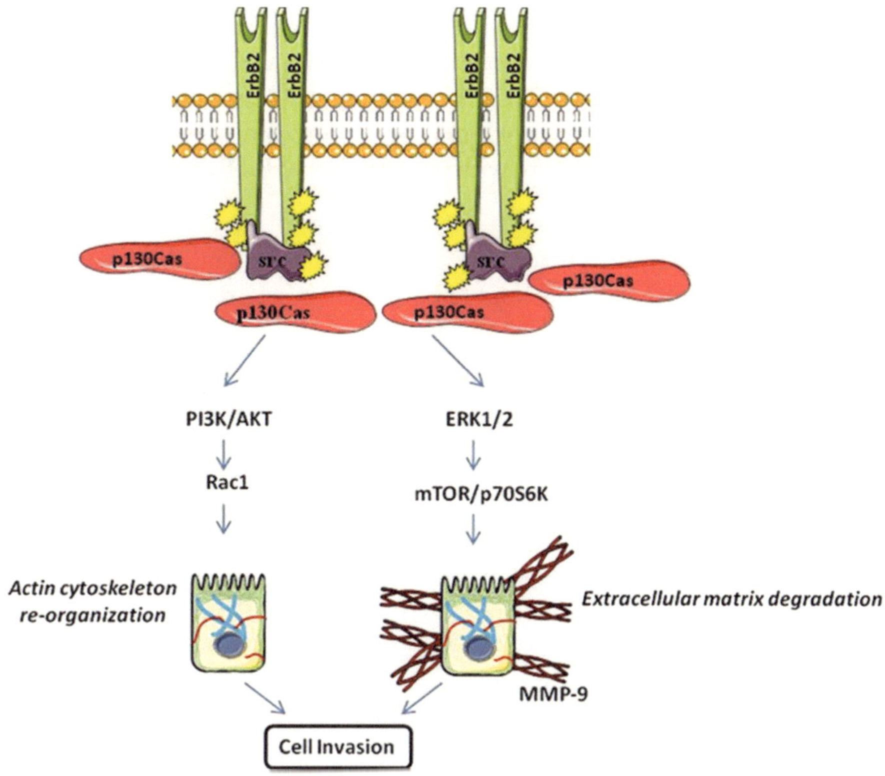

Figure 2. ErbB2 signaling mediated by the adaptor proteins p130Cas. In a 3D cell model, concomitant p130Cas overexpression and ErbB2 activation enhance PI3K/Akt and Erk1/2 MAPK signaling pathways, both signaling cascades are required for the invasive behavior of p130Cas overexpressing and ErbB2 activated acini. Erk1/2 MAPK and PI3K/Akt signaling promote invasion through distinct downstream effectors involving mTOR/p70S6K and Rac1 activation, respectively.

2.3. MicroRNA in ErbB2-overexpressing cancer

The discovery of microRNAs (miRNAs) has provided new perspectives to study cancer at the molecular level. These noncoding regulatory RNA molecules of ~22 nucleotides have emerged as important cancer biomarkers, effectors and targets. Alteration of miRNAs expression has been correlated with a variety of human diseases, including breast cancer [27].

It was initially demonstrated that the overexpression of miR-125a and miR-125b in human breast cancer cell line SKBR3 overexpressing ErbB2 was sufficient to lower ErbB2 and ErbB3 mRNA and protein levels, with consequent inhibition of anchorage-dependent growth, migration and invasion. Consistently, activation of canonical ErbB2 downstream signaling such as MAPK and PI3K/Akt pathways was severely impaired [28]. Two subsequent studies identified by using different methodologies two miRNA signatures of ErbB2 positive breast cancer. In particular, miR-520d, miR-181c, miR-302c, miR-376b, miR-30e were identified as miRNA associated with HER2 status to be added to the previously found let-7f, let-7g, miR-107, mir-10b, miR-126, miR-154 and miR-195 as miRNA characterizing HER2 status [29, 30]

These data highlight the relevance of microRNA signatures as novel breast cancer biomarkers. The consequences of the association of ErbB2 and miRNAs are still under investigation but three possible scenarios can be identified. The first one envisages the regulation of miRNAs as a consequence of ErbB2 activation. The second possibility is that miRNAs contributes to the activation of ErbB2 and to its capacity to trigger downstream-signaling pathways. The last option is that miRNAs can interfere with the response to ErbB2 targeted-therapy thereby mediating the onset of resistance.

Further investigations are needed to identify which is the crucial miRNAs implicating in the different responses to ErbB2 activation and to develop new selective anticancer therapy.

3. Role of Erbb2 in breast cancer invasion and metastasis

From the physiological point of view, ErbB2 represents an important molecule implicated in the regulation of cell proliferation, differentiation, survival and migration during embryonic development and in adults, during tissue maintenance. Importantly, during pathological conditions, ErbB2 aberrant expression and activation in breast cancer have been extensively linked to invasive, aggressive phenotype and poor prognosis [31]. Acquirement of migratory properties allow cancer cell to invade the surrounding tissues and reach the blood vessels to generate metastasis. At the cellular level, the transition from noninvasive to invasive status is characterized by loss of the epithelial characteristics such as expression of cytokeratins and E-cadherin and gain of mesenchymal traits like vimentin, fibronectin and N-cadherin through a process that is known as epithelial to mesenchymal transition (EMT) [32]. EMT promotes cancer progression by allowing cancer cells to acquire invasive properties, to metastasize and also to acquire stem cell properties [33, 34]. Interestingly, these cells that have acquired stem cell properties are characterized by increased expression of EMT genes, such as FoxC2, Zeb and N-cadherin [35, 36]. Moreover, it has been demonstrated that ErbB2 overexpression in breast cancer cell lines can enhance the stem cell population which is responsible for breast cancer progression [37].

3.1. Erbb2 invasive signaling signature

For the past years, extensive investigations have been performed in order to understand the precise mechanisms implicated in the regulation of cell invasion and metastasis as the result of ErbB2 activation. Several *in vitro* studies have pointed out the requirement of additional

http://dx.doi.org/10.5772/66902

molecular hits in order to induce malignant transformation mediated by ErbB2 overexpression. For example, in nontransformed MCF10A breast epithelial three-dimensional cell cultures, ErbB2-mediated cell transformation occurs upon the activation of the TGFβ signaling [38]. Additional studies in 3D MCF10A cultures have led to the identification of signaling proteins already implicated in cytoskeletal organization and cancer cell invasion. In particular, these studies suggest that p21-activated protein kinase (PAK) family of serine/threonine kinases that function as effectors of Cdc42 and Rac, by activating the Raf/Mek/Erk and Akt pathways, cooperates with ErbB2 in transforming mammary epithelial cells [39]. More recently, using the same in *vitro* cell model, it was shown that the ErbB2-driven invasive phenotype requires both cathepsins B and L. Cathepsins B and L are lysosomal cysteine cathepsins that upon secretion to the extracellular space can cleave and activate urokinase plasminogen activator, heparanase and various matrix metalloproteases as well as E-cadherin and, thus, contribute to invasion and metastasis [40]. In MCF10A cells engineered to express a chimeric form of ErbB2 that can be induced to dimerize by treatment with a synthetic ligand [41], it was reported that the adaptor molecule p130Cas controls ErbB2-dependent invasion. Indeed, the overexpression of p130Cas in ERbB2-transformed mammary acini leads to activation of PI3K/Akt and Erk1/2 MAPK signaling pathways and promote invasion of mammary acini. It was further demonstrated that Erk1/2 MAPK and PI3K/Akt-signaling triggers invasion through distinct downstream effectors involving mTOR/p70S6K and Rac1 activation [25]. The relevance of p130Cas in ErbB2-dependent invasion was further assessed by identifying the coding and noncoding genes that are differentially expressed in p130Cas overexpressing and ErbB2 transformed invasive acini compared to ErbB2 transformed noninvasive multiacinar structures [42].

The study of the consequences ErbB2/Neu activation in *in vivo* mouse models has shown that overexpression of ErbB2 seems to be enough for the induction of metastatic mammary cancer

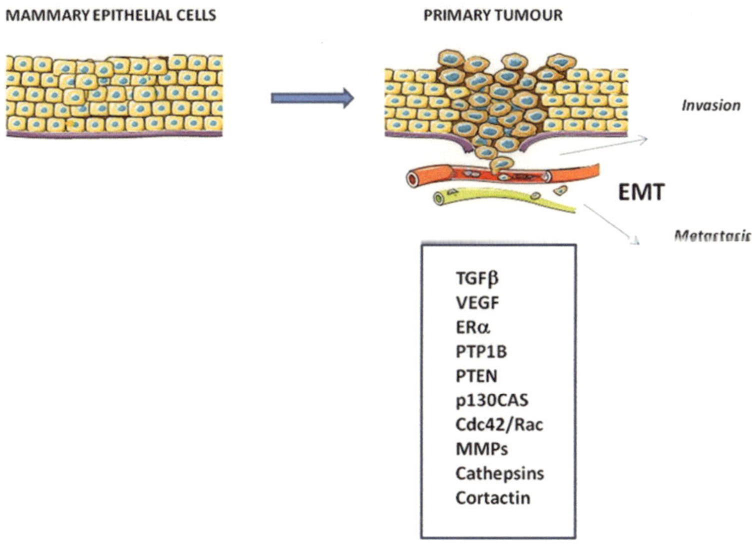

Figure 3. Erbb2 invasive signaling signature. ErbB2 activation impacts on EMT and cell invasion through the activation of a variety of downstream effectors.

[43]. However, there are several data demonstrating that ErbB2 cooperation with additional signaling effectors is crucial for cell transformation and invasion [22]. More recently, *in vivo* studies combining ErbB2/Neu with overexpression or knockout of different genes have led to the identification of several molecular targets that contribute to ErbB2-induced metastasis. These include molecules such as protein tyrosine phosphatase 1B (PTP1B), tensing homolog (PTEN), vascular adapter protein (VEGF), Gab2, EphA2 receptor tyrosine kinase, Rho GTPase activating protein p190B, receptor activator of nuclear factor- KB (RANK), estrogen receptor α, semaphorin receptor plexin-B1 and Rac-specific guanidine nucleotide exchange factor DOCK1. Altogether these studies reflect the complexity of the molecular mechanisms implicated in the regulation of invasion and metastasis by ErbB2 [31] (**Figure 3**).

4. Mechanisms of Erbb2—breast cancer therapy resistance

The assessment that ErbB2 overexpression correlates with aggressive breast cancer and poor survival has led to the development of targeted therapies to inhibit the receptor. Among them, the monoclonal antibody is trastuzumab and pertuzumab and the tyrosine kinase inhibitor is lapatinib [44]. Although ErbB2 overexpression identifies patients who are likely to respond to targeted therapy, not all of them benefit from the treatment. Indeed, many patients relapse after therapy due to the acquirement of primary or acquired resistance. Primary resistance might occur because of lack of target dependency or activation of compensatory pathways [45, 46]. Acquired resistance, which develops in most patients with advanced disease, may be due to the loss of the expression of the target because of continuous therapy, or to additional mutations that occur either in the target or on downstream signaling pathways that ultimately result in enhanced cell proliferation [47].

Many factors can contribute to resistance to ErbB2-targeted therapies. Among them, loss of ErbB2 amplification, compensatory mechanisms such as ErbB3 activation or the presence of p95ErbB2, a fragment of ErbB2 that cannot bind to trastuzumab as it lacks the extracellular part but can still activate the downstream pathways by retaining the ability to associate with ErbB2-signaling partners [44]. Additional factors that might be responsible for resistance to ErbB2-targeted therapies include aberrant activation of downstream signaling pathways due to mutations occurring during therapy, for example in the PI3K pathway [48, 49] or the activation of crosstalk with other receptor tyrosine kinases leading to compensatory mechanisms [50, 51].

In addition, poor internalization of ErbB2 resulting in a long half-life at the plasma membrane has been described as an important mechanism implicated in ErbB2 therapy resistance. In this context, it has been shown that Hsp90 inhibition can induce ErbB2 ubiquitination followed by its downregulation [52], however the mechanisms underlying ErbB2 downregulation are still obscure. Recently it has been demonstrated that molecular association between p130Cas and ErbB2 protects the receptor from degradation through autophagy [53]. On this regard, increasing evidence points out that ubiquitination is an important mechanism driving autophagic degradation. Interestingly, in breast cancer cells overexpressing ErbB2, p130Cas protects ErbB2 from autophagy-mediated degradation by interfering with its ubiquitination, thus suggesting that high levels of p130Cas expression might be crucial to promote resistance to trastuzumab treatment by protecting ErbB2 from degradation [53].

http://dx.doi.org/10.5772/66902

In conclusion, the unraveling of the molecular mechanisms responsible for resistance would greatly contribute to improve prognosis and outcomes for patients with ErbB2 tumors allowing a better selection of patients who are likely to respond to ErbB2-targeted therapies. Moreover, the dissection of the molecular pathways might reveal new insights for the development of strategies to overcome resistance.

4.1. Overcoming resistance to targeted therapy

Two main strategies have been adopted to try to overcome resistance to trastuzumab therapy. One strategy is still based on targeting ErbB2 either by maintaining trastuzumab therapy beyond progression, since it has been demonstrated that some patients could benefit of trastuzumab therapy with progressive disease [54, 55], or by treatment with TKI inhibitor lapatinib in combination with chemotherapy [56]. Another option is to treat trastuzumab resistant patients with the T-DM1. T-DM1 consists of an antibody (trastuzumab) conjugated with a microtubule inhibitor (maytansine derivative) with cytotoxic activity (developed by Genentech, Inc.).

At present, many new drugs targeting ErbB2 are undergoing clinical investigation in patients with ErbB2-resistant breast cancer overexpression. Since resistance to ErbB2-targeted therapy might occur as a result of aberrant activation of signaling pathways downstream to the receptor, the other strategy adopted to overcome resistance to trastuzumab is to target downstream signaling pathways known to be activated by ErbB2.

A major effort has been undertaken to inhibit the PI3K/Akt/mTOR pathway that, as mentioned before, is one of the most relevant downstream signaling activated by ErbB2. Indeed, alterations of PI3K/Akt pathway result in the upregulation of the mTOR pathway that in turn promotes translation and increased cellular proliferation [57, 58]. These signaling events have been characterized in breast cancer models in which the PI3K/Akt/mTOR axis is constitutively activated and responsible for the acquirement of resistance to ErbB2-targeted therapy [59]. It has been also described that the deregulation of this pathway accounts for gain of function mutations *PIK3CA* gene and/or mutations in AKT1, amplification of AKT2 and loss of PTEN [60]. The correlation between PTEN loss and trastuzumab and lapatinib resistance has also been reported [49, 61]. *PIK3CA* gene mutations acquired during disease progression are likely to reflect increased activation of the PI3K pathway and therefore suggest possible implications in resistance [47]. Consistently with this hypothesis, in vitro data show that ErbB2 gene amplification and *PI3KCA* gene mutations are associated with resistance to ErbB2-targeted agents [49, 62, 63] and PTEN loss or *PIK3CA* gene mutations have been linked to resistance to ErbB2 targeted therapy [48]. Since the serine/threonine kinase mTOR represents the final sensor of the ErbB2-dependent activation of the PI3K/AKT pathway and it is negatively regulated by PTEN, it is conceivable that targeting mTOR might be more efficacious than targeting multiple pathways with different strategies [48, 64] to interfere with tumor progression and to prevent resistance to ErbB2-targeted therapy. Consequently, several inhibitors of mTOR have been developed and tested in *in vitro* and *in vivo* models of trastuzumab resistance showing that the combined therapy (trastuzumab + mTOR inhibitor) was efficacious in inhibiting tumor growth [65]. The mTOR inhibitor everolimus is currently being tested in combination with trastuzumab and with different chemotherapeutic drugs in clinical studies to evaluate its potential in overcoming resistance to ErbB2-targeted therapy [66–68]. Besides inhibitors of the PI3K/Akt/mTOR pathways, additional inhibitors against other pathways or molecules known to play a role in ErbB2-resistance to targeted therapy have been developed. Among them IGFR, Hsp90, VEGF and telomerase inhibitors whose mechanisms of action and ongoing preclinical and clinical studies have been reviewed in [69].

Further ongoing characterization of the key effectors implicated in the resistance of ErbB2-targeted therapy might provide new efficacious pharmaceutics to improve or to overcome trastuzumab resistance.

5. Conclusion

Many progresses have been made in the understanding of the molecular mechanisms leading to the activation of ErbB2 and its downstream signaling pathways. Further studies are needed for a better comprehension of the mechanisms that lead to resistance to ErbB2-targeted treatment and especially to identify the crucial molecules deserving a therapeutic approach. New efforts have to be undertaken to see whether new modulators of ErbB2 such as miRNAs and adaptor proteins like p130Cas can be used as new therapeutic targets.

Acknowledgements

Research support to Sara Cabodi from AIRC IG11346, MIUR (FIRB giovani 2008 RBFR08F2FS) and Ricerca Sanitaria Finalizzata GR-20091543842. Maria del Pilar Camacho Leal is supported by an Umberto Veronesi Foundation Fellowship.

Abbreviations

AKT	protein kinase B (PKB)
DCIS	ductal carcinomas in situ
EGF	**R**epidermal growth factor receptor
EphA2	EPH receptor A2
ERK1/2	extracellular signal–regulated kinase 1/2
EMT	epithelial–mesenchymal transition
FAK	focal adhesion kinase
FoxC2	forkhead box protein C2
Gab2	GRB2-associated-binding protein 2

GRB2	growth factor receptor-bound protein 2
IGFR	insulin growth factor receptor
MAPK	mitogen-activated protein kinase 1
mTOR	mammalian target of rapamycin complex 1
PI3K	phosphoinositide 3-kinase
PTP1B	protein tyrosine phosphatase 1B
PTEN	phosphatase and tensin homolog
PLXNB1	plexin-B1
RANK	receptor activator of nuclear factor- KB
Rac	Ras-related C3 botulinum toxin substrate 1**RAF**
Rho	Ras homolog gene family, member A
Src	proto-oncogene tyrosine-protein kinase
SOS	adaptor protein son of sevenless
TGFbeta	transforming growth factor beta
TGFR-beta	transforming growth beta receptor
VEGF	vascular endothelial growth factor
ZEB1	zinc finger E-box-binding homeobox 1

Author details

Maria del Pilar Camacho-Leal*, Marianna Sciortino and Sara Cabodi

*Address all correspondence to: mariadelpilar.camacholeal@unito.it

Department of Molecular Biotechnology and Health Sciences, Molecular Biotechnology Center (MBC), University of Turin, Turin, Italy

References

[1] Kamangar F, Dores GM, Anderson WF: Patterns of cancer incidence, mortality and prevalence across five continents: defining priorities to reduce cancer disparities in different geographic regions of the world. *J Clin Oncol* 2006, **24**(14):2137–2150.

[2] Slamon DJ, Godolphin W, Jones LA, Holt JA, Wong SG, Keith DE, Levin WJ, Stuart SG, Udove J, Ullrich A et al.: Studies of the HER-2/neu proto-oncogene in human breast and ovarian cancer. *Science* 1989, **244**(4905):707–712.

[3] Feng C, Neumeister V, Ma W, Xu J, Lu L, Bordeaux J, Maihle NJ, Rimm DL, Huang Y: Lin28 regulates HER2 and promotes malignancy through multiple mechanisms. *Cell Cycle* 2012, **11**(13):2486–2494.

[4] Moody SE, Sarkisian CJ, Hahn KT, Gunther EJ, Pickup S, Dugan KD, Innocent N, Cardiff RD, Schnall MD, Chodosh LA: Conditional activation of Neu in the mammary epithelium of transgenic mice results in reversible pulmonary metastasis. *Cancer Cell* 2002, **2**(6):451–461.

[5] Raven JF, Williams V, Wang S, Tremblay ML, Muller WJ, Durbin JE, Koromilas AE: Stat1 is a suppressor of ErbB2/Neu-mediated cellular transformation and mouse mammary gland tumor formation. *Cell Cycle* 2011, **10**(5):794–804.

[6] Tan M, Yao J, Yu D: Overexpression of the c-erbB-2 gene enhanced intrinsic metastasis potential in human breast cancer cells without increasing their transformation abilities. *Cancer Res* 1997, **57**(6):1199–1205.

[7] Liu E, Thor A, He M, Barcos M, Ljung BM, Benz C: The HER2 (c-erbB-2) oncogene is frequently amplified in in situ carcinomas of the breast. *Oncogene* 1992, **7**(5):1027–1032.

[8] Feigin ME, Muthuswamy SK: ErbB receptors and cell polarity: new pathways and paradigms for understanding cell migration and invasion. *Exp Cell Res* 2009, **315**(4):707–716.

[9] Baselga J: Treatment of HER2-overexpressing breast cancer. *Ann Oncol* 2010, **21 Suppl 7**:vii36–40.

[10] Emde A, Kostler WJ, Yarden Y: Therapeutic strategies and mechanisms of tumorigenesis of HER2-overexpressing breast cancer. *Crit Rev Oncol Hematol* 2012, **84 Suppl 1**: e49–57.

[11] Valabrega G, Montemurro F, Aglietta M: Trastuzumab: mechanism of action, resistance and future perspectives in HER2-overexpressing breast cancer. *Ann Oncol* 2007, **18**(6):977–984.

[12] Schulz R, Streller F, Scheel AH, Ruschoff J, Reinert MC, Dobbelstein M, Marchenko ND, Moll UM: HER2/ErbB2 activates HSF1 and thereby controls HSP90 clients including MIF in HER2-overexpressing breast cancer. *Cell Death Dis* 2014, **5**:e980.

[13] Kufe DW: MUC1-C oncoprotein as a target in breast cancer: activation of signaling pathways and therapeutic approaches. *Oncogene* 2013, **32**(9):1073–1081.

[14] Eisenberg A, Biener E, Charlier M, Krishnan RV, Djiane J, Herman B, Gertler A: Transactivation of erbB2 by short and long isoforms of leptin receptors. *FEBS Lett* 2004, **565**(1–3):139–142.

[15] Dittrich A, Gautrey H, Browell D, Tyson-Capper A: The HER2 signaling network in breast cancer--like a spider in its web. *J Mammary Gland Biol Neoplasia* 2014, **19**(3–4):253–270.

[16] Lemmon MA, Schlessinger J: Cell signaling by receptor tyrosine kinases. *Cell* 2010, **141**(7):1117–1134.

[17] Aksamitiene E, Kiyatkin A, Kholodenko BN: Cross-talk between mitogenic Ras/MAPK and survival PI3K/Akt pathways: a fine balance. *Biochem Soc Trans* 2012, **40**(1):139–146.

[18] De Luca A, Maiello MR, D'Alessio A, Pergameno M, Normanno N: The RAS/RAF/MEK/ERK and the PI3K/AKT signaling pathways: role in cancer pathogenesis and implications for therapeutic approaches. *Expert Opin Ther Targets* 2012, **16 Suppl 2**:S17–27.

[19] Romeo Y, Zhang X, Roux PP: Regulation and function of the RSK family of protein kinases. *Biochem J* 2012, **441**(2):553–569.

[20] Fruman DA, Rommel C: PI3K and cancer: lessons, challenges and opportunities. *Nat Rev Drug Discov* 2014, **13**(2):140–156.

[21] Castaneda CA, Cortes-Funes H, Gomez HL, Ciruelos EM: The phosphatidyl inositol 3-kinase/AKT signaling pathway in breast cancer. *Cancer Metastasis Rev* 2010, **29**(4):751–759.

[22] Cabodi S, del Pilar Camacho-Leal M, Di Stefano P, Defilippi P: Integrin signaling adaptors: not only figurants in the cancer story. *Nat Rev Cancer* 2010, **10**(12):858–870.

[23] Defilippi P, Di Stefano P, Cabodi S: p130Cas: a versatile scaffold in signaling networks. *TrenWds Cell Biol* 2006, **16**(5):257–263.

[24] Cabodi S, Tinnirello A, Bisaro B, Tornillo G, del Pilar Camacho-Leal M, Forni G, Cojoca R, Iezzi M, Amici A, Montani M *et al*: p130Cas is an essential transducer element in ErbB2 transformation. *FASEB J* 2010, **24**(10):3796–3808.

[25] Tornillo G, Bisaro B, Camacho-Leal Mdel P, Galie M, Provero P, Di Stefano P, Turco E, Defilippi P, Cabodi S: p130Cas promotes invasiveness of three-dimensional ErbB2-transformed mammary acinar structures by enhanced activation of mTOR/p70S6K and Rac1. *Eur J Cell Biol* 2011, **90**(2–3):237–248.

[26] Cabodi S, Tinnirello A, Di Stefano P, Bisaro B, Ambrosino E, Castellano I, Sapino A, Arisio R, Cavallo F, Forni G *et al*: p130Cas as a new regulator of mammary epithelial cell proliferation, survival and HER2-neu oncogene-dependent breast tumorigenesis. *Cancer Res* 2006, **66**(9):4672–4680.

[27] Wang SE, Lin RJ: MicroRNA and HER2-overexpressing cancer. *Microrna* 2013, **2**(2):137–147.

[28] Scott GK, Goga A, Bhaumik D, Berger CE, Sullivan CS, Benz CC: Coordinate suppression of ERBB2 and ERBB3 by enforced expression of micro-RNA miR-125a or miR-125b. *J Biol Chem* 2007, **282**(2):1479–1486.

[29] Lowery AJ, Miller N, Devaney A, McNeill RE, Davoren PA, Lemetre C, Benes V, Schmidt S, Blake J, Ball G et al.: MicroRNA signatures predict oestrogen receptor, progesterone receptor and HER2/neu receptor status in breast cancer. *Breast Cancer Res* 2009, **11**(3):R27.

[30] Mattie MD, Benz CC, Bowers J, Sensinger K, Wong L, Scott GK, Fedele V, Ginzinger D, Getts R, Haqq C: Optimized high-throughput microRNA expression profiling provides novel biomarker assessment of clinical prostate and breast cancer biopsies. *Mol Cancer* 2006, **5**:24.

[31] Brix DM, Clemmensen KK, Kallunki T: When good turns bad: regulation of invasion and metastasis by ErbB2 receptor tyrosine kinase. *Cells* 2014, **3**(1):53–78.

[32] Lamouille S, Xu J, Derynck R: Molecular mechanisms of epithelial-mesenchymal transition. *Nat Rev Mol Cell Biol* 2014, **15**(3):178–196.

[33] Appert-Collin A, Hubert P, Cremel G, Bennasroune A: Role of ErbB Receptors in Cancer Cell Migration and Invasion. *Front Pharmacol* 2015, **6**:283.

[34] Mallini P, Lennard T, Kirby J, Meeson A: Epithelial-to-mesenchymal transition: what is the impact on breast cancer stem cells and drug resistance. *Cancer Treat Rev* 2014, **40**(3):341–348.

[35] Creighton CJ, Li X, Landis M, Dixon JM, Neumeister VM, Sjolund A, Rimm DL, Wong H, Rodriguez A, Herschkowitz JI *et al*: Residual breast cancers after conventional therapy display mesenchymal as well as tumor-initiating features. *Proc Natl Acad Sci U S A* 2009, **106**(33):13820–13825.

[36] Morel AP, Lievre M, Thomas C, Hinkal G, Ansieau S, Puisieux A: Generation of breast cancer stem cells through epithelial-mesenchymal transition. *PLoS One* 2008, **3**(8):e2888.

[37] Korkaya H, Paulson A, Iovino F, Wicha MS: HER2 regulates the mammary stem/progenitor cell population driving tumorigenesis and invasion. *Oncogene* 2008, **27**(47):6120–6130.

[38] Wang SE, Shin I, Wu FY, Friedman DB, Arteaga CL: HER2/Neu (ErbB2) signaling to Rac1-Pak1 is temporally and spatially modulated by transforming growth factor beta. *Cancer Res* 2006, **66**(19):9591–9600.

[39] Arias-Romero LE, Villamar-Cruz O, Pacheco A, Kosoff R, Huang M, Muthuswamy SK, Chernoff J: A Rac-Pak signaling pathway is essential for ErbB2-mediated transformation of human breast epithelial cancer cells. *Oncogene* 2010, **29**(43):5839–5849.

[40] Rafn B, Nielsen CF, Andersen SH, Szyniarowski P, Corcelle-Termeau E, Valo E, Fehrenbacher N, Olsen CJ, Daugaard M, Egebjerg C et al.: ErbB2-driven breast cancer cell invasion depends on a complex signaling network activating myeloid zinc finger-1-dependent cathepsin B expression. *Mol Cell* 2012, **45**(6):764–776.

[41] Muthuswamy SK, Li D, Lelievre S, Bissell MJ, Brugge JS: ErbB2, but not ErbB1, reinitiates proliferation and induces luminal repopulation in epithelial acini. *Nat Cell Biol* 2001, **3**(9):785–792.

[42] Pincini A, Tornillo G, Orso F, Sciortino M, Bisaro B, Leal Mdel P, Lembo A, Brizzi MF, Turco E, De Pitta C et al.: Identification of p130Cas/ErbB2-dependent invasive signatures in transformed mammary epithelial cells. *Cell Cycle* 2013, **12**(15):2409–2422.

[43] Ursini-Siegel J, Schade B, Cardiff RD, Muller WJ: Insights from transgenic mouse models of ERBB2-induced breast cancer. *Nat Rev Cancer* 2007, **7**(5):389–397.

[44] Wilks ST: Potential of overcoming resistance to HER2-targeted therapies through the PI3K/Akt/mTOR pathway. *Breast* 2015, **24**(5):548–555.

[45] Higgins MJ, Baselga J: Targeted therapies for breast cancer. *J Clin Invest* 2011, **121**(10):3797–3803.

[46] Rexer BN, Arteaga CL: Intrinsic and acquired resistance to HER2-targeted therapies in HER2 gene-amplified breast cancer: mechanisms and clinical implications. *Crit Rev Oncog* 2012, **17**(1):1–16.

[47] Hurvitz SA, Hu Y, O'Brien N, Finn RS: Current approaches and future directions in the treatment of HER2-positive breast cancer. *Cancer Treat Rev* 2013, **39**(3):219–229.

[48] Berns K, Horlings HM, Hennessy BT, Madiredjo M, Hijmans EM, Beelen K, Linn SC, Gonzalez-Angulo AM, Stemke-Hale K, Hauptmann M et al.: A functional genetic approach identifies the PI3K pathway as a major determinant of trastuzumab resistance in breast cancer. *Cancer Cell* 2007, **12**(4):395–402.

[49] Eichhorn PJ, Gili M, Scaltriti M, Serra V, Guzman M, Nijkamp W, Beijersbergen RL, Valero V, Seoane J, Bernards R *et al*: Phosphatidylinositol 3-kinase hyperactivation results in lapatinib resistance that is reversed by the mTOR/phosphatidylinositol 3-kinase inhibitor NVP-BEZ235. *Cancer Res* 2008, **68**(22):9221–9230.

[50] Bender LM, Nahta R: Her2 cross talk and therapeutic resistance in breast cancer. *Front Biosci* 2008, **13**:3906–3912.

[51] Nahta R, Yuan LX, Zhang B, Kobayashi R, Esteva FJ: Insulin-like growth factor-I receptor/human epidermal growth factor receptor 2 heterodimerization contributes to trastuzumab resistance of breast cancer cells. *Cancer Res* 2005, **65**(23):11118–11128.

[52] Bertelsen V, Stang E: The mysterious ways of ErbB2/HER2 trafficking. *Membranes (Basel)* 2014, **4**(3):424–446.

[53] Bisaro B, Sciortino M, Colombo S, Camacho Leal MP, Costamagna A, Castellano I, Montemurro F, Rossi V, Valabrega G, Turco E et al.: p130Cas scaffold protein regulates ErbB2 stability by altering breast cancer cell sensitivity to autophagy. *Oncotarget* 2016, **7**(4):4442–4453.

[54] Mannocci A, De Feo E, de Waure C, Specchia ML, Gualano MR, Barone C, Ricciardi W, La Torre G: Use of trastuzumab in HER2-positive metastatic breast cancer beyond disease progression: a systematic review of published studies. *Tumori* 2010, **96**(3):385–391.

[55] Petrelli F, Barni S: A pooled analysis of 2618 patients treated with trastuzumab beyond progression for advanced breast cancer. *Clin Breast Cancer* 2013, **13**(2):81–87.

[56] Geyer CE, Forster J, Lindquist D, Chan S, Romieu CG, Pienkowski T, Jagiello-Gruszfeld A, Crown J, Chan A, Kaufman B et al.: Lapatinib plus capecitabine for HER2-positive advanced breast cancer. *N Engl J Med* 2006, **355**(26):2733–2743.

[57] Burris HA, 3rd: Overcoming acquired resistance to anticancer therapy: focus on the PI3K/AKT/mTOR pathway. *Cancer Chemother Pharmacol* 2013, **71**(4):829–842.

[58] Yuan R, Kay A, Berg WJ, Lebwohl D: Targeting tumorigenesis: development and use of mTOR inhibitors in cancer therapy. *J Hematol Oncol* 2009, **2**:45.

[59] Keck S, Glencer AC, Rugo HS: Everolimus and its role in hormone-resistant and trastuzumab-resistant metastatic breast cancer. *Future Oncol* 2012, **8**(11):1383–1396.

[60] Mayer I: Role of mTOR inhibition in preventing resistance and restoring sensitivity to hormone-targeted and HER2-targeted therapies in breast cancer. *Clin Adv Hematol Oncol* 2013, **11**(4):217–224.

[61] O'Brien NA, Browne BC, Chow L, Wang Y, Ginther C, Arboleda J, Duffy MJ, Crown J, O'Donovan N, Slamon DJ: Activated phosphoinositide 3-kinase/AKT signaling confers resistance to trastuzumab but not lapatinib. *Mol Cancer Ther* 2010, **9**(6):1489–1502.

[62] Kataoka Y, Mukohara T, Shimada H, Saijo N, Hirai M, Minami H: Association between gain-of-function mutations in PIK3CA and resistance to HER2-targeted agents in HER2-amplified breast cancer cell lines. *Ann Oncol* 2010, **21**(2):255–262.

[63] Rexer BN, Chanthaphaychith S, Dahlman K, Arteaga CL: Direct inhibition of PI3K in combination with dual HER2 inhibitors is required for optimal antitumor activity in HER2+ breast cancer cells. *Breast Cancer Res* 2014, **16**(1):R9.

[64] Whenham N, D'Hondt V, Piccart MJ: HER2-positive breast cancer: from trastuzumab to innovatory anti-HER2 strategies. *Clin Breast Cancer* 2008, **8**(1):38–49.

[65] Miller TW, Forbes JT, Shah C, Wyatt SK, Manning HC, Olivares MG, Sanchez V, Dugger TC, de Matos Granja N, Narasanna A *et al*: Inhibition of mammalian target of rapamycin is required for optimal antitumor effect of HER2 inhibitors against HER2-overexpressing cancer cells. *Clin Cancer Res* 2009, **15**(23):7266–7276.

[66] Andre F, Campone M, O'Regan R, Manlius C, Massacesi C, Sahmoud T, Mukhopadhyay P, Soria JC, Naughton M, Hurvitz SA: Phase I study of everolimus plus weekly paclitaxel and trastuzumab in patients with metastatic breast cancer pretreated with trastuzumab. *J Clin Oncol* 2010, **28**(34):5110–5115.

[67] Hurvitz SA, Dalenc F, Campone M, O'Regan RM, Tjan-Heijnen VC, Gligorov J, Llombart A, Jhangiani H, Mirshahidi HR, Tan-Chiu E *et al*: A phase 2 study of everolimus combined with trastuzumab and paclitaxel in patients with HER2-overexpressing advanced breast cancer that progressed during prior trastuzumab and taxane therapy. *Breast Cancer Res Treat* 2013, **141**(3):437–446.

http://dx.doi.org/10.5772/66902

[68] Jerusalem G, Fasolo A, Dieras V, Cardoso F, Bergh J, Vittori L, Zhang Y, Massacesi C, Sahmoud T, Gianni L: Phase I trial of oral mTOR inhibitor everolimus in combination with trastuzumab and vinorelbine in pre-treated patients with HER2-overexpressing metastatic breast cancer. *Breast Cancer Res Treat* 2011, **125**(2):447–455.

[69] Brufsky AM: Current approaches and emerging directions in HER2-resistant breast cancer. *Breast Cancer (Auckl)* 2014, **8**:109–118.

Chapter 9

Analysis of 10086 Microarray Gene Expression Data Uncovers Genes that Subclassify Breast Cancer Intrinsic Subtypes

I-Hsuan Lin and Ming-Ta Hsu

Additional information is available at the end of the chapter

http://dx.doi.org/10.5772/66161

Abstract

Breast cancer is a complex disease comprising molecularly distinct subtypes. The prognosis and treatment differ between subtypes; thus, it is important to distinguish one subtype from another. In this chapter, we make use of high-throughput microarray dataset to perform breast cancer subtyping of 10086 samples. Aside from the four major subtypes, that is, Basal-like, HER2-enriched, luminal A, and luminal B, we defined a normal-like subtype that has a gene expression profile similar to that found in normal and adjacent normal breast samples. Also, a group of luminal B-like samples with better prognosis was distinguished from the high-risk luminal B breast cancer. We additionally identified 33 surface-protein encoding genes whose gene expression profiles were associated with survival outcomes. We believe these genes are potential therapeutic targets and diagnostic biomarkers for breast cancer.

Keywords: breast cancer, intrinsic subtypes, gene expression, microarray, survival analysis

1. Introduction

In many countries, breast cancer remains the most common cancer among women and one of the top leading causes of cancer death in women. Multiple efforts and studies have been directed toward the understanding of the cause and mechanisms leading to breast cancer and to improve the diagnosis and treatment of this disease. To aid its identification and treatment, breast cancer is divided into four major molecular subtypes [luminal A (LumA), luminal B

(LumB), HER2-enriched (HER2E), and basal-like (BasalL)] according to hormone receptor status assessed by immunohistochemistry (IHC) [1, 2].

The luminal types are estrogen receptor positive cancers, and their gene expression patterns are similar to the luminal epithelial cells that line the breast ducts and glands. They can be treated with endocrine therapy and chemotherapy. Luminal A is a low-grade cancer that has the best prognosis, high survival rates and low recurrence rates compared to other subtypes [3]. Patients with luminal B cancer tend to have poorer prognosis and lower survival rates than those with luminal A cancer. In HER2-enriched cancer, the HER2 gene is often overexpressed due to gene duplication. This type of breast cancer is high-grade and fast-growing. Before the discovery of anti-HER2 drugs such as trastuzumab and lapatinib [4, 5], the treatment for patent of this subtype is limited to chemotherapeutic approaches. The other major subtype is the basal-like breast cancer. The gene expression pattern of basal-like breast cancer is similar to cells in the basal layers of the breast ductal epithelium. Many cases of basal-like breast cancer are also triple-negative breast cancer, which lack estrogen or progesterone receptors and without elevated expression of *HER2*. The basal-like breast cancer is also high-grade and fast-growing. Patients diagnosed with this subtype have poorer prognosis and are treated with combination of surgery, radiotherapy and anthracycline/taxane-based chemotherapy [6].

After the launch of microarray in the early 2000s as an affordable solution to high-throughput quantification of genome-wide gene expression, many research projects begin to use this technology to study breast cancer [7–9]. Findings derived from microarray studies provide useful biological, prognostic, and predictive information in basic science and clinical practice. One of the applications resulting from microarray analysis is the reclassification of breast cancer samples according to the gene expression patterns of multiple genes [10].

In this chapter, we present our method of analyzing large public breast cancer microarray datasets and discuss our findings concerning breast cancer subtyping using gene expression signatures. By thoroughly gathering of microarray datasets, we collected gene expression results of 10086 normal breast and breast cancer samples from public depositories. We took advantage of the large sample size to explore the similarities and differences among and within breast cancer subtypes. Through the clustering of this large breast cancer dataset, our aim is to update the subtype labels of these samples and re-define the intrinsic subtypes of breast cancer, as well as to identify genes whose expression profiles are not subtype-specific but can subclassify samples within a given subtype and with prognostic values. By analyzing the functional subgroups of human genes through consensus clustering, we identified specific genes that can subdivide breast cancer subtype and provided useful prognostic information as well as possible genetic clues for breast carcinogenesis.

2. Processing of gene expression microarray datasets

We explored the two largest public repositories, NCBI GEO (https://www.ncbi.nlm.nih.gov/geo) and EBI ArrayExpress (http://www.ebi.ac.uk/arrayexpress) for gene expression microarray datasets relating to normal breast tissues and breast cancers. Different microarray platforms produce variations in the final interpretation of gene expression levels due to differences in probe design and detection methods. We chose to obtain experiment conducted using the Human Genome U133A (HG-U133A) and Human Genome U133 Plus 2.0 (HG-U133 Plus 2.0) arrays, as these are the most widely used platforms we found in the databases. Overall, we identified 41 HG-U133A and 62 HG-U133 Plus 2.0 datasets relating to our topic of interest. Redundant and irrelevant arrays were identified and removed. 4952 HG-U133A and 5134 HG-U133 Plus 2.0 arrays, representing 165 normal breast, 193 adjacent disease-free, 5 proliferative breast lesions, and 9723 breast cancer samples, were selected for downstream analysis. The clinicopathological data associated with the samples were also retrieved at the same time if available. In **Supplementary Table 1**, we list the accession numbers associated with the dataset we collect and used in this study.

Accession No.	HG-U133A	HG-U133 Plus 2.0
E-MEXP-882	0	24
E-MEXP-3688	0	8
E-MTAB-365	0	536
E-MTAB-566	0	36
E-MTAB-748	0	46
E-MTAB-1006	0	96
E-MTAB-1547	0	208
E-MTAB-2501	0	32
E-TABM-43	35	0
E-TABM-66	0	6
E-TABM-276	0	60
E-TABM-854	0	73
GSE1456	159	0
GSE1561	46	0
GSE2034	286	0
GSE2109	0	346
GSE2603	99	0
GSE3494	251	0
GSE3744	0	47
GSE4611	216	0
GSE4922	287	0

Accession No.	HG-U133A	HG-U133 Plus 2.0
GSE5327	58	0
GSE5462	54	0
GSE5764	0	18
GSE5847	92	0
GSE6532	327	87
GSE6596	26	0
GSE6883	7	0
GSE7307	0	10
GSE7390	196	0
GSE7904	0	62
GSE8977	0	22
GSE9195	0	77
GSE9574	3	0
GSE10780	0	177
GSE11121	198	0
GSE12093	134	0
GSE12276	0	204
GSE12763	0	30
GSE16391	0	55
GSE16446	0	112
GSE16873	11	0
GSE17705	293	0
GSE17907	0	53
GSE18864	0	2
GSE19615	0	115
GSE20086	0	5
GSE20194	265	0
GSE20271	174	0
GSE20437	25	0
GSE20685	0	326
GSE20711	0	88

Accession No.	HG-U133A	HG-U133 Plus 2.0
GSE21422	0	19
GSE21653	0	254
GSE21947	10	0
GSE22035	0	43
GSE22093	102	0
GSE22513	0	16
GSE22544	0	18
GSE23177	0	116
GSE23720	0	191
GSE23988	59	0
GSE24185	100	0
GSE25011	11	0
GSE25066	506	0
GSE26910	0	11
GSE26971	277	0
GSE28796	0	14
GSE28821	0	10
GSE29431	0	38
GSE31448	0	29
GSE31519	67	0
GSE32072	28	0
GSE36771	0	107
GSE36772	96	0
GSE36773	48	0
GSE37946	49	0
GSE38506	0	13
GSE42568	0	112
GSE43358	0	57
GSE43365	0	111
GSE43502	0	10
GSE45255	134	0

Accession No.	HG-U133A	HG-U133 Plus 2.0
GSE46184	74	0
GSE46222	0	46
GSE46928	50	0
GSE47389	0	47
GSE48390	0	80
GSE50567	0	40
GSE50948	0	5
GSE54002	0	418
GSE55594	0	10
GSE58812	0	107
GSE61304	0	61
GSE63626	0	6
GSE65194	0	162
GSE68892	99	0
GSE70233	0	22

Supplementary Table 1. Gene expression microarray datasets used.

Due to the different array design and number of probes of HG-U133A and HG-U133 Plus 2.0, the raw data files (.CEL) of the two platforms were imported into the R environment separately. The raw data were normalized using the justRMA function from the affy Bioconductor package with the Robust Multiarray Averaging (RMA) normalization method [11]. The default hgu133a and hgu133plus2 annotation were used to obtain probe-level expression intensities. The intensity of a probe is used to represent the corresponding gene-level expression value. For any given gene detected by more than one probe sets, the probe set with the highest Jetset score is selected to represent its gene-level expression [12]. Then, inSilicoMerging package was used to combine expression intensities from the two microarray platforms and remove batch effect to obtain log2-normalized intensities [13].

3. Identification of differentially expressed genes among subsets of samples

Some of the samples were provided with relevant clinicopathological data. We used this information to perform differential expression analysis using the limma Bioconductor package in R [14]. Specifically, we used disease status (normal vs. cancer), receptor status assessed by IHC, and the subtype classification to subset samples and performed differential expression analysis. The aim was to identify a list of candidate genes from these comparisons to be used in breast cancer subtyping. Seven categories of differentially expressed genes sets were defined. They are:

a. Normal versus cancer: *ABCA8, ADH1B, ASPM, AURKA, BUB1B, CCNB1, CCNB2, CDC20, CDK1, CENPA, CEP55, CKS2, COL10A1, CXCL10, CXCL11, CXCL2, CXCL9, DLGAP5, DTL, FABP4, FOSB, GABRP, ID4, KRT14, KRT15, KRT5, MELK, MMP1, NEK2, NUSAP1, OXTR, PBK, PRC1, PTN, RRM2, S100P, SFRP1, SPP1, SYNM, TGFBR3, TOP2A, TPX2, UBE2C*, and *WIF1*.

b. Basal-like: *AGR2, CA12, DHRS2, ELF5, EN1, ESR1, FABP7, FOXA1, GABRP, GATA3, KRT6B, MLPH, NAT1, PIP, PROM1, ROPN1B, SCGB1D2, SCGB2A2, SCNN1A, TFF1, TFF3, TOX3*, and *VGLL1*.

c. HER2-enriched: *CALML5, CEACAM6, CLCA2, CRISP3, ERBB2, ESR1, FGG, GRB7, KMO, KYNU, NPY1R, PGAP3, PNMT, S100A8, S100A9, S100P, SCUBE2, STARD3*, and *TFAP2B*.

d. Luminal A: *ABAT, AGR2, AGTR1, BMPR1B, CA12, CPB1, DACH1, ERBB4, ESR1, FABP7, GATA3, GFRA1, GREB1, IGF1R, MMP1, NAT1, NPY1R, PGR, PROM1, RARRES1, S100A8, SCUBE2, SERPINA3, STC2, TBC1D9, TFF1*, and *TFF3*.

e. Luminal B: *AGR2, ARMT1, CA12, DHRS2, ESR1, FABP7, GABRP, GATA3, KRT6B, NAT1, PROM1, SFRP1, SLPI, TFF1*, and *TFF3*.

f. Luminal C: *COL10A1, CXCL9, ESR1, FABP7, GABRP, GATA3, IFI44L, SCGB2A2*, and *TFF1*.

g. Apocrine: *CALML5, CLCA2, CPB1, CRISP3, ERBB4, ESR1, IGF1R, KYNU, MMP1, NPY1R, S100A8, S100A9, SERPINA3*, and *TFF1*.

Some of the genes were identified in more than one category, for example the estrogen receptor 1 (*ESR1*) was found in six of the seven categories. The redundant genes were removed, and the remaining 100 unique genes were used to perform sample subtyping with consensus clustering.

4. Consensus hierarchical clustering using subtype-specific genes

The ConsensusClusterPlus Bioconductor package was used to perform consensus hierarchical clustering on the 10086 samples using the expression intensities of the 100 genes discovered in the previous step [15]. The distance metric used in the clustering was calculated as one minus the Pearson correlation coefficient. The parameters used were: maxK = 6, reps = 1000, pItem = 0.8, pFeature = 1, whereby the clustering was performed 1000 times using the expression of all the genes of randomly selected samples consisting of 80% of the total sample size and with a maximum of six clusters. **Figure 1** shows the cumulative distribution functions (CDFs) of the consensus matrix for each number of clusters (i.e. $k = 2$ to $k = 6$) on the left and relative change in area under the CDF curves on the right. Both plots were used to help determine the appropriate number of clusters to be selected.

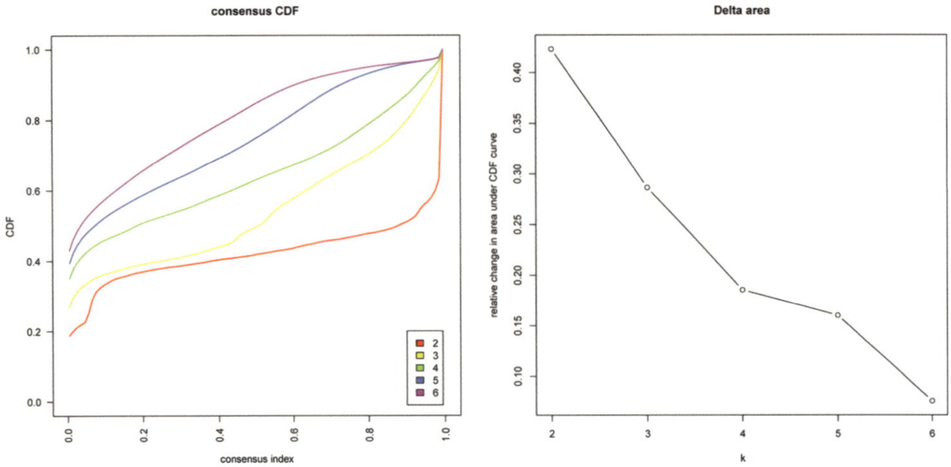

Figure 1. Analysis of breast cancer gene expression cluster stability. The optimum partitioning of breast cancers is determined with (left) consensus CDF and (right) Delta area plots for cluster between $k = 2$ and $k = 6$. The optimal choice of cluster number is 6 whereby the CDF curve is reaching a plateau and has minimal relative change in area under CDF curves.

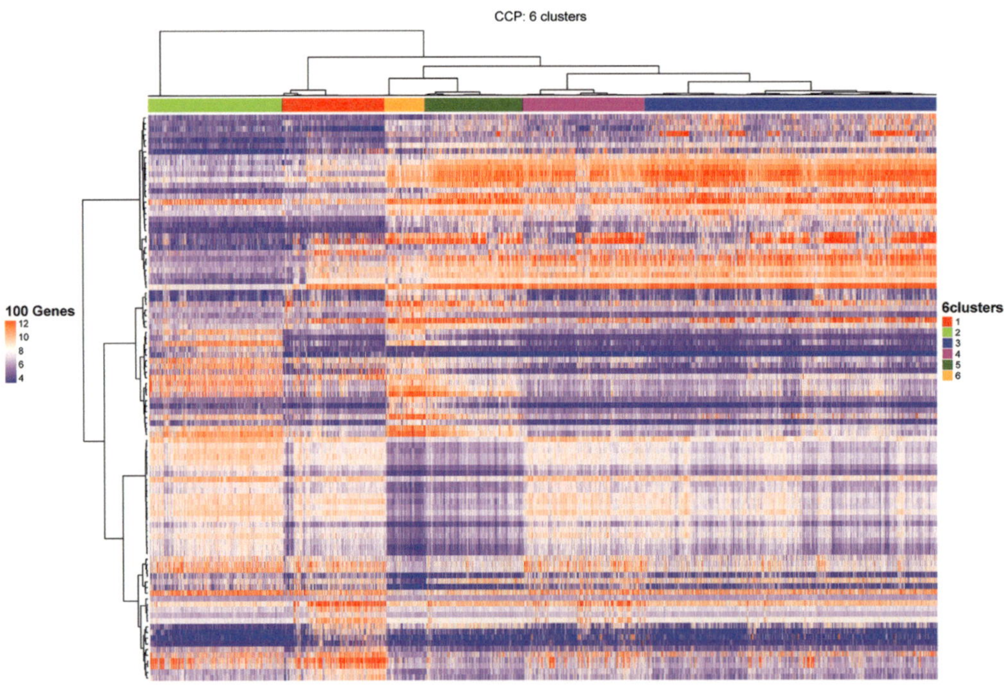

Figure 2. Consensus clustering of 10086 samples using the expression profile of 100 genes. The color of each cell of the matrix represents the gene expression intensity a sample (column) of a given genes (row). The red and blue colors reflect high and low expression levels, respectively, as indicated in the color bar. Samples with similar gene expression profiles are grouped together and distributed into six clusters (colored bars).

We assigned the six clusters with names correspond to convention breast cancer subtypes. To visualize the classification result, we used the ComplexHeatmap Bioconductor package to produce heatmap representation of the clustering result [16]. The six clusters were represented with different colors in the heatmap shown in **Figure 2**, and they are HER2-enriched (HER2E; leftmost), basal-like (BasalL), normal-like (NormL), luminal A (LumA), luminal B (LumB), and mixed luminal (LumMix; rightmost). The clinical features of the six clusters were presented in **Table 1**. The mixed luminal cancer has the most number of samples, and the normal-like cancer has the fewest samples. The patients of the basal-like cancer were significantly younger (median age at diagnosis 49; *t* test *P*-value < 2.2e−16), and the mixed luminal patients were significantly older (median age at diagnosis 56; *t* test *P*-value = 4.3e−15). These are consistent with previous reports [17–19].

	BasalL	HER2E	LumA	LumB	LumMix	NormL
No. of samples	1727	1330	1251	1533	3735	510
Age range	24–84	26–90	27–88	24–93	24–91	21–86
Median age	49	55	54	53	56	51
ER status by IHC						
No. of ER+	106	157	710	831	2271	101
No. of ER−	1085	614	83	114	77	73
ER+:ER−	1:10.24	1:3.91	1:0.12	1:0.14	1:0.03	1:0.72
Missing ER data	536 (31.0%)	559 (42.0%)	458 (36.6%)	588 (38.4%)	1387 (37.1%)	336 (65.9%)
PR status by IHC						
No. of PR+	44	60	383	315	1061	56
No. of PR−	657	436	104	200	219	48
PR+:PR−	1:14.93	1:7.27	1:0.27	1:0.63	1:0.21	1:0.86
Missing PR data	1026 (59.4%)	834 (62.7%)	764 (61.1%)	1018 (66.4%)	2455 (65.7%)	406 (79.6%)
HER2 status by IHC						
No. of HER2+	49	302	35	174	100	14
No. of HER2−	861	222	285	391	1050	93
HER2+:HER2−	1:17.57	1:0.74	1:8.14	1:2.25	1:10.50	1:6.64
Missing HER2 data	817 (47.3%)	806 (60.6%)	931 (74.4%)	968 (63.1%)	2585 (69.2%)	403 (79.0%)

Table 1. Clinical features of the six clusters.

We compared the subtype assignment by ConsensusClusterPlus with the molecular subtyping by PAM50, SSP2006 and AIMS models using the genefu Bioconductor package (see **Tables 2–4**) [20]. The comparisons showed the four major breast cancer subtypes were present in our analysis. The concordances between different methods on the HER2-enriched and basal-like subtype were higher than other subtypes. The classification of luminal subtypes and normal-like samples were more inconsistent. Based on the heatmap and structure of the dendrogram shown in **Figure 2**, the transcriptome profiles of HER2-enriched and basal-like breast cancers were more distinctive compared to other subtypes. Hence, the clustering results of these two subtypes were more consistent than other subtypes using different methods. The ConsensusClusterPlus assignment is most similar to that produced by the PAM50 model, whereas SSP2006 and AIMS models have classified many samples as HER2-enriched but were determined as luminal B subtype using our method. The major difference between the ConsensusClusterPlus and PAM50 assignment is that our method identified a large subgroup within the luminal subtypes, which we defined it as mixed luminal, that were classified as either luminal A or luminal B by the PAM50 model. We think the increase in the number of samples, as well as selection of different gene candidates, used in our study helped to distinguish and define three luminal subtypes rather than two. The implication of this distinction is rather profound. Although the mixed luminal breast cancers have similar gene expression profile to the luminal B subtype as seen in **Figure 2**, we showed in the next section that the two subgroups vary in their survival outcomes.

Subtype comparison		**PAM50**				
		BasalL	**HER2E**	**LumA**	**LumB**	**NormL**
ConsensusClusterPlus	**HER2E**	141	909	58	127	51
	BasalL	1686	7	0	3	25
	LumMix	3	22	1686	2004	15
	LumB	6	175	81	1269	2
	LumA	3	1	1187	12	41
	NormL	7	0	73	0	134

Table 2. Comparison of molecular subtyping by ConsensusClusterPlus and PAM50.

Subtype comparison		**SSP2006**				
		BasalL	**HER2E**	**LumA**	**LumB**	**NormL**
ConsensusClusterPlus	**HER2E**	263	833	53	6	131
	BasalL	1695	2	0	0	24
	LumMix	10	109	2882	625	104
	LumB	23	541	441	505	23
	LumA	5	1	1036	0	202
	NormL	0	0	40	0	174

Table 3. Comparison of molecular subtyping by ConsensusClusterPlus and SSP2006.

Subtype comparison		**AIMS**				
		BasalL	**HER2E**	**LumA**	**LumB**	**NormL**
ConsensusClusterPlus	**HER2E**	384	789	4	1	108
	BasalL	1699	3	0	0	19
	LumMix	9	400	1511	1489	321
	LumB	27	936	30	526	14
	LumA	5	10	275	5	949
	NormL	1	0	0	0	213

Table 4. Comparison of molecular subtyping by ConsensusClusterPlus and AIMS.

5. Survival analysis of breast cancer subtypes

We used the Kaplan-Meier method to estimate the survival curves of overall survival (OS), relapse-free survival (RFS) and distant metastasis-free survival (DMFS). The gene expression values were converted to expression status using a modified R script taken from the Kaplan Meier-plotter website (http://kmplot.com/). The survival probabilities were calculated using the survival package [21]. The log-rank test was used to assess the statistical significance of the survival differences. The prognostic significance of our classification relating to breast cancer survival was analyzed using the Cox proportional regression model. The Kaplan-Meier curves were produced using a modified R script taken from http://biostat.mc.vanderbilt.edu/wiki/Main/TatsukiRcode#kmplot.

We showed in **Figure 3** the Kaplan-Meier plots of the OS, RFS, and DMFS of the six subtypes that we determined using consensus clustering. In all three survival endpoints, the luminal A patients had highest survival rates (5-year OS = 86.8%, 5-year RFS = 83.8%, 5-year DMFS = 87.4%), whereas the HER2-enriched had worse outcomes (5-year OS = 67.3%, 5-year RFS = 56.8%, 5-year DMFS = 62.2%). The luminal B breast cancers are widely recognized as high risk [22–24], and our analysis showed equivalent results. Similar to basal-like and HER2-enriched breast cancers that had poorer prognosis, the luminal B subtype had greater relative risk of locoregional and distant breast cancer recurrence.

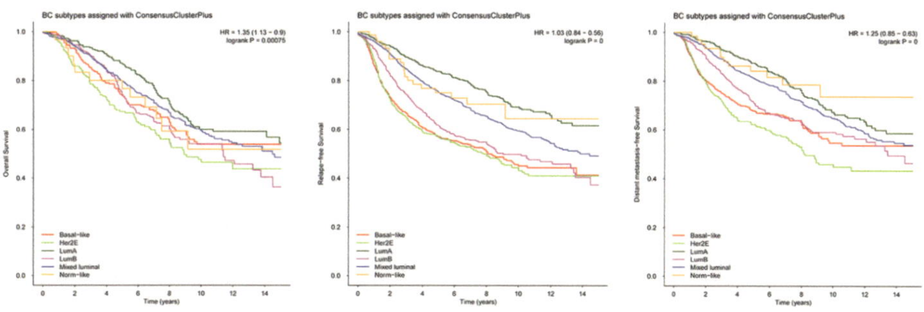

Figure 3. Kaplan-Meier plots showing the relation between subtypes determined with ConsensusClusterPlus and clinical outcome in breast cancer patients. Overall survival (OS; left), relapse-free survival (RFS; middle), and distant metastasis-free survival (DMFS; right) for samples in the six subtypes based on the consensus clustering with 100 genes.

6. Consensus hierarchical clustering using function-specific genes and survival analysis

Besides classifying samples according to the expression of genes relating to breast cancer subtypes, we also aimed to identify subsets of patients that might harbor specific expression profiles that could affect their survival outcome. To do this, we used the current knowledge about protein functions and the participation of genes in biological pathways to select specific functions and pathways that might have an effect or are affected by the development and progression of breast cancer. We used databases such as Ingenuity Pathway Analysis (http://www.ingenuity.com/products/ipa), KEGG (http://www.genome.jp/kegg/), and HGNC (http://www.genenames.org/) to gather genes participates and/or of the following functions: cadherins, zinc fingers, C2 domain-containing, ion channels, solute carriers, integrins, chemokine receptors, chemokine ligands, receptor kinases, immunoglobulins, CD molecules, homeoboxes, interferons, interferon receptors, interleukins, interleukin receptors, intermediate filaments, histones, chromatin-modifying enzymes, ATPases, glycosyltransferases, phosphatases, metallopeptidases, apoptosis, autophagy, unfolded protein response, oxidative stress response, and epithelial-mesenchymal transition pathway. Consensus clustering was performed as before using ConsensusClusterPlus with same parameters to determine at most six clusters from each or collections of gene sets. Then, these clusters were analyzed for their associations with survival.

Using a *P*-value cutoff of 0.01, we identified two collections of genes that were statistically significantly associated with survivals: the CD molecules and the cytokines and cytokine receptors. **Figure 4** shows the Kaplan-Meier plots of OS, RFS, and DMFS for each of the six CD molecules clusters. In both RFS and DMFS, Cluster 2 (lime green colored) had the best survival outcome, and is made up of mixed luminal, luminal A, HER2-enriched, and normal-like breast cancers as shown in **Table 5**. Cluster 3 (dark green colored), which are mainly HER2-enriched and luminal B cancers, and Cluster 4 (magenta colored) consists of basal-like cancers had worse outcomes. We looked into the CD molecules that showed greater expression differences between Cluster 2 (best survival) and Clusters 3 and 4 (worse survival) by computing the Cohen's *d* effect size statistics [25]. Of the 317 CD molecules analyzed, the 20 genes that had large effect size ($d > 1$) are: *ACKR1, BCAM, CD248, CD34, CD36, EPCAM, FUT3, HMMR, IGF1R, IL6ST, JAM2, LAMP3, LEPR, LRP1, PDGFRA, PDGFRB, SLC7A5, TEK, TFRC*, and *TSPAN7*. **Figure 5** showed their respective expression distributions in Clusters 2, 3, and 4.

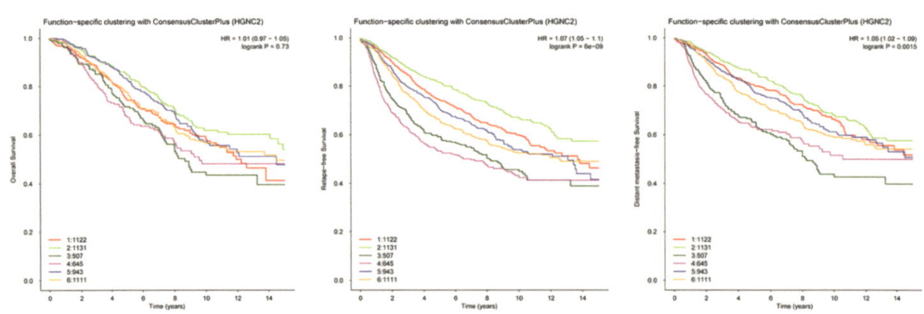

Figure 4. Kaplan-Meier estimates of breast cancer survival of clusters determined using CD molecules. Overall survival (OS; left), relapse-free survival (RFS; middle), and distant metastasis-free survival (DMFS; right) for samples in the six subtypes based on the consensus clustering with 317 genes encoding for CD molecules.

Comparison		Subtypes					
		BasalL	Her2E	LumA	LumB	LumMix	NormL
Clustering using expression profiles of CD molecules	1	4	9	69	248	1666	0
	2	16	173	913	48	469	482
	3	34	704	26	221	64	1
	4	1132	49	3	14	6	5
	5	539	325	57	524	447	16
	6	2	70	183	478	1083	6

Table 5. Comparison of sample assignment between subtype-specific genes and CD molecules.

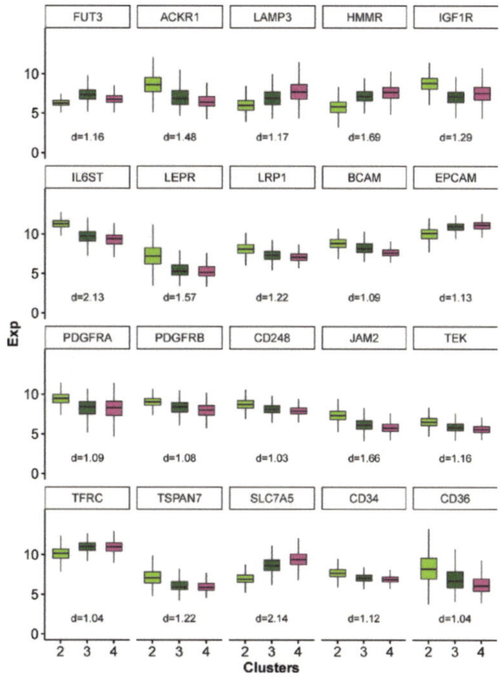

Figure 5. Box plots of the distribution of gene expression values of 20 CD molecules with large effect size between samples with best and worse outcomes. Cluster 2 (best outcome), 3 and 4 (worse outcomes) are chosen to demonstrate the difference in gene expression levels between samples from these three clusters. The box plots of Clusters 2, 3 and 4 are colored in light green, dark green, and magenta, respectively.

The second collection of genes consists of 113 cytokines and cytokine receptors. In **Figure 6**, the Kaplan-Meier plots showed that Cluster 6 (orange colored) had the worst survival outcome. It consists of Basal-like, HER2-enriched, and some luminal cancers (see **Table 6**). We again used Cohen's d as a measure to assess whether the expression profiles of Cluster 6 and the two clusters with better survival (Clusters 2 and 4) are significantly different in gene expression for each gene in this collection. We identified 15 genes that had large effect size ($d > 1$). They are: *ACKR1, CCL19, CCL20, CCL7, CX3CR1, CXCL1, CXCL12, CXCL14, CXCL8, IL12RB2, IL13RA1, IL1R1, IL1R2, IL6ST,* and *PITPNM3*, and their respective expression distributions in Clusters 2, 4 and 6 are shown in **Figure 7**.

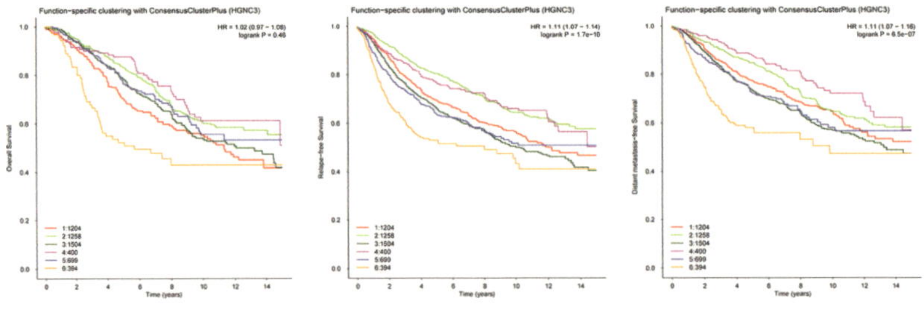

Figure 6. Kaplan-Meier estimates of breast cancer survival of clusters determined using chemokine ligands, chemokine receptors, interferons, interferon receptors, interleukins, and interleukin receptors. Overall survival (OS; left), relapse-free survival (RFS; middle), and distant metastasis-free survival (DMFS; right) for samples in the six subtypes based on the consensus clustering with 113 genes encoding for cytokines and cytokine receptors.

Comparison		Subtypes					
		BasalL	HER2E	LumA	LumB	LumMix	NormL
Clustering using expression profiles of cytokines and cytokine receptors	1	68	102	77	341	1585	2
	2	33	153	830	62	764	444
	3	350	477	166	758	809	21
	4	4	30	174	47	409	10
	5	750	268	0	219	47	0
	6	522	300	4	106	121	33

Table 6. Comparison of sample assignment between subtype-specific genes and cytokines and cytokine receptors.

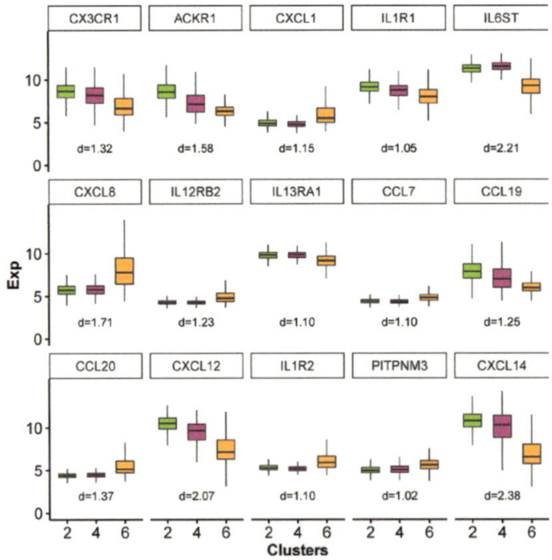

Figure 7. Box plots of the distribution of gene expression values of 15 cytokines and cytokine receptors with large effect size between samples of better and worst outcomes. Cluster 6 (worse outcome), 2 and 4 (best outcomes) are chosen to demonstrate the difference in gene expression levels between samples from these three clusters. The box plots of Clusters 2, 4, and 6 are colored in light green, magenta, and orange, respectively.

7. Conclusion and perspectives

Breast cancer is a complex disease comprising different subtypes that may be characterized by the change in expression patterns and/or mutations of few candidate genes. The ability to distinguish breast cancer subtypes using these underlying differences has significant clinical implications as it is one of the variables that affect prognosis and treatment of the disease. There were many studies with goals to classify breast cancer based on the amount of literatures and gene expression datasets available in public domain. However, there is a lack of recent meta-analysis to utilize this collection of data generated by various research groups and institutes over the past 15 years. In this chapter, we presented our effort to employ these high-throughput microarray dataset to perform breast cancer subtyping of 10086 samples.

The breast cancer subtypes that we characterized using consensus clustering of 100 genes and 10086 samples not only confirmed the existence of the four major intrinsic subtypes, that is, Basal-like, HER2-enriched, luminal A, and luminal B, but we also defined a normal-like subtype that consists of cancer samples with similar gene expression profile as that found in normal and adjacent normal breast samples. In addition, we distinguished a group of luminal B–like samples with better prognosis (that we term mixed luminal) from the high-risk luminal B breast cancer.

In addition, consensus clustering of the expression signatures of CD molecules and cytokines and cytokine receptors were associated with survival outcomes. Thirty-three genes showed significant differential gene expression between the classes with best and worse survival rates were identified. The *ACKR1* (Atypical Chemokine Receptor 1, CD234 Antigen) and *IL6ST* (Interleukin 6 Signal Transducer, CD130 Antigen) were found in both gene sets. Kaplan-Meier analysis showed patients with higher expression of either one gene had longer survival time. Others includes *CX3CR1* (C-X3-C motif chemokine receptor 1), *CXCL12* (C-X-C motif chemokine ligand 12), *CXCL14* (C-X-C motif chemokine ligand 14), *IGF1R* (insulin-like growth factor 1 receptor), *IL13RA1* (interleukin 13 receptor subunit alpha 1), *IL6ST* (interleukin 6 signal transducer), *JAM2* (junctional adhesion molecule 2), and *LEPR* (leptin receptor) are also genes that had higher expression associating with better outcomes. On the other end of the spectrum are *CCL7* (C-C motif chemokine ligand 7), *CXCL1* (C-X-C motif chemokine ligand 1), *CXCL8* (C-X-C motif chemokine ligand 8), *FUT3* (fucosyltransferase 3 (Lewis blood group)), *HMMR* (hyaluronan mediated motility receptor), and *SLC7A5* (solute carrier family 7 member 5) that were overexpressed in patients with lower survival rates. We believe these genes are potential therapeutic targets and diagnostic biomarkers for breast cancer.

Acknowledgements

The authors acknowledge financial support from the Ministry of Science and Technology, Taiwan (MOST 103-2811-B-010-020 and MOST 104-2811-B-010-007). We also thank the National Center for High-performance Computing of National Applied Research Laboratories of Taiwan and National Research Program for Biopharmaceuticals (MOST 104-2325-B-492-001) for providing computational biology platform. The funders had no role in study design, data collection and analysis, decision to publish, or preparation of the manuscript.

Author details

I-Hsuan Lin[1,2] and Ming-Ta Hsu[1*]

*Address all correspondence to: mth@ym.edu.tw

1 Institute of Biochemistry and Molecular Biology, School of Life Science, National Yang-Ming University, Taipei, Taiwan

2 The Center of Translational Medicine, Taipei Medical University, Taipei, Taiwan

References

[1] Hammond ME, Hayes DF, Dowsett M, Allred DC, Hagerty KL, et al. American Society of Clinical Oncology/College Of American Pathologists guideline recommendations for immunohistochemical testing of estrogen and progesterone receptors in breast cancer. Journal of Clinical Oncology. 2010;28:2784-95. DOI: 10.1200/JCO.2009.25.6529

[2] Blows FM, Driver KE, Schmidt MK, Broeks A, van Leeuwen FE, et al. Subtyping of breast cancer by immunohistochemistry to investigate a relationship between subtype and short and long term survival: a collaborative analysis of data for 10,159 cases from 12 studies. PLoS Medicine. 2010;7:e1000279. DOI: 10.1371/journal.pmed.1000279

[3] Onitilo AA, Engel JM, Greenlee RT, Mukesh BN. Breast cancer subtypes based on ER/PR and Her2 expression: comparison of clinicopathologic features and survival. Clinical Medicine & Research. 2009;7:4-13. DOI: 10.3121/cmr.2009.825

[4] Slamon DJ, Leyland-Jones B, Shak S, Fuchs H, Paton V, et al. Use of chemotherapy plus a monoclonal antibody against HER2 for metastatic breast cancer that overexpresses HER2. The New England Journal of Medicine. 2001;344:783-92. DOI: 10.1056/NEJM200103153441101

[5] Geyer CE, Forster J, Lindquist D, Chan S, Romieu CG, et al. Lapatinib plus capecitabine for HER2-positive advanced breast cancer. The New England Journal of Medicine. 2006;355:2733-43. DOI: 10.1056/NEJMoa064320

[6] Brewster AM, Chavez-MacGregor M, Brown P. Epidemiology, biology, and treatment of triple-negative breast cancer in women of African ancestry. The Lancet Oncology. 2014;15:e625-34. DOI: 10.1016/S1470-2045(14)70364-X

[7] Perou CM, Sorlie T, Eisen MB, van de Rijn M, Jeffrey SS, et al. Molecular portraits of human breast tumours. Nature. 2000;406:747-52. DOI: 10.1038/35021093

[8] Sorlie T, Perou CM, Tibshirani R, Aas T, Geisler S, et al. Gene expression patterns of breast carcinomas distinguish tumor subclasses with clinical implications. Proceedings of the National Academy of Sciences of the United States of America. 2001;98:10869-74. DOI: 10.1073/pnas.191367098

[9] Reis-Filho JS, Pusztai L. Gene expression profiling in breast cancer: classification, prognostication, and prediction. Lancet. 2011;378:1812-23. DOI: 10.1016/S0140-6736(11)61539-0

[10] Norum JH, Andersen K, Sorlie T. Lessons learned from the intrinsic subtypes of breast cancer in the quest for precision therapy. The British Journal of Surgery. 2014;101:925-38. DOI: 10.1002/bjs.9562

[11] Gautier L, Cope L, Bolstad BM, Irizarry RA. affy—analysis of AffymetrixGeneChip data at the probe level. Bioinformatics. 2004;20:307-15. DOI: 10.1093/bioinformatics/btg405

[12] Li Q, Birkbak NJ, Gyorffy B, Szallasi Z, Eklund AC. Jetset: selecting the optimal microarray probe set to represent a gene. BMC Bioinformatics. 2011;12:474. DOI: 10.1186/1471-2105-12-474

[13] Taminau J, Meganck S, Lazar C, Steenhoff D, Coletta A, et al. Unlocking the potential of publicly available microarray data using inSilicoDb and inSilicoMerging R/Bioconductor packages. BMC Bioinformatics. 2012;13:335. DOI: 10.1186/1471-2105-13-335

[14] Ritchie ME, Phipson B, Wu D, Hu Y, Law CW, et al. limma powers differential expression analyses for RNA-sequencing and microarray studies. Nucleic Acids Research. 2015;43:e47. DOI: 10.1093/nar/gkv007

[15] Wilkerson MD, Hayes DN. ConsensusClusterPlus: a class discovery tool with confidence assessments and item tracking. Bioinformatics. 2010;26:1572-3. DOI: 10.1093/bioinformatics/btq170

[16] Gu Z, Eils R, Schlesner M. Complex heatmaps reveal patterns and correlations in multidimensional genomic data. Bioinformatics. 2016. DOI. 10.1093/bioinformatics/btw313

[17] Kwan ML, Kushi LH, Weltzien E, Maring B, Kutner SE, et al. Epidemiology of breast cancer subtypes in two prospective cohort studies of breast cancer survivors. Breast Cancer Research. 2009;11:R31. DOI: 10.1186/bcr2261

[18] Rakha EA, Ellis IO. Triple-negative/basal-like breast cancer: review. Pathology. 2009; 41:40-7. DOI: 10.1080/00313020802563510

[19] Jenkins EO, Deal AM, Anders CK, Prat A, Perou CM, et al. Age-specific changes in intrinsic breast cancer subtypes: a focus on older women. The Oncologist. 2014;19:1076-83. DOI: 10.1634/theoncologist.2014-0184

[20] Gendoo DM, Ratanasirigulchai N, Schroder MS, Pare L, Parker JS, et al. Genefu: an R/Bioconductor package for computation of gene expression-based signatures in breast cancer. Bioinformatics. 2015. DOI: 10.1093/bioinformatics/btv693

[21] Therneau TM, Grambsch PM. Modeling Survival Data: Extending the Cox Model. 1st ed. New York: Springer-Verlag; 2000. DOI: 10.1007/978-1-4757-3294-8

[22] Hu Z, Fan C, Oh DS, Marron JS, He X, et al. The molecular portraits of breast tumors are conserved across microarray platforms. BMC Genomics. 2006;7:96. DOI: 10.1186/1471-2164-7-96

[23] Cheang MC, Chia SK, Voduc D, Gao D, Leung S, et al. Ki67 index, HER2 status, and prognosis of patients with luminal B breast cancer. Journal of the National Cancer Institute. 2009;101:736-50. DOI: 10.1093/jnci/djp082

[24] Tran B, Bedard PL. Luminal-B breast cancer and novel therapeutic targets. Breast Cancer Research. 2011;13:221. DOI: 10.1186/bcr2904

[25] Cohen J. Statistical power analysis for the behavioral sciences. 2nd ed. Hillsdale, N.J.: L. Erlbaum Associates; 1988.

Chapter 10

Jab1/Csn5 Signaling in Breast Cancer

Yunbao Pan and Francois X. Claret

Additional information is available at the end of the chapter

http://dx.doi.org/10.5772/66174

Abstract

c-Jun activation domain-binding protein1 (Jab1), also known as a monomer or the fifth component of the constitutive photomorphogenesis 9 signalosome (Csn5) complex, regulates cell proliferation, cell-cycle progression, and apoptosis and affects a series of pathways. Jab1/Csn5 also promotes cell transformation and tumorigenesis, and its overexpression in many tumor types suggests it is involved in cancer progression and closely associated with poor cancer prognosis. Jab1/Csn5 dysregulation contributes to oncogenesis by deactivating several tumor suppressors. Increasing evidence of the role of Jab1/Csn5 overexpression in breast and other cancers has spurred interest in Jab1/Csn5 inhibitors for cancer therapy. In this chapter, we summarize the evidence demonstrating the importance of Jab1/Csn5 expression in breast and other cancers and review recent advances in dissecting the Jab1/Csn5 signaling pathway along with its potential as a therapeutic target for cancer.

Keywords: breast cancer, Jab1/Csn5, biomarker, DNA damage, therapeutic approach

1. Introduction

c-Jun activation domain-binding protein 1 (Jab1), primarily identified as a c-Jun coactivator [1], is the fifth member of the constitutive photomorphogenesis 9 signalosome (Csn5) complex. Specifically, Jab1/Csn5 is an evolutionarily conserved multifunctional protein involved in developmental processes in eukaryotic organisms and primarily identified as an inhibitor of light-dependent growth and transcription in *Arabidopsis* [2, 3]. Jab1/Csn5 participates in deneddylation of neural precursor cell expressed developmentally downregulated gene 8 (NEDD8), transcription factor specificity, and binding of several key molecules. Increasing evidence indicates that dysregulation of Jab1/Csn5 activity contributes to tumorigenesis, which is functionally inactivating several tumor suppressors and key negative regulatory proteins, including the cyclin-dependent kinase (CDK) inhibitor p27Kip1 (p27), p53, and SMAD4/7 [4]. Jab1/Csn5 is aberrantly expressed in different tumor types and lines of evidence support that it is a proto-oncogene. In this chapter, we describe some mechanisms by which Jab1/Csn5 is involved in cancer progression to provide perspective with the hope that these mechanisms will lay the foundation for future therapeutic intervention.

2. Structural features of Jab1/Csn5

CSN is a conserved protein complex that typically comprises eight subunits $^{1/m}$CSN1–CSN8$^{1/m}$ in descending order according to molecular weight [5]. Six of these subunits contain a proteasome, constitutive photomorphogenesis 9 signalosome, initiation factor 3 domain or PINT domain, that serves as a structural scaffold for the assembly of the constitutive photomorphogenesis 9 signalosome, and the other two subunits contain an MPR1 and PAD1 N-terminal (MPN) domain [5, 6]. Although both CSN5 and CSN6 have MPN domains; only the CSN5 MPN domain contains an embedded Jab1/MPN domain metalloenzyme motif (also named as an MPN + motif), which is the catalytic center for CSN isopeptidase activity [5]. Jab1/Csn5 contains 334 amino acids and assembles a nuclear export signal (NES) domain near the p27-binding domain at the end of the C-terminus [7]. This is a rich blend of leucine nuclear export signal sequences, which are highly conserved among different species. Through interaction with the NES domain, CRM1, which exports factors from the nucleus, combines with Jab1/Csn5 via an LMB-sensitive method and then carries the p27 protein out of the nucleus. When the leucine residues of Jab1/Csn5 are replaced by alanine residues, the NES can reduce Jab1 and CRM1 interaction, which impacts LMB-dependent nuclear cytoplasmic output process as well as the degradation of p27 in cells.

The catalytic activity of the CSN complex resides in the deneddylation of the CRLs, that is, the hydrolysis of the cullin-neural precursor cell expressed developmentally downregulated gene 8 (Nedd8) isopeptide bond. Although CSN-dependent Jab1/Csn5 has isopeptidase activity, it is intrinsically inactive in other physiologically conditions. Although the Jab1/Csn5 active site is catalytically competent and compatible with di-isopeptide binding, the Ins-1 segment obstructs access to its substrate-binding site, and structural rearrangements are necessary for the Nedd8-binding pocket formation. Detailed study of Jab1/Csn5 by molecular dynamics discovered the flexibility and plasticity of the Ins-1 segment [8]. These studies resulted in the identification of a molecular trigger implicated in the active/inactive switch that is sufficient to impose on Jab1/Csn5 an active isopeptidase state. Additionally, a dynamic monomer-dimer equilibrium exists both in vitro and in vivo and may be functionally relevant [8].

3. Jab1/Csn5 overexpression in breast cancer and other cancer types

Jab1/Csn5 regulates the transcriptional activity of activator protein 1 (AP-1) and also modulates cell signal transduction, regulating genetic transcription and the stability of the protein [1]. Importantly, Jab1/Csn5, alongside with Myc, was found to act as a master regulator of a wound gene expression signature in breast cancer cells. This study suggests that Jab1/CSN5 plays an important role in translating the cell stress response to transcription of response genes that are involved in proliferation and matrix invasiveness [9]. Aberrant overexpression of Jab1/Csn5 is implicated to play a role in the pathogenesis of several types of human malignancies and tends to correlate with poor cancer prognosis. Adler et al. [10] provided the first evidence that Jab1/Csn5 isopeptidase activity is essential for human and murine mammary epithelial transformation and progression. In another study, Jab1/Csn5 expression was low in or absent from normal breast tissue, but it was aberrantly expressed in 57% (125 of 220) of node-negative breast tumors and 90% (9 of 10) of metastatic lesions [11]. Importantly, breast cancer patients with Jab1/Csn5-negative tumors had neither relapse nor disease progression at a median follow-up time of 70 months [12]. Additionally, Jab1/Csn5 was overexpressed in 33% (11 of 33) of benign ovarian tumors and 68% (32 of 47) of malignant ovarian tumors and correlated with poor overall survival of ovarian cancer [13]. Additionally, aberrant expression of Jab1/Csn5 has been positively associated with hepatitis C virus infection and negatively correlated with hepatitis B virus infection in hepatocellular carcinoma patients, indicating a possible mechanism that promotes hepatocarcinogenesis [14]. In a study of non-small cell lung cancer patients, those with elevated Jab1/Csn5 expression had a poorer overall survival rate (44%) after 5 years than did patients with lower Jab1 expression levels (63%) [15]. Jab1/Csn5 expression also is closely linked with histological differentiation, clinical stage, and lymph node metastasis in oral squamous cell carcinoma cases [16]. Patients with oral squamous cell carcinoma, nasopharyngeal carcinoma, and laryngeal squamous cell carcinomas, as well as those with thyroid carcinomas and Jab1/Csn5 overexpression, tend to have poor overall survival, indicating a critical role in cancer progression [16–19]. Furthermore, Jab1/Csn5 plays a role in cancer therapy. In particular, depletion of Jab1/Csn5 enhanced the antitumor effects of cisplatin and ionizing radiation in NPC cells [20, 21].

Researchers have made substantial progress in deciphering the critical role of Jab1/Csn5 in diverse cellular and developmental processes. However, little is known about the underlying regulatory principles that promote Jab1/CSN5 overexpression in cancer. Jab1/Csn5 overexpression may result from *Jab1/Csn5* gene amplification. The *Jab1/Csn5* locus is located on 8q13.1, which is always amplified in breast cancer and other cancer patients [9, 22]. As we described above, several other signaling pathways may also contribute to overexpression of Jab1/Csn5, such as interleukin 6/signal transducer and activator of transcription 3 (Stat 3), human epidermal growth factor receptor 2 (EGFR) (HER–2)/AKT, and Bcr/Abl. For example, the protein psoriasin (S100A7) enhances Jab1/Csn5 as well as activator protein 1 activity and promotes tumorigenesis [23]. Moreover, expression of Jab1/Csn5 is related to degradation of p57 protein [24] and contributes to tumor recurrence [19]. These findings provided a new opportunity to make Jab1/Csn5 a tumor target. Identifying the underlying mechanisms of Jab1/Csn5 in cancer still requires further exploration, but Jab1/Csn5 has proven to be a useful diagnostic and prognostic marker for cancer.

4. Jab1/Csn5-associated signaling

A number of studies have demonstrated that Jab1 lies at the intersection of several important signal transduction pathways that are believed to be important in the progression of breast cancer (**Figure 1**). Elucidating the regulatory mechanism of Jab1/Csn5 expression in these pathways will enhance our understanding of breast tumorigenesis.

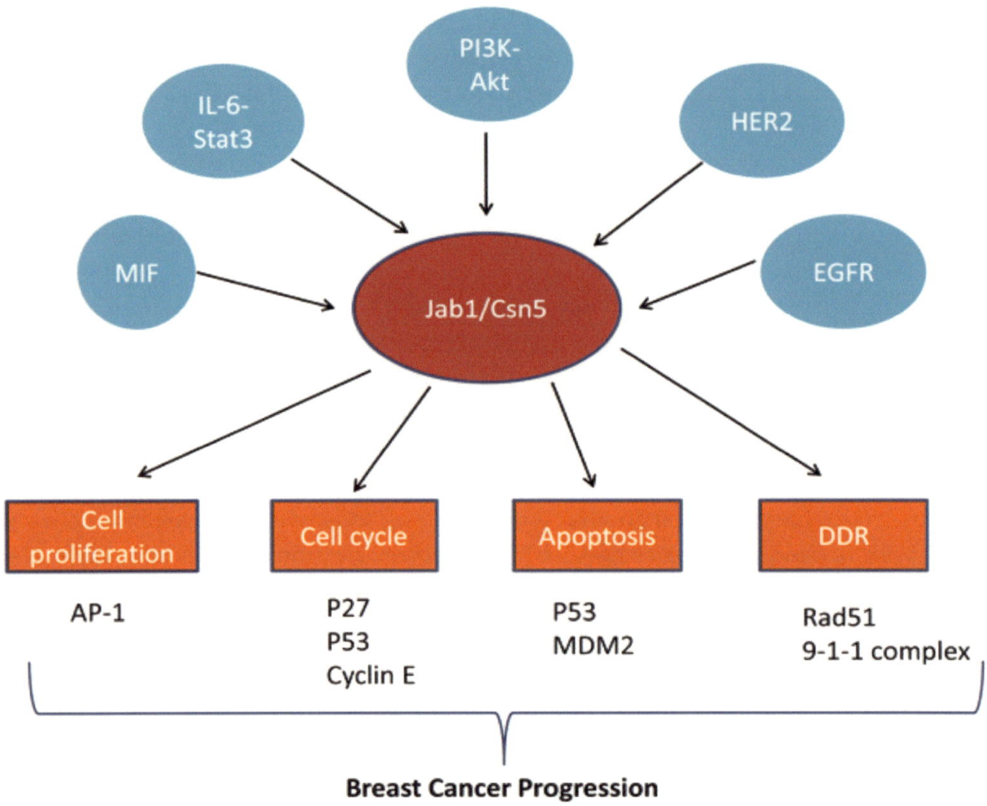

Figure 1. Jab1/Csn5 regulatory network in breast cancer cases. Jab1/Csn5 plays an essential role in breast cancer progression. On the one hand, Jab1/Csn5 activity and expression can be regulated by several typical oncogenic signaling pathways, such as MIF, phosphoinositide 3-kinase/AKT, interleukin-6/Stat3, HER-2/AKT, and EGFR. On the other hand, Jab1/Csn5 regulates a myriad of proteins involved in cell proliferation, cell cycle, apoptosis, and DDR.

4.1. Jab1/p27 signaling

Increasingly, studies have demonstrated that Jab1/Csn5 overexpression is negatively associated with p27 expression and poor prognosis [25] for many human cancers. p27 is a member of the cell-cycle inhibitor family of proteins, which is a primary driving force for cell-cycle progression through ubiquitination of G1 cyclins and CDK inhibitors, such as cyclinE-CDK2 and cyclinD1-CDK4 [25]. Eventually, p27 causes cell-cycle arrest during G1 phase and inhibits cell proliferation. Jab1/Csn5 directly binds to p27 and mediates its shuttling from the nucleus to cytoplasm in a CRM1-dependent manner via the NES sequence [7]. Furthermore, researchers have observed cytoplasmic translocalization of p27 in human cancers and that it correlates with poor survival [26]. Many studies have demonstrated that Jab1/Csn5 expression increases along with p27 nuclear translocation, thereby accelerating p27 degradation via the ubiquitin-proteasome pathway [27]. Also, depletion of Jab1/Csn5 by small interfering RNA substantially increases p27 expression, including that of the p27/cyclin E/Cdk2 complex, and nuclear accumulation of p27 and inhibits the cell-cycle transition from G1 to S phase [27]. In addition, Jab1/Csn5 may degrade p27 through a Skp2-independent mechanism [28]. Investigators found that Skp2-mediated degradation of p27 mainly occurred in cells undergoing DNA replication [29]. Interestingly, evidence suggests that elevated AKT (a protein kinase B) expression leads to decreased p27 expression in the nucleus. AKT-mediated phosphorylation of p27 at Thr187 is known to inactivate p27 and restrain the translocation of p27 into the nucleus. Subsequently, degradation of p27 by the ubiquitin-proteasome system is associated with dysregulation of the cell cycle and promotes tumor formation [30]. Hsu et al. [31] provided the first evidence that Jab1/Csn5 expression may be regulated by HER-2/neu via the AKT signaling pathway. Whether Jab1 is directly related to AKT or the underlying mechanism of action between them is currently unknown.

4.2. HER-2 and EGFR signaling

Jab1/Csn5 is linked with EGFR and HER-2/neu receptor signaling in breast tumorigenesis. Jab1/Csn5 is a downstream target of HER-2/neu, and Jab1/Csn5 overexpression is correlated with HER-2/neu in breast cancer [32]. HER-2/neu directly activates Jab1/Csn5 promoter activity and upregulates Jab1/Csn5 mRNA expression via AKT/β-catenin signaling [31]. Suppression of HER-2/neu by treatment with trastuzumab (Herceptin) decreases Jab1/Csn5 expression in different types of cancer cells [33]. Furthermore, Jab1/Csn5 is a target of EGFR signaling, and its expression correlates with EGFR expression in estrogen receptor-alpha-negative breast cancer cell lines. EGFR activation increases the translocation of Jab1/Csn5 to the nucleus and regulates p27 downstream from Jab1 [34]. These findings suggested that Jab1/Csn5 is involved in the development and progression of breast cancer.

4.3. Migration inhibitory factor/phosphoinositide 3-kinase/AKT signaling

Jab1/Csn5 controls autocrine macrophage migration inhibitory factor (MIF)-mediated activation of phosphoinositide 3-kinase/AKT signaling, a novel, indirect mechanism between the Jab1/Csn5 and phosphoinositide 3-kinase/AKT pathways, by inhibiting MIF secretion and its autocrine prosurvival activities [35]. In turn, MIF negatively regulates Jab1/Csn5, as MIF can specifically interact with Jab1/Csn5 and inhibit Jab1/Csn5-enhanced activator protein 1 and c-Jun N-terminal kinase activity [36].

4.4. Interleukin-6/STAT3 signaling

Jab1/Csn5 interacts with protein to regulate unphosphorylated Stat3 DNA-binding activity. Loss of Jab1/Csn5 expression markedly decreases unphosphorylated Stat3 DNA-binding activity as well as expression of Stat3 target genes but tends to increase nuclear Stat3 in human colon cancer cells [37]. This interesting phenomenon must be studied further to elucidate how Jab1/Csn5 determines the fate of transcription factors as its binding partners. Does it do so by binding to target DNA or via protein degradation? In contrast, another study demonstrated that Stat3 binds to the Jab1/Csn5 promoter, enhances its promoter activity, and increases Jab1/Csn5 transcription in breast cancer cells. Depletion of Stat3 dramatically decreases Jab1/Csn5 promoter activity and Jab1/Csn5 mRNA and protein expression [38]. Moreover, upstream activators of Stat3, such as interleukin-6 and Src, also contribute to activation of Jab1/Csn5 transcription and expression via Stat3.

4.5. Jab1/Csn5 in DNA damage response

In recent years, owing to rapid advances in knowledge of DNA damage repair signal mechanisms and the study of epigenetic molecular mechanisms, researchers have made great progress in understanding the principle and mechanism of tumorigenesis after DNA damage response (DDR). Inactivation of DDR genes increases the risk of accumulating genetic mutations, which may greatly promote cancer development [4]. Increasing evidence supports that Jab1/Csn5 affects both the activity and stability of DDR proteins [20]. Jab1/Csn5 is essential for tumor survival and enhances tumor resistance to chemotherapy and radiotherapy [20]. Importantly, Jab1/Csn5 can mediate the nuclear export and degradation of several nuclear proteins, including those involved in DDR [4]. Study results have demonstrated that Jab1/Csn5 deletion during meiosis can activate the DNA damage checkpoint in *Drosophila melanogaster* [39]. CSNs regulate the ubiquitin ligase activity of the damage DNA-binding protein 1 or DNA-binding protein 2 and Cockayne syndrome group A complexes in response to exposure to DNA-damaging agents. The authors report that Jab1/Csn5 deficiency decreased the repair vitality of DNA-binding protein 2 by 50% [40]. Additionally, Cdc10-dependent transcript 1, a licensing factor for the prereplication complex, is regulated by Jab1/Csn5. Cdc10-dependent transcript 1 is degraded after DNA damage, and Jab1/Csn5 deficiency may lead to accumulation of Cdc10-dependent transcript 1 [41]. Also, the Rad9/Rad1/Hus1 complex is a DNA damage sensor that transduces DNA damage and plays an important role in initiation of cellular responses to DNA damage. This complex promotes ATR-mediated phosphorylation and activation of Chk1, a protein kinase that regulates progression to S phase, cell-cycle arrest at G2/M, and replication fork stabilization [42]. Because Jab1/Csn5 is involved in regulating the stability and translocation of the Rad9/Rad1/Hus1 complex in cells, it likely provides information about Jab1/Csn5 in checkpoint and DDR [4].

In eukaryotes, Rad51, a key DNA-repair protein, plays a primary role in DNA damage repair using emerging nucleoprotein filaments and mediation of strand conversion among DNA duplexes [43]. Rad51 is vital for embryo survival in response to exogenous DNA-damaging stimulation for the repair of spontaneous chromosome breaks during cell development [44]. In accordance with these findings, Jab1/Csn5 has been discovered the function with Rad51 in the homologous recombination repair pathway [43]. Furthermore, Jab1/Csn5 deficiency has not only decreased Rad51 expression but also affected its activity, and the

http://dx.doi.org/10.5772/66174

absence of Rad51 has caused a large number of chromosome breaks, leading to increased apoptosis. Decreased Rad51 expression in Jab1/Csn5 knockdown cells is at least partly dependent on p53 expression [20].

5. Predictive and therapeutic roles of Jab1 in cancer cases

Increasingly, studies have demonstrated that overexpressed Jab1/Csn5 is involved in cancer pathogenesis and correlates with poor cancer prognosis [25]. The authors reported that Jab1+/p27− patients had poor overall survival of many cancers [13, 25]. Lin Guo's group recently provided the first evidence that NCoR is a target of Jab1/Csn5 and mediates endocrine resistance in breast cancer [45]. Jab1/Csn5 might involve in multiple stages of breast cancer progression by regulating different protein targets. Further identification and elucidation of the E3 ligase that connects Jab1/Csn5 and NCoR are of importance to understand the precise mechanisms underlying endocrine resistance and identify additional druggable molecular targets. Thus, Jab1/Csn5 is an attractive therapeutic target for cancer given its multiple prominent functions in many stages of tumorigenesis.

Downregulation of Jab1/Csn5 expression has inhibited growth of and induced apoptosis in breast cancer [31] and nasopharyngeal carcinoma cells [27]. Furthermore, researchers found that Jab1/Csn5-deficient mice had an embryonically lethal phenotype, indicating that Jab1/Csn5 is critical for fetal development and survival [46]. In that study, Jab1/Csn5-null embryos were smaller than wild-type embryos and displayed delayed growth [46].

Also, the development of Jab1/Csn5-specific inhibitors has had major effects on cancer treatment. For example, curcumin is a yellow plant pigment that directly inhibits the activity of Jab1/Csn5-associated kinases, causing cell-cycle arrest in tumor cells during the mitotic phase and making them more prone to apoptosis by inhibiting Jab1/Csn5 [47]. A recent study demonstrated that PEGylated curcumin, a water-soluble compound, inhibited the growth of pancreatic cancer cells and sensitized them to gemcitabine-induced apoptosis [48]. Another study demonstrated that the curcumin analog T83 markedly induced cell-cycle arrest and apoptosis in nasopharyngeal carcinoma cells. In addition, T83 effectively inhibited Jab1/Csn5 expression in these cells and sensitized them to radiotherapy [49].

Another potential Jab1/Csn5-targeted drug is troglitazone, a peroxisome proliferator-activated receptor γ ligand that directly suppresses Jab1/Csn5 promoter activity by inhibiting Sp1- and Tcf4-mediated transcription [32]. A number of in vitro and in vivo studies have demonstrated that treatment with troglitazone effectively attenuated tumor growth and upregulated p27 expression in tumor cells in a time- and dose-dependent manner [50]. Animal studies verified that intratumoral or intraperitoneal injection of troglitazone attenuated hepatocellular carcinoma cell growth and reduced Jab1/Csn5 expression in hepatocellular tumors [14].

Although increasing evidence demonstrates that Jab1/Csn5 can be used as a therapeutic target for cancer, much work is still needed to develop a Jab1/Csn5-specific inhibitor for cancer treatment. The degree, duration, and cell specificity required for Jab1/Csn5 blockade to attenuate tumor growth should be studied further.

6. Conclusion and perspective

Jab1/Csn5 is a master regulator of a myriad of protein interactions involved in signaling pathways, cell survival, apoptosis, and DNA damage repair via ubiquitin-dependent proteolysis (**Figure 1**). Although Jab1/Csn5 function has a different role in each tumor type, overexpressed Jab1/Csn5 is associated with the whole process of carcinogenesis and cancer progression, and further studies of Jab1/Csn5 as a therapeutic target will provide new insight into cancer treatment. Considering the pivotal role of Jab1/Csn5 signaling, a reasonable assumption is that Jab1/Csn5 is a promising diagnostic, prognostic, and therapeutic biomarker for cancer.

Acknowledgements

This work was supported in part by the National Natural Science Foundation of China (81372816), Fundamental Research Funds for the Central Universities (JUSRP115A31) (to Y.P) ,NIH grant (RO1-CA90853), and the Cancer Prevention Research Institute of Texas (RP120451) (to FXC). We thank Brandon Carl Strubberg and Ann Sutton at the Department of Scientific Publications in MD Anderson Cancer Center for editing this manuscript.

Conflict of interest

None.

Author details

Yunbao Pan[1] and Francois X. Claret[2*]

*Address all correspondence to: fxclaret@mdanderson.org

1 Department of Pathology, Affiliated Hospital, Wuxi Medical School, Jiangnan University, Wuxi, People's Republic of China

2 Department of Systems Biology, The University of Texas MD Anderson Cancer Center, Houston, TX, USA

http://dx.doi.org/10.5772/66174

References

[1] Claret FX, Hibi M, Dhut S, Toda T and Karin M. A new group of conserved coactivators that increase the specificity of AP-1 transcription factors. Nature 1996; 383: 453–457.

[2] Wei N, Chamovitz DA and Deng XW. Arabidopsis COP9 is a component of a novel signaling complex mediating light control of development. Cell 1994; 78: 117–124.

[3] Wei N and Deng XW. The COP9 signalosome. Annu Rev Cell Dev Biol 2003; 19: 261–286.

[4] Pan Y, Yang H and Claret FX. Emerging roles of Jab1/CSN5 in DNA damage response, DNA repair, and cancer. Cancer Biol Ther 2014; 15: 256–262.

[5] Wei N, Serino G and Deng XW. The COP9 signalosome: more than a protease. Trends Biochem Sci 2008; 33: 592–600.

[6] Cope GA, Suh GS, Aravind L, Schwarz SE, Zipursky SL, Koonin EV and Deshaies RJ. Role of predicted metalloprotease motif of Jab1/Csn5 in cleavage of Nedd8 from Cul1. Science 2002; 298: 608–611.

[7] Tomoda K, Kubota Y, Arata Y, Mori S, Maeda M, Tanaka T, Yoshida M, Yoneda-Kato N and Kato JY. The cytoplasmic shuttling and subsequent degradation of p27Kip1 mediated by Jab1/CSN5 and the COP9 signalosome complex. J Biol Chem 2002; 277: 2302–2310.

[8] Echalier A, Pan Y, Birol M, Tavernier N, Pintard L, Hoh F, Ebel C, Galophe N, Claret FX and Dumas C. Insights into the regulation of the human COP9 signalosome catalytic subunit, CSN5/Jab1. Proc Natl Acad Sci U S A 2013; 110: 1273–1278.

[9] Adler AS, Lin M, Horlings H, Nuyten DS, van de Vijver MJ and Chang HY. Genetic regulators of large-scale transcriptional signatures in cancer. Nat Genet 2006; 38: 421–430.

[10] Adler AS, Littlepage LE, Lin M, Kawahara TL, Wong DJ, Werb Z and Chang HY. CSN5 isopeptidase activity links COP9 signalosome activation to breast cancer progression. Cancer Res 2008; 68: 506–515.

[11] Esteva FJ, Sahin AA, Rassidakis GZ, Yuan LX, Smith TL, Yang Y, Gilcrease MZ, Cristofanilli M, Nahta R, Pusztai L and Claret FX. Jun activation domain binding protein 1 expression is associated with low p27(Kip1)levels in node-negative breast cancer. Clin Cancer Res 2003; 9: 5652–5659.

[12] Kouvaraki MA, Rassidakis GZ, Tian L, Kumar R, Kittas C and Claret FX. Jun activation domain-binding protein 1 expression in breast cancer inversely correlates with the cell cycle inhibitor p27(Kip1). Cancer Res 2003; 63: 2977–2981.

[13] Sui L, Dong Y, Ohno M, Watanabe Y, Sugimoto K, Tai Y and Tokuda M. Jab1 expression is associated with inverse expression of p27(kip1) and poor prognosis in epithelial ovarian tumors. Clin Cancer Res 2001; 7: 4130–4135.

[14] Hsu MC, Huang CC, Chang HC, Hu TH and Hung WC. Overexpression of Jab1 in hepatocellular carcinoma and its inhibition by peroxisome proliferator-activated receptor{gamma} ligands in vitro and in vivo. Clin Cancer Res 2008; 14: 4045–4052.

[15] Osoegawa A, Yoshino I, Kometani T, Yamaguchi M, Kameyama T, Yohena T and Maehara Y. Overexpression of Jun activation domain-binding protein 1 in nonsmall cell lung cancer and its significance in p27 expression and clinical features. Cancer 2006; 107: 154–161.

[16] Gao L, Huang S, Ren W, Zhao L, Li J, Zhi K, Zhang Y, Qi H and Huang C. Jun activation domain-binding protein 1 expression in oral squamous cell carcinomas inversely correlates with the cell cycle inhibitor p27. Med Oncol 2012; 29: 2499–2504.

[17] Ahn J, Hong SA, Lee SE, Kim J, Oh YS, Park SJ and Chung YJ. Cytoplasmic localization of Jab1 and p27 Kip1 might be associated with invasiveness of papillary thyroid carcinoma. Endocr J 2009; 56: 707–713.

[18] Dong Y, Sui L, Watanabe Y, Yamaguchi F, Hatano N and Tokuda M. Prognostic significance of Jab1 expression in laryngeal squamous cell carcinomas. Clin Cancer Res 2005; 11: 259–266.

[19] Xu T, Su B, Wang C, Wang S, Huang H, Pan Y, Wang D, Wei W, Claret FX and Yang H. Molecular markers to assess short-term disease local recurrence in nasopharyngeal carcinoma. Oncol Rep 2015; 33: 1418–1426.

[20] Pan Y, Zhang Q, Atsaves V, Yang H and Claret FX. Suppression of Jab1/CSN5 induces radio- and chemo-sensitivity in nasopharyngeal carcinoma through changes to the DNA damage and repair pathways. Oncogene 2013; 32: 2756–2766.

[21] Wang S, Pan Y, Zhang R, Xu T, Wu W, Zhang R, Wang C, Huang H, Calin CA, Yang H and Claret FX. Hsa-miR-24-3p increases nasopharyngeal carcinoma radiosensitivity by targeting both the 3'UTR and 5'UTR of Jab1/CSN5. Oncogene PMID: 27157611 or DOI: 10.1038/onc.2016.147.

[22] Dimova I, Orsetti B, Negre V, Rouge C, Ursule L, Lasorsa L, Dimitrov R, Doganov N, Toncheva D and Theillet C. Genomic markers for ovarian cancer at chromosomes 1, 8 and 17 revealed by array CGH analysis. Tumori 2009; 95: 357–366.

[23] Emberley ED, Niu Y, Leygue E, Tomes L, Gietz RD, Murphy LC and Watson PH. Psoriasin interacts with Jab1 and influences breast cancer progression. Cancer Res 2003; 63: 1954–1961.

[24] Guo H, Jing L, Cheng Y, Atsaves V, Lv Y, Wu T, Su R, Zhang Y, Zhang R, Liu W, Rassidakis GZ, Wei Y, Nan K and Claret FX. Down-regulation of the cyclin-dependent

kinase inhibitor p57 is mediated by Jab1/Csn5 in hepatocarcinogenesis. Hepatology 2016; 63: 898–913.

[25] Shackleford TJ and Claret FX. JAB1/CSN5: a new player in cell cycle control and cancer. Cell Div 2010; 5: 26.

[26] Masciullo V, Sgambato A, Pacilio C, Pucci B, Ferrandina G, Palazzo J, Carbone A, Cittadini A, Mancuso S, Scambia G and Giordano A. Frequent loss of expression of the cyclin-dependent kinase inhibitor p27 in epithelial ovarian cancer. Cancer Res 1999; 59: 3790–3794.

[27] Pan Y, Zhang Q, Tian L, Wang X, Fan X, Zhang H, Claret FX and Yang H. Jab1/CSN5 negatively regulates p27 and plays a role in the pathogenesis of nasopharyngeal carcinoma. Cancer Res 2012; 72: 1890–1900.

[28] Kouvaraki MA, Korapati AL, Rassidakis GZ, Tian L, Zhang Q, Chiao P, Ho L, Evans DB and Claret FX. Potential role of Jun activation domain-binding protein 1 as a negative regulator of p27kip1 in pancreatic adenocarcinoma. Cancer Res 2006; 66: 8581–8589.

[29] Kamura T, Hara T, Matsumoto M, Ishida N, Okumura F, Hatakeyama S, Yoshida M, Nakayama K and Nakayama KI. Cytoplasmic ubiquitin ligase KPC regulates proteolysis of p27(Kip1) at G1 phase. Nat Cell Biol 2004; 6: 1229–1235.

[30] Zhang Q, Tian L, Mansouri A, Korapati AL, Johnson TJ and Claret FX. Inducible expression of a degradation-resistant form of p27Kip1 causes growth arrest and apoptosis in breast cancer cells. FEBS Lett 2005; 579: 3932–3940.

[31] Hsu MC, Chang HC and Hung WC. HER-2/neu transcriptionally activates Jab1 expression via the AKT/beta-catenin pathway in breast cancer cells. Endocr Relat Cancer 2007; 14: 655–667.

[32] Hsu MC, Chai CY, Hou MF, Chang HC, Chen WT and Hung WC. Jab1 is overexpressed in human breast cancer and is a downstream target for HER-2/neu. Mod Pathol 2008; 21: 609–616.

[33] Le XF, Pruefer F and Bast RC, Jr. HER2-targeting antibodies modulate the cyclin-dependent kinase inhibitor p27Kip1 via multiple signaling pathways. Cell Cycle 2005; 4: 87–95.

[34] Wang J, Barnes RO, West NR, Olson M, Chu JE and Watson PH. Jab1 is a target of EGFR signaling in ERalpha-negative breast cancer. Breast Cancer Res 2008; 10: R51.

[35] Lue H, Thiele M, Franz J, Dahl E, Speckgens S, Leng L, Fingerle-Rowson G, Bucala R, Luscher B and Bernhagen J. Macrophage migration inhibitory factor (MIF) promotes cell survival by activation of the Akt pathway and role for CSN5/JAB1 in the control of autocrine MIF activity. Oncogene 2007; 26: 5046–5059.

[36] Kleemann R, Hausser A, Geiger G, Mischke R, Burger-Kentischer A, Flieger O, Johannes FJ, Roger T, Calandra T, Kapurniotu A, Grell M, Finkelmeier D, Brunner H and Bernhagen J. Intracellular action of the cytokine MIF to modulate AP-1 activity and the cell cycle through Jab1. Nature 2000; 408: 211–216.

[37] Nishimoto A, Kugimiya N, Hosoyama T, Enoki T, Li TS and Hamano K. JAB1 regulates unphosphorylated STAT3 DNA-binding activity through protein-protein interaction in human colon cancer cells. Biochem Biophys Res Commun 2013; 438: 513–518.

[38] Shackleford TJ, Zhang Q, Tian L, Vu TT, Korapati AL, Baumgartner AM, Le XF, Liao WS and Claret FX. Stat3 and CCAAT/enhancer binding protein beta (C/EBP-beta) regulate Jab1/CSN5 expression in mammary carcinoma cells. Breast Cancer Res 2011; 13: R65.

[39] Doronkin S, Djagaeva I and Beckendorf SK. CSN5/Jab1 mutations affect axis formation in the Drosophila oocyte by activating a meiotic checkpoint. Development 2002; 129: 5053–5064.

[40] Groisman R, Polanowska J, Kuraoka I, Sawada J, Saijo M, Drapkin R, Kisselev AF, Tanaka K and Nakatani Y. The ubiquitin ligase activity in the DDB2 and CSA complexes is differentially regulated by the COP9 signalosome in response to DNA damage. Cell 2003; 113: 357–367.

[41] Higa LA, Mihaylov IS, Banks DP, Zheng J and Zhang H. Radiation-mediated proteolysis of CDT1 by CUL4-ROC1 and CSN complexes constitutes a new checkpoint. Nat Cell Biol 2003; 5: 1008–1015.

[42] Parrilla-Castellar ER, Arlander SJ and Karnitz L. Dial 9-1-1 for DNA damage: the Rad9-Hus1-Rad1 (9-1-1) clamp complex. DNA Repair (Amst) 2004; 3: 1009–1014.

[43] Shinohara A, Ogawa H and Ogawa T. Rad51 protein involved in repair and recombination in *S. cerevisiae* is a RecA-like protein. Cell 1992; 69: 457–470.

[44] Sonoda E, Sasaki MS, Buerstedde JM, Bezzubova O, Shinohara A, Ogawa H, Takata M, Yamaguchi-Iwai Y and Takeda S. Rad51-deficient vertebrate cells accumulate chromosomal breaks prior to cell death. EMBO J 1998; 17: 598–608.

[45] Lu R, Hu X, Zhou J, Sun J, Zhu AZ, Xu X, Zheng H, Gao X, Wang X, Jin H, Zhu P and Guo L. COPS5 amplification and overexpression confers tamoxifen-resistance in ER[alpha]-positive breast cancer by degradation of NCoR. Nat Commun 2016; 7: 12044.

[46] Tian L, Peng G, Parant JM, Leventaki V, Drakos E, Zhang Q, Parker-Thornburg J, Shackleford TJ, Dai H, Lin SY, Lozano G, Rassidakis GZ and Claret FX. Essential roles of Jab1 in cell survival, spontaneous DNA damage and DNA repair. Oncogene 2010; 29: 6125–6137.

[47] Fullbeck M, Huang X, Dumdey R, Frommel C, Dubiel W and Preissner R. Novel curcumin- and emodin-related compounds identified by in silico 2D/3D conformer screening induce apoptosis in tumor cells. BMC Cancer 2005; 5: 97.

[48] Li J, Wang Y, Yang C, Wang P, Oelschlager DK, Zheng Y, Tian DA, Grizzle WE, Buchsbaum DJ and Wan M. Polyethylene glycosylated curcumin conjugate inhibits pancreatic cancer cell growth through inactivation of Jab1. Mol Pharmacol 2009; 76: 81–90.

[49] Pan Y, Wang M, Bu X, Zuo Y, Wang S, Wang D, Liu Q, Su B, Xu T, Wang C, Claret FX and Yang H. Curcumin analogue T83 exhibits potent antitumor activity and induces radiosensitivity through inactivation of Jab1 in nasopharyngeal carcinoma. BMC Cancer 2013; 13: 323.

[50] Yu J, Qiao L, Zimmermann L, Ebert MP, Zhang H, Lin W, Rocken C, Malfertheiner P and Farrell GC. Troglitazone inhibits tumor growth in hepatocellular carcinoma in vitro and in vivo. Hepatology 2006; 43: 134–143.

Chapter 11

Splicing Factors in Breast Cancer: Drivers of the Breast Tumor Fate

Felipe A. C. da Luz, Paula C. Brígido,
Alberto S. Moraes, Rogério A. Araújo and
Marcelo J. B. Silva

Additional information is available at the end of the chapter

http://dx.doi.org/10.5772/66162

Abstract

Splicing is a critical step in gene expression, responsible for the excision of introns, producing the mature form of mRNA. Also, the possible arrangements of exons enlarge the proteome in 80%, enabling one gene to encode more than one protein isoform, thus increasing proteome. Growing data show deregulation of splicing events in cancer, being breast cancer the most studied. This aberrant pattern of splicing has an important role in breast tumor progression. These alterations are mainly caused by misexpression of some critical alternative splicing factors. The behavior of these splicing factors is implicated with important clinical features, such as chemoresistance, aggressiveness, and also metastases. In this chapter, the role of five splicing factors is discussed in the light of relevant data about *in vitro*, *in vivo*, and *ex vivo* studies to construct a representative scheme of their behavior in breast cancer progression. Although the presented five splicing factors have important role in breast cancer, only three of them (ESRP1, RBFOX2, and SRSF1) have a more prominent role in tumorigenesis and tumor progression. These concepts will elucidate their role in tumorigenesis and a prospective use as biomarkers in breast cancer.

Keywords: breast cancer, aberrant splicing, tumor progression, splicing program, splicing factors

INTECH
open science | open minds

1. Introduction

1.1. Breast cancer: subtypes and epidemiology

Breast cancer is the most frequently diagnosed cancer and the leading cause of cancer death among women worldwide, with an estimated 1.7 million cases and 521,900 deaths in 2012 and accounts for 25% of all cancer cases and 15% of all cancer deaths among women [1]. The USA government expected 232,670 new cases of breast cancer in 2014, representing 29% of all cancers in women. Also, breast cancer represents 15% of all women cancer deaths [2].

If diagnosed in the initial stage, breast cancer is curable. However, at advanced stage, it is almost incurable. Actually, late diagnosis is one of the main factors that contribute to the poor prognosis of breast cancer patients [2].

Clinically, this heterogeneous disease is divided in three basic therapeutic categories: hormonal receptor-positive (ER/PR-positive; luminal A and luminal B), the most common and numerous, with several prognostic tests for hormonal-based therapy-treated patients; HER2/neu+ or ERBB2^{+}, with poor prognostic, but with target therapy, there is an improve in survival; and the triple-negative breast cancers (ER-negative, PR-negative, and HER2/neu-negative), with seven subtypes, the majority is aggressive, its treatment is more limited principally with chemotherapy, and has an incidence associated with mutated BRCA1 lineage or African ascendancy [3]. Another category, recently classified, was denominated as claudin-low, which is also triple-negative, but with low expression of proteins of cell-to-cell junctions, especially tight junctions, making it a highly infiltrating tumor [4].

1.2. Spliceosome and splicing: molecular basis of a critical event

All eukaryotic genes contain intragenic regions (introns), that usually not encode expression sequence to produce proteins, and expression regions (exons), that are the responsible for encoding expression sequence to produce proteins. Therefore, when expressing a gene, it is important to remove (excising) introns and the constitutive splicing is the event responsible for this event. In addition, approximately 95% of human genes encodes more than one protein isoform. This is achieved by differentially splicing the exons of the gene, called alternative exons, by alternative splicing. Importantly, alternative splicing is responsible for about 80% of gene variability [5].

Splicing is performed by the spliceosome, a core complex formed by five subcomplexes of snRNPs (small nuclear ribonucleoproteins), called U1, U2, U4/5 (always present as a bi-subcomplex), and U6 (U from **uracil** rich), and they participate in different steps during splicing. Several spliceosome-associated proteins, named splicing factors, coordinate the constitutive and alternative splicing. Alternative and constitutive splicing operate through a combination of positive and negative signals, called silencers and enhancers (*cis*-acting signals), present in the pre-mRNA (premature RNA) that are recognized by several splicing factors (*trans*-acting factors). In addition to *cis*-acting signals and *trans*-acting factors to splicing be exerted, the integrity of DNA and epigenetic changes (e.g. histone post-translational modifications) are important for physiological splicing as they can alter, or dictate, transcription rate and interaction of a splicing core complex and splicing factors, with the transcript and nucleosome [6, 7].

The most studied alternative splicing factors are the proteins of the SR (serine/arginine rich proteins) family, and hnRNP (heterogeneous nuclear ribonucleoproteins). These two types of proteins have RNA recognition motifs (RRM) and other domains that allow protein-protein and RNA-protein interactions during splicing [5].

1.3. Understanding the splicing factor stoichiometric relationship

As mentioned above, splicing factors can interact with proteins and RNA. Each splicing factor can recognize a different RNA sequence, therefore each splicing factor participates in the pre-mRNA excision (splicing) of a specific group of genes. Thus, the action spectra of each splicing factor are limited [5].

Many splicing factors are involved in the alternative splicing of a same pre-mRNA. For example, *FGFR2* (fibroblast growth factor receptor 2 gene) pre-mRNA has a UGCAUG sequence in the exon IIIc; this sequence is recognized by the splicing factor RBFOX2 in the exon IIIc, but, upstream to exon IIIc exists another sequence (CUGGGA) the SRSF1 splicing factor. The resulting interaction will dictate the resulting isoform: the IIIc (mesenchymal) or IIIb (epithelial) transcript isoform of *FGFR2*. Notwithstanding, the splicing factor hnRNP H/F recognizes the GGG sequence that is within the sequence (CUGGGGA) that SRSF1 recognizes, and inhibits the alternative splicing (exon IIIc inclusion). In addition, RBFOX2 interacts with hnRNP H/F. Thus, an interactive network is formed by these four splicing factors in a stoichiometric and competitive manner, depending on the expression levels of each splicing factor. Also, these splicing factors that compete by the same RNA region (SRSF1, hnRNP F/H) bind with different affinities [8].

Not only is the stoichiometric relationship important to dictate production of transcript isoform production but the localization of the splicing factor network is critical to alternative splicing. In the cited example (*FGFR2* alternative splicing), when the RBFOX2-hnRNP H/F network associates downstream of the exon IIIc, the splicing factors act toward alternative splicing, but they act as alternative splicing suppressors when associated upstream of the exon [8].

In summary, the association site of splicing factors determines the transcript destiny (constitutive, alternative or even aberrant, truncated, or degraded) [5]. However, how the splicing pattern of a cell is governed? Some studies elucidated whether splicing program is specific for each cell. The knowledge about this matter may help to understand why cancer cell presents such an aberrant splicing pattern.

1.4. Regulating the expression and activity of splicing factors

The relationship between splicing factors is mainly stoichiometric, and the expression levels of the splicing factors determine the expression of a dominant isoform of a transcript. Thus, one important question is raised: how the expression and activity of the splicing factors determined? Like other proteins by specific stimuli. For example, the activation and activity level of SR splicing factors are determined by their phosphorylation state (hypo- or hyper-phosphorylation) [14, 15], and the splicing activity depends on proper *de novo* phosphorylation and dephosphorylation [16–18]. One well-known stimulus is the activation of Ser/Arg-rich protein kinase 1 by AKT [19]. The AKT signaling pathway is activated by epidermal growth factor signaling [20]. Another example is the phosphorylation of SAM68 by MAPK, which regulates the CD44 alternative splicing [21]. Similar stimuli are important for regulating the levels of splicing factors and for noncoding RNA, mainly miRNA [22–25]. Therefore, regulation of splicing factor expression and activity, according to their own properties, is similar to other genes and proteins.

1.5. Understanding the splicing programs in physio(patho)logical contexts

The knowledge about the cellular splicing pattern (splicing program), that is, the production of cell-specific transcript isoform, consequently cell-specific protein isoforms, help to understand cell programming and fate, and, by extension, tumor fate.

The splicing pattern of pluripotent cells differs from a differentiated cell. During differentiation, the transcripts are differentially spliced, generating different isoforms (splicing shift). In addition, some splicing factors are differentially expressed. Nevertheless, induction of pluripotent cells from adult cells reverts the splicing program features. Also, the ectopic regulation of the splicing factors that govern the splicing shift results in an effectively splicing program shift [9].

These characteristics, that is, the regulation of cellular differentiation-specific splicing program by specific splicing factors, also occur in tissue-specific cells. It is now understood that the major cell types (epithelial, endothelial, and mesenchymal cells) have a common splicing program among these cell types of different organs, but a different splicing program among these cell types, and at least one main splicing factor governs each splicing program (ESRP1, PTBP1, and RBFOX2 for epithelial, endothelial, and mesenchymal cells, respectively). Notwithstanding, the cell type-specific splicing programs observed in these cell types may be controlled by a balanced expression of antagonist splicing factors, as well as antagonistic interactions between these three main splicing factors (ESRPs, RBFOX2, and PTBP1) [10].

Another important characteristic in physiologic splicing program regulation is the splicing shift and balance in cellular reprogramming, such as EMT (epithelial-to-mesenchymal transition). When EMT is triggered in epithelial cells, which have a high epithelial splicing program/low mesenchymal splicing program ratio, a balance is created by a splicing program switch. These cells express higher levels of RBFOX2 and have several splicing features similar to mesenchymal cells [11].

In carcinoma cells, a similar pattern is observed. These cells commonly have an epithelial splicing program/mesenchymal splicing program ratio resembling their phenotype, that is, a cell with lower epithelial features and high mesenchymal features has a lower epithelial splicing program/mesenchymal splicing program ratio, that is, their splicing program prone to a mesenchymal splicing program [11]. In addition, growing data point to a common splice program in cancer, considering its cellular type (epithelial, endothelial, or mesenchymal), despite its origin, with the main governing splicing factors as in healthy cells [12]. Understanding these common splicing program features shared among tumors allows us to predict tumor behavior during tumor progression in breast cancer according to their differentiation state.

1.6. Epithelial-to-mesenchymal transition (EMT)

Epithelial-to-mesenchymal transition (EMT) is the most important mechanisms that allow epithelial malignant cell to migrate, leading to metastases. During EMT, epithelial cells that are naturally attached to their tissue lose their epithelial markers and gain mesenchymal characteristics, being able to move away from tissue and migrate to a distant site, where they settle and return to an epithelial state by the reverse event mesenchymal-to-epithelial transition (MET) [12–14]. Several transcription factors regulate EMT, and other, different, regulate MET. As example, proteins of the Twist, Snail, and Zeb families, the well-known transcription factors of EMT, recognize specific DNA sequences (regulatory regions) near the promoters of genes, repressing genes of epithelial markers. Also, these transcription factors are involved in the expression of genes related to extracellular matrix degradation and migration [13, 14].

Important, misregulation of splicing factors has been observed during this event, and they are involved with a switch to the production of mesenchymal isoforms of several genes [11, 15–17].

1.7. Aberrant splicing in breast cancer

In cancerous cells, it is possible to observe an aberrant, thus different, pattern of splicing of several genes, even without DNA sequence change (mutations) or epigenetic changes [16, 18]. Actually, these alterations are due to the expression of misregulated splicing factors.

Several studies observed the misregulated expression of splicing factors in cancer, mainly breast cancer, although suggesting that the aberrant splicing is caused by an unbalanced stoichiometric relationship of splicing factors, compared to normal cells, leading to malignant features. Thus, many studies summarized the misregulated splicing factors observed in cancer and/or the consequences of aberrant splicing, including breast cancer [18–20]. For example, upregulation of RBFOX2, SRSF1, SF3B1, hnRNP A1, hnRNP F, and hnRNP H and downregulation of ESRPs are involved with tumor aggressiveness in breast cancer and other cancers [9, 11, 17, 21–38].

The growing evidence of splicing misregulations in cancer prompted several studies to understand the impact in splicing by these misregulations.

2. Misregulated splicing factors: directing the tumor fate

Aberrant splicing program in cancer cells is altered in comparison to healthy cells, but still is governed by splicing factors. In breast cancer, aberrant splicing is intricate with alternative and constitutive splicing factors. However, only the most relevant and most studied splicing factors in breast cancer are presented to understand the splicing behavior during breast cancer tumor progression. These splicing factors are representative of main types: SF3B1, component of spliceosomal core complex; SRSF1, a member of SR family; ESRP1 and ESRP2, alternative splicing factors with main role in tissue-specific (epithelial) splice program; and RBFOX2, the main alternative splicing factor that governs tissue-specific (mesenchymal) splice program.

Complementary data related to these splicing factors in other cancers will be presented for a greater understand of the tumor progression process in breast cancer.

2.1. SF3B1

SF3B1 (also known as Sap155, Sf3b155), from the SF1 complex, is responsible for the spliceosome core assembly in the pre-mRNA [5]. It is a constitutive splicing factor and is critical to the event. The SF3B1 protein complex is responsible for mis-spliced mRNA retention, performing quality control, which is the inspection of the intron excision and exon junction [39].

Despite the fact that this splicing factor is mostly studied in hematologic malignances [40] and its role in solid tumors is still being elucidated [41]. Some breast cancer patients showed a mutation in SF3B1 that was associated with the alternative splicing of key genes in ER-positive breast cancer, such as genes involved with cell metabolism, cell cycle, cell motility, protein degradation, apoptosis, and other cell events [42].

One extensive study showed upregulation of SF3B1 and SF3B3, associated with endocrine resistance in breast cancer samples, as well as two important correlations: in ER-positive breast cancer, the aggressiveness was associated with higher expression of SF3B3, while the aggressiveness of ER-negative breast cancer was associated with lower expression of SF3B1. Thus, researchers were able to correlate the levels, high or low, of SF3B3 and SF3B1, respectively, with prognosis in breast cancer patients, according to their ER status [32].

Although some studies reported impairment in the expression levels of constitutive splicing factors, such as SF3B1, other studies observed different behaviors. In one study, overexpression of some core complex splicing factors was observed in MYC-overexpressing breast cancer. Inhibition, or knockdown, of SF3B1 or BUD31, another component of the splicing core complex, but not of other core complex splicing factor, led to impaired tumor growth, reduced metastases, and apoptosis resistance abolishment in MYC-overexpressing breast cancer, without the substantial effect in normal cells. Studies also found that the overexpression of these splicing factors is related to the increased transcription rate caused by MYC-overexpression [33].

In brief, deregulation of SF3B1 as well as **constitutive** splicing factors is implicated with cell transcription rate rather than an oncoprotein *per se*.

2.2. SRSF1

SRSF1 is involved, additionally to splicing, with mRNA transport (nuclear exporting) and translation (in association with elF4E) [43]. It has one SR domain, in which the main regulatory function occurs, and two RRM domains that interact with RNA and other splicing factors [44].

The important role of SRSF1 was intensively analyzed in several studies. Overexpression of SRSF1 in mammary epithelial cells conferred apoptosis resistance by alternative splicing of apoptosis proteins BIM and BIN, high proliferative rate, invasion of skin and muscle, slight necrosis, high angiogenesis, and well-defined borders *in vivo* [30]. Upregulation of SRSF1 was responsible for conferring cell motility in several human adenocarcinoma cell lines by regulating alternative splicing of *RON* (a tyrosine kinase receptor), generating an alternative isoform that confers motility properties [31]. Similar results were obtained by other researchers [25]. Also, chemotherapy resistance was observed due to SRSF1 overexpression concomitant to EMT [45]. The role of SRSF1 upregulation in tumorigenesis was corroborated by other studies. Knockdown of SRSF1, or one of its products, in SRSF1-overexpressing cancer cells reverted the tumor features to a normal phenotype [25, 46].

Regarding the activity of SRSF1, very important results have been obtained. In one study, it was observed a differential expression of SRSF1 in cancer cell lines: it is highly expressed in the mesenchymal-like cells (low-density culture) when compared to the epithelial-like cells (high-density culture). The difference in the expression levels is related to an EMT alternative splicing profile: EMT cells produce a full-length mRNA of *SRSF1*, while epithelial cells produce an mRNA with a premature stop codon, leading to degradation of *SRSF1* mRNA. The main cause of that striking difference was analyzed: mesenchymal-like cells have highly phosphorylated ERK1/ERK2 pathway proteins compared to epithelial-like cells, and inhibition of the phosphorylation status in this pathway led to a hypophosphorylated status of Sam68, another splicing factor that mediates the splicing of *SRSF1* results in the production of an isoform with a premature stop codon, decreasing SRSF1 levels [47]. Thus, SRSF1 levels depend on signaling pathways in cancer cells too, and extracellular signals that led to EMT are also responsible for SRSF1 upregulation. This is corroborated by inhibition of proteins' intricate in important pathways that led, or sustain, EMT. For example, inhibition GSK3 kinase, as well as knockdown of AKT and GSK3beta kinase, led to SRSF1 downregulation, with a loss of apoptosis resistance and colony formation impairment [48]. In addition, inhibition of SRK1, a kinase of several SR proteins, led to reduced tumor growth *in vivo* through inhibition of angiogenesis [49]. Therefore, the activation of SR splicing factors by phosphorylation is crucial in the tumor context.

SRSF1 upregulation was observed not only in *in vitro* and *in vivo* models, but also in *ex vivo* samples. SRSF1 upregulation is observed in malignant tissue, but not in nonmalignant lesions [49]. SRSF1 upregulation was observed in several tumors, if compared to normal surrounding tissue, concomitant with antiapoptotic isoform of *BIN1* and oncogenic isoform of transcript targets of SRSF1 were observed in *in vitro* studies [25]. Moreover, SRSF1 upregulation was found to be correlated with tumor invasiveness only in some malignant lesions [45]. The tumorigenic role of SRSF1 is corroborated by the synergistic correlation between the oncogene *MYC*. A high expression of *SRSF1* occurs significantly more often in tumors that overexpress *MYC*, and positively correlated with a high histological grade compared to low *SRSF1* and/or low *MYC*-expressing breast tumors [30].

In summary, SRSF1 is an oncoprotein *per se*, as its overexpression causes tumor promotion, EMT, aggressive phenotypes, and chemoresistance. Nevertheless, signaling pathways directly regulate its activity and expression level. In addition, it is intricately related to the cell transcription rate, as seen in the overexpression of *MYC* in breast cancer.

2.3. ESRP1 and ESRP2

Epithelial splicing regulatory proteins (ESRPs) 1 and 2 participate in the epithelial-specific splicing program, downregulated during EMT [50]. ESRP1 knockout is lethal in embryos, and several developmental genes are regulated by these splicing factors [51].

As ESRPs are involved in the splice program in epithelial cells and play an important role in EMT. EMT transcription factors downregulate ESRPs, impacting the production of several protein isoforms coded by different genes, such as *FGFR2* and *CD44*, as well as adhesion molecules, surface receptors, and cytoskeleton [50, 52–56], independently of the stimuli that trigger EMT [34, 36, 57], resulting in predominance of mesenchymal splice program, mainly by ESRP1 downregulation [17, 34]. Otherwise, ESRP1 overexpression abrogates EMT [36, 54, 56, 58, 59], and the inverse phenomenon—the induction of MET—upregulates ESRP1 and reverts EMT [60].

The intricate role and behavior of ESRP1 in EMT seem to be orchestrated by upstream regulators, and indeed it is. ESRP1 expression is directly inhibited by some EMT transcription factors that recognize specific sequences near ESRP1 promoter, repressing its expression during EMT [54, 59].

Although all data appoint to ESRP1 downregulation in tumorigenesis and tumor progression, ESRP1 overexpression can contribute to the tumoral process and metastasis too [61]. However, ESRP1 downregulation is more expected in tumor progression than its upregulation. ESRP1 upregulation can be found within tumor lesion and can correlate with tumor progression, but ESRP1 downregulation is observed in the invasive front, mainly in invasive tumors with EMT features [34]. That phenomenon can be found concomitant with downstream products of ESRP1, like FGFR2-IIIc expression in function of ESRP1 downregulation, but not necessarily with metastases [37]; also can be found in poorly differentiated cancer and correlate with poor prognosis [36]. Also, ESRP1 downregulation is intricate with advent of cancer stem-like cell features in breast cancer [55].

In brief, upstream effectors that dictate cell phenotype and behavior, mainly EMT/MET-TFs, also regulate ESRP expression, the main **alternative** splicing factor that governs the epithelial splice program. Other transcription factors, such as stem transcription factors, may also regulate ESRPs, as ESRP upregulation was observed concomitantly with stemness. The low expression level of ESRPs led to the production of alternative transcript isoforms of key genes involved with cell metabolism, cell cycle, motility, invasiveness, and robustness.

2.4. RBFOX2

RBFOX2 (also known as Fox2 and Rbm9, and formerly known as the repressor of tamoxifen transcriptional activity—RTA) is a tissue-specific splicing factor [11]. It is directly associated with the production of alternative protein isoforms and rarely to constitutive isoforms [62].

The first study that described RBFOX2 as an RRM-containing protein observed that it inhibits the partial ERβ agonistic activity of tamoxifen through this domain. Moreover, this splicing factor is intricately related to the repression of ERβ, PR (progesterone receptor), and GR (glucocorticoid receptor) activities. With these data, it is inductive to think that RBFOX2 is a repressor of activity in the steroid receptor family [63]

The role of RBFOX2 in EMT has been partially elucidated and has been intensively studied in breast cancer. Different cancer cell lines have high expression of RBFOX2 [11]. This splicing factor is associated with a mesenchymal identity, since depletion of RBFOX2 in breast cancer with mesenchymal features induced MET, thus reverting EMT [11, 17]. Similar events occur in mouse breast cancer cells. EMT causes Rbfox2 (mouse homolog of RBFOX2) overexpression, and abolishment of EMT reestablishes the expression levels of Rbfox2. Also, Rbfox2 is important to maintain invasive features [15].

RBFOX2 expression and splicing activity are regulated by some EMT transcription factors, leading to a similar splicing pattern to that of breast cancer cells, which is associated with the expression of distinct isoforms of several genes that govern EMT [17]. RBFOX2 expression is altered in some cancer in comparison to their normal counterparts [64]. In addition, RBFOX2 has an important role in the overall splicing patter in breast cancer [65] and is more expressed in claudin-low and basal-like cancers than in luminal A and B, leading to the aberrant inclusion of alternative exons observed in cancer [35]. These aggressiveness of these breast cancer subtypes (claudin-low and basal-like) could be partially explained by the resultant splicing events of RBFOX2 upregulation [35].

In summary, RBFOX is the primary **alternative** splicing factor that governs the mesenchymal splice program, mainly EMT/MET-TFs. Other transcription factors, such as stem transcription factors, may regulate RBFOX2. The expression level of RBFOX2 leads to the production of alternative transcript isoforms of key genes involved with cell metabolism, cell cycle, motility, invasiveness, and robustness.

3. Lessons from alternative splicing misregulation

Albeit few splicing factors were presented in the last section, though the most important splicing factors, to date, in breast cancer, the understanding of their role in tumor promotion and progression in breast cancer allows us to construct and predict the behavior of these splicing factors, according to clinical features and molecular subtype. Several splicing markers can discriminate ER^+ from ER^- breast cancer and correlate with a tumor grade, demonstrating that the ER status impacts the splicing program [11, 35, 56, 66, 67]. Therefore, the splicing factors play a role in a key and basic event (alternative splicing) that dictates several features and phenotype of cells.

The main impact of splicing observed in cancer is due to alternative splicing factor misregulation rather than the constitutive splicing factor, as mentioned in the previous section. In addition, not all alternative splicing factors have an expressive role in alternative splicing, but only few main splicing factors. ESRP1 and RBFOX2, splicing factors that govern splicing programs, are responsible for general aggressive phenotypic features of breast cancer, and SRSF1 plays a critical role in breast cancer tumorigenesis and malignancy. These findings allow us to predict general features of breast cancer according to the behavior (expression) of these splicing factors. Current data about these three splicing factors in breast cancer let the construction of a hypothetical scheme of well- and poor-differentiated breast cancer, starting from tumor promotion [30, 43], following tumor progression [15, 25, 30, 31, 43, 45–47, 52], metastasis, and acquired resistance (clone selection) [11, 15, 31, 34, 38, 47, 50, 53, 54, 61], regarding the behavior of these splicing factors (**Figure 1**). Summarizing these findings in one figure opens a door to an important practical use of that knowledge: a potential power as diagnostic and prognostic markers.

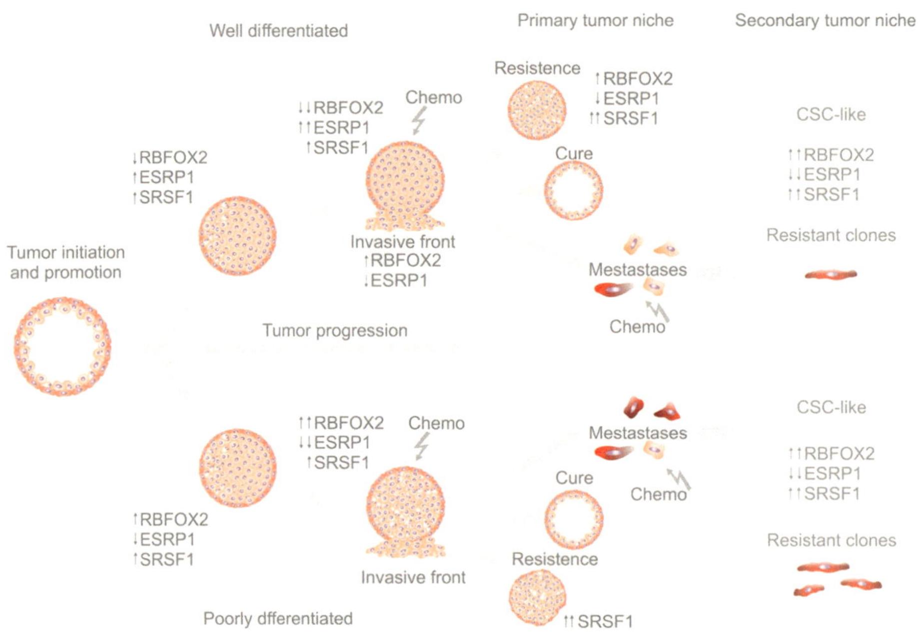

Figure 1. SRSF1, ESRP1, and RBFOX2 participation in tumor progression. Expression patterns of splicing factors according to the pathological status of tumors. Well-differentiated tumor (upper side): according to the literature, well-differentiated tumors express higher levels of ESRP1 and SRSF1 and lower levels of RBFOX2 compared to normal surrounding tissue, and these characteristics are most striking with tumor progression. However, the invasive front has an inverse pattern that is similar to EMT cells. The majority of metastatic cells that originate from these tumors do not have CSC features. Poorly differentiated tumor (lower side): according to the literature, poorly differentiated tumors express higher levels of RBFOX2 and SRSF1 and lower levels of ESRP1 compared to normal surrounding tissue, and these characteristics are most striking with tumor progression. As these cells have EMT features (mesenchymal-like), the invasive front is derived from the tumor pool in the primary niche. The majority of metastatic cells that originate from these tumors have CSC features. These two tumors have two fates in response to chemotherapy: cure and resistance. Although well-differentiated tumors are more sensitive to chemotherapy, with a higher cure index, resistant clones in the primary tumor niche, mainly EMT cells, can be selected and expanded, originating a poorly differentiated tumor; the metastatic cells and secondary tumor cells are cleared with chemotherapy, but CSCs, when present, are selected and expanded. Resistant cells (CSCs) express even higher levels of RBFOX2 and SRSF1 and even lower levels of ESRP1 with an EMT phenotype.

4. Concluding remarks

Although the prognostic and diagnostic value of splicing factors is not well understood, some studies have shown that an expression pattern of some splicing factors is observable in breast cancer. In addition, analysis of splicing factors related to splicing programs help to understand other processes involved in tumor progression, like aggressiveness. Also, other splicing factors are related to chemoresistance and hormonal status, mainly estrogen. Thus, the behavior of splicing factors could be used, at least, as prognostic markers for breast cancer and could help to choice, or direct, therapy in a near future.

Acknowledgements

We gratefully acknowledge financial support from the Brazilian Agencies CAPES, FAPEMIG and MCT/CNPq, and NUPPEC-Cancer Hospital of Uberlândia/Grupo Luta pela Vida.

Abbreviations

ESRP1	Epithelial splicing regulatory protein 1
RBFOX2	RNA binding protein fox-1 homolog 2
SRSF1	Serine/arginine rich splicing factor 1
SF3B1	Splicing factor 3B subunit 1
PTBP1	Polypyrimidine tract binding protein 1
ER	Estrogen receptor
PR	Progesterone receptor
ERBB2	ERB-b receptor tyrosine kinase 2
FGFR2	Fibroblast growth factor receptor 2
hnRNP	Heterogeneous ribonucleoprotein particle
MAPK	Mitogen activated protein kinase
EMT	Epithelial mesenchymal transition
MET	Mesenchymal epithelial transition
ERK	Extracellular signal-regulated kinases

Author details

Felipe A. C. da Luz[1], Paula C. Brígido[2], Alberto S. Moraes[3], Rogério A. Araújo[4] and Marcelo J. B. Silva[1*]

*Address all correspondence to: majbsilva@gmail.com

1 Laboratório de Osteoimunologia e Imunologia dos Tumores, Instituto de Ciências Biomédicas (ICBIM), Universidade Federal de Uberlândia (UFU), Uberlândia, MG, Brazil

2 Laboratório de Tripanossomatídeos, Instituto de Ciências Biomédicas (ICBIM), Universidade Federal de Uberlândia (UFU), Uberlândia, MG, Brazil

3 Department ode Biologia Celular, Histologia e Embriologia, Instituto de Ciências Biomédicas, Universidade Federal de Uberlândia, Uberlândia, MG, Brazil

4 Hospital do Câncer, HC, UFU, MG, Brazil

References

[1] Torre LA, Bray F, Siegel RL, Ferlay J, Lortet-Tieulent J, Jemal A. Global cancer statistics, 2012. CA Cancer J Clin. 2015;2:87–108. Doi: 10.3322/caac.21262.

[2] Siegel R, Ma J, Zou Z, Jemal A. Cancer statistics, 2014. CA Cancer J Clin. 2014;1:9–29. Doi: 10.3322/caac.21208.

[3] Schnitt SJ. Classification and prognosis of invasive breast cancer: from morphology to molecular taxonomy. Mod Pathol. 2010; 23:S60–64. Doi: 10.1038/modpathol.2010.33.

[4] Network TCGA. Comprehensive molecular portraits of human breast tumours. Nature. 2012;7418:61–70. Doi: 10.1038/nature11412.

[5] Wahl MC, Will CL, Luhrmann R. The spliceosome: design principles of a dynamic RNP machine. Cell. 2009;4:701–718. Doi: 10.1016/j.cell.2009.02.009.

[6] de la Mata M, Lafaille C, Kornblihtt AR. First come, first served revisited: factors affecting the same alternative splicing event have different effects on the relative rates of intron removal. RNA. 2010;5:904–912. Doi: 10.1261/rna.1993510.

[7] Sims RJ, 3rd, Millhouse S, Chen CF, Lewis BA, Erdjument-Bromage H, Tempst P, et al. Recognition of trimethylated histone H3 lysine 4 facilitates the recruitment of transcription postinitiation factors and pre-mRNA splicing. Mol Cell. 2007;4:665–676. Doi: 10.1016/j.molcel.2007.11.010.

[8] Mauger DM, Lin C, Garcia-Blanco MA. hnRNP H and hnRNP F complex with Fox2 to silence fibroblast growth factor receptor 2 exon IIIc. Mol Cell Biol. 2008;17:5403–5419. Doi: 10.1128/MCB.00739-08.

[9] Venables JP, Lapasset L, Gadea G, Fort P, Klinck R, Irimia M, et al. MBNL1 and RBFOX2 cooperate to establish a splicing programme involved in pluripotent stem cell differentiation. Nat Commun. 2013:248010.1038/ncomms3480.

[10] Mallinjoud P, Villemin JP, Mortada H, Polay Espinoza M, Desmet FO, Samaan S, et al. Endothelial, epithelial, and fibroblast cells exhibit specific splicing programs independently of their tissue of origin. Genome Res. 2014;3:511–521. Doi: 10.1101/gr.162933.113.

[11] Venables JP, Brosseau JP, Gadea G, Klinck R, Prinos P, Beaulieu JF, et al. RBFOX2 is an important regulator of mesenchymal tissue-specific splicing in both normal and cancer tissues. Mol Cell Biol. 2013;2:396–405. Doi: 10.1128/MCB.01174-12.

[12] Danan-Gotthold M, Golan-Gerstl R, Eisenberg E, Meir K, Karni R, Levanon EY. Identification of recurrent regulated alternative splicing events across human solid tumors. Nucleic Acids Res. 2015;10:5130–5144. Doi: 10.1093/nar/gkv210.

[13] Chou YS, Yang MH. Epithelial-mesenchymal transition-related factors in solid tumor and hematological malignancy. J Chin Med Assoc. 2015;8:438–445. Doi: 10.1016/j.jcma.2015.05.002.

[14] Cichon MA, Nelson CM, Radisky DC. Regulation of epithelial-mesenchymal transition in breast cancer cells by cell contact and adhesion. Cancer informatics. 2015;Suppl 3:1–13. Doi: 10.4137/CIN.S18965.

[15] Braeutigam C, Rago L, Rolke A, Waldmeier L, Christofori G, Winter J. The RNA-binding protein Rbfox2: an essential regulator of EMT-driven alternative splicing and a mediator of cellular invasion. Oncogene. 2014;9:1082–1092. Doi: 10.1038/onc.2013.50.

[16] Germann S, Gratadou L, Dutertre M, Auboeuf D. Splicing programs and cancer. J Nucleic Acids. 2012; 2012, Article ID: 269570. Doi: 10.1155/2012/269570.

[17] Shapiro IM, Cheng AW, Flytzanis NC, Balsamo M, Condeelis JS, Oktay MH, et al. An EMT-driven alternative splicing program occurs in human breast cancer and modulates cellular phenotype. PLoS Genet. 2011;8:e1002218. Doi: 10.1371/journal.pgen.1002218.

[18] Venables JP. Aberrant and alternative splicing in cancer. Cancer Res. 2004;21:7647–7654. Doi: 10.1158/0008-5472.CAN-04-1910.

[19] Fackenthal JD, Godley LA. Aberrant RNA splicing and its functional consequences in cancer cells. Dis Model Mech. 2008;1:37–42. Doi: 10.1242/dmm.000331.

[20] Silipo M, Gautrey H, Tyson-Capper A. Deregulation of splicing factors and breast cancer development. J Mol Cell Biol. 2015; 7: 388–401. Doi: 10.1093/jmcb/mjv027.

[21] Patry C, Bouchard L, Labrecque P, Gendron D, Lemieux B, Toutant J, et al. Small interfering RNA-mediated reduction in heterogeneous nuclear ribonucleoparticule A1/

A2 proteins induces apoptosis in human cancer cells but not in normal mortal cell lines. Cancer Res. 2003;22:7679–7688.

[22] He Y, Brown MA, Rothnagel JA, Saunders NA, Smith R. Roles of heterogeneous nuclear ribonucleoproteins A and B in cell proliferation. J Cell Sci. 2005;Pt 14:3173–3183. Doi: 10.1242/jcs.02448.

[23] David CJ, Manley JL. Alternative pre-mRNA splicing regulation in cancer: pathways and programs unhinged. Genes Dev. 2010;21:2343–2364. Doi: 10.1101/gad.1973010.

[24] Li S, Xu H, Ding H, Huang Y, Cao X, Yang G, et al. Identification of an aptamer targeting hnRNP A1 by tissue slide-based SELEX. J Pathol. 2009;3:327–336. Doi: 10.1002/path. 2543.

[25] Karni R, de Stanchina E, Lowe SW, Sinha R, Mu D, Krainer AR. The gene encoding the splicing factor SF2/ASF is a proto-oncogene. Nat Struct Mol Biol. 2007;3:185–193. Doi: 10.1038/nsmb1209.

[26] Zhou ZJ, Dai Z, Zhou SL, Fu XT, Zhao YM, Shi YH, et al. Overexpression of HnRNP A1 promotes tumor invasion through regulating CD44v6 and indicates poor prognosis for hepatocellular carcinoma. Int J Cancer. 2013;5:1080–1089. Doi: 10.1002/ijc.27742.

[27] Honore B, Baandrup U, Vorum H. Heterogeneous nuclear ribonucleoproteins F and H/ H′ show differential expression in normal and selected cancer tissues. Experiment Cell Res. 2004;1:199–209. Doi: 10.1016/j.yexcr.2003.11.011.

[28] Rauch J, Ahlemann M, Schaffrik M, Mack B, Ertongur S, Andratschke M, et al. Allogenic antibody-mediated identification of head and neck cancer antigens. Biochem Biophys Res Commun. 2004;1:156–162. Doi: 10.1016/j.bbrc.2004.08.071.

[29] Rauch J, O'Neill E, Mack B, Matthias C, Munz M, Kolch W, et al. Heterogeneous nuclear ribonucleoprotein H blocks MST2-mediated apoptosis in cancer cells by regulating A-Raf transcription. Cancer Res. 2010;4:16791688. Doi: 10.1158/0008-5472.CAN-09-2740.

[30] Anczukow O, Rosenberg AZ, Akerman M, Das S, Zhan L, Karni R, et al. The splicing factor SRSF1 regulates apoptosis and proliferation to promote mammary epithelial cell transformation. Nat Struct Mol Biol. 2012;2:220–228. Doi: 10.1038/nsmb.2207.

[31] Ghigna C, Giordano S, Shen H, Benvenuto F, Castiglioni F, Comoglio PM, et al. Cell motility is controlled by SF2/ASF through alternative splicing of the Ron protooncogene. Mol Cell. 2005;6:881–890. Doi: 10.1016/j.molcel.2005.10.026.

[32] Gokmen-Polar Y, Neelamraju Y, Goswami CP, Gu X, Nallamothu G, Janga SC, et al. Expression levels of SF3B3 correlate with prognosis and endocrine resistance in estrogen receptor-positive breast cancer. Mod Pathol. 2014;28:677–685. Doi: 10.1038/ modpathol.2014.146.

[33] Hsu TY, Simon LM, Neill NJ, Marcotte R, Sayad A, Bland CS, et al. The spliceosome is a therapeutic vulnerability in MYC-driven cancer. Nature. 2015;7569:384–388. Doi: 10.1038/nature14985.

[34] Ishii H, Saitoh M, Sakamoto K, Kondo T, Katoh R, Tanaka S, et al. Epithelial splicing regulatory proteins 1 (ESRP1) and 2 (ESRP2) suppress cancer cell motility via different mechanisms. J Biol Chem. 2014;40:27386–27399. Doi: 10.1074/jbc.M114.589432.

[35] Lapuk A, Marr H, Jakkula L, Pedro H, Bhattacharya S, Purdom E, et al. Exon-level microarray analyses identify alternative splicing programs in breast cancer. Mol Cancer Res. 2010;7:961–974. Doi: 10.1158/1541-7786.MCR-09-0528.

[36] Ueda J, Matsuda Y, Yamahatsu K, Uchida E, Naito Z, Korc M, et al. Epithelial splicing regulatory protein 1 is a favorable prognostic factor in pancreatic cancer that attenuates pancreatic metastases. Oncogene. 2014;36:4485–4495. Doi: 10.1038/onc.2013.392.

[37] Zhao Q, Caballero OL, Davis ID, Jonasch E, Tamboli P, Yung WK, et al. Tumor-specific isoform switch of the fibroblast growth factor receptor 2 underlies the mesenchymal and malignant phenotypes of clear cell renal cell carcinomas. Clin Cancer Res. 2013;9:2460–2472. Doi: 10.1158/1078-0432.CCR-12-3708.

[38] Zheng X, Carstens JL, Kim J, Scheible M, Kaye J, Sugimoto H, et al. Epithelial-to-mesenchymal transition is dispensable for metastasis but induces chemoresistance in pancreatic cancer. Nature. 2015;7579:525–530. Doi: 10.1038/nature16064.

[39] Lo CW, Kaida D, Nishimura S, Matsuyama A, Yashiroda Y, Taoka H, et al. Inhibition of splicing and nuclear retention of pre-mRNA by spliceostatin A in fission yeast. Biochem Biophys Res Commun. 2007;3:573–577. Doi: 10.1016/j.bbrc.2007.10.029.

[40] Hahn CN, Venugopal P, Scott HS, Hiwase DK. Splice factor mutations and alternative splicing as drivers of hematopoietic malignancy. Immunol Rev. 2015;1:257–278. Doi: 10.1111/imr.12241.

[41] Scott LM, Rebel VI. Acquired mutations that affect pre-mRNA splicing in hematologic malignancies and solid tumors. J Natl Cancer Inst. 2013;20:1540–1549. Doi: 10.1093/jnci/djt257.

[42] Maguire SL, Leonidou A, Wai P, Marchio C, Ng CK, Sapino A, et al. SF3B1 mutations constitute a novel therapeutic target in breast cancer. J Pathol. 2014;235:571–580. Doi: 10.1002/path.4483.

[43] Li X, Manley JL. Inactivation of the SR protein splicing factor ASF/SF2 results in genomic instability. Cell. 2005;3:365–378. Doi: 10.1016/j.cell.2005.06.008.

[44] Ngo JC, Giang K, Chakrabarti S, Ma CT, Huynh N, Hagopian JC, et al. A sliding docking interaction is essential for sequential and processive phosphorylation of an SR protein by SRPK1. Mol Cell. 2008;5:563–576. Doi; 10.1016/j.molcel.2007.12.017.

[45] Gout S, Brambilla E, Boudria A, Drissi R, Lantuejoul S, Gazzeri S, et al. Abnormal expression of the pre-mRNA splicing regulators SRSF1, SRSF2, SRPK1 and SRPK2 in

non small cell lung carcinoma. PLoS One. 2012;10:e46539. Doi: 10.1371/journal.pone.0046539.

[46] Ben-Hur V, Denichenko P, Siegfried Z, Maimon A, Krainer A, Davidson B, et al. S6K1 alternative splicing modulates its oncogenic activity and regulates mTORC1. Cell Reports. 2013;1:103–115. Doi: 10.1016/j.celrep.2012.11.020.

[47] Valacca C, Bonomi S, Buratti E, Pedrotti S, Baralle FE, Sette C, et al. Sam68 regulates EMT through alternative splicing-activated nonsense-mediated mRNA decay of the SF2/ASF proto-oncogene. J Cell Biol. 2010;1:87–99. Doi: 10.1083/jcb.201001073.

[48] Yadav AK, Vashishta V, Joshi N, Taneja P. AR-A 014418 Used against GSK3beta Downregulates expression of hnRNPA1 and SF2/ASF splicing factors. J Oncol. 2014; 2014:9 Article ID 695325. Doi: 10.1155/2014/695325.

[49] Mavrou A, Brakspear K, Hamdollah-Zadeh M, Damodaran G, Babaei-Jadidi R, Oxley J, et al. Serine-arginine protein kinase 1 (SRPK1) inhibition as a potential novel targeted therapeutic strategy in prostate cancer. Oncogene. 2015;33:4311–4319. Doi: 10.1038/onc.2014.360.

[50] Warzecha CC, Shen S, Xing Y, Carstens RP. The epithelial splicing factors ESRP1 and ESRP2 positively and negatively regulate diverse types of alternative splicing events. RNA Biol. 2009;5:546–562.

[51] Bebee TW, Park JW, Sheridan KI, Warzecha CC, Cieply BW, Rohacek AM, et al. The splicing regulators Esrp1 and Esrp2 direct an epithelial splicing program essential for mammalian development. eLife. 2015; 4: 10.7554/eLife.08954.

[52] Brown RL, Reinke LM, Damerow MS, Perez D, Chodosh LA, Yang J, et al. CD44 splice isoform switching in human and mouse epithelium is essential for epithelial-mesenchymal transition and breast cancer progression. J Clin Invest. 2011;3:1064–1074. Doi: 10.1172/JCI44540.

[53] Warzecha CC, Jiang P, Amirikian K, Dittmar KA, Lu H, Shen S, et al. An ESRP-regulated splicing programme is abrogated during the epithelial-mesenchymal transition. EMBO J. 2010;19:3286–3300. Doi: 10.1038/emboj.2010.195.

[54] Reinke LM, Xu Y, Cheng C. Snail represses the splicing regulator epithelial splicing regulatory protein 1 to promote epithelial-mesenchymal transition. J Biol Chem. 2012;43:36435–36442. Doi: 10.1074/jbc.M112.397125.

[55] Goel HL, Gritsko T, Pursell B, Chang C, Shultz LD, Greiner DL, et al. Regulated splicing of the alpha6 integrin cytoplasmic domain determines the fate of breast cancer stem cells. Cell reports. 2014;3:747–761. Doi: 10.1016/j.celrep.2014.03.059.

[56] Di Modugno F, Iapicca P, Boudreau A, Mottolese M, Terrenato I, Perracchio L, et al. Splicing program of human MENA produces a previously undescribed isoform associated with invasive, mesenchymal-like breast tumors. Proc Natl Acad Sci U S A. 2012;47:19280–19285. Doi: 10.1073/pnas.1214394109.

[57] Ranieri D, Belleudi F, Magenta A, Torrisi MR. HPV16 E5 expression induces switching from FGFR2b to FGFR2c and epithelial-mesenchymal transition. Int J Cancer. 2015;1:61–72. Doi: 10.1002/ijc.29373.

[58] Leontieva OV, Ionov Y. RNA-binding motif protein 35A is a novel tumor suppressor for colorectal cancer. Cell cycle. 2009;3:490–497.

[59] Horiguchi K, Sakamoto K, Koinuma D, Semba K, Inoue A, Inoue S, et al. TGF-beta drives epithelial-mesenchymal transition through deltaEF1-mediated downregulation of ESRP. Oncogene. 2012;26:3190–3201. Doi: 10.1038/onc.2011.493.

[60] Roca H, Hernandez J, Weidner S, McEachin RC, Fuller D, Sud S, et al. Transcription factors OVOL1 and OVOL2 induce the mesenchymal to epithelial transition in human cancer. PLoS One. 2013;10:e76773. Doi: 10.1371/journal.pone.0076773.

[61] Yae T, Tsuchihashi K, Ishimoto T, Motohara T, Yoshikawa M, Yoshida GJ, et al. Alternative splicing of CD44 mRNA by ESRP1 enhances lung colonization of metastatic cancer cell. Nat Commun. 2012;3:883. Doi: 10.1038/ncomms1892.

[62] Damianov A, Black DL. Autoregulation of Fox protein expression to produce dominant negative splicing factors. RNA. 2010;2:405–416. Doi: 10.1261/rna.1838210.

[63] Norris JD, Fan D, Sherk A, McDonnell DP. A negative coregulator for the human ER. Mol Endocrinol. 2002;3:459–468. Doi: 10.1210/mend.16.3.0787.

[64] Venables JP, Klinck R, Koh C, Gervais-Bird J, Bramard A, Inkel L, et al. Cancer-associated regulation of alternative splicing. Nat Struct Mol Biol. 2009;6:670–676. Doi: 10.1038/nsmb.1608.

[65] Wen J, Toomer KH, Chen Z, Cai X. Genome-wide analysis of alternative transcripts in human breast cancer. Breast Cancer Res Treat. 2015;2:295–307. Doi: 10.1007/s10549-015-3395-2.

[66] Venables JP, Klinck R, Bramard A, Inkel L, Dufresne-Martin G, Koh C, et al. Identification of alternative splicing markers for breast cancer. Cancer Res. 2008;22:9525–9531. Doi: 10.1158/0008-5472.CAN-08-1769.

[67] Cen YL, Qi ML, Li HG, Su Y, Chen LJ, Lin Y, et al. Associations of polymorphisms in the genes of FGFR2, FGF1, and RBFOX2 with breast cancer risk by estrogen/progesterone receptor status. Mol Carcinog. 2013, 52:E52–59. Doi: 10.1002/mc.21979.

Chapter 12

The Role of Stem Cells in Breast Cancer

Joanna Magdalena Zarzynska

Additional information is available at the end of the chapter

http://dx.doi.org/10.5772/66904

Abstract

A significant progress has been made in describing cellular hierarchy and the stem cell niche in the human mammary gland. Mammary stem and progenitor cells exist in two different states: epithelial-like and mesenchymal-like. Several features of the mammary stem cells predispose them to play a critical role in breast cancer initiation, progression and metastasis. Signaling pathways contributing to the self-renewal, such as Wnt, Notch, Hh and BMP, have been shown to be linked with breast cancer stem cells. Furthermore, biomarkers connected with stemness, such as CD44, CD24, EpCAM and ALDH1, have been identified and used to characterize these cells. Additionally, many different miRNA families and microenvironmental factors were shown to regulate a lot of cancer stem cells properties and maintain their stemness. All these findings have started a new era of breast cancer research. In present breast cancer, stem cells have become the targets of breast cancer therapy, although the tests are mainly on the basic stage level. Since the cancer stem cells are able to escape chemotherapy and are resistant to drugs, radiotherapy and apoptotic processes, the therapeutic targeting is mostly concentrated on the disruption of survival signaling pathways and the use of modern technology, like nanotechnology.

Keywords: cancer stem cells, breast cancer, MaSC, BCSCs, stem cell niche, miRNA, EMT

1. Introduction

As most epithelia, mammary epithelium continuously replaces dead or damaged cells during the whole life of an animal and this process called tissue homeostasis is critical for adult tissues maintenance. Typically, epithelial tissue homeostasis is maintained through the presence of stem cells (SC). They are functionally defined in connection with their ability to self-renew and differentiate into cell lineages of their original tissue [1–3]. Mammary stem cells (MaSC) are capable of generating the complex bilayer system of the mammary epithelium composed of basal (myoepithelial) and luminal (secretory) epithelial cells. In addition, there are mesenchymal stem cells (MSCs), representing the stromal (fat pad) part of this organ [1]. According to current knowledge, scientists had made the model of SC mitotic division, which can be symmetric or asymmetric. During symmetric division, stem cell gives two daughter stem cells and it allows for the expansion of stem cell population. When a stem cell undergoes asymmetric division, one stem cell is obtained maintaining the self-renewal properties, whereas the another cell is called a progenitor cell. Progenitor cells have a more restricted potential in terms of their renewal and differentiation. Progenitor cells also have limited proliferation capacity and can undergo senescence [1, 2].

Several features of MaSC make them plausible sites for breast cancer (BC) initiation. Breast cancer is a potentially life-threatening malignant tumor that still causes high mortality among women. Decreasing mortality rates has been achieved, that is, by efficient screening strategies [4]. Still, BC is ranked on the second place among cancer types regarding mortality [5]. It has been estimated that approximately 1.3 million females develop BC each year with around 465,000 expected to succumb to the disease [6–8]. MaSC have been postulated to underlie the cellular heterogeneity observed in human breast cancers due to their preserved replicative capacity and differentiation potential, resulting in prolonged life span and thus increased probability of harboring and accumulation of mutations [9, 10]. The cancer stem cell (CSC) fraction typically constitutes 1–5% of the tumor size [8, 11]. In the healthy human mammary gland, SC account for approximately 8% of the cells [12]. The concept of CSC has led to the development of new theoretical models explaining the cellular origin of cancer [13, 14]. One theory, called the stochastic theory, claims that every single cell can potentially become cancerous in the appropriate microenvironment. However, differentiated cells are probably unable to accumulate a sufficient number of mutations in order to become neoplastic because of their shorter life span. Second theory, called the hierarchy (CSC) theory, suggests that CSC are more likely to initiate the tumor, as they have longer life span, increased migratory and proliferative potential and advanced DNA repair mechanisms. Since it is more probable that these two models coexist, a dynamic version of the CSC model has been developed, suggesting that within the tumor hierarchy, differentiated tumor cells may undergo dedifferentiation as a result of microenvironmental influences. In addition to the generation of cells with stem-like properties, the tumor microenvironment is also involved in the preservation of the established CSC subpopulation [15, 16].

Increasing evidence demonstrates that CSC play a critical role not only in BC initiation, but also in progression and metastasis [13]. Accumulating evidence indicates that the local recurrent and/or distant metastatic tumors, which constitute the major causes of lethality in the clinic, are related to the aggressive phenotype of a small fraction of cancer stem cells, tumor-initiating cells (TICs) or cancer metastasis-initiating cells (CMICs) [17].

Breast cancer stem cells (BCSCs) are able to escape chemotherapy due to elevated expression of ABC transporters that enable them to efflux some chemotherapeutic drugs [13]. They are resistant to apoptosis (they also express high levels of anti-apoptotic proteins, such as survivin and Bcl-2) and show drug resistance [11]. In addition, the activity of BCSCs can enhance and the ratio of side population can increase after radiation treatment. Furthermore, BC has capability to resist radiotherapy [17–19]. Therefore, it has been suggested that BCSCs might be responsible for tumor regrowth and the development of drug resistance [2, 13, 17].

http://dx.doi.org/10.5772/66904

Identification of BCSCs represents a major step forward in elucidation of the BC tumor hierarchy and has started a new era of breast cancer research. Still, in present, there is no uniform approach, which would allow for a quick and simple detection of BCSCs in solid tumors. Therefore, a lot of scientific studies are focused on targeting BCSCs in BC therapy in different ways, using the current knowledge about those cells. For example, BCSCs are characterized by the activation of stemness-related pathways, such as the Notch and Wnt pathways and by the expression of certain stem cell markers. Since CSC are highly resistant to chemotherapy, additional treatment of BC patients with BCSC-specific drugs and inhibitors, which target the Wnt or Notch pathway, respectively, will be required [2].

2. The concept of stem cell hierarchy in the mammary gland

The mammary epithelial tissue forms a highly organized branched bilayered ductal network consisting of basal myoepithelial cells and luminal (secretory) epithelial cells [1, 20]. Distinct markers characterize luminal and basal cells. Luminal cells express cytokeratins (CKs) 8/18 and 19, as well as other molecular markers, such as MUC1, GATA3 and CD24. Basal myoepithelial cells express CK14 (50 kDa), CK5 (58 kDa) and CK17 (46 kDa), as well as smooth muscle actin (SMA) and vimentin [21]. Numerous scientific reports have provided evidence of existence of a much more complex mammary epithelial hierarchy, which is responsible for tissue growth and maintenance during periods of development and homeostasis [20]. Mammary cell proliferation, turnover and tissue regeneration are functions of MaSC [21, 22]. To present the idea in a simplified model, progenitor cell lineages are derived strictly from bi-potent or multi-potent stem cells. Then, they divide and differentiate into the epithelium of adult mammary gland composed of both matured luminal and basal cells [23] (**Figure 1A**). The scientists have identified different subpopulations of cells in human and mouse mammary gland, using cell sorting techniques [20]. Subsets of mammary epithelial cells (MEC) were characterized using different surface markers. Accordingly, CD24 and EpCAM are known to be the luminal cell markers and CD49f and CD29 are the basal cell markers. This diversification is invariably used in classifying of luminal and basal MEC populations.

The perspective of MaSC isolation, which then were be able to give rise to an entire mammary epithelial tree upon transplantation of a single stem cell [24, 25] and the phenotypic identification of several mammary epithelial progenitor cell (MaPC) populations [26, 27], has enhanced our current understanding of the differentiation hierarchy [28]. Furthermore, *in vivo* genetic tracing experiments have shown that both cell types contribute to morphogenesis in puberty and pregnancy and ductal maintenance in the adult gland [28].

To characterize MaSC, a clear distinction between normal stem cells and tumor stem cells must be made. Emerging evidence suggests that normal breast cells, as well as breast cancer stem and progenitor cells, exist in two different states, epithelial-like and mesenchymal-like [27, 29, 30] (**Figure 1B**). Recent studies revealed that in the case of human BCSCs, epithelial-like stem cells express aldehyde dehydrogenase ($ALDH^{+}$), whereas mesenchymal-like stem cells are characterized by $CD44^{+}/CD24^{-}$ surface expression [29, 31–33].

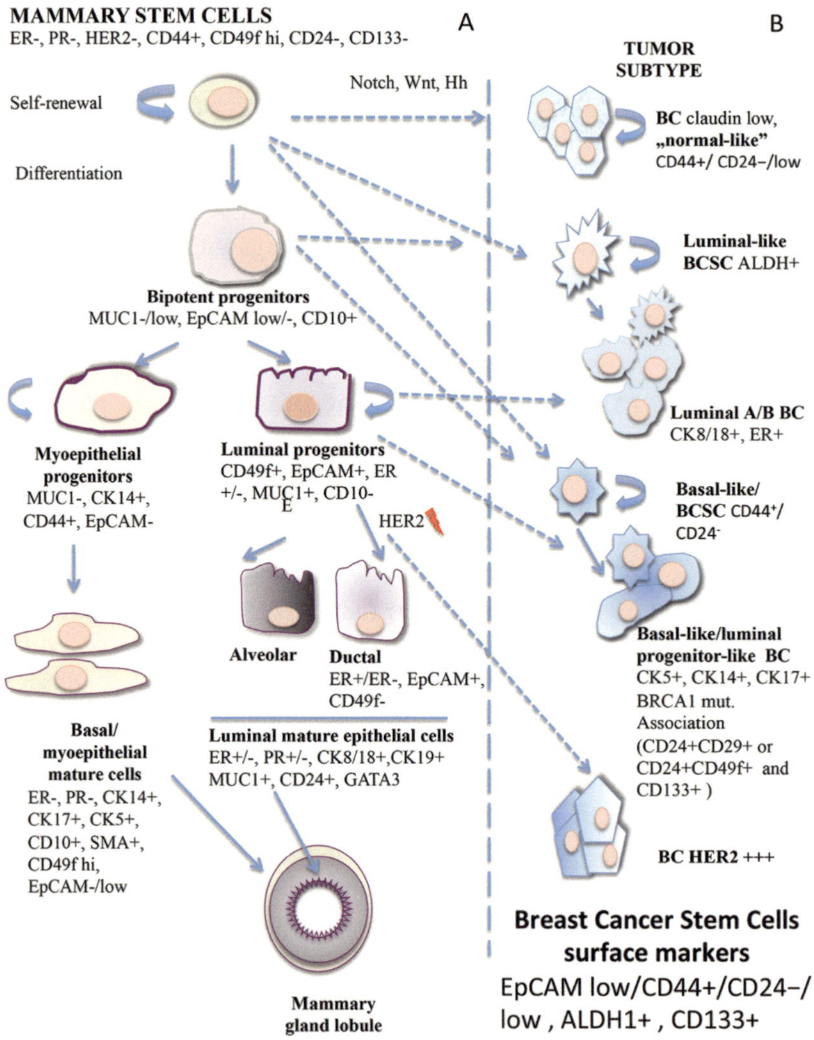

Figure 1. The simplistic draft of hierarchical model of human mammary gland stem cells (A) and correlation of stem cells with breast cancer (BC) subtypes (B). Bi-potent or multi-potent stem cells (with self-renewal ability) give rise to lineage-restricted bi-potent progenitor cells. These progenitors then divide and differentiate into the mature luminal (ductal and alveolar) and basal cells of the adult mammary epithelium. Cells are characterized with expression of different surface markers—which allow for phenotypic identifying of the subpopulations. Normal mammary stem cells (MSC) must be distinguished from tumor stem cells (BCSCs). Deregulation of MaSC self-renewal may contribute to preneoplasia of mammary gland. In particular, deregulation of conserved signaling pathways, such as Wnt, Notch and hedgehog, is linked with oncogenesis. Breast tumors are divided into hypothetical subtypes according to different profiles and different origins of cells. We can find following subtypes: normal-like/claudin low, luminal and basal-like and overexpressing HER2. Luminal progenitors cells (A and B) are mostly associated with good prognosis, those with HER2 overexpressing, also with luminal features, but usually associated with poor survival. Basal-like (the most heterogeneous) origin from luminal progenitors cells and those tumors are the most aggressive and with tendency to exhibit triple-negative phenotype. Additionally, those tumors are highly associated with BRCA1 gene mutations.

3. MaSC and BCSC markers

The approaches to BCSC isolation at present include the following: surface marker sorting, aldehyde dehydrogenase activity assay, flow cytometry sorting side population, etc. [8]. CD44, CD24 and ALDH1 are the most commonly used biomarkers to identify the BCSC fraction [31]. Two proteins, CD44 and CD24, were found in 2003 to be useful markers to distinguish tumor-initiating cells (TICs) from non-tumorigenic cells in BC [2].

CD44 (hyaluronan-binding transmembrane protein) is expressed in different isoforms and can have different glycosylation patterns [34]. Its smallest form (CD44s) is expressed in many cells, whereas its variant forms (CD44v) are particularly found in cancer cells. CD44v is involved in EMT, cellular migration, transendothelial migration and extravasation and it supports many cellular activities required to initiate tumor growth and metastasis [2, 34]. CD24 (heavily glycosylated membrane protein) downregulation may be required to prevent its interference with CD44-dependent invasiveness [35], though the underlying mechanism is not clear since CD24 also has tumor-promoting effects [2, 36]. The gene expression profile associated with $CD44^{+}/CD24^{-}$ cells was demonstrated to correlate with a worse prognosis in BC [33] and approximately one-third of all circulating BC cells in the blood of BC patients is $CD44^{+}/CD24^{-}$ [37]. $CD44^{+}/CD24^{-}$ phenotype of cell surface markers has an increased ability to form tumors in immunosuppressed mice than the bulk of the tumor cells [38]. Maycotte et al. had analyzed CD24 and CD44 expression in MCF7 and MDA-MB-468 cell lines using assay based on flow cytometry. Analysed cells showed different levels of autophagic flux ("autophagic flux" is defined as the activity of autophagic degradation, which comprises autophagosomes formation, transportation of substartes and lysosomic degradation) [39]. CD24 expression was decreased in cells with low autophagic flux in both cancer cell lines. Similar results were obtained in cells expressing shRNA for ATG7 or BECN1, as these cells also showed low expression of CD24, whereas the expression of CD44 remained stable. Presented results indicate that cells with decreased autophagic activity have declined CD24 expression. These results suggest that autophagy can selectively regulate CSC maintenance in autophagy-dependent breast cancer cells. It has been widely predicted that a quality control mechanism, like autophagy, is important for maintaining normal and cancer stem cell homeostasis [7, 38].

Palmer et al. [40] proposed a stem gene pluripotentiality signature as an indicator of the tumor grade in a variety of solid tumors, including BC. In addition to tissue samples, BCSC subpopulations have also been identified *ex vivo* within individual cultured BC cell lines. In triple-negative BC cell lines, $CD44^{+}/CD24^{-/low}$ BCSCs were further classified into two subcategories: the $CD44^{high}/CD24^{-}$ mesenchymal-like basal B and the $CD44^{high}/CD24^{low}$ epithelioid basal A, which displayed stronger tumor-initiating properties [15].

Recent data suggest that CD44 and CD24 may not be sufficient to distinguish the cancer cell subpopulation with CSC/TIC activity, so other proteins, like ALDH1 (aldehyde dehydrogenase 1) and EpCAM (epithelial cell adhesion molecule), may also be required for cancer cells to develop tumor-initiating potential [2]. Members of ALDH1 family ALDH1A1 and ALDH1A3 are thought to be the most important for stem cell activity in cancer cells [41]. Recently, ALDH1 expression has been linked to the expression of RhoC [15, 42], a GTPase known to be involved in metastasis. ALDH1-positive breast cancer cells could be identified by the ALDEFLUOR assay and they showed stem-like and tumor-initiating activities [15]. In the abovementioned experiment of Palmer et al. [40], distinct ALDEFLUOR-positive subgroups with stem cell characteristics have been shown to exist in eight BC cell lines and a 413 gene-specific molecular signature characterizing these BCSCs was determined by microarray analysis.

EpCAM, a transmembrane protein, was considered to be a cellular adhesion molecule until it was discovered that it is able to activate c-myc involved in maintenance of stemness [36]. The level of EpCAM expression may be critical for defining stem cells. Recent reports demonstrated that BCSC activity is associated with low EpCAM expression, whereas luminal or basal cells showed either high or no expression of EpCAM, respectively [43].

The aforementioned epithelial-like and mesenchymal-like BCSCs have been shown to interconvert from one type to another, presumably depending on the tumor phase and requirements [31]. The use of CD49f as an additional marker for the detection of BC cells lacking CK8/18/19 expression has been shown to possibly enhance the detection of circulating tumor cells (CTCs) involved in EMT-associated processes, such as drug resistance and metastasis [44]. $CD44^+/CD24^-$ cells express epithelial-mesenchymal transition (EMT) genes [17], display a quiescent phenotype and are localized in the tumor periphery, possibly promoting tumor spreading. The characteristic pattern of surface markers expression ($CD44^+/CD24^{-/low}$) was found mostly in molecular subtype of breast tumors presenting low expression of claudin. It is accompanied by EMT-associated genes, like N-cadherin, FoxC2 and Zeb [17]. In contrast, ALDH1+ cells are situated within the tumor. They are typical epithelial cells, expressing mesenchymal-epithelial transition (MET) genes and high rate of proliferation, which can influence tumor progression. All these subpopulations are similarly expressing a large number of genes, which were confirmed by high-throughput gene expression profiling (microarray analyses). BCSCs are suggested to have hallmarks of both types of normal MaSCs, epithelial (EpCAM+/CD49f+) and mesenchymal (EpCAM−/CD49f+). According to research results, BCSCs with phenotype ALDH1+/CD44+/CD24- are more aggressive and exhibit big metastatic potential. In the immunosuppressed mice, it was possible to induce tumor growth using just a few ALDH1+/CD44+/CD24- cells [31].

In human breast tumor cells, phenotype $CD44^+/CD24^{low}$ is connected with basal-like tumors, in particular with inherited BRCA1 BC. Additionally, the cells are expressing the CD49f marker and their status is $CK5/14^{high}$ $EGFR^{high}$ and ER^{low}, PR^{low}, HER-2^{low}. It is worth noting that basal-like tumors are often linked to poorer prognosis. The occurrence of the $CD44+/CD24^{low}$ phenotype was found to be lower in tumors of luminal type and particularly HER-2+ tumors, irrespective of ER status [11]. Results of a different study demonstrated the presence of BCSC subtypes in a CTCs population, in peripheral blood samples taken from 30 patients. In total number of 1439 CTCs, 35% of the CTCs in 2/3 patients displayed the $CD44^+/CD24^{-/low}$ phenotype, while 17.7% CTCs selected in seven patients revealed phenotype $ADLH1^{high}/CD24^{-/low}$ [45].

β1-integrin subunit (CD29) has also been implicated in the phenotypic characterization of BCSCs. It has been shown that BRCA1 mutant cancer cell lines contain $CD24^+CD29^+$ or $CD24^+CD49f^+$ cells, with increased proliferation and colony-forming ability [15].

In BCTCs epithelial markers expression is routinely detected and therefore, many isolation techniques are based on the use of specific antibodies, like EpCAM and MUC1. For example, for EpCAM identification, the most popular tests are Cellsearch™ system (Veridex LLC, Raritan, NJ, USA) approved by the US Food and Drug Administration, the herringbone chip, the AdnaTest breast cancer detection kit, fluorescence-activated cell sorting (FACS) analysis and the microfluidic technology. Apart from the peripheral blood, BCSCs have also been isolated directly from the primary or metastatic tumors of breast cancer patients [31].

Other techniques used for stem cell isolation are 3D cultivation in cell cultures spheroids. Stem cells are detectable by light microscopy as small and light cells (SLC) and have the ability to maintain DNA staining (using BrdU) due to their low proliferative activity [46]. However, it was shown that only 15% of [^{3}H] thymidine-positive cells are also positive for one of the two stem cell markers $p21^{CIP1}$ or Musahi-1 (MSi-1) [47].

The next marker worth mentioning is CD133 (prominin-1). Hematopoietic progenitors and adult stem cells normally express this transmembrane glycoprotein. It is a well-established melanoma and brain CSC marker. In addition, the expression of CD133 has been also detected in BCSCs and has been associated with resistance to chemotherapy in BC biopsies [48]. Furthermore, distinct $CD44^+/CD24^-$ and $CD133^+$ subpopulations with CSC characteristics have been detected in BRCA1 breast tumors, while $CD44^{pos}CD49f^{hi}CD133/2^{hi}$ cells were characterized by xenograft-initiating capacity in estrogen receptor–negative BC [15]. Co-expression of stem (ALDH1) and EMT (TWIST) markers has been demonstrated in CTCs from patients with early and metastatic BC. The majority of CTCs expressing the SC marker CD133 also co-expressed the EMT marker N-cadherin and vice versa. The expression of CD133 in CTCs of BC patients has been suggested to promote chemoresistance [15]. Basal-type breast tumors with elevated SLUG expression were shown to overexpress stem-like genes, including CD133 [20]. Additional studies revealed that BC overexpressing SLUG display increased proportions of $CD44^+/CD24^-$ CSCs, suggesting that transcriptional programs induced by SLUG promote stemness [49].

Activation of some genes is proposed to be associated with stem cell phenotypic characteristics, for example, *Sox2* gene (a transcription factor involved in the maintenance of pluripotency of undifferentiated embryonic stem cells) [15]. Activation of this gene is typical for early steps of BC development and characterizes tumors with basal-like phenotype. Increased expression of Sox2 is analyzed as prognostic predictor of BC. Also, mutations in p53 are representative for BC with stem cell-like patterns. It is suggested that loss of p53 function promotes dedifferentiation and is positively selected during tumor progression [15, 50].

4. The role of microenvironment in BC progression: stem cell niche

Stem cell niche refers to a microenvironment in which stem cells reside. The anatomical niche for SC is composed of different compartments [51]. Signals from surrounding cells (stromal cells, a specific type of fibroblast which interacts with the stem/progenitor cells via surface receptors, gap junctions, cytokines, growth factors, hormones, etc.) and extracellular matrix

(ECM) seem to be involved in regulation of SC activity, regulation of SC renewal and survival [1]. Since mammary gland is an endocrine-responsive organ, many hormonal factors are analyzed also in connection with stem cells, for example, the biological influence of E2 and P on the compartment of stem and progenitor cells is largely unknown. However, it is assumed that the stem cells are estrogen receptor (ER) negative, whereas the progenitor cells are ER positive [2]. The role of BRCA1 gene in human ER^- stem/progenitor cell differentiation into ER + luminal epithelial cells has been revealed in the latest scientific findings [11]. ER^- stem cell transition into ER^+ progenitor cells is precluded by BRCA1 deletion. Studies demonstrated that women with heterozygous mutations in the BRCA1 gene are more susceptible to breast and ovarian cancers and the tumors formed were mostly of basal-like phenotype, showing characteristic deficiency of ER, PR and HER-2 receptors.

As mentioned above, deregulation of the microenvironmental homeostasis of normal SC is suggested to contribute to their neoplastic transformation [52]. The activation of the EMT program has been associated with the acquisition of SC traits by normal and neoplastic cells [15]. Transcription factors involved in EMT (*e.g.* Snail, Twist and Zeb) have also been found to induce SC properties in human mammary carcinoma cells [15]. Environmental cues from signaling molecules, which induce EMT in BC such as IL-6, can promote pluripotency in breast cancer cells *via* a positive feedback loop including NF-kB, Lin28 and Let-7 miRNA [15].

5. miRNA and stem cells in breast cancer

MicroRNAs are negative regulators of genes, repressing expression at the posttranscriptional level [53]. They also regulate various properties of CSC, including self-renewal, differentiation, proliferation and fate determination, by affecting several key signaling pathways at the molecular level. Many different miRNA families have already been connected with suppressing/promoting cancer cells. For example, miR-125a is known tumor suppressor in bulk tumor cells of BC origin [53, 54]; however, it has been shown that miR-125a plays a different role in breast epithelial SC, which is cancer promotion [53]. MicroRNA profiling of BCCSs indicated that miR-200c, miR-203 and miR-375 expression was significantly inhibited, whereas the expression of miR-125b, miR-100, miR-221 and miR-222 was most notably enhanced [55]. Expression analysis of miRNAs in both normal mouse and human mammary tissue has revealed three conserved clusters of miRNAs, miR-200C-141, miR-200b-200a-429 and miR-183-96-182, that appear to be downregulated in MaSC and putative BCSCs [56, 57]. In humans, miR-93 level was significantly higher in luminal progenitor cells than in the MaSC-enriched population and overexpression of this miRNA biased these cells toward a luminal fate [58].

MiR-200 family serves as a key mediator of CSC due to its prominent role as an EMT regulator. These family members are downregulated in BCCSs due to epigenetic alternation, in comparison with non-tumorgenic cancer cells [59]. Downregulation of miR-200 expression expands the SC compartment and promotes BC progression. The tumor suppressor p53, which can activate miR-200c by direct binding to miR-200c promoter sites, is reported to regulate both EMT and CSCs [60]. Similar results were obtained in the case of miR-22, a strong inhibitor of miR-200 promoter demethylation, which is connected with tumor invasiveness and metastatic properties [59]—therefore, miR-22 is a crucial epigenetic modifier and promoter of EMT and cancer stemness toward metastasis [61]. In addition to miR-200 family, miR-21 and MiR-302/369 have also been proposed to regulate EMT and CSC. In BC, the depletion of miR-21 expression leads to reversal of EMT and decreased CSC numbers through inactivation of AKT/ERK pathway [60]. MiR-302/369 cluster members can directly target EMT genes, like TGF-beta receptors or the RhoC and the downregulation of miR-302/369 promotes the switch of fibroblasts into somatic stem cells [60].

miRNAs can also regulate the breast cancer cell interactions with other cells by affecting certain genes, for example, Tac1 gene, linked to BC, regulates breast cancer cell interaction with the mesenchymal stem cells. Three miRNAs—miR-130a, miR-206 and miR-302a—have been shown to regulate Tac1 expression and their action against Tac1 may affect quiescence of breast cancer cells in the marrow cavity [11].

6. Signaling pathways regulating MaSC and contributing to the etiology of breast cancer

Wnt (wingless), Hh (hedgehog), Notch and BMP/TGF-β (bone morphogenetic proteins/transforming growth factor β) signaling pathways contribute to the self-renewal of stem and/or progenitor cells in a variety of organs. When deregulated, these pathways can contribute to oncogenesis [59].

The Notch pathway has been shown to play a particular role in MaSC expansion [62, 63] and promotes BC progression by supporting EMT [11, 64]. Overexpression of the Notch pathway components has been linked to decreased survival of BC patients [65]. In a large proportion of BCs, epigenetic mechanisms that activate Notch signaling were related to the role of miR-146a, which targets NUMB, a negative regulator of Notch [59]. Inhibition of Notch1 with specific antibodies significantly reduced the $CD44^{+}CD24^{-/low}$ subpopulation (BCSCs) and diminished the incidence of brain metastases from BCC.

β-Catenin, a downstream target of Wnt signaling pathway, has been identified as a crucial survival signal for MaSC and a balance modulator between differentiation and stemness in adult stem cell niche in the mammary gland [59]. Overexpression of Wnt in mouse mammary glands can also lead to increased mammary tumor formation. Such tumors contain cells of both basal/myoepithelial and luminal phenotypes, suggesting an origin from a common precursor [11, 59].

In the hedgehog pathway, Patched (PTCH) transmembrane protein is a receptor for the hedgehog family of signaling molecules (Sonic-Shh, Indian-Ihh and Desert-Dhh) [59] and has been connected to early embryonic tumorigenesis [11]. PTCH constitutively represses Hh pathway activity through its interaction with a transmembrane protein Smoothened (SMO) [59]. Overexpression of these pathway components, that is, Shh, Ptch1 and Gli1, has been found in majority of human BCs.

Furthermore, studies demonstrated that EMT stimulation by TGF-β co-occurs with BCSC formation [66]. BCSCs with $CD44^{+}/CD24^{-/low}$ phenotype show increased expression of many genes which are known to be TGF-β targets and they are typical for mesenchymal and migratory cell type. In one of the experiments, when MDA-MB-231 cells (model of BC) were injected to athymic mice, the change in TGF-β actions was observed. The cancer-promoting actions (tumorgenic and metastatic) of TGF-β were counteracted by BMP7 or BMP2/7 heterodimer [59], which diminished Smad signaling pathway activity and increased cancer cell invasiveness. Additionally, the activity of pro-survival and anti-apoptotic pathways is often increased in CSCs. Typically, for example, JAK/STAT pathway is highly activated [59].

7. Ways of targeting cancer stem cells: pharmacological agents

Although targeting BCSCs brings hope for future treatment of BC and is widely tested on the basic research level, a disproportionally limited number of clinical trials evaluating the effect of treatment on the expression of BCSC biomarkers are in progress [31].

Among the tested treatment approaches are those regulating the activity of signaling pathways. The targeting of BCSCs involves the disruption of BCSC survival signaling pathways (i.e., Notch, HER2, hedgehog, Wnt, PI3K/Akt/mTOR, interleukin 8, TGF-beta) [31]. Targeting Notch signaling has become a promising field in the treatment of stem cells in breast cancer. By inhibiting the Notch pathway, the CSC population can be reduced along with improved responses to chemotherapy [67]. Several inhibitors of Wnt signaling molecules are under investigation with reference to several cancers [68]. For example, inhibition of the Notch signaling pathway by γ-secretase inhibitors (GSI) has been shown to reduce the pool of BCSCs [15, 62]. GSI and other drugs that interfere with the Notch pathway are currently under consideration as new options to treat BC [65]. Because there is a link between the Notch and Her2-dependent pathways [69], blocking either of them was found to affect CSC survival. Hence, Her2 inhibitors, such as trastuzumab, may be potential additional drugs suitable for targeting CSC [70]. Several scientific groups have exploited cyclopamine (SMO signaling inhibitor), to inhibit the Hh cascade, thereby inhibiting the growth, invasion and metastasis of breast, prostatic, pancreatic and brain malignancies both *in vitro* and *in vivo* [71]. PKF118-310, an inhibitor of Wnt signaling pathway, was recently reported to eliminate BCSCs in a HER2 overexpressing mouse model. Vismodegib, GDC-0449, a hedgehog inhibitor, can block tumor growth in tamoxifen-resistant BC xenografts [31]. Everolimus (RAD001), an inhibitor of PI3K/Akt/mTOR pathway, halted tumor growth of SC in primary breast cancer cells and cell lines and was particularly effective when administered in combination with docetaxel [72].

The resistance of BCSCs to chemotherapeutic drugs leads to the reconstitution of the initial tumor cell population and disease progression [15]. Conventional therapies targeting the tumor bulk have proven insufficient for the eradication of CSC. For example, conventional therapies based on mitotic interference of taxanes (paclitaxel and docetaxel) [73] do not target the subpopulation of quiescent CSC in a tumor. Bhola et al. [74] reported that paclitaxel increased IL-8 expression by autocrine TGF-β signaling and enriched CSC. Interestingly, Gupta et al. reported that SAL, a polyether antibiotic widely used in veterinary medicine, is a potent agent able to selectively target BCSCs and to inhibit mammary tumor growth in vivo [43]. Since autophagy promotes the maintenance of BCSCs [75], SAL can inhibit autophagy and lysosomal proteolytic activity in both BCSCs and cancer cells [76]. It also acts as an inhibitor of potassium ionophore in Wnt signaling.

Another therapeutic approach is blocking the ABC transporters expressed in most CSC [13]. For instance, tyrosine kinase inhibitors (TKIs) act by binding to ATP and preventing it from binding to the ATP-binding site of several oncogenic tyrosine kinases. It has been reported that some TKIs, such as nilotinib (Tasigna), can efficiently reduce the activity of ABCB1 and ABCG2 transporters. Apatinib (YN968D1) was tested on breast cancer cell lines and in xenograft models of breast cancers overexpressing ABCG2 and/or ABCB1. In combination with paclitaxel, it significantly increased the activity of paclitaxel in the animal models. The therapeutic use of ABC transporters inhibitors has failed so far because of the toxicity issues [13].

One of the most recent innovative approaches in breast cancer therapy is the recruitment of normal stem cells for the eradication of tumor cells. It has been pointed that mesenchymal stem cells (MSCs) have "tumor tropism," which means that they show the ability of migration not only toward the sites of inflammation or injury, but also importantly to the tumor microenvironment.

Other tested options include the following: targeting of CSC metabolic pathways, the use of miRNAs, the use of small inhibitors as salinomycin, cancer immunotherapy, drugs involved in the treatment of noncancer diseases and nanotechnology (nanodrugs can easily accumulate within tumor sites due to their enhanced vascular permeability) [31].

8. Conclusions

Scientific findings from breast cancer studies have revealed that the SC content in breast tumor correlates with its invasiveness and the outcome of the disease. The resistance of BCSCs to chemotherapeutic drugs and other conventional BC therapies has led scientists to move toward establishment of novel therapeutic approaches. Current knowledge about BCSC characteristics and regulators still allows only for evaluation of those therapies on an experimental level of preclinical studies. The most efficient cancer treatment protocols remain to be established on the basis of simultaneous targeting of BCSCs and bulk tumor cells. Therefore, there is still a great need for profound studies, which would extend our knowledge about stem cells and the interplay between these cells and tumor microenvironment. Looking at the practical aspects of BCSC usage one of the biggest challenges that still need to be resolved is the isolation of their population from the patients' blood.

Abbreviations List

ABC transporters	ATP-binding cassette transporters
AKT/ERK	Protein kinase B/extracellural signal-regulated kinase
ALDH	Aldehyde dehydrogenase

ATG7	Autophagy-related protein 7
BC	Breast cancer
Bcl-2	B-cell lymphoma 2 protein
BCSCs	Breast cancer stem cell
BECN1	Beclin1
BMP/TGF-β	Bone morphogenetic proteins/transforming growth factor β signaling pathway
BMP2	Bone morphogenetic protein 2
BMP7	Bone morphogenetic protein 7
BRCA1	Breast cancer 1 gene
CD133	Prominin-1
CD24	Cluster of differentiation 24
CD29	Integrin beta 1
CD44	Cell surface glycoprotein/hyaluronan-binding transmembrane protein
CD49f	Integrin alpha 6
CK	Cytokeratin
CMIC	Cancer metastasis-initiating cell
CSC	Cancer stem cells
Dhh	Desert signaling molecule (hedgehog family)
E2	Estrogen
ECM	Extracellular matrix
EGFR	Epidermal growth factor receptor
EMT	Epithelial-mesenchymal transition
EpCAM	Epithelial cell adhesion molecule
ER	Estrogen receptor
FACS	Fluorescence-activated cell sorting
FoxC2	Forkhead box protein C2
GATA3	Trans-acting T-cell-specific transcription factor GATA-3
Gli1	Glioma-associated oncogene homolog 1 (zinc finger protein)/glioma-associated oncogen1

http://dx.doi.org/10.5772/66904

GSI	γ-Secretase inhibitors
HER-2	Human epidermal growth factor receptor2/ERBB2
Hh	Hedgehog signaling pathway
Ihh	Indian signaling molecule (hedgehog family)
IL-6	Interleukin 6
JAK	Janus kinase
Let-7	Let-7 family, microRNA precursors
Lin28	Lin28-homolog A
MaPC	Mammary epithelial progenitor cell
MaSC	Mammary stem cells
MCF7	Human breast adenocarcinoma cell line (Michigan Cancer Foundation-7)
MDA-MB-468	Breast adenocarcinoma cell line/ATCC HTB-132; triple negative
MEC	Mammary epithelial cells
MET	Mesenchymal-epithelial transition
MSi-1	Musahi-1
mTOR	Mammalian target of rapamycin kinase
MUC1	Mucin 1
NF-kB	Nuclear factor kappa light-chain-enhancer of activated B cells
P	Progesterone
PR	Progesterone receptor
PI3K	Phosphoinositide 3-kinase
PTCH	Patched transmembrane protein
RhoC	Small signaling G protein, Ras homolog gene family, member C
SC	Stem cells
Shh	Sonic signaling molecule (hedgehog family)
shRNA	Small hairpin RNA
SLC	Small and light cells
SLUG	Snail2 and zink finger protein
SMA	Smooth muscle actin

SMO	Smoothened transmembrane protein
Sox2	SRY—(sex determining region Y)—box2
Src	Protooncogene non-receptor tyrosine-protein kinase Src
STAT	Signal transducers and activators of transcription
TGF-beta	Transforming growth factor beta
TIC	Tumor-initiating cells
TKIs	Tyrosine kinase inhibitors
TWIST	Twist-related protein and transcription factor
Wnt	Wingless signaling pathway
Zeb	Zink finger transcription factor

Author details

Joanna Magdalena Zarzynska

Address all correspondence to: joanna_zarzynska@sggw.pl

Department of Food Hygiene and Public Health Protection, Faculty of Veterinary Medicine, Warsaw University of Life Sciences-SGGW, Warsaw, Poland

References

[1] Capuco AV, Choudhary RK, Daniels KM, Li RW, Evock-Clover CM. Bovine mammary stem cells: cell biology meets production agriculture. Animal. 2012; **6**(3): 382–393. doi:10.1017/S1751731111002369

[2] Dittmer J, Rody A. Cancer stem cells in breast cancer. Histol Histopathol. 2013; **28**(7): 827–838.

[3] Reya T, Morrison SJ, Clarke MF, Weissman IL. Stem cells, cancer and cancer stem cells. Nature. 2001; **414**: 105–111.

[4] Howard JH, Bland KI. Current management and treatment strategies for breast cancer. Curr Opin Obstet Gynecol. 2012; **24**(1): 44–48.

[5] Gomes LR, Terra LF, Wailemann AM, Labriola L, Sogayar. TGF-β1 modulates the homeostasis between MMPs and MMP inhibitors through p38 MAPK and ERK1/2 in highly invasive breast cancer cells. BMC Cancer. 2012; **12**:26.

[6] Shah NR, Chen H. MicroRNAs in pathogenesis of breast cancer: implications in diagnosis and treatment. World J Clin Oncol. 2014; **5**(2): 48–60.

[7] Zarzynska J. Targeting the Autophagy Process in Breast Cancer Development and Treatment. Chapter 4. Cell Death—Autophagy, Apoptosisi and Necrosis. 2015; 63–81. In Tech Open, Rjeka, Croatia doi:10.5772/61181

[8] Chen H, Wang Y, Wang T, Shi D, Sun Z, Xia C, Wang B. Application prospective of nano-probes with MRI and FI dual-modality imaging on breast cancer stem cells in tumor. J Nanobiotechnol. 2016; **14**(1): 52. doi:10.1186/s12951-016-0195-8

[9] Magee JA, Piskounova E, Morrison SJ. Cancer stem cells: impact, heterogeneity and uncertainty. Cancer Cell. 2012; **21**(3): 283–296.

[10] Dontu G, Al-Hajj M, Abdallah WM, Clarke MF, Wicha MS: Stem cells in normal breast development and breast cancer. Cell Prolif. 2003; **36**(Suppl 1): 59–72.

[11] Nigam A. Breast cancer stem cells, pathways and therapeutic perspectives 2011. Indian J Surg. 2013; **75**(3): 170–180. doi:10.1007/s12262-012-0616-3

[12] Dontu G, Abdallah WM, Foley JM, Jackson KW, Clarke MF, Kawamura MJ, Wicha MS. *In vitro* propagation and transcriptional profiling of human mammary stem/progenitor cells. Genes Dev. 2003; **17:** 1253–1270.

[13] Mallini P, Lennard T, Kirby J, Meeson A. Epithelial-to-mesenchymal transition: what is the impact on breast cancer stem cells and drug resistance. Cancer Treat Rev. 2014; **40**(3): 341–348. doi:10.1016/j.ctrv.2013.09.008

[14] Graziano A, d'Aquino R, Tirino V, Desiderio V, Rossi A, Pirozzi G. The stem cell hypothesis in head and neck cancer. J Cell Biochem. 2008; **103:** 408–412.

[15] Chiotaki R, Polioudaki H, Theodoropoulos PA. Cancer stem cells in solid and liquid tissues of breast cancer patients: characterization and therapeutic perspectives. Curr Cancer Drug Targets. 2015; **15**(3): 256–269.

[16] Vermeulen L, de Sousa E Melo F, Richel DJ, Medema JP. The developing cancer stem-cell model: clinical challenges and opportunities. Lancet Oncol. 2012; **13**(2): e83–e89.

[17] Geng SQ, Alexandrou AT, Li JJ. Breast cancer stem cells: multiple capacities in tumor metastasis. Cancer Lett. 2014; **349**(1): 1–7. doi:10.1016/j.canlet.2014.03.036

[18] Dick JE. Breast cancer stem cells revealed. Proc Natl Acad Sci U S A. 2003; **100**: 3547–3549.

[19] Tiffany MP, William HM, Frank P. The response of CD24(-/low)/CD44 + breast cancer—initiating cells to radiation. J Natl Cancer I. 2006; **98**(24): 1777–1785.

[20] Phillips S, Kuperwasser C. SLUG: critical regulator of epithelial cell identity in breast development and cancer. Cell Adhes Migr. 2014; **8**(6): 578–587.

[21] Petersen OW, Polyak K. Stem cells in the human breast. Cold Spring Harb Perspect Biol. 2010; **2:** a003160.

[22] Luo J, Yin X, Ma T, Lu J. Stem cells in normal mammary gland and breast cancer. Am J Med Sci. 2010; **339**: 366–370.

[23] Visvader JE. Keeping abreast of the mammary epithelial hierarchy and breast tumorigenesis. Genes Dev. 2009; **23**: 2563–2577.

[24] Shackleton M, Vaillant F, Simpson KJ, Stingl J, Smyth GK, Asselin- Labat ML, Wu L, Lindeman GJ, Visvader JE. Generation of a functional mammary gland from a single stem cell. Nature. 2006; **439**: 84–88.

[25] Stingl J, Eirew P, Ricketson I, Shackleton M, Vaillant F, Choi D, Li HI, Eaves CJ. Purification and unique properties of mammary epithelial stem cells. Nature. 2006; **439**: 993–997.

[26] Asselin-Labat ML, Shackleton M, Stingl J, Vaillant F, Forrest NC, Eaves CJ, Visvader JE, Lindeman GJ. Steroid hormone receptor status of mouse mammary stem cells. J Natl Cancer Inst. 2006; **98**: 1011–1014.

[27] Van Keymeulen A, et al. Distinct stem cells contribute to mammary gland development and maintenance. Nature. 2011; **479**(7372): 189–193.

[28] Sheridan JM, Ritchie ME, Best SA, Jiang K, Beck TJ, Vaillant F, Liu K, Dickins RA, Smyth GK, Lindeman GJ, Visvader JE. A pooled shRNA screen for regulators of primary mammary stem and progenitor cells identifies roles for Asap1 and Prox1. BMC Cancer. 2015; **3**(15): 221. doi:10.1186/s12885-015-1187-z

[29] Liu S, et al. Breast cancer stem cells transition between epithelial and mesenchymal states reflective of their normal counterparts. Stem Cell Rep. 2013; **2**(1): 78–91.

[30] Colacino JA, McDermott SP, Sartor MA, Wicha MS, Rozek LS. Transcriptomic profiling of curcumin-treated human breast stem cells identifies a role for stearoyl-coa desaturase in breast cancer prevention. Breast Cancer Res Treat. 2016; **158**(1): 29–41. doi:10.1007/s10549-016-3854-4

[31] Chiotaki R, Polioudaki H, Theodoropoulos PA. Stem cell technology in breast cancer: current status and potential applications. Stem Cells Cloning. 2016; **26**(9): 17–29. doi:10.2147/SCCAA.S72836

[32] Sheridan C, Kishimoto H, Fuchs RK, Mehrotra S, Bhat-Nakshatri P, Turner CH, Goulet R Jr, Badve S, Nakshatri H. CD44+/CD24- breast cancer cells exhibit enhanced invasive properties: an early step necessary for metastasis. Breast Cancer Res. 2006; **8:** R59.

[33] Shipitsin M, Campbell LL, Argani P, Weremowicz S, Bloushtain-Qimron N, Yao J, Nikolskaya T, Serebryiskaya T, Beroukhim R, Hu M, Halushka MK, Sukumar S, Parker LM, Anderson KS, Harris LN, Garber JE, Richardson AL, Schnitt SJ, Nikolsky Y, Gelman RS, Polyak K. Molecular definition of breast tumor heterogeneity. Cancer Cell. 2007; **11**: 259–273.

[34] Zoller M. CD44: can a cancer-initiating cell profit from an abundantly expressed molecule? Nat Rev Cancer. 2011; **11**: 254–267.

[35] Meyer MJ, Fleming JM, Ali MA, Pesesky MW, Ginsburg E, Vonderhaar BK . Dynamic regulation of CD24 and the invasive, CD44posCD24neg phenotype in breast cancer cell lines. Breast Cancer Res. 2009; **11**: R82.

[36] Gires O. Lessons from common markers of tumor-initiating cells in solid cancers. Cell Mol Life Sci. 2011; **68**: 4009–4022.

[37] Bednarz-Knoll N, Alix-Panabieres C, Pantel K. Clinical relevance and biology of circulating tumor cells. Breast Cancer Res. 2011; **13**: 228.

[38] Guan JL, Simon AK, Prescott M, Menendez JA, Liu F, Wang F, et al. Autophagy in stem cells. Autophagy. 2013; **9**(6): 830–849.

[39] Maycotte P, Gearheart CM, Barnard R, Aryal S, Mulcahy Levy JM, Fosmire SP, et al. STAT3-mediated autophagy dependence identifies subtypes of breast cancer where autophagy inhibition can be efficacious. Cancer Res. 2014; **74**(9): 2579–2590.

[40] Palmer NP, Schmid PR, Berger B, Kohane IS. A gene expression profile of stem cell pluripotentiality and differentiation is conserved across diverse solid and hematopoietic cancers. Genome Biol. 2012; **13**(8): R71.

[41] Marcato P, Dean CA, Giacomantonio CA, Lee PW. Aldehyde dehydrogenase: its role as a cancer stem cell marker comes down to the specific isoform. Cell Cycle. 2011; **10**: 1378–1384.

[42] Rosenthal DT, Zhang J, Bao L, Zhu L, Wu Z, Toy K, Kleer CG, Merajver SD. RhoC impacts the metastatic potential and abundance of breast cancer stem cells. PLoS One. 2012; **7**: e40979.

[43] Gupta PB, Onder RA, Lander ES. Identification of selective inhibitors of cancer stem cells by high-throughput screening. Cell. 2009; **138**: 645–659.

[44] Mostert B, Kraan J, Sieuwerts AM, van der Spoel P, Bolt-de Vries J, Prager-van der Smissen WJ, Smid M, Timmermans AM, Martens JW, Gratama JW, Foekens JA, Sleijfer S. CD49f-based selection of circulating tumor cells (CTCs) improves detection across breast cancer subtypes. Cancer Lett. 2012; **319**(1): 49–55.

[45] Theodoropoulos PA, Polioudaki H, Agelaki S, Kallergi G, Saridaki Z, Mavroudis D, Georgoulias V. Circulating tumor cells with a putative stem cell phenotype in peripheral blood of patients with breast cancer. Cancer Lett. 2010; **288**: 99–106.

[46] Molyneux G, Regan J, Smalley MJ. Mammary stem cells and breast cancer. Cell Mol Life Sci. 2007; **64**: 3248–3260.

[47] Clarke RB, Spence K, Anderson E, Howell A, Okano H, Potten CS. A enriched for steroid receptor-positive cells. Dev Biol. 2005; **277**: 443–456.

[48] Aomatsu N, Yashiro M, Kashiwagi S, Takashima T, Ishikawa T, Ohsawa M, Wakasa K, Hirakawa K. CD133 is a useful surrogate marker for predicting chemosensitivity to neoadjuvant chemotherapy in breast cancer. PLoS One. 2012; **7**(9): e45865.

[49] Guo W, Keckesova Z, Donaher JL, Shibue T, Tischler V, Reinhardt F, Itzkovitz S, Noske A, Zurrer-Hardi U, Bell G, et al. Slug and Sox9 cooperatively determine the mammary stem cell state. Cell. 2012; **148**: 1015–1028. PMID:22385965; doi:10.1016/j.cell.2012.02.008

[50] Mizuno H, Spike BT, Wahl GM, Levine AJ. Inactivation of p53 in breast cancers correlates with stem cell transcriptional signatures. Proc Nat Acad Sci U S A. 2010; **107**(52): 22745–22750.

[51] Jones DL, Wagers AJ. No place like home: anatomy and function of the stem cell niche. Nat Rev Mol Cell Biol. 2008; **9**: 11–21.

[52] Li L, Neaves WB. Normal stem cells and cancer stem cells: the niche matters. Cancer Res. 2006; **66**(9): 4553–4557.

[53] Nandy SB, Arumugam A, Subramani R, Pedroza D, Hernandez K, Saltzstein E, Lakshmanaswamy R. MicroRNA-125a influences breast cancer stem cells by targeting leukemia inhibitory factor receptor which regulates the Hippo signaling pathway. Oncotarget. 2015; **6**(19): 17366–17378.

[54] O'Day E, Lal A. MicroRNAs and their target gene networks in breast cancer. Breast Cancer Res. 2010; **12**: 201.

[55] Wang L, Zhang D, Zhang C, et al. A microRNA expression signature characterizing the proper- ties of tumor-initiating cells for breast cancer. Oncol Lett. 2012; **3**: 119–24.

[56] Shimono Y, Zabala M, Cho RW, Lobo N, Dalerba P, Qian D, et al. Down-regulation of miRNA-200c links breast cancer stem cells with normal stem cells. Cell. 2009; **138**: 592–603.

[57] Fu N, Lindeman GJ, Visvader JE. The mammary stem cell hierarchy. Curr Top Dev Biol. 2014; **107**: 133–160. doi:10.1016/B978-0-12-416022-4.00005-6

[58] Liu S, Patel SH, Ginestier C, Ibarra I, Martin-Trevino R, Bai S, et al. MicroRNA93 regulates proliferation and differentiation of normal and malignant breast stem cells. PLoS Genet. 2012; **8**: e1002751.

[59] Czerwinska P, Kaminska B. Regulation of breast cancer stem cell features. Contemp Oncol (Pozn). 2015; **19**(1A): A7–A15. doi:10.5114/wo.2014.47126

[60] Hao J, Zhang Y, Deng M, Ye R, Zhao S, Wang Y, Li J, Zhao Z. MicroRNA control of epithelial-mesenchymal transition in cancer stem cells. Int J Cancer. 2014; **135**(5): 1019–1027. doi:10.1002/ijc.28761

[61] Song SJ, Poliseno L, Song MS, et al. MicroRNA-antagonism regulates breast cancer stemness and metastasis via tet-family-dependent chromatin remodeling. Cell. 2013; **154**: 311–324.

[62] Bouras T, Pal B, Vaillant F, Harburg G, Asselin-Labat ML, Oakes SR, Lindeman GJ, Visvader JE. Notch signaling regulates mammary stem cell function and luminal cell-fate commitment. Cell Stem Cell. 2008; **3**: 429–441.

[63] Harrison H, Farnie G, Brennan KR, Clarke RB. Breast cancer stem cells: something out of notching? Cancer Res. 2010; **70**: 8973–8976.

[64] Sethi N, Kang Y. Notch signalling in cancer progression and bone metastasis. Br J Cancer. 2011; **105**: 1805–1810.

[65] Han J, Hendzel MJ, Allalunis-Turner J. Notch signaling as a therapeutic target for breast cancer treatment? Breast Cancer Res. 2011; **13**: 210.

[66] Mani SA, Guo W, Liao MJ, et al. The epithelial-mesenchymal transition generates cells with properties of stem cells. Cell. 2008; **133**: 704–15.

[67] Qiu M, Peng Q, Jiang I, Carroll C, Han G, Rymer I, Lippincott J, Zachwieja J, Gajiwala K, Kraynov E, Thibault S, Stone D, Gao Y, Sofia S, Gallo J, Li G, Yang J, Li K and Wei P. Specific inhibition of Notch1 signaling enhances the antitumor efficacy of chemotherapy in triple negative breast cancer through reduction of cancer stem cells. Cancer Lett. 2013; **328**: 261–270.

[68] Vermeulen L, De Sousa E Melo F, van der Heijden M, et al. Wnt activity defines colon cancer stem cells and is regulated by the microenvironment. Nat Cell Biol. 2010; **12**: 468–476.

[69] Korkaya H, Wicha MS. HER-2, notch and breast cancer stem cells: targeting an axis of evil. Clin Cancer Res. 2009; **15**: 1845–1847.

[70] Liu S, Wicha MS. Targeting breast cancer stem cells. J Clin Oncol. 2010; **28**: 4006–4012.

[71] Ramaswamy B, Lu Y, Teng KY, Nuovo G, Li X, Shapiro CL, Majum-der S. Hedgehog signaling is a novel therapeutic target in tamoxifen-resistant breast cancer aberrantly activated by PI3K/AKT pathway. Cancer Res. 2012; **72**: 5048–5059.

[72] Zhang X, Zhang S, Liu Y, Liu J, Ma Y, Zhu Y, Zhang J. Effects of the combination of RAD001 and docetaxel on breast cancer stem cells. Eur J Cancer. 2012; **48**(10): 1581–1592.

[73] Hernandez-Vargas H, Palacios J, Moreno-Bueno G. Telling cells how to die: docetaxel therapy in cancer cell lines. Cell Cycle. 2007; **6**(7): 780–783.

[74] Bhola NE, Balko JM, Dugger TC, Kuba MG, Sanchez V, Sanders M, Stanford J, Cook RS, Arteaga CL. TGF-beta inhibition enhances chemotherapy action against triple-negative breast cancer. J Clin Invest. 2013; **123**(3): 1348–1358.

[75] Gong C, Bauvy C, Tonelli G, Yue W, Delomenie C, Nicolas V, et al. Beclin 1 and autophagy are required for the tumorigenicity of breast cancer stem-like/progenitor cells. Oncogene. 2012; **32**: 2261–2272.

[76] Yue W, Hamai A, Tonelli G, Bauvy C, Nicolas V, Tharinger H, Codogno P, Mehrpour M. Inhibition of the autophagic flux by salinomycin in breast cancer stem-like/progenitor cells interferes with their maintenance. Autophagy. 2013; **9**(5): 714–729.

Chapter 13

Ion Channels in Breast Cancer: From Signaling to Therapy

Dowd Jonathan, Hendin Josh,
Daniela F. Fukushiro-Lopes, David Laczynski and
Saverio Gentile

Additional information is available at the end of the chapter

http://dx.doi.org/10.5772/66172

Abstract

Breast cancer consists of an assortment of illness and therapeutic failure is mostly due to the complex and heterogeneous phenotype of the disease. Recently, changes in expression of several ion channels have been associated with malignancy including breast cancers. This suggests that breast cancer cells might gain a selective advantage by controlling ion channel expression/activity and that ion channels can contribute to the hallmarks of cancer. Due to the growing body of research demonstrating that ion channels are key factors in breast cancer biology. In this chapter, we discuss the role of specific ion channels in contributing to hallmarks of breast and whether these ion channels can be used as potential pharmacologic targets for breast cancer.

Keywords: breast cancer, ion channels, hallmarks of cancer, therapeutic targets

1. Introduction

Breast cancer is the most diagnosed cancer in women affecting more than 1.7 million women worldwide. Once metastasis has been detected, the average survival is 2 years and it is estimated that in 2016 about 250,000 women will be diagnosed with invasive breast cancer in the USA, and about 41,000 women under the age of 68 will die from the disease [1].

Molecular characterization of different breast cancer types offered the opportunity to separate breast cancers into two large groups that include luminal type [express estrogen receptors (ER); relatively good response to treatment] and the less common but more aggressive basal-like subtype (do not express ER; poor response to treatment). Innovations in targeted therapy are being rapidly developed for the treatment of breast cancer, but the lack of suitable targets, limited drug availability, side effects, and drug resistance have severely hindered efforts toward improving outcomes in breast cancer patients [2].

Ion channels are pore-forming integral membrane proteins that create ionic concentration gradients by allowing flow of ions such as K^+, Ca^{2+}, Cl^- and Na^+ down their electrochemical gradients. There are at least 232 genes that encode for a variety of ion channel families that are organized according to ion channels function (IUPHAR: e.g., Kv potassium (K^+) voltage-gated) or gene name (HUGO: KCNH; K^+ voltage-gated channel subfamily H) [3, 4].

Variation in ionic gradients across cellular membranes plays a fundamental role in virtually all cellular events including electrical conductance, transcriptional regulation, contraction, secretion, motility, cell death, and proliferation [5, 6]. Activity of different families of ion channels can be gated by a variety of stimuli that range from changes in voltage (voltage-gated) and intracellular molecules to mechanical cues. In addition, ion channel activity can be modulated by a variety of events that are independent of their protein synthesis such as posttranslational modification (e.g., reversible phosphorylation) or epigenetically making ion channels one of the most abundant and functionally versatile classes of proteins. Therefore, ion channels are central in maintaining homeostasis and in pathological conditions.

Remarkably, recent research revealed that the expression level of several ion channels has been found altered in different types of breast cancers but not in healthy surrounding tissues [7–11]. Expression profiling of genes encoding for ion channels in breast cancers has provided evidence that the presence of specific ion channels can predict clinical outcome [12]. These studies indicate that changes in the activity of these proteins can potentially contribute to several of the hallmark of cancer and, therefore, to malignant transformation of breast cells.

2. Ion channels in cell proliferation

Cell proliferation is a complex, well-synchronized event that is stringently regulated by a number of ions, molecules, and proteins including K^+, Ca^{++}, ATP, cyclins, cyclin-dependent kinases, and many other cell cycle regulators that are associated with the cell-cycle machinery [13–19]. All cells present an intracellular negative electrical charge called transmembrane potential (V_m) that arises from the combined activities of a variety of ion channels/transporters, which create ionic gradients across the cell surface [20]. Transient decrease of this electrical charge (depolarization) followed by transient increase (repolarization) corresponds to key cell cycle checkpoints and it is critical for cell cycle progression of different cell types [21–27]. Several studies have established that in breast cancer cells, transient depolarization is a potent signal to initiate DNA synthesis causing ectopic reentry in the cell cycle, which is pivotal for malignant proliferation [22, 28]. In the MCF-7 breast cancer cell line, it has been observed that the Vm during a cell cycle progression correlates with the transition in each phase, such that, the pharmacological arrest of MCF-7 cells in G1/S or G2/M transition enriches cells with hyperpolarized Vm while cells arrested in the G0/G1 and M phases were enriched with depolarized Vm [10, 29].

Preservation of the oscillatory nature of membrane potential is necessary for cell proliferation. For example, chronic inhibition or chronic activation of a K^+ channel such as Kv11.1 produces persistent depolarization or hyperpolarization, which in either case can result in cell death or inhibition of proliferation (**Figure 1**) [30].

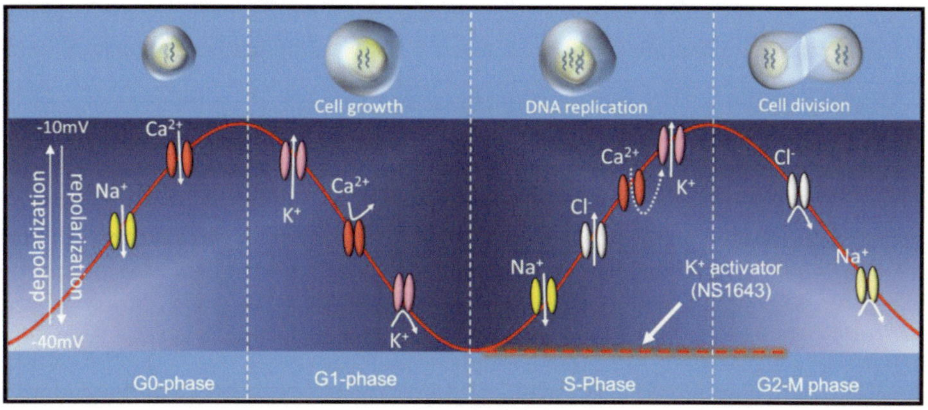

Figure 1. Schematic representation of ion channel activities during the cell cycle. Opening of the voltage-gated K^+ channels (e.g., Kv11.1) move positive charges from the intracellular to the extracellular space causing repolarization (red line). This event is required to promote transition from the G0/G1 to the S-phase of the cell cycle. In contrast, membrane potential during the S phase tends to depolarize due to opening of Na^+, some Ca^{2+}, and/or Na^+ channels. Mitosis is associated with more activity of Na^+ and/or Ca^{2+} that again depolarize the cell until duplication and return to repolarization in the G0/G1. Chronic application of a K^+ channel activator produces persistent repolarization. Conversely, K^+ blocker produces persistent depolarization. Both stop the cell cycle. ↓ = inward ionic flux; ↑ = outward ionic flux; ↺ = no ionic flux (Adapted from reference [10]).

3. Ion channels and the hallmark of breast cancer

Clinical differences of breast cancers are manifested by their histopathological characteristics, outcomes, and response to therapeutics. Nevertheless, the heterogeneity of breast cancers appears to be driven by the "classical" hallmarks of cancer identified by Hanahan and Weinberg which include: sustaining proliferative signaling, enabling replicative immortality, evading growth suppressors, resisting cell death, activating invasion and metastasis, evading immunodestruction, inducing angiogenesis, and reprogramming of energy [31–33].

3.1. Ion channels and proliferation of breast cancer cells

A growing body of experimental and clinical data supports the notion that ion channels can play a major role in contributing to these hallmarks in breast cancers [34].

It has been well established that a calcium ion is the universal signaling molecule in both physiological and pathological conditions [35, 36]. The intracellular concentration of calcium is kept at roughly 100 nM; however, cytoplasmic calcium can increase 100-fold upon specific cellular events. Calcium gradients are finely controlled by a sophisticated set of calcium permeant ions that are localized on the cell surface and intracellular membranes and can regulate ionic fluxes from two major calcium stores: the extracellular space and the endoplasmic reticulum. Although calcium signaling plays a role in diverse cellular processes such as gene expression, cell growth, proliferation, apoptosis, migration, and among others, very little is still known about the role and functions of calcium channel in cancer biology.

The transient receptor potential (TRP) channels are a group of nonselective surface membrane cation channels that mediate a variety of sensations including taste, temperature, and taste [37, 38]. In addition, these channels can act as sensors for osmotic pressure, volume, stretch, or pressure.

TRPC6 (canonical) is elevated in breast carcinoma tissue compared to normal breast tissue and is functional, but it is not correlated with tumor grade, ER expression, or lymph node metastasis [39]. TRPV6 channel (activated by vanilloids and capsaicin) in breast cancer cells has been shown to provide cytoplasmic calcium necessary to promote downstream signaling for cell proliferation [40]. Pharmacologic inhibition of TRPV6 has been shows to sensitize breast cancer cells to apoptosis as well as decrease proliferation [41].

Furthermore, it has been found that activation of store-operated Ca entry (SOCE) in breast cancer cells leads to augmented expression of cyclins and suppresses cyclin-dependent kinase inhibitors, which ultimately leads to progression through the cell cycle.

Thus, abnormal expression of an ion channels family such as calcium channels in cancer cells could be considered as an adaptive mechanism by which the cells increase the frequency with which they proliferate [9].

K^+ is the most abundant intracellular ion and increased or decreased variation in $[K^+]$ significantly contributes to changes of Vm during the cell cycle [10, 42]. Opening of K^+ channels allows K^+ to leave the cell resulting in depletion of positive charges from the cytoplasm, which contributes to repolarization. Temporary increased expression and/or activity of a K^+ channel drive a faster repolarization. This event can result in shortening the G1 phase of the cell cycle and increased proliferation [43].

Several voltage-gated K^+ channels (VGKC) such as Kv10.1, Kv11.1, and Kv1.3, the G-protein-coupled inwardly rectifying potassium channels (Kir3.1; GIRK1) or the two-pore potassium channel KCNK9 have been found to be overexpressed in different types of breast tumors suggesting that transcription of these K^+ channel genes is upregulated independently of the molecular characterization of breast cancers [12, 44, 45].

In contrast, other channels such as the potassium calcium-activated channel $K_{Ca}3.1$ have been found overexpressed mostly in high-grade breast tumors while an isoform of $K_{Ca}3.1$, $K_{Ca}1.1$ (or BK for short) has been found to be mostly expressed in tumors with lower grade [12]. Furthermore, breast cancer cells that metastasized to brain present higher expression of the BK channels compared to cells that metastasized in other body compartments [46, 47].

3.2. Control of ion channels activity in breast cancer

The expression level of potassium channels in breast cancers has been found to be controlled by a variety of factors, for example, mitogen-activated biochemical signaling. Estrogen can control protein synthesis of several ion channels such as potassium channels [48], calcium channels, and sodium channels (via the novel membrane-bound G-protein-estrogen receptor (GPER) [49] or proteins that directly alter activity of ion channels such as the potassium channel tetramerization domain containing 11 (e.g., KCTD11) [50]. Furthermore, the β-adrenoreceptor (a G–protein-coupled receptor) can promote the growth of breast cancer cells by activating the GIRK potassium channel [51]. This indicates that these channel proteins might play a key role in sustaining proliferative signaling in luminal breast cancer cells.

The contribution of ion channel activity to proliferation can be finely controlled by a variety of cellular events including translational, reversible posttranslational, and epigenetic mechanisms. For example, it has been shown that the abundance of Kv11.1 mRNA encoded by the human ether-a-go-go-related gene 1 (hERG1) oscillates during the cell cycle and reaches its highest concentration in the G1 phase [52].

A timely increased expression of Kv11.1 translates into an increased exit of potassium ions from the cell which produces a faster repolarization. This event results in shortening the G1 to S transitions during the cell cycle and initiates a carcinogenic event [43]. Furthermore, it has been shown that hERG1 gene can undergo abnormal epigenetic regulation in breast cancer tumors which results in a considerably decrease Kv11.1 mRNA by gene promoter methylation [53]. Furthermore, mass spectrometry investigations revealed that Kv11.1 protein is among the 10 most phosphorylated proteins expressed in the breast tumors of MMTV-PyMT transgenic mouse [54]. Although the specific effect of this posttranslational modification has been characterized yet, it is well known that phosphorylation and dephosphorylation of Kv11.1 can drive dramatic changes in its activity [55–57] and it has been proposed that phosphorylated Kv11.1 channel might be the part of a not-yet-identified oncogenic signature [54].

Overall, these studies indicate that the contribution of ion channels to bypass the effect of growth suppression factors could be a consequence of a fine regulation of their activity via a reversible posttranslational and epigenetic mechanism.

4. Ion channels and apoptosis of breast cancer cells

Interestingly, ion channel activity has also been involved in suppressing proliferation by mediating apoptotic events or by activating a cellular senescence program in breast cancer cells.

Apoptosis is a cellular death mechanism controlled by a series of biochemical cascades that are activated by intrinsic (cellular stress) or extrinsic (signaling molecules from other cells) pathways. In both pathways, calcium is a necessary factor for the maintenance of the adequate signaling required for the effective execution of cell death [58, 59].

For example, it has been shown that the transient receptor potential-melastatin-like 7 (TRPM7) channels can be a target of caspase-8 and its cleavage mediates an inward calcium flux current during apoptosis [60]. In addition, suppression of TRPV6 functions by gene silencing reduces proliferation and activates apoptosis in breast cancer cells [41].

Furthermore, overexpression of the voltage-gated calcium channel $Ca_V3.1$ suppressed cell proliferation in luminal breast cancer cells while knockdown of the *CACNA1G* gene encoding for Cav3.1 promoted the cell proliferation. In contrast, overexpression of another member of the Cav3 family, $Ca_V3.2$, did not affect the cell proliferation [61, 62]. In their study, the authors showed convincing evidence of a differential distribution of $Ca_V3.1$ and $Ca_V3.2$ channels at plasma membranes of apoptotic and nonapoptotic cells, respectively.

In addition, the calcium-activated chloride channel CLCA2 has been found downregulated in breast cancers and it is considered as a candidate tumor suppressor [63].

Cellular senescence is characterized by a permanent arrest of the cell cycle without activation of cell death pathways. Senescence can arise as response to hyperactivity of oncogenes and it is considered an important tumor-suppressor mechanism [64–66]. Increased expression of the Kv1.1 potassium channel in human mammary epithelial cells appears to mediate oncogene-induced senescence while reduction of Kv1.1 protein level associates with augmented cancer aggressiveness [67]. Additionally, hyperactivity of the Kv11.1 channel produced cellular senescence in different human breast cancer cell lines independently of their molecular characterization [30, 68, 69]. Therefore, activation of Kv11.1 channel can reprogram breast cancer cells from replicative to nonreplicative immortality.

5. Ion channels in breast cancer metastasis

Metastasis is a multistep process in which cancer cells detach from the primary tumor and spread to other body compartments (secondary foci). The metastatic cascade can be summarized in three main steps including: (1) loss of cell-cell contact, (2) invasion of surrounding stroma and vasculature, and (3) extraversion into the tissue of the organ host. Activation of each steps of the metastatic cascade is controlled by a numerous signaling molecules including hormones such as epidermal growth factor (EGF) and transforming growth factor (TGFβ) [70]. Metastatic cells retain most of the hallmarks of cancer including proliferation, and they are able to form new tumors in distant parts of the body. Changes in expression and activity of ion channel proteins have been associated with each step of the metastatic phenotype.

5.1. Ion channels in loss of breast cancer cell-cell contact

It has been well established that cell-cell contact is guaranteed by a high expression level of adhesive molecules such as E-cadherin (epithelial cadherin) and loss of E-cadherin and/or increased vimentin expression promote the transitioning of cancer cells from an epithelial to mesenchymal phenotype (epithelial to mesenchymal transition; EMT) in which cells present an enhanced migratory behavior [70]. Changes in calcium dynamics play a major role in the EMT process as intracellular calcium chelation can strongly affect transcription of several EMT markers [71]. TRPM7 calcium channel mRNA is prognostic of disease recurrence and distant metastasis in breast cancer. In addition, suppression of TRPM7 activity inhibits the expression of EGF-dependent vimentin in metastatic breast cancer cells [71, 72], while TGFβ-dependent

EMT is directly associated with enhanced activity of two major components of the store-operated calcium entry channels, STIM1 and Orai1 [73].

In contrast, the activity of the chloride channel cystic fibrosis transmembrane conductance regulator (CFTR) plays a role in suppressing EMT in breast adenocarcinoma and metastatic cell lines. Suppression of CFTR is associated with reduction of E-cadherin protein level producing a weakened cell-cell contact [74].

5.2. Ion channels in breast cancer cell invasion

Invasion of cancer cells into surrounding tissues relies on the ability of cells to move through biological and physical barriers (e.g., extracellular matrix (ECM) and basement membranes). This process occurs by formation of membrane protrusions (e.g., lamellipodia and/or invadopodia/filopodia), which are driven by actin polymerization after cell polarization and formation of focal contact points between ECM and cytoskeleton. These processes are regulated by biochemical pathways that include a set of important proteins such as the focal adhesion kinase (Fak).

The increased expression level of TRPM7 in breast cancers correlates with metastatic phenotype [75, 76]. In ER-ductal adenocarcinomas, TRPM7 is increased in invasive cells and knockdown of TRPM7 impairs MDA-MB-231 cell migration *in vitro* and metastasis *in vivo* [77]. Interestingly, the TRPM7 contains both a calcium channel and a kinase. Rapid, local calcium permeability (calcium flickers) through TRPM7appears to play a role mostly at the leading lamella of migrating cells while its kinase activity has been directly involved in changing focal adhesion sites to generate the necessary driving force for movement [78].

Ectopic expression of the voltage-gated sodium channel Nav1.5 has been directly associated with the ability of breast cancer cells to migrate and invade surrounding organs [79]. Suppression of Nav1.5 activity by using blockers or siRNAs in breast cancers produced a strong inhibition of outgrowth/extension processes, migration, and invasion without affecting proliferation.

During the process of invadopodia formation, outgrowth is guaranteed by digestion of the surrounding ECM by secretion of cathepsins-like enzymes and metalloproteases such as MMP2 and MMP9. Activity of Nav1.5 has been correlated with increased cathepsin secretion [80]. Upregulation of both MMP2 and MMP9 enzymatic activity requires calcium [81]. Interestingly, in metastatic breast cancer cell lines, suppression of voltage-gated calcium channel activity inhibits MMP9 expression level [82] and stimulation of the purinoceptor calcium channel P2X7 (ATP-gated calcium channel) increases secretion of cathepsins and accelerates invasion [83].

Interestingly, analyses of the MMP23 enzyme (which is abundantly expressed in breast cancer cells) protein structure revealed the presence of a particular domain (TxD) that inhibits the activity of several voltage-gated potassium channels (Kv1.6, Kv1.3, Kv1.1, Kv3.2, and Kv1.4) by directly blocking ionic fluxes and inhibiting trafficking of these channels to the surface membrane of T cells [84, 85]. Activity of these channels in T cells is fundamental for proliferation as well as production of cytokines. Therefore, it has been proposed that dual activity of MMP23 in breast cancer cells can favor invasion and suppress antitumor immunity.

5.3. Ion channels in breast cancer extravasation

In malignant cancer metastasis, extravasation refers to the ability of cancer cells to exit the capillaries and enter tissues. Typically, upregulation of the calcium channel transient receptor potential cation channel subfamily V member 4 (TRPV4) has been found strongly correlated with metastatic status of breast cancers [86]. Interestingly, increased activity of TRPV4 produced a softening of breast cancer cells and it has been associated with an extravasation trait in a murine breast cancer model, while suppression of the trpv4 gene significantly reduced lung metastasis.

6. Repurposing drugs targeting ion channels for breast cancer therapy

The body of research on the role of ion channels in breast cancer biology is growing and with the large availability of pharmacologic agents targeting the vast majority of ion channels, there is an interest in considering these proteins as potential novel therapeutic targets.

A study in which calcium channel blockers that have been already used in the clinic (e.g., antihypertensives such as verapamil) were tested for their effects on breast cancer biology showed that these compounds could increase the risk of intraductal and intralobular breast cancer. However, other studies showed no increased risk indicating that using these molecules as antibreast cancer agents is still debated [87, 88].

The nonvoltage-operated calcium channel blocker carboxyamidotriazole that is at this time in clinical trial shows antineoplastic potential [89] as it can produce decreased endothelial proliferation and angiogenesis in breast cancer cell lines.

More recently, the focus has moved to looking for agents that will specifically target the upregulated calcium channels seen in breast cancer cells. One such agent is lidocaine, a well-known anesthetic that inhibits sodium channels was found to reduce calcium influx through the TRPV6 channel and decrease the migration of breast cancer cells [90].

Several sodium channel blockers have revealed antitumor properties. Riluzole and carbamazepine, which are used for the treatment of neurodegenerative diseases, respectively, amyotrophic lateral sclerosis and epilepsy, have shown promising antitumor properties in metastatic breast cancer cells [91, 92]. Although the biochemical mechanism linking riluzole to inhibition of cell proliferation has been clarified yet, it has been established that inhibition of the sodium channel by carbamazepine produces an enhancement of proteasome-mediated degradation of ER alpha and human epidermal growth factor 2 (HER-2) [92, 93] indicating that these drugs might offer a therapeutic opportunity for both luminal and basal breast cancers. Furthermore, the anticonvulsant phenytoin can suppress migration and invasion of metastatic breast cancer cells [94].

Interestingly, some focus has moved from inhibiting the calcium channels to upregulating them with the idea being that the cancer cells, which already have more channels, become overwhelmed with the influx. Capsaicin was discovered to activate the TRPV1 channel in cancer cells. Administration of capsaicin was found to induce cell death in cancer cells [95].

7. Concluding remarks and perspectives

As ion channels play a fundamental role in virtually every cellular event, uncovering the contribution of these proteins in each of the hallmarks of breast cancer is important for understanding potential treatment for this heterogeneous collection of diseases. Ion channels are recognized as one the most important therapeutic targets and a large collection of molecules that can "correct" ion channel behavior have been traditionally employed to treat a vast variety of human diseases. Nevertheless, more research aiming to understand ion channel-dependent biochemical pathways, improve drug selectivity, and assess side effects is needed to convert promising discoveries on the use of molecules targeting ion channels as a therapeutic approach against breast cancer is needed.

Author details

Dowd Jonathan, Hendin Josh, Daniela F. Fukushiro-Lopes, David Laczynski and Saverio Gentile*

*Address all correspondence to: sagentile@luc.edu

Loyola University Chicago, Maywood, Illinois, USA

References

[1] Breast Cancer Facts & Figures 2016. Atlanta: American Cancer Society Inc.; 2016.

[2] Tinoco G, Warsch S, Gluck S, Avancha K, Montero AJ. Treating breast cancer in the 21st century: emerging biological therapies. J Cancer. 2013;4(2):117–132.

[3] Hugo Gene Nomenclature Committee. Ion Channels. 2016 [updated 2016; cited 24 August 2016]. Available from: http://www.genenames.org/genefamilies/IC.

[4] Pharmacology IUoBaC. Ion Channels. 2016 [updated 2016; cited 24 August 2016]. Available from: http://www.guidetopharmacology.org/GRAC/ReceptorFamiliesForward?type=IC.

[5] Nature. Ion Channels: structure and function. Nature. 2016 [cited 24 August 2016]. Available from: http://www.nature.com/nature/focus/ionchannel/#resource.

[6] Aldrich RW. A new standard: a review of handjournal of ion channels. J Gen Physiol. 2015;146(2):119–121.

[7] Arcangeli A, Crociani O, Lastraioli E, Masi A, Pillozzi S, Becchetti A. Targeting ion channels in cancer: a novel frontier in antineoplastic therapy. Curr Med Chem. 2009;16(1):66–93.

[8] Kunzelmann K. Ion channels and cancer. J Membr Biol. 2005;205(3):159–173.

[9] Prevarskaya N, Skryma R, Shuba Y. Ion channels and the hallmarks of cancer. Trends Mol Med. 2010;16(3):107–121.

[10] Rao VR, Perez-Neut M, Kaja S, Gentile S. Voltage-gated ion channels in cancer cell proliferation. Cancers (Basel). 2015;7(2):849–875.

[11] Roger S, Potier M, Vandier C, Besson P, Le Guennec JY. Voltage-gated sodium channels: new targets in cancer therapy? Curr Pharm Des. 2006;12(28):3681–3695.

[12] Ko JH, Ko EA, Gu W, Lim I, Bang H, Zhou T. Expression profiling of ion channel genes predicts clinical outcome in breast cancer. Mol Cancer. 2013;12(1):106.

[13] O'Grady SM, Lee SY. Molecular diversity and function of voltage-gated (Kv) potassium channels in epithelial cells. Int J Biochem Cell Biol. 2005;37(8):1578–1594.

[14] Pardo LA. Voltage-gated potassium channels in cell proliferation. Physiology (Bethesda). 2004;19:285–292.

[15] Wang XT, Nagaba Y, Cross HS, Wrba F, Zhang L, Guggino SE. The mRNA of L-type calcium channel elevated in colon cancer: protein distribution in normal and cancerous colon. Am J Pathol. 2000;157(5):1549–1562.

[16] Gray LS, Perez-Reyes E, Gomora JC, Haverstick DM, Shattock M, McLatchie L, et al. The role of voltage gated T-type Ca2+ channel isoforms in mediating "capacitative" Ca2+ entry in cancer cells. Cell Calcium. 2004;36(6):489–497.

[17] Munaron L, Antoniotti S, Lovisolo D. Intracellular calcium signals and control of cell proliferation: how many mechanisms? J Cell Mol Med. 2004;8(2):161–168.

[18] Kapur N, Mignery GA, Banach K. Cell cycle-dependent calcium oscillations in mouse embryonic stem cells. Am J Physiol Cell Physiol. 2007;292(4):C1510–8.

[19] DeCoursey TE, Chandy KG, Gupta S, Cahalan MD. Voltage-gated K+ channels in human T lymphocytes: a role in mitogenesis? Nature. 1984;307(5950):465–468.

[20] Wright SH. Generation of resting membrane potential. Adv Physiol Educ. 2004;28(1–4):139–142.

[21] Cone CD, Jr. Electroosmotic interactions accompanying mitosis initiation in sarcoma cells in vitro. Trans N Y Acad Sci. 1969;31(4):404–427.

[22] Cone CD, Jr. Variation of the transmembrane potential level as a basic mechanism of mitosis control. Oncology. 1970;24(6):438–470.

[23] Cone CD, Jr. Unified theory on the basic mechanism of normal mitotic control and oncogenesis. J Theor Biol. 1971;30(1):151–181.

[24] Binggeli R, Weinstein RC. Membrane potentials and sodium channels: hypotheses for growth regulation and cancer formation based on changes in sodium channels and gap junctions. J Theor Biol. 1986;123(4):377–401.

[25] Tokuoka S, Morioka H. The membrane potential of the human cancer and related cells. I. Gan. 1957;48(4):353–354.

[26] Johnstone BM. Micro-electrode penetration of ascites tumour cells. Nature. 1959;183(4658):411.

[27] Marino AA, Morris DM, Schwalke MA, Iliev IG, Rogers S. Electrical potential measurements in human breast cancer and benign lesions. Tumour Biol. 1994;15(3):147–152.

[28] Lobikin M, Chernet B, Lobo D, Levin M. Resting potential, oncogene-induced tumorigenesis, and metastasis: the bioelectric basis of cancer in vivo. Phys Biol. 2012;9(6): 065002.

[29] Klimatcheva E, Wonderlin WF. An ATP-sensitive K(+) current that regulates progression through early G1 phase of the cell cycle in MCF-7 human breast cancer cells. J Membr Biol. 1999;171(1):35–46.

[30] Lansu K, Gentile S. Potassium channel activation inhibits proliferation of breast cancer cells by activating a senescence program. Cell Death Dis. 2013;4:e652.

[31] Dai X, Xiang L, Li T, Bai Z. Cancer hallmarks, biomarkers and breast cancer molecular subtypes. J Cancer. 2016;7(10):1281–1294.

[32] Hanahan D, Weinberg RA. The hallmarks of cancer. Cell. 2000;100(1):57–70.

[33] Hanahan D, Weinberg RA. Hallmarks of cancer: the next generation. Cell. 2011;144(5): 646–674.

[34] Litan A, Langhans SA. Cancer as a channelopathy: ion channels and pumps in tumor development and progression. Front Cell Neurosci. 2015;9:86.

[35] Clapham DE. Calcium signaling. Cell. 2007;131(6):1047–1058.

[36] Berridge MJ. Calcium signalling remodelling and disease. Biochem Soc Trans. 2012;40(2):297–309.

[37] Zheng J. Molecular mechanism of TRP channels. Compr Physiol. 2013;3(1):221–242.

[38] Billeter AT, Hellmann JL, Bhatnagar A, Polk HC, Jr. Transient receptor potential ion channels: powerful regulators of cell function. Ann Surg. 2014;259(2):229–235.

[39] Guilbert A, Dhennin-Duthille I, Hiani YE, Haren N, Khorsi H, Sevestre H, et al. Expression of TRPC6 channels in human epithelial breast cancer cells. BMC Cancer. 2008;8:125.

[40] Kim SY, Yang D, Myeong J, Ha K, Kim SH, Park EJ, et al. Regulation of calcium influx and signaling pathway in cancer cells via TRPV6-Numb1 interaction. Cell Calcium. 2013;53(2):102–111.

[41] Bolanz KA, Hediger MA, Landowski CP. The role of TRPV6 in breast carcinogenesis. Mol Cancer Ther. 2008;7(2):271–279.

[42] Accardi A. Cell signaling. Lipids link ion channels and cancer. Science. 2015;349(6250): 789–790.

[43] Lam D, Schlichter LC. Expression and contributions of the Kir2.1 inward-rectifier K(+) channel to proliferation, migration and chemotaxis of microglia in unstimulated and anti-inflammatory states. Front Cell Neurosci. 2015;9:185.

[44] Ouadid-Ahidouch H, Ahidouch A. K+ channel expression in human breast cancer cells: involvement in cell cycle regulation and carcinogenesis. J Membr Biol. 2008;221(1):1–6.

[45] Stringer BK, Cooper AG, Shepard SB. Overexpression of the G-protein inwardly rectifying potassium channel 1 (GIRK1) in primary breast carcinomas correlates with axillary lymph node metastasis. Cancer Res. 2001;61(2):582–588.

[46] Khaitan D, Sankpal UT, Weksler B, Meister EA, Romero IA, Couraud PO, et al. Role of KCNMA1 gene in breast cancer invasion and metastasis to brain. BMC Cancer. 2009;9:258.

[47] Oeggerli M, Tian Y, Ruiz C, Wijker B, Sauter G, Obermann E, et al. Role of KCNMA1 in breast cancer. PLoS One. 2010;7(8):e41664.

[48] Alvarez-Baron CP, Jonsson P, Thomas C, Dryer SE, Williams C. The two-pore domain potassium channel KCNK5: induction by estrogen receptor alpha and role in proliferation of breast cancer cells. Mol Endocrinol. 2011;25(8):1326–1336.

[49] Fraser SP, Ozerlat-Gunduz I, Onkal R, Diss JK, Latchman DS, Djamgoz MB. Estrogen and non-genomic upregulation of voltage-gated Na(+) channel activity in MDA-MB-231 human breast cancer cells: role in adhesion. J Cell Physiol. 2010;224(2):527–539.

[50] Williams C, Edvardsson K, Lewandowski SA, Strom A, Gustafsson JA. A genome-wide study of the repressive effects of estrogen receptor beta on estrogen receptor alpha signaling in breast cancer cells. Oncogene. 2008;27(7):1019–1032.

[51] Plummer HK, 3rd, Yu Q, Cakir Y, Schuller HM. Expression of inwardly rectifying potassium channels (GIRKs) and beta-adrenergic regulation of breast cancer cell lines. BMC Cancer. 2004;4:93.

[52] Crociani O, Guasti L, Balzi M, Becchetti A, Wanke E, Olivotto M, et al. Cell cycle-dependent expression of HERG1 and HERG1B isoforms in tumor cells. J Biol Chem. 2003;278(5):2947–2955.

[53] Kuznetsova EB, Kekeeva TV, Larin SS, Zemliakova VV, Babenko OV, Nemtsova MV, et al. Novel methylation and expression markers associated with breast cancer. Mol Biol (Mosk). 2007;41(4):624–633.

[54] Ali NA, Wu J, Hochgrafe F, Chan H, Nair R, Ye S, et al. Profiling the tyrosine phosphoproteome of different mouse mammary tumour models reveals distinct, model-specific signalling networks and conserved oncogenic pathways. Breast Cancer Res. 2014;16(5): 437.

[55] Gentile S. Ion channel phosphorylopathy: a link between genomic variation and human disease. ChemMedChem. 2012;7(10):1757–1761.

[56] Gentile S, Darden T, Erxleben C, Romeo C, Russo A, Martin N, et al. Rac GTPase signaling through the PP5 protein phosphatase. Proc Natl Acad Sci U S A. 2006;103(13): 5202–5206.

[57] Gentile S, Martin N, Scappini E, Williams J, Erxleben C, Armstrong DL. The human ERG1 channel polymorphism, K897T, creates a phosphorylation site that inhibits channel activity. Proc Natl Acad Sci U S A. 2008;105(38):14704–14708.

[58] Elmore S. Apoptosis: a review of programmed cell death. Toxicol Pathol. 2007;35(4): 495–516.

[59] Orrenius S, Zhivotovsky B, Nicotera P. Regulation of cell death: the calcium-apoptosis link. Nat Rev Mol Cell Biol. 2003;4(7):552–565.

[60] Desai BN, Krapivinsky G, Navarro B, Krapivinsky L, Carter BC, Febvay S, et al. Cleavage of TRPM7 releases the kinase domain from the ion channel and regulates its participation in Fas-induced apoptosis. Dev Cell. 2012;22(6):1149–1162.

[61] Ohkubo T, Yamazaki J. T-type voltage-activated calcium channel Cav3.1, but not Cav3.2, is involved in the inhibition of proliferation and apoptosis in MCF-7 human breast cancer cells. Int J Oncol. 2012;41(1):267–275.

[62] Taylor JT, Huang L, Pottle JE, Liu K, Yang Y, Zeng X, et al. Selective blockade of T-type Ca2+ channels suppresses human breast cancer cell proliferation. Cancer Lett. 2008;267(1):116–124.

[63] Bustin SA, Li SR, Dorudi S. Expression of the Ca2+-activated chloride channel genes CLCA1 and CLCA2 is downregulated in human colorectal cancer. DNA Cell Biol. 2001;20(6):331–338.

[64] Munoz-Espin D, Serrano M. Cellular senescence: from physiology to pathology. Nat Rev Mol Cell Biol. 2014;15(7):482–496.

[65] Campisi J. Cellular senescence as a tumor-suppressor mechanism. Trends Cell Biol. 2001;11(11):S27–S31.

[66] McCormick A, Campisi J. Cellular aging and senescence. Curr Opin Cell Biol. 1991;3(2): 230–234.

[67] Lallet-Daher H, Wiel C, Gitenay D, Navaratnam N, Augert A, Le Calve B, et al. Potassium channel KCNA1 modulates oncogene-induced senescence and transformation. Cancer Res. 2013;73(16):5253–5265.

[68] Perez-Neut M, Rao VR, Gentile S. hERG1/Kv11.1 activation stimulates transcription of p21waf/cip in breast cancer cells via a calcineurin-dependent mechanism. Oncotarget. 2015;7(37):58893–58902.

[69] Perez-Neut M, Shum A, Cuevas BD, Miller R, Gentile S. Stimulation of hERG1 channel activity promotes a calcium-dependent degradation of cyclin E2, but not cyclin E1, in breast cancer cells. Oncotarget. 2015;6(3):1631–1639.

[70] Valastyan S, Weinberg RA. Tumor metastasis: molecular insights and evolving paradigms. Cell. 2011;147(2):275–292.

[71] Davis FM, Azimi I, Faville RA, Peters AA, Jalink K, Putney JW, Jr., et al. Induction of epithelial-mesenchymal transition (EMT) in breast cancer cells is calcium signal dependent. Oncogene. 2014;33(18):2307–2316.

[72] Davis FM, Peters AA, Grice DM, Cabot PJ, Parat MO, Roberts-Thomson SJ, et al. Non-stimulated, agonist-stimulated and store-operated Ca2+ influx in MDA-MB-468 breast cancer cells and the effect of EGF-induced EMT on calcium entry. PLoS One. 2012;7(5):e36923.

[73] Hu J, Qin K, Zhang Y, Gong J, Li N, Lv D, et al. Downregulation of transcription factor Oct4 induces an epithelial-to-mesenchymal transition via enhancement of Ca^{2+} influx in breast cancer cells. Biochem Biophys Res Commun. 2011;411(4):786–791.

[74] Zhang JT, Jiang XH, Xie C, Cheng H, Da Dong J, Wang Y, et al. Downregulation of CFTR promotes epithelial-to-mesenchymal transition and is associated with poor prognosis of breast cancer. Biochim Biophys Acta. 2013;1833(12):2961–2969.

[75] Guilbert A, Gautier M, Dhennin-Duthille I, Rybarczyk P, Sahni J, Sevestre H, et al. Transient receptor potential melastatin 7 is involved in oestrogen receptor-negative metastatic breast cancer cells migration through its kinase domain. Eur J Cancer. 2013;49(17):3694–3707.

[76] Meng X, Cai C, Wu J, Cai S, Ye C, Chen H, et al. TRPM7 mediates breast cancer cell migration and invasion through the MAPK pathway. Cancer Lett. 2013;333(1):96–102.

[77] Middelbeek J, Kuipers AJ, Henneman L, Visser D, Eidhof I, van Horssen R, et al. TRPM7 is required for breast tumor cell metastasis. Cancer Res. 2012;72(16):4250–4261.

[78] Wei C, Wang X, Chen M, Ouyang K, Song LS, Cheng H. Calcium flickers steer cell migration. Nature. 2009;457(7231):901–905.

[79] Nelson M, Yang M, Millican-Slater R, Brackenbury WJ. Nav1.5 regulates breast tumor growth and metastatic dissemination in vivo. Oncotarget. 2015;6(32):32914–32929.

[80] Brisson L, Driffort V, Benoist L, Poet M, Counillon L, Antelmi E, et al. NaV1.5 $Na^{(+)}$ channels allosterically regulate the NHE-1 exchanger and promote the activity of breast cancer cell invadopodia. J Cell Sci. 2013;126(Pt 21):4835–4842.

[81] Makowski GS, Ramsby ML. Autoactivation profiles of calcium-dependent matrix metalloproteinase-2 and -9 in inflammatory synovial fluid: effect of pyrophosphate and bisphosphonates. Clin Chim Acta. 2005;358(1–2):182–191.

[82] Kohn EC, Jacobs W, Kim YS, Alessandro R, Stetler-Stevenson WG, Liotta LA. Calcium influx modulates expression of matrix metalloproteinase-2 (72-kDa type IV collagenase, gelatinase A). J Biol Chem. 1994;269(34):21505–21511.

[83] Xia J, Yu X, Tang L, Li G, He T. P2X7 receptor stimulates breast cancer cell invasion and migration via the AKT pathway. Oncol Rep. 2015;34(1):103–110.

[84] Chhabra S, Chang SC, Nguyen HM, Huq R, Tanner MR, Londono LM, et al. Kv1.3 channel-blocking immunomodulatory peptides from parasitic worms: implications for autoimmune diseases. FASEB J. 2014;28(9):3952–3964.

[85] Nguyen HM, Galea CA, Schmunk G, Smith BJ, Edwards RA, Norton RS, et al. Intracellular trafficking of the KV1.3 potassium channel is regulated by the prodomain of a matrix metalloprotease. J Biol Chem. 2013;288(9):6451–6464.

[86] Lee WH, Choong LY, Mon NN, Lu S, Lin Q, Pang B, et al. TRPV4 Regulates breast cancer cell extravasation, stiffness and actin cortex. Sci Rep. 2015;6:27903.

[87] Azoulay L, Soldera S, Yin H, Bouganim N. Use of calcium channel blockers and risk of breast cancer: a population-based cohort study. Epidemiology. 2016;27(4):594–601.

[88] Brandenburg NA, Backstrom JT, Hinkle RL. Calcium channel blockers and cancer: the evidence against an association. Am J Hypertens. 1996;9(10 Pt 1):1049–1050, author reply 51 53.

[89] Guo L, Li ZS, Wang HL, Ye CY, Zhang DC. Carboxyamido-triazole inhibits proliferation of human breast cancer cells via G(2)/M cell cycle arrest and apoptosis. Eur J Pharmacol. 2006;538(1–3):15–22.

[90] Martin F, Ufodiama C, Watt I, Bland M, Brackenbury WJ. Therapeutic value of voltage-gated sodium channel inhibitors in breast, colorectal, and prostate cancer: a systematic review. Front Pharmacol. 2015;6:273.

[91] Speyer CL, Nassar MA, Hachem AH, Bukhsh MA, Jafry WS, Khansa RM, et al. Riluzole mediates anti-tumor properties in breast cancer cells independent of metabotropic glutamate receptor-1. Breast Cancer Res Treat. 2016;157(2):217–228.

[92] Meng QW, Zhao CH, Xi YH, Cai L, Sun LC, Sui GJ. Inhibitory effect of carbamazepine on proliferation of estrogen-dependent breast cancer cells. Ai Zheng. 2006;25(8):967–973.

[93] Meng Q, Chen X, Sun L, Zhao C, Sui G, Cai L. Carbamazepine promotes Her-2 protein degradation in breast cancer cells by modulating HDAC6 activity and acetylation of Hsp90. Mol Cell Biochem. 2011;348(1–2):165–171.

[94] Nelson M, Yang M, Dowle AA, Thomas JR, Brackenbury WJ. The sodium channel-blocking antiepileptic drug phenytoin inhibits breast tumour growth and metastasis. Mol Cancer. 2015;14:13.

[95] Azimi I, Roberts-Thomson SJ, Monteith GR. Calcium influx pathways in breast cancer: opportunities for pharmacological intervention. Br J Pharmacol. 2014;171(4):945–960.

Section 3

Diagnosis and Treatment of Breast Cancer

Chapter 14

Modern Radiotherapy Era in Breast Cancer

Yasemin Bolukbasi and Ugur Selek

Additional information is available at the end of the chapter

http://dx.doi.org/10.5772/66906

Abstract

Radiation therapy (RT) is one of the major treatment modalities that are used in breast cancer treatment, and depending on the chest-wall anatomy, RT fields have to be customized. Techniques used in planning have been evolving since last two decades from two dimensional (2D) to three-dimensional (3D), while intensity modulated radiotherapy (IMRT), volumetric modulated arc therapy (VMAT) and even proton therapy have been an option in daily approach. In addition, technological hardware and software advances in delivery and planning systems, total treatment duration of breast RT have been shortened in last decades along with recent hypofractionated radiotherapy schemes or emerging partial-breast irradiation protocols. The other attractive approach—accelerated partial breast irradiation (APBI) could be a reasonable option for highly selected subpopulation of early-stage breast cancer patients out of a clinical trial. Long-term follow-up results have emerged heart and coronary sparing with maximum safety and efficacy. The most important advance could be named as cardiac sparing—deep breath-hold approach—in all the modern technique improvement. Although most advanced techniques in management of breast cancer have not been verified to increase survival, we suggest recommending resource stratified advanced in order to provide best technical and clinical care in this long-term survivor candidates.

Keywords: radiotherapy, IMRT, VMAT, breath hold

1. Introduction

Radiation therapy (RT) has become an essential component of breast cancer treatment, and depending on the anatomic structure of the region to be irradiated (breast, chest wall or regional lymphatics), RT can be technically challenging and varying from one patient to another.

Breast RT has evolved from two-dimensional (2D) to three-dimensional (3D), while intensity modulated radiotherapy (IMRT), volumetric modulated arc therapy (VMAT) and even proton therapy have been options to discuss with our patients in daily practice. Besides technological hardware and software advances in delivery and planning systems, total treatment duration of breast RT has been changing dramatically in last decades along with recent hypofractionated radiotherapy schemes or emerging partial-breast irradiation protocols. As modern RT allowed us a successive reduction in the treatment-related complications such as fibrosis and long-term cardiac toxicity in addition to improving the locoregional control rates, rationale of as low as possible is appealing to focus more on heart and coronary sparing with four-dimensional (4D) breath-hold techniques. Modern radiotherapy techniques and fundamentals need to be implemented in routine clinical care with maximum safety and efficacy in order to maximize the benefit of locoregional treatment and to minimize the risks of late complications.

We aim to summarize the advances of modern radiotherapy in breast cancer through clinical approaches and routine treatment indications based on present knowledge and evidence-based recommendations.

2. Simulation and immobilization techniques

2.1. Supine

Radiotherapy has been widely used as a part of breast cancer in partial or total mastectomy. Radiotherapy technique can be difficult and variable depending on the anatomy of the patient such as chest-wall concavity, depth of axilla. The first step of radiation treatment is to perform CT simulation to obtain a reproducible detailed anatomy for planning conformal or intensity-modulated radiotherapy with using heart-sparing techniques such as breath hold or heart blocking, especially for left breast cancer patients. Adjuvant therapy for breast cancer starts early 4–6 weeks after surgery or after chemotherapy and was delivered with 6 or 18 MV photons using usually wedged tangent fields, or field and field, 3DCRT and IMRT at 1.8–2.67 cGy doses ranged from 40 to 60 Gy.

Treatment fields are a composite of adjacent whole breast or chest wall, mammaria interna, supraclavicular and axillary fields. The main purpose of the breast radiotherapy fields is to avoid hot and cold dose regions between contiguous fields while minimizing the dose of organs at risk such as lung and heart. RT fields have to be modified according to patient's chest wall and breast anatomy due to its irregular surface, which can cause dose inhomogeneity. At the same time, setup has to be easily applicable and reproducible. Immobilization devices, specially designed for breast cancer treatments, are commercially widely available and are frequently used in daily practice. The best known devices are listed as follows: inclined plane, breast boards, Board-wing butterfly Board, Vac-fix bag-Vacuum Cradle Bed and alpha cradle. The most common, preferred and basic set-up has been performed by a breast board having an inclined plane with an arm support, in supine position. The head of the patient has been pointed to the opposite side, and arm has been abducted (90°–120°) and externally rotated. Skin folds in supraclavicular field and soft tissue of arm has to be modified if required. The patient is positioned on her back on a stable breast board, and board is angled to ensure the sternum—chest parallel to table. This angle can be adjusted according to clinical needs, but larger angels can cause increased dose in lungs in patients requiring the supraclavicular field. The border between the chest wall and supraclavicular field is usually placed at the bottom of clavicular head. Radiopaque wires must be used to define incisions and breast borders [1].

Supine positioning has been used for breast cancer patient's alignment for several decades over the world. It provides patient comfort and position reproducibility for the whole treatment period, while ensures better axillary coverage in comparison to prone positioning. When setup errors in supine position were studied with three-dimensional cone-beam computed tomography (CBCT), the average magnitude of error was found to be generally less than 5 mm across a number of studies [2]. Sethi et al. compared both prone and supine positioning for 3DCRT and IMRT plans; traditional three- or four-field planning has inadequate nodal coverage, especially performed in prone setup compared to supine (29 and 42% vs. 50 and 59%), and this disadvantage has been altered by CT-based planning and coverage varied from 92 to 97% depending on IMRT or 3DCRT independent from positioning [3].

2.2. Prone

Rarely, in case of a very large pendulous breast, lateral decubitus or prone position can help. Prone position has been proposed for especially large breasted patient as this volume can cause dose homogeneity due to hot spots and also overlapping breast tissue could create an auto bolus effect, which can abbreviate skin toxicity [4, 5]. While prone setup has also been proposed to increase the lung and heart tissue sparing, the literature has conflicting results in terms of normal tissue dose reduction [6, 7]. Wurschmidt et al. stated that the prone position increasing incidental dose of LAD coronary artery to a mean dose of 33.5 Gy in comparison with supine setup with a mean dose of 25.6 Gy in left whole breast irradiation, without any significant differences in the average mean dose to heart between two different setups [6]. In contrast, Kirby et al. also documented prone positioning to reduce cardiac doses in almost 64% of 30 patients treated whole breast irradiation with a median reduction in LAD mean = 6.2 Gy and 24% of the 30 cases treated with partial breast irradiation (median reduction in LAD max = 29.3 Gy) in addition to reducing ipsilateral-lung (mean) in all whole breast and 61 of 65 partial irradiation cases, and chest wall V (50 Gy) in all whole breast irradiation cases. They concluded that prone positioning is likely to benefit left-breast-affected women of larger breast volume both for whole or partial breast irradiation, and right-breast-affected women regardless of breast volume [7]. Despite the improvement of dose homogeneity, prevention of hot spot regions and lower lung and heart doses, prone position for whole breast irradiation has not been applied in routine clinical practice. Prone setup has been considered to be more problematic to reproduce than supine position and to be less precise. In Varga et al.'s randomized study, the range of displacement was greater in prone position as well as the prone relocation precision presented an expansion over time without any correlation to any patient-related parameters [8]. Patient treatment-related comfort and inadequate target coverage of tumors especially extending down to chest wall were also mentioned as main concerns [9, 10].

Main concern about prone position as setup errors and reproducibility in comparison with the international standard supine position in women undergoing whole-breast radiotherapy was justified by Kirby et al., matching chest wall and clips on cone-beam CT (CBCT) images acquired prior to the fractions 1, 4, 7, 8, 11 and 14. Setup errors were greater using prone technique than for supine technique as follows: systematic errors: 1.3–1.9 mm (supine) and 3.1–4.3 mm (prone) ($p = 0.02$) and random errors: 2.6–3.2 mm (supine) and 3.8–5.4 mm (prone) ($p = 0.02$). Even patient-comfort-scores and treatment times were similar, calculated CTV-PTV margins were calculated to be larger for prone (12–16 mm) than for supine treatment (10 mm) [11].

2.3. Lateral decubitus position

Lateral decubitus position is a side-lying setup especially generated for large-sized and pendulous breasted patients. In experienced clinics, this setup has been used especially for only breast irradiated cases as lymphatic coverage could be problematic in this position. Campana et al. presented their isocentric lateral decubitus technique at the Institute Curie where almost 500 patients were treated at 50 Gy whole beast radiotherapy [12]. Thin carbon fiber supports and special patient positioning devices have been developed especially for this technique. Their techniques have been proven to show good homogeneity of the dose in breast treatment volume, with extremely low dose to the underlying lung and heart [12]. Despite applicable single center results, this technique has not been spread out and accepted for the routine clinical work flow.

2.4. Thermoplastic bra

Use of thermoplastic bra has been investigated with the objective of minimizing organ at risk doses, as it moves the breast widely lateral. It has been found to provide shallower beam arrangement for left breast (medial: 288°–315° with bra vs. 302°–325° without bra) and to decrease lung doses by 30.6% without any dedicated selection criteria for daily clinical use [13]. The main concern on thermoplastic mask users related with the skin dose and possible associated clinical exacerbation of side effects turned out to be not significant.

3. Planning and delivery methods

3.1. 3DCRT

Conventional two dimensional wedge compensators have been used to shape the treatment fields for many decades. After integration of CT and more sophisticated planning programs in radiotherapy clinical routine, target location can be defined precisely and dose distribution can be obtained more homogenously. The target and critical structure volumes for three-dimensional conformal radiotherapy (3DCRT) have been defined according to ICRU reports 50 and 62 [14]. A major challenge to improve dose uniformity is the irregular shape and size of the breast while minimizing the risk of treatment-related complications. In recent years, conformal RT, particularly, forward or inverse intensity modulated RT (IMRT), which is a more advanced and sophisticated form of 3DCRT, is becoming popular for breast irradiation as it provides reduced inhomogeneity and/or better normal tissue sparing [15]. Additionally, lately accessible image-guided RT (IGRT) can significantly increase precision of conformal treatment delivery.

3DCRT is based on patient's simulation CT with pertinent anatomical data for target definition as the first and most important step of this advanced planning system. Target delineation and consistency of target volumes have been accepted as priority, RTOG and EORTC have published breast cancer-specific atlases easily reachable on websites for uniformity among interobservers [16, 17] (http://www.rtog.org/CoreLab/ContouringAtlases/BreastCancerAtlas.aspx). In addition to atlas-based contouring publications, quantification of the multi-institutional, multi-observer variability of target and organ-at-risk (OAR) delineation for breast cancer radiotherapy and its dosimetric impacts has been an attractive topic. Li et al. assembled nine radiation oncologists specializing in breast RT from eight institutions to individually delineate lumpectomy cavity, boost planning target volume, breast, supraclavicular, axillary and internal mammary nodes, chest wall and OARs (e.g., heart, lung) on the same CT images of three demonstrative patients with breast cancer [18]. The variability in contouring the targets and OARs was as low as 10% while the volume variations had standard deviations up to 60%. These inter-observer differences can easily end up in significant changes in dosimetry in for breast radiotherapy planning. Further work is warranted to obtain a systematic consensus, especially in the era of IMRT/IGRT, which could be used and easily adapted by the institutions. In similar standardization attempts to minimize the variation in substructure delineation for organs at risk, a detailed cardiac CT atlas have been developed by University of Michigan [19]. If patient has supraclavicular positive lymph node present, additional dose to supraclavicular region will bring into the question of brachial plexus dose. Brachial plexus contouring is mostly thought as a part of head and neck or lung IMRT, so breast radiation oncologists are encouraged to follow contouring guidelines for the brachial plexus (BP) using anatomically validated cadaver data set and head and neck case series [20, 21]. An average margin of 4.7 mm around the anatomically validated brachial plexus contour is instructed to cover and compensate all the anatomic variations of brachial plexus [20].

Many irradiation techniques such as single isocentric 3D conformal whole breast irradiation, prone position technique, four or five field irradiation technique for peripheral lymphatic were described and widely used all over the world and details will not be given as it is not in the scope of this chapter. For each CT data (2–5-mm slices), the dosimetric plans were created by appropriately adjusting the beam apertures such as beam angle, collimator angle, couch angle, wedges, energies, weights and multi-leaf collimators by virtual simulation through digitally reconstructed radiographs (DRR); therefore, the planning goals on coverage and OAR sparing can be achieved. Beam apertures were selected to fully cover the targets for each set of contours. Photon beams of 6 and/or high energy 15–18 MV were used to irradiate breasts, chest wall and boost PTVs tangentially, supraclavicular and axillary nodes. Electron beams with or without a combination of 6 MV photons were used for internal mammary nodes.

As the treatment plan evaluation starts with all axial slices to be checked whether bearing hot or cold regions or not. Next step is the evaluation of dose volume histograms (DVH), which is a graphic expression of dose distribution volume in target or OAR. The planning goals are recommended to cover the breast or chest wall with ≥95% with maximal point dose but ≤110%, while OAR doses are limited with contralateral breast ≤3.30 Gy, ≤20% of ipsilateral lung ≥20%, ≤5% of heart ≥20% for left-sided breast cancer and 0% of heart ≥25% for right-sided breast patients, and mean heart dose ≤5 Gy [22].

Transition from 2D to 3D has been promising under dosimetric studies revealing an improvement. When conventional 2D and mono-isocentric 3D techniques were dosimetrically compared in terms of coverage and normal tissue doses, Guillert et al. stated that homogeneity, regional lymphatic irradiation and heart and spinal cord protection were better with the mono-isocentric 3D technique [23]. Leite et al. dosimetrically assessed incidental irradiation of the internal mammary lymph nodes (IMLNs) with using opposed tangential fields with 45–50.4 Gy conventional two-dimensional (2D) or 3DCRT techniques in their cohort of 80 breast cancer patients and documented the mean dose to the IMLNs as 7.93 Gy in the 2D cohort in comparison with 20.64 Gy in the 3D cohort [24]. Even all dosimetric parameters were higher in 3DCRT plans, still we need to improve coverage. These results from the studies analyzed above have proven that more attempts have to be taken to cover target volume without increasing dose to normal organs.

3.2. IMRT

Breast has been one of the complex radiation delivery areas due to the complex anatomical geometry and differences of depth of regional nodal areas. Two-dimensional and 3DCRT have been used safely and with high local control rates, but homogeneity and normal tissue doses have been the two problematic topics until advanced radiation delivery techniques based on image guidance has been established. IMRT can be designed as a forward or inverse planning technique [25]. The forward planning is more common in clinical practice, uses similar beam angles without old school wedges, but manually created field in fields decreasing the hot high dose regions to optimize the dose distribution [26, 27]. Forward planning follows optimization algorithms to provide dose homogeneity and coverage [27].

The use of IMRT in breast cancer radiotherapy has been investigated in couple of fundamental prospective clinical studies [28, 29]. First was the Royal Marsden study comparing 2D wedge based, 3D and IMRT techniques in terms of acute and long-term side effects. The primary end point was objective change in breast appearance based on serial photographs of 306 patients obtained before treatment, at 1-, 2- and 5-year follow-up. The conventional treatment arm patients were 1.7 times more likely to have a change in breast appearance compared to IMRT arm patients, suggesting that minimization of dose inhomogeneity in the breast reduces late adverse effects, whereas there were no significant differences on the patient reported breast discomfort and quality of life between 2SD and IMRT arms [28]. Second randomized trial by the Canadian group has supported the findings and concluded that 4–7 segmented IMRT decreased moist desquamation rates which was also related with the breast cup size [30]. Third prospective trial from Cambridge has focused selective forward IMRT planning on the patients if inhomogeneity exceeds 107% with standard planning and concluded that improved plan parameters with forward IMRT were obtained [29]. Dosimetrically reduction in surface doses using IMRT technique has been shown to be almost 20%, and this has been turned to be a reduction in skin acute side effects from 52 to 39% in clinical experience without compromising local regional control success [26]. All pertinent studies have supported the value of early breast cancer treatment with IMRT providing lesser acute skin toxicities, which would effect long-term cosmetics [31, 32].

The next question was whether more homogenous dose distribution will turn into survival advantage compared to conventional 2D or 3DCRT. Yang et al. retrospectively reviewed 234 patients treated for stage 0–III breast cancer (conventional:131 vs. IMRT: 103) and documented locoregional failure-free survival and disease-free survival at 8 years as 96.7 vs. 97.6% and 91.2 vs. 93.1% for conventional RT and IMRT, respectively [33], while less frequent acute skin toxicity by IMRT did not translate into a significant decrease in late toxicity rates in follow-up.

IMRT can add benefit when hypofractionation is prescribed. Hardee et al. compared toxicity of patients treated according to the Canadian hypofractionation regimen (40 patients with 3DCRT and 57 with IMRT) [34] and demonstrated IMRT reducing the maximum dose (Dmax median, 109.96% for 3DCRT vs. 107.28% for IMRT; $p < 0.0001$) and improving median dose homogeneity in comparison with 3D-CRT. Besides, grade 2 dermatitis decreased from 13% in the 3DCRT group to 2% in the IMRT group, and decreasing rates of acute pruritus and grade 2–3 sub-acute hyperpigmentation were noted in IMRT group [34].

The use of more sophisticated treatment techniques will be more critical especially for organ at risk—lung and heart—doses in more complex treatment fields for locally advanced breast cancer patients. A dosimetric study by Lohr et al. evaluated the effect of IMRT on cardiac doses compared to 3DCRT at their CT data set of 14 patients [35]. Plans were generated by two conformal beam angles chosen to minimize heart and lung doses for 3DCRT and nine beams (0°–335°, 25° apart) over left hemi-thorax in a coplanar fashion for IMRT [35], where IMRT had provided superior dosimetric parameters for maximal dose to heart, V30 and V40 of heart and left ventricle except mean and median dose of heart which increased from 6.8 to 8.5 Gy and from 1.02 to 2.77 Gy, respectively. In the light of these results, Lohr et al. stated that mean risk of excess cardiac mortality significantly decreased from 6.03 to 0.25% according to their relative seriality model [35].

Conventional irradiation of regional nodal irradiation was known to deliver inadequate homogeneity and to be usually a challenge depending on the patients' geometry, location close to the normal organs and patient-dependent variation of depth [3, 36]. In a dosimetric study, three field, four field, CT-based 3D and forward IMRT treatment options were compared and superior nodal coverage has been achieved by both CT-based 3D and IMRT techniques, despite the fact that contralateral breast and ipsilateral lung V5 and V20 doses increased by 3–4 field IMRT [3]. The recent rotational form of IMRT, volumetric arc therapy, has also been studied dosimetrically for locally advanced breast cancer patients requiring regional lymph node irradiation with conflicting results [37, 38]. Ma et al. replanned left-sided, locally advanced patients with 3DCRT-field in field, five field IMRT (2 tangents, 2 anterior and 1 supraclavicular field) and two coplanar partial arc VMAT to a prescription dose of 50 Gy [37], the planning goals were defined as follows: PTV:[D95 (95% of PTV receiving a prescription dose or higher) = 50 Gy, V47.5 Gy ≥95%, V53.5 Gy ≤5%]; heart: [Dmean ≤10 Gy, V10Gy ≤20%,V20Gy ≤15%]; left lung: [Dmean ≤15 Gy, V10Gy ≤30%, V20Gy ≤20%, V30Gy ≤10%]; right breast:[Dmax ≤3 Gy]; spinal cord: [Dmax ≤45 Gy]; left humeral head: [Dmean ≤50 Gy]. Both 5F-IMRT and 2P-VMAT plans demonstrated comparable PTV coverage (V95%), hotspot areas (V110%) and conformity (all $p > 0.05$) which were significantly superior to 3DCRT-FinF, and 5F-IMRT plans provided significantly less heart and left lung dose than 2P-VMAT (all $p < 0.05$); therefore, Ma et al. specified that 5F-IMRT has dosimetrical advantages compared with the other two techniques in comprehensive breast irradiation for left-sided breast cancer based on balance between PTV coverage and normal organ sparing [37]. Tyran et al. evaluated arc therapy and a forward-planned multi-segment technique with a mono-isocenter technique for left-sided breast treatment, involving lymph node irradiation including the internal mammary chain [38]. VMAT improved PTV coverage and dose homogeneity but distributed low doses to a larger volume which blurred the clinical benefits. In another preclinic study revealed that VMAT achieved similar PTV coverage and sparing of organs at risk, with fewer monitor units and shorter delivery time than cIMRT with conventional modified wide-tangent (MWT) techniques for locoregional radiotherapy of breast cancer [39]. Based on the conflicting dosimetric studies and without any published clinical study, no general recommendations for VMAT could be drawn for its use in daily clinical practice, leaving the decision to the institutional decision based on the planner's experience, expectations and required quality assurance.

Especially forward IMRT, using tangential bream angels and creating multiple segment, can be accepted as standard approach in clinical practice taking into the considerations of acute toxicity [40, 41]. The published literature of forward or inverse IMRT use in clinical practice of breast cancer, has mainly focusing on toxicities and have short follow-up time. In Canadian guidelines, based on the similar local control and overall survival results, IMRT has not been recommended over tangential radiotherapy field design [42]. Of course, the cost of using new technologies needs to considered as if they only reduce toxicity profile due to treatment. In USA, systematic analysis of Medicare reimbursement data during 2012–2015, for prostate, anal, gynecological and head-neck cancers, declared that IMRT has been more costly than 3DCRT approximately 12.834$ per patients and this cost can go up to 19.113$ and breast IMRT has been named as the least expensive IMRT depending on the less complex structure compared to a head and neck workload [43].

3.3. Tomotherapy

Lately, an innovative method of IMRT has been developed as a combination of helical IMRT with CT image guidance at the University of Wisconsin-Madison named as TomoTherapy® Hi•Art® [44]. A small megavoltage X-ray source was built in an analogous to that of a CT X-ray source, and the geometry provided the chance to deliver treatment applying the 360° rotation of the CT gantry and the couch moving the patient slowly through the center of the ring, with the mounted megavoltage linear accelerator around the gantry ring in a spiral fashion to direct the beam at a slightly different plane at the each rotation of gantry. TomoTherapy Hi•Art can also accomplish a quick CT scan before each treatment starts for image guidance in the era of modern linear accelerators [45].

TomoTherapy has been used to treat other sites than breast such as prostate, brain, head and neck, lung, prostate, etc. [44], and when considered for breast cancer treatment, the format of helical tomotherapy sound unsuitable based on the use of all gantry angles delivering low doses to areas such as contralateral lung and breast in comparison with conventional standard tangents field design which would only deliver a scatter dose to these organs. Starting point of clinical experience of helical tomotherapy for breast cancer has been a treatment of complicated case scenarios such as bilateral breast cancer to be irradiated for the bilateral breasts/chest wall and regional nodes. Kaidar-Person et al. reviewed nine-cased treated for breast and regional nodal irradiation with Helical tomotherapy in their institute in 5 years of period [46]. The average lung V20, lung V5 and heart mean dose was 29%, 66% and 20 G, respectively. Clinical significant acute toxicity was observed such as dysphagia (5/9), fatigue (4/9), nausea and weight loss (1/9) and skin desquamation (9/9) [46]. Goddu et al. also estimated the practicability of using helical tomotherapy for locally advanced left-sided breast cancer in a dosimetric planning study on 10 CT data sets comparing a multifield three-dimensional technique with the tomotherapy treatment planning for 50.4 Gy dose [47] and found tomotherapy to increase the minimal dose to the planning target volume and improve the dose homogeneity. While decreasing the mean percentage of the left lung volume receiving 20 Gy in the tomotherapy plans decreased from 32.6% to 17.6 ± 3.5%, while increasing lower dose levels as V5 from 25 to46%. The same observation was present for heart such tomotherapy decreased V35 Gy from 5.6 to 2.2% with an increase from 7.5 to 12.2 Gy for mean heart dose levels [47]. These dosimetric studies confirmed that tomotherapy plans provided better dose conformity and homogeneity than three-dimensional radiotherapy, while the disadvantage of tomotherapy seems to be low dose bath and higher lower dose parameters for the normal tissue bearing an unpredictable effect for the long-term effects. In a case presentation from Institue Curie, comparison of 3DCRT dorsal decubitus and 3DCRT lateral isocentric decubitus with tomotherapy plan for T2N0M0 breast cancer patient revealed that tomotherapy plan has been preferred as it could deliver optimal coverage to the planning target volumes while also providing tolerable doses to the patient's heart and lungs [48].

The use of the tomotherapy unit in fixed gantry positions with the beam intensity modulated by the micro collimators as the patient is moved through a stationary gantry could be the best approach in breast cancer treatment. This design can limit the low dose bath effect and created an almost a tangential approach. This form of tomotherapy has been used by O'Donnell and they present their case solutions for bilateral disease, left breast irradiation, pectus excavatum, prominent contralateral prosthesis and internal mammary chain disease [49]. Their planning results with a more limited number and angle of beams than standard helical tomotherapy technique results reassured better conformity of treatment with improved coverage of the planning target volume, including regional nodes, without field junction problems [49].

The major two important concerns in tomotherapy similar to IMRT and VMAT are time-consuming planning and quality assurance than standard breast irradiation and increasing low dose 'bath' as a major concern on late oncogenesis. Published comparative studies of conformal radiotherapy and IMRT have revealed generally better target volume coverage and organ-at-risk dose reductions and worse risk of secondary cancer induction based on increased out-of-field leakage radiation with higher number of fields and used monitor units in IMRT plans; the overall estimation of lifetime attributable risk of the radiation-induced cancer risk was lower with 3DCRT than with IMRT or VMAT [50, 51]. Comparison of five treatment modalities including tomotherapy, 3D conformal radiotherapy, field in field, IMRT and VMAT in breast cancer patients, tomotherapy plans provided better dose homogeneity in the target volume, as IMRT and VMAT plans created better dose coverage and dose conformity; the V20Gy of the ipsilateral lung was the lowest in the single isocentric IMRT plan, followed by the 3–4 arc VMAT, 3D-CRT, TOMO, and Field in field plans, and the V10Gy was the highest for the VMAT plan among the five modalities [52]. Keeping in mind that lifetime attributable risk of secondary cancers depends on organ's distance from the primary beam and the used modality, risk of secondary malignancies expected in the ipsilateral lung, thyroid, contralateral lung and contralateral breast were found to be the highest for the VMAT plans, followed by the IMRT plans [34], and remarkably, the risk of the Tomotherapy was comparable to or lower than those of the 3DCRT and Field in field plans [52]. This study clarified one of the major concerns of tomotherapy and can reflect more common use of tomotherapy in breast cancer treatment.

3.4. Proton therapy

Proton radiation is a particle radiation which has a capability of depositing therapeutic radiation at a fixed point with sparing of tissues beyond the target. Although proton therapy is prescribed in fractions similar to photons, its radiobiological effect rate is higher than (1.1) photons [53]. The use of protons in treatment has been evaluated primarily for tumors requiring high doses or located in close proximity to critical structures such as prostate cancer, brain tumors and childhood cancer. Despite dosimetric advantages, extensive cost of equipment and maintenance has been defined as an important barrier fact for protons to become widespread in clinical use. Nowadays, 61 centers are operating over the world, and in 2020, the estimated number of proportional proton radiotherapy centers will be 91 [54]. Clinically, proton has limited use in breast cancer, although it has an exclusive capability to archive full coverage of the breast or chest wall with a rapid fall-off of dose beyond the target which would be a great contribution for acute and late cardiopulmonary toxicities. Hence, greater data were present for accelerated partial breast irradiation (APBI) with longer follow-up.

Galland-Girodet et al. compared photon-based and proton-based APBI in phase 1 study and 7 year ipsilateral breast recurrence rate 11 vs. 4%, respectively. The physician assessment of overall cosmesis was good or excellent for 62% of proton patients, compared with 94% for photon patients depending on more skin toxicities such as telangiectasia, pigmentation changes, fibrosis and patchy atrophy [55]. Loma Linda Medical center has the largest proton-based APBI experience including 100 patients treated with 40 Gy (RBE) in 10 daily fractions, with patient and physician reported cosmesis, tumor recurrence and dermatitis rates of 90, 3 and62% at 5 years, respectively [56]. Proton-based APBI, therefore, is accepted as a non-inferior treatment option for early-stage breast cancer patients.

There are few single-center case series that presented the use of proton for treating peripheral lymphatics, especially for locally advanced breast cancer with short follow-up periods. In a dosimetric comparison of proton in combination with 3DCRT to 3DCRT (photon + electron) and IMRT, proton have improved coverage and has decreased dose exposure to normal tissue adjacent to target [57]. First clinical report from Massachusetts General Hospital consists for 12 locally advanced breast cancer and they based their prospective trial on a dosimetric comparison of 11 patients plans with protons, partially wide tangent photon fields (PWTF) and photon/electron (P/E) fields. Proton therapy achieved superior coverage with a more homogeneous plan compared to PWTF and P/E fields, also considerable cardiac and pulmonary sparing was achieved with proton therapy as compared to PWTF and P/E [58]. They afterwards reported feasibility of proton delivery of post-mastectomy proton radiation to a dose of 50.4 Gy [relative biological effectiveness (RBE)] to the chest wall and 45–50.4 Gy (RBE) to the regional lymphatics with or without reconstruction. With maximum grade 2 skin toxicity (75%) and no radiation pneumonitis reported, proton RT for post-mastectomy RT was found to be feasible and well-tolerated. They noted that mean heart dose was as low as 0.44 Gy and this was the strongest argument for using protons for extensive chest-wall irradiation.

The second report by Memorial Sloan Kettering, including 30 patients, supported the positive results of early toxicity and normal tissue sparing shown by the previous literature [59]. They have used uniform scanning beams with anterior orientation for delivery. Supraclavicular field and chest-wall field were matched anteriorly, a set of beams with same orientation has been shifted 1-cm superior/inferiorly for feathering to minimize hot spots. Similar to previous report, mean heart dose was 1 Gy (RBE) and grade 2 skin toxicity rate was 71.4%, also 29% of the patient experienced moist desquamation [59]. Uniform scanning proton therapy provides100% dose at the skin without using a bolus for post-mastectomy patients. This effect depends on the technique, selective skin sparing can be obtained by pencil beam scanning with proximal range modulation advantage.

University of Florida recently published a prospective pilot study including 18 women (stage IIA-IIIB, 10 patients with proton therapy, 8 patients with proton-photon combination) requiring comprehensive breast radiation [60]. Proton therapy was shown to improve target coverage for the internal mammary nodes and level 2 axilla while median cardiac V5 was 0.6% with PT and 16.3% with conventional radiation ($p < 0.0001$). Within median 20-month follow-up, only grade 3 toxicity developed was dermatitis in four patients (22%) [60].

The most important advantage of proton treatment was almost none 'low dose bath' dose compared to IMRT techniques as high integral doses of heart, lung and coronary arteries could be associated with increased long-term complications and secondary cancers for especially young population. This philosophy behind using proton therapy in breast cancer treatment has been an attractive research area.

Another repeatedly cited concern concerning about the use of proton radiation is cost. Although the dosimetry serves for advantage dose distribution and superior normal organ sparing compared to standard RT, clearly more long-term and superior clinical results are also warranted to rationalize the higher cost of proton therapy. Lundkvist et al., accomplished a cost analysis demonstrating that proton therapy could be cost-effective if main aim is primarily heart sparing [61]. As a conclusion, proton radiotherapy dose distribution of radiation to chest wall/breast and regional lymphatics has been proven to provide excellent coverage with improved sparing of adjacent normal structures but until the cost of proton therapy decreases, we have to select eligible patients carefully.

3.5. Hypofractionation

Conventionally, radiation treatment after breast surgery has prescribed to the whole breast with total doses of 45–50 Gy delivered in 1.8- to 2-Gy daily fractions, and in many cases followed by an additional 10- to 15-Gy boost dose to the tumor bed, for a total of 5–6 weeks of daily treatment. The cost and travel distance to radiotherapy centers for multiple weeks are the most known barriers to the administration of radiotherapy. One of the solution was using increased daily fractions to lessen the total treatment time. Radiobiologic studies have proposed that breast cancer cells have a alpha-beta ratio which is similar to late reacting normal irradiated tissues [62] and the Royal Marsden Hospital/Gloucestershine Oncology Center trial based on the alpha-beta ratio of almost 4 Gy aiming equivalent tumor control with shorter hypofractionated schedules to a lower total dose randomized 1410 women with invasive breast cancer to receive 50 Gy radiotherapy given in 25 fractions, 39 Gy given in 13 fractions, or 42.9 Gy given in 13 fractions, all given over 5 weeks [63, 64]. After a median follow-up of 9.7 years, the risk of ipsilateral tumor relapse after 10 years was 12.1% in the 50 Gy group, 14.8% in the 39 Gy group, and 9.6% in the 42.9 Gy group [64]. Hypofractionation schemes were confirmed to be safe, effective and encouraged shorter course for early-stage breast cancer patients without compromising local recurrence or survival end points.

Hypofractionated regimens of irradiation to the whole breast have been studied by Canadian and English radiation oncology groups. Initially, Canadian trial enrolled 1234 women with invasive, lymph node-negative breast cancer treated by lumpectomy with negative pathologic margins and small to moderate breast size (breast separation ≤ 25 cm) to randomize to receive hypofractionated whole breast irradiation of 42.5 Gy in 16 fractions over 22 days versus standard whole breast irradiation of 50 Gy in 25 fractions over 35 days [65]. Acute toxicity was recorded similar between the arms, with only grade 2 or 3 radiation skin toxicity observed in 3% of patients in each arm. Additionally, long-term outcomes also were comparable between treatment schemas, the 10-year risk of local recurrence was 6.2% in the hypofractionated arm and 6.7% in the standard arm, as well as the rate of good or excellent cosmesis was 69.8% in the hypofractionated arm and 71.3% in the standard arm [65]. The following supporting hypofractionation randomized trial presented by START Trialists' Group-START-A enrolled 1410 patients to either standard fractionated whole breast irradiation or hypofractionated schedules of 42.9 or 39 Gy in 13 fractions over 5 weeks [66, 67]. Disease-free survival and overall survival were found to be similar in all arms except more moderate or marked skin toxicities were recorded at 39 Gy such as breast induration, telangiectasia and breast edema [66, 67]. The START B trial randomized 50 Gy in 25 fractions over 5 weeks versus 40 Gy in 15 fractions over 3 weeks in 2215 women (pT1-3a pN0-1 M0), and after a median follow-up of 6.0 years, reported lower local-regional tumor relapse (2.2 vs. 3.3%) and also lower rates of late adverse effects by photographic and patient assessments at 5 years in the accelerated hypofractionated arm [68]. Combining these START trials have suggested that use of 40 Gy in 15 fractions schema with fewer fractions of larger dose per fraction is at least as safe and effective as the historical standard regimen (50 Gy in 25 fractions) for women after primary surgery for early breast cancer [68].

An unplanned subgroup analysis of Ontario study proposed that the hypofractionated regimen was less effective in patients with high-grade tumors, having 10 years of cumulative recurrence incidence of 4.7% for standard RT and 15.6% for the hypofractionated RT with high-grade tumors [65]. In contrast, START A and B studies did not demonstrate a significant outcome measure respective to grade [67]. The proportion of patients with high grade tumors were 19, 28% and 23% in the Canadian, START A and START B trials implying insufficient numbers for appropriate conclusions as well as not calculated for a proper hypothesis. Therefore, the American Society for Radiation Oncology (ASTRO) task force could not reach a strict conclusion for comfortably advising use of HF-WBI for women with high-grade tumors until other studies clarified the outcome [69]. Bane et al. reexamined molecular and pathological features of 989 patients whose tumor blocks were present and checked thoroughly the association between tumor classifications and local recurrence rates [70]. The 10-year cumulative incidence was 4.5% for luminal A and basal-like, 7.9% for luminal B and 16.9% for HER-2 enriched tumors ($p < 0.01$); albeit tumor grade, molecular subtype or hypoxia did not predict any correlation between local recurrence and hypofractionation. Accordingly, hypofractionated radiotherapy is now considered appropriate regimens as a first treatment option for all grades and molecular subtypes of breast cancer; ASTRO published an evidence-based guideline for the use of hypofractionation and whom to prescribe in clinical practice [69]. Mainly, the routine suitable group for hypofractionation was defined as follows: age older than 50 years, stage T1–T2, no use of chemotherapy and central axis dose of 93–107%. The recommended schedules were 42.5 Gy in 16 fractions (Canadian trail), 41.6 Gy in 16 fractions over 5 weeks (START A), 40 Gy in 15 fractions over 3 weeks (START B). As the clinical approach spread all over the radiation oncology world, the suitable group criteria's expanded and nowadays this scheme is suitable for all ductal carcinoma in situ or T1–T2 invasive ductal carcinoma tumors with N0 status above 40-year old without any restriction. In case of regional lymph node irradiation, the literature has low toxicity rates in retrospective analysis regarding brachial plexopathy with the use of hypofractionation.

There is an increasing attention to more intensified hypofractionation in the treatment of breast cancer which has ground for randomized UK FAST Trial, published in 2001 with first results [71]. They have compared 50 Gy in 25 fractions, 30 Gy in 5 fractions or 28.5 Gy in 5 fractions, all over 5 weeks, and based on adverse effects in the breast with 3-year median follow-up, 28.5 Gy in 5 fractions was found to be comparable to 50 Gy in 25 fractions and was significantly better than ultra-short schema 30 Gy in 5 fractions [71]. Further studies are ongoing to build upon these findings including questions for assessing the values of concomitant boost with IMRT.

3.6. Accelerated partial breast radiotherapy

The role of partial breast irradiation (PBI) has been based on the knowledge that whole breast radiotherapy does not appear to prevent the development of new primary cancer in elsewhere localization in breast other than primary tumor quadrant being true recurrences. Pathological studies have examined specimens, and it revealed that residual tumor is detected in 15 mm or less in more than 90% of the cases [72]. PBI is the limited volume irradiation of breast tissue covering just around the tumor bed with a margin. PBI delivers a larger fraction dose in shorter total treatment time to reduce RT waiting period. Today, this technique can be applied by either intracavitary brachytherapy or MammoSite, interstitial brachytherapy, intra-operative techniques using electrons or X-rays at 50 kVp or external beam radiotherapy.

In order to select proper patients for these modalities, three different groups have been described where only minor differences were present between the set criteria's. American

Society of Therapeutic Radiation Oncology (ASTRO) recommendations are divided into three categories labeled as 'suitable' [≥60 years, tumor size ≤2 cm, pN0(i+/i−), no LVSI, invasive ductal carcinoma (IDC), margin (−), unifocal], 'cautionary' [50–59 years old, tumor size 2.1–3.0 cm, limited/focal LVSI, invasive lobular carcinoma (IlC), close margin (<2 mm), unifocal, DCIS ≤3 cm] 'unsuitable' [≤50 years, tumor size ≥3 cm, DCIS ≥3 cm, positive margin, multifocal, LVSI (+), ≥pN1] groups. American Society of Breast Surgeons (ASBS) has defined as age 45-year old or older for invasive cancer, age 50 years or older for DCIS, invasive carcinoma or ductal carcinoma in situ, Total tumor size less than or equal to 3 cm in size, negative microscopic surgical margins, pN0 [73]. American Brachytherapy Society (ABS) APBI criteria's based on a review of clinical and pathologic factors by the clinician [age (≥50 years old), tumor size (≤3 cm), all invasive subtypes and ductal carcinoma in situ, surgical margins (negative), LVSI (not present) and nodal status (negative)] [74]. To clarify the patient selecting for APBI depending on the clinicopathological features, a nomogram detecting the locoregional recurrence in patients treated with accelerated partial-breast irradiation has been developed. The nomogram was established on the results of a total of 2000 breasts (1990 women) treated with APBI at William Beaumont Hospital (n = 551) and in the American Society of Breast Surgeons MammoSite Registry Trial (n = 1449). Almost all APBI types were prescribed (multiplanar interstitial catheters, 98; balloon-based brachytherapy, 1689; and three-dimensional conformal radiation therapy, 213). Univariate analysis found that age <50 years, pre-/perimenopausal status, close/positive margins, estrogen receptor negativity and high grade were associated with a higher frequency of LRR [75].

Interstitial brachytherapy is the first technique used to treat only a partial amount of breast tissue. At that time, electron beam therapy was not available, so boosts were delivered to tumor bed using low dose rate (LDR) interstitial brachytherapy. With the advent of high-energy linear accelerators, electron beam boosts for the most part replaced interstitial brachytherapy with better dose homogeneity and improved overall cosmesis parallel to the experience [76]. To date, numerous single-arm and some randomized studies have been published examining multi-catheter interstitial brachytherapy [77–80]. Commonly, these studies registered patients with early-stage low-risk invasive and in situ carcinoma of, T1 or T2, with some allowing up to three positive axillary lymph nodes (N1) with negative surgical margins. Interstitial catheters were placed with a free-hand technique or a breast template with the placed surgical clips between 4 and 8 weeks after surgery. Earlier studies tend to use LDR or pulsed dose rate (PDR) sources, but the majority of the more recent series have been using 192Iridium (192Ir) high dose rate (HDR) brachytherapy. Generally, the target volume has been defined as the tumor bed plus 1–2 cm, 45–50 Gy with LDR and 30–36 Gy (using twice daily fractionation) with HDR. Local recurrence rates were ranged form0 to 8.9% [77, 79–81]. Usually, the rates of recurrence were low except the Guy's Hospital experience which stated an ipsilateral breast tumor recurrence rate of 18% [82]. GEC-ESTRO published 5-year follow-up results of randomized trial comparing interstisyel brachytherapy to whole breast radiotherapy for patients aged 40 years or more, small T1-2N0-miM0 (less than 3 cm) with negative margins and no lympho-vascular invasion (LVI) and excluded women with multifocal tumors. This trial has been conducted in 16 different centers in Europe. Planning and dose limits were as follows: The maximum skin dose less than 70% of the prescribed dose, the dose nonuniformity ratio

(V100/V150) below 0.35, 100% of the prescribed dose covered at least 90% of the target volume (coverage index ≥0.9). APBI was delivered a total dose of 32.0 Gy in eight fractions (8 × 4.0 Gy) or 30.3 Gy in seven fractions (7 × 4.3 Gy), with fractionation twice a day, was used for HDR brachytherapy. A total dose of 50 Gy with pulses of 0.60–60.80 Gy/h (one pulse per h, 24 h/day) was given by PDR brachytherapy. Analysis of 1184 patients with low-risk invasive and ductal carcinoma in situ treated with breast-conserving surgery has demonstrated that the cumulative incidence of local recurrence was 1.44% with APBI and 0.92% with whole-breast irradiation. The five-year risk of grade 2–3 late side-effects to the skin was 3.2% with APBI versus 5.7% with whole-breast irradiation, and grade 3 fibrosis at 5 years was noted as 0.2% with whole-breast irradiation and 0% with APBI. Polgar et al., randomized 258 pT1N0-1miM0, grade 1 or 2; T1N0-N1miM0, grade 1 or 2 patients with invasive breast cancer (unifocal tumors, tumor size less than 20 mm, clinically or pathologically N0, or single microscopic nodal metastasis) after wide local excision of tumor and negative pathological margins (greater than 2 mm and less than 2.0 mm) to receive either 50 Gy whole-breast irradiation (n = 130), APBI with multi-catheter HDR brachytherapy (n = 88), or APBI with electron beam irradiation (n = 40). The local recurrence at 10 years was 5.9% after APBI and 5.1% with whole-breast irradiation (p = 0.767) after median follow-up of 10.2 years. Excellent-to-good cosmetic results were 81% with APBI and 63% with whole-breast irradiation (p < 0.01) [77]. The literature has confirming results showing that the overall cosmesis scores were good to excellent for the majority of the patients with low rates of late complications [77, 80, 83]. Recently, phase 2 study of NRG Oncology/Radiation Therapy Oncology Group 9517 published 10-year rates of oncological outcome measures of accelerated partial breast irradiation using multi-catheter brachytherapy including 98 stage I/II unifocal breast cancer patients (tumor size <3 cm, negative surgical margins and 0–3 positive axillary nodes without extracapsular extension). High dose rate group received 34 Gy in 10 twice-daily fractions over 5 days and low dose rate (LDR) brachytherapy had 45 Gy in 3.5–5 days. Only five regional recurrences were defined. The 10-year disease-free survival, overall survival and contralateral breast event rates were 69.8, 78.0 and 4.2%, respectively [84]. Despite the encouraging results of the literature and long years' experience, interstitial brachytherapy stayed limited to selected institutes owing to the requirements of dedicated team, experience, skills and specific equipment.

External-beam XRT is the other option for APBI administration with an advantage of noninvasive nature, widespread availability of required resources, and knowledge of final pathology before the treatment planning. External APBI is most frequently administered in a 38.5-Gy regimen divided into 10 fractions given twice per day for 5 days. Rodríguez et al. reported on the 5-year outcomes of 102 patients with features of pT1-2pN0M0 invasive ductal carcinoma, tumor size 3 cm or less, negative margins and grade 1 or 2 histology randomized to receive whole breast irradiation (48 Gy/with or without boost) using three-dimensional conformal external beam radiation therapy (37.5 Gy in 3.75 Gy per fraction) or APBI [85]. Beam weights were manually optimized to cover the PTV by the 95% isodose line while maintaining a hot spot of <105%. For imaging, portal images of each beam and an orthogonal (anteroposterior) images were obtained for the first and second fractions. At a median 5 years of follow-up, aside from no local recurrences, APBI also reduced acute side effects and radiation doses to healthy tissues compared with WBI. Physician assessment showed that >75% of patients in the APBI arm had excellent or good cosmesis similar to whole breast group, and these outcomes has not changed at the follow-up [85].

An interim analysis of the RAPID (randomized trial of APBI) trial was important in terms of cosmetic results in which 1108 patients (invasive ductal carcinoma or ductal carcinoma in situ with tumors <3 cm, negative margins and no involved axillary nodes) were randomized to either 3D external beam APBI or WBRT. RAPID trial used 3DCRT in 38.5 Gy/10 fractions over 5–8 days (with a minimum 6 h gap between fractions given on the same day) and two fractionation schemas for WBRT: 50 Gy/25 fractions or 42.5 Gy/16 fractions. Baseline post-treatment nurse assessment for adverse cosmesis was 19% in the APBI arm and 17% in the WBRT arm and at the third year evaluation, these rates were increased in APBI arm to 29% and remains stable −17% for WBRT [86]. The worsening cosmetic results have been shown previously reported by single institute reports of Michigan University and Tufts University. Despite the good cosmetic outcome results in the non-randomized, multicenter studies, external beam-based APBI has been used with caution in practice [87–90]. The National Surgical Adjuvant Breast and Bowel Project (NSABP) B-39/Radiation Therapy Oncology Group (RTOG) 0413 trial that randomized 3000 patients to WBXRT or partial breast irradiation (PBI) finished patient recruiting but will be completed at April 2020. As most of the patients on the non-WBXRT arm have received 3D-CRT, the results will help to enlighten the cosmetic results and routine use of external beam as an option [91].

Catheter-based radiation therapy (brachytherapy) has been performed with MammoSite™ (Hologic, Marlborough, MA, USA) as the first balloon-based catheter and following with single and multi-lumen catheters Contura®, and SAVI™, in historical order. These catheters can be found in different sizes and shapes. All placement for insertion shared the same protocols where placement can be performed at either at the time of lumpectomy or as a postponed procedure up to 2–6 weeks after operation. Ultrasound guidance is the key device to detect the seroma and guide the catheter insertion along the longest axis diameter of the cavity. The device can be inserted through the surgical scar or a separate incision pathway could be chosen depending on Ultrasound guidance or the cavity evaluation CT of the patients that was obtained at radiation oncology clinic before placement. This cavity evaluation CT also serves for detecting proper size of the catheter. If the APBI decision was already given before surgery, a 'placer' can be put in the cavity and the balloon placer is then inflated with sterile saline to a diameter of 4.0–5.0 as it is described above and after evaluating the final pathology, it can be replaced by the selected size of the catheter. After insertion, a new CT scan is then obtained to assess the conformance of the balloon to the cavity and the presence of air or fluid gaps. A ratio of air or fluid in the cavity to balloon surface of less than 10% is usually acceptable, and also just for single lumen catheters a balloon-skin distance equal or greater than 5 mm is warranted. The lumpectomy cavity is then delineated and expanded by 1 cm to define the PTV. The most commonly prescribed dose is 3.4 Gy BID to a total of 34 Gy. Recommended dose constraints and contouring recommendations are given in **Table 1**. It is recommended that the placement and the position of the catheter has to be checked before each treatment.

MammoSite is the first developed balloon-based single-lumen device and major disadvantage is the minimum distance of skin required from skin to cavity which is about 7 mm. After

http://dx.doi.org/10.5772/66906

new developments, MammoSite also changed its single lumen form and a multi-lumen catheter released similar to Contura and SAVI.

Contura™ (SenoRx, Inc. Aliso Viejo, CA, USA) is a similar balloon catheter that has multiple catheters within the balloon and also comes in different sizes to fit the cavity. The multiple catheters offer optimization of the plan to that better normal tissue and skin sparing meaning that skin cavity distance has no more importance for patient selection, allow more precise

Contouring	
-Excision cavity	Outlined based on either *visualization* on CT, or if placed, contouring around the surgical clips
Clinical target volume CTV)	**CTV = Excision cavity + 15 mm** CTV limited to 5 mm *from the skin surface* and by the *posterior breast tissue* (chest wall and pectoralis muscles are not to be included)
PTV	**PTV = CTV + 10 mm** PTV is used to generate the beam aperture with an additional margin for penumbra
PTV_EVAL	PTV_EVAL = PTV—anything outside the ipsilateral breast, the first 5 mm of tissue under the skin (in order to remove most of the buildup region), and any PTV expansion beyond the posterior extent of breast tissue (chest wall, pectoralis muscle, and lung)
Normal tissue	Skin Thyroid Ipsilateral lung Contralateral lung Heart
Dose volume histogram Acceptable criteria's:	-Dose volume histogram analysis of target coverage will confirm ≥90% of the prescribed dose covering ≥90% of the PTV_EVAL -The actual volume of tissue receiving 150% (V150) and 200% (V200) of the prescribed dose will be limited to ≤70 cc and ≤20 cc, respectively. -Critical normal tissue DVHs within 5% specified value (uninvolved normal breast: ideally, <60% of the whole breast reference volume should receive ≥50% of the prescribed dose.) -Dose delivered twice a day for a total of 10 treatments over a period of 5–10 days

Unacceptable:	-Dose volume analysis of the target volume confirms <90% of the prescribed dose and/or <90% coverage of the PTV_EVAL -Critical normal structure DVH exceeds 5% of the specified value (uninvolved normal breast: ideally, <60% of the whole breast reference volume uninvolved normal breast: ideally, <60% of the whole breast reference volume should receive ≥50% of the prescribed dose and <35% of the whole breast reference volume should receive the prescribed dose)
Normal tissue	• **Contralateral breast**: The contralateral breast reference volume, contoured using the same methods described for the ipsilateral breast reference volume, should receive <3% of the prescribed dose to any point • **Ipsilateral lung**: <15% of the lung can receive 30% of the prescribed dose • **Contralateral lung**: <15% of the lung can receive 5% of the prescribed dose • **Heart (right-sided lesions)**: <5% of the heart should receive 5% of the prescribed dose • Heart (left-sided lesions): The volume of the heart receiving 5% of the prescribed dose (V5) should be less than the 40% • Thyroid: maximum point dose of 3% of the prescribed dose. Should receive ≥50% of the prescribed dose.) • The maximum skin dose at any point is ≤145% of prescription dose, assuring that the skin dose does not exceed acceptable limits the maximum allowable skin dose is kept below 100% of the prescription. If the balloon-skin distance is 5–7 mm, up to 145% of the prescribed dose is also acceptable

Table 1. Recommendations for APBI contouring and DVH evaluation based on RTOG NSABP PROTOCOL B-39 [91].

treatment planning. The other advantage of this catheter is the vacuum ports which helps to remove fluid and air if needed.

The **SAVI**™ (Cianna Medical, Inc., Aliso Viejo, CA, USA) device has also multi-catheter (6, 8 or 10) body in an elliptic shape. The catheter body of the device does not have a balloon around the catheters and can be opened and closed like an umbrella which helps fit easily the fat tissue of the cavity. As it locked in the lumpectomy cavity, the rotation and the problems with the delivery will be ruled out. ClearPath™ (Renata Medical, Irvine, CA, USA) is a single entry multi-catheter device which allows both HDR- and LDR-based APBI treatment. If the patient carries Ir125 seeds placed in ClearPath device, they have to wear a fully shielded bra during the low dose rate APBI treatment. Axxent® (Sunnyvale, CA, USA) is a novel electronic brachytherapy system that is developed to simplify the brachytherapy technique. In its form, there is an iridium seed-based single catheter balloon, also it does not require a high dose rate afterloader unit or a shielded vault and can be turned on and off such that it can be used in the office setting [92]. The balloon is radiolucent to improve visibility on breast radiographs and CT images. In a dosimetric evaluation, electronic brachytherapy plans were stated as providing comparable target coverage, increased high-dose regions, and a significantly reduced dose to the ipsilateral breast and lungs as well as the heart compared with the iridium-192 treatment plans [93]. Also, the intersocietal Electronic Xoft Intersocietal Brachytherapy Trial (EXIBT) registry recruited 400 patients and at 1-year follow-up demonstrated that breast infection occurred in two (2.9%) patients, and no tumor recurrences were reported. Cosmetic outcomes were excellent or good in 83.9–100% of evaluable patients at 1, 6 months and 1 year [94].

The MammoSite Registry of the American Society of Breast Surgeons has the biggest number of patients with this device with a median follow of 63.1 months. The registry data had 1449 patients with a five-year actuarial IBTR rate is 3.8% and axillary recurrence rate is 0.6%. Excellent/good cosmetic results at 60, 72 and 84 months were as follows: 91.3, 90.5 and 90.6%. The overall rates of fat necrosis, symptomatic seroma and infections remained low at 2.5, 13.4 and 9.6% with few late toxicity events beyond 2 years. These results have been found to be comparable to the rates for whole breast irradiation and other forms of APBI. Mann et al. retrospectively examined the long-term results of 111 patients treated with MammoSite APBI and revealed that the incidence of ipsilateral breast tumor recurrence was 2.7%. The incidence of ipsilateral axilla nodal recurrence was low as well (1.8%). Excellent to good cosmesis rate was 98.1% of the patients. The cosmetic results were found to be paralleled to the mean value of maximum skin dose: excellent, good and fair cosmesis were 88.9, 92.7 and 109.5% of the prescription dose, respectively [95]. These results also confirmed by Northwest University prospective MammoSite study (n:33), which noted that local recurrence is 100%, and cosmetic results were good to excellent in 94% of the patients [96]. Gitt et al. used MammoSite brachytherapy as a boost (15 Gy in 2.5-Gy fractions) after whole breast radiotherapy for carefully selected early-stage pT1-2, pN0-1, M0 disease 107 patients were treated with breast-conserving therapy and adjuvant radiotherapy with MammoSite followed by WBI (median = 50.4 Gy). In a short follow-up period of 21 months, no ipsilateral breast-tumor recurrences have been observed with an acceptable toxicity profile of 28% asymptomatic and 10% symptomatic seroma in 90 days after treatment [97]. Another retrospective long-term single institute (N:157) results confirmed that rate of ipsilateral breast recurrence was low as 2.5% at a median follow-up time of 5.5 years (range 0–10.0 years). Good to excellent cosmetic outcomes were achieved in 93.4% of patients and proved that skin dose >100% significantly projected the development of telangiectasia (50 vs. 14%, $p < 0.0001$) [98].

In Mayo clinic, a prospective protocol for completing all locoregional treatment (surgery and APBI) within 10 days with acceptable complication rates and cosmesis. Intraoperative multi-lumen strut-based device was placed for 123 women [age 50 years or older with clinical T1 estrogen receptor positive (ER+) sentinel lymph node (SLN)-negative invasive ductal cancer or pure ductal carcinoma in situ]. Analyzing the procedure, 110 (90%) of these patient underwent intraoperative catheter placement, whereas 13 did not due to intraoperative pathology findings. Prescribed radiotherapy was completed within 5 days at 109 APBI patients (99%), for all patients, this duration was 9 days with 6% 30-day complication rate. The local recurrence rate was 1.8% (two patients), and excellent or good cosmesis was achieved in 88% of patients [99]. Evaluating early toxicity in a prospective manner in 132 patients treated with strut-adjusted volume implant (SAVI) for early-stage breast cancer, SAVI has been observed as a safe treatment option with one acute and three late skin infections (two were grade 3), besides grade 1 or 2 late toxicities of hyperpigmentation (44%), telangiectasia (0.8%), seroma (9%), fat necrosis (5%), and fibrosis (12%). Crude local recurrence rate was 4% at a median follow-up time of 20 months [100]. It has to be noted that the literature studying new catheters except MammoSite are mostly presenting early results for feasibility and toxicity profile. Wobb et al. recently documented late side effects of 1034 patients treated with brachytherapy-based APBI (interstitial 40%, applicator-based 60%) and whole breast irradiation using intensity modulated radiotherapy [101], and stated that though brachytherapy-based APBI was associated with higher rates of ≥grade 2 seroma formation (14.4 vs. 2.9%, $p < 0.001$), telangiectasia (12.3 vs. 2.1%, $p = 0.002$) and symptomatic fat necrosis (10.2 vs. 3.6%, $p < 0.001$), there was no difference between rates of fair or poor cosmesis [101].

The use of partial irradiation in the treatment of ductal carcinoma in situ was tested in a prospective multicenter trial consisting 41 patients (42 breasts) with the eligibility criteria's of a diagnosis of DCIS confirmed by core needle biopsy, unicentric disease _<3 cm in size by mammogram, and an estimated life expectancy of >5 years [102], where the mean tumor size was 0.82 cm with comedo necrosis in 21.4%, and estrogen receptor positivity was 52.4%. Abbott et al. documented four patients (9.8%) developing an IBTR (all DCIS) outside the treatment field with a 3.2 years mean time of recurrence, and the actuarial recurrence rate at 5 years of 11.3%. It has to be noted that all patients with recurrence had at least one normal mammogram after treatment and before recurrence. Even all the recurrences were DCIS and occurred outside of the treatment field, prospective randomized trials have to waited before recommending routine use of APBI for DCIS [102].

In a meta-analysis of nine randomized trials comparing APBI vs. whole breast radiotherapy, the overall mortality was 4.9% and as no difference was observed in the proportion of breast cancer-related deaths, both non-breast cancer mortality with a difference of 1.1% ($p = 0.023$) and total mortality with a difference of 1.3% ($p = 0.05$) were found to be significantly lower in PBI than WBI cohorts which encourages PBI in selected patients with a 25% reduction in five-year non-breast cancer and overall mortality in comparison with WBI [103]. The most criticized study in APBI practice was the population-based retrospective analyses by Smith et al. based on Medicare billing codes rather than actual clinical outcomes defining the rate of mastectomy after APBI or whole breast radiotherapy [104], which analyzed 6952 breast cancer patients treated with brachytherapy and 85,783 with whole breast radiotherapy over 67-year old. Mastectomy was required in more women treated with brachytherapy (3.95%) than WBI (2.18%), and though five-year overall survival was similar on both group 87.66% with brachytherapy vs. 87.04% WBI, brachytherapy was shown to be linked with more frequent infectious (16.20 vs. 10.33%) and noninfectious (16.25 vs. 9.00%) postoperative complications such as breast pain (14.55 vs. 11.92%), fat necrosis (8.26 vs. 4.05%) and rib fracture (4.53 vs. 3.62%; p ≤

0.01 for all) [104]. These rates contradicted with the ones by Wobb et al. with mastectomy rates due to local recurrence (3.1% for WBI–IMRT and 1.2% for APBI, p = 0.06), or other reasons (0.8 and 0.6%, p = 0.60) [101]. In another series by Mann et al., the salvage mastectomy rate was 2.7% for patient treated with APBI which is not as high in Medicare data [95]. Although single institute results favored APBI, Medicare-based data slowed down the use of APBI which nowadays is recommended mainly in prospective protocols.

Intraoperative radiotherapy is the delivery of a single fraction of radiotherapy at the time of surgery directed to only tumor cavity. This can help to reduce long treatment duration for patient; but in today's practice, it is still expensive due to additional staffing, workload and specific equipment requirements. The available methods of delivering IORT are low-energy X-ray systems, electron beam radiation therapy and high dose rate afterloaders.

The Intrabeam® device (Carl Zeiss, Oberkochen, Germany) is a low-energy X-ray IORT device that has solid and rounded applicators in different sizes. After the lumpectomy is performed, Tungsten-impregnated sheets are used to shield the wound, and afterwards, applicator fixing in the tumor cavity is placed. A 20-Gy one-time dose is delivered at the surface of the applicator decreasing to a dose of 5 Gy at a depth of 1 cm from the cavity. Treatment time varies from 20 to 40 min. Shielding is essential to reduce radiation scatter, operation room walls will often provide sufficient shielding for the low-energy X-rays but measure environmental radiation dose rates around the theatre is essential.

There are three commercially available mobile linear accelerators, which can deliver electron beam radiation therapy the Novac7® (Hitesys S.p.A., Aprilia, Latina, Italy), the Liac® (Sordina, Padova, Italy) and the Mobetron® (IntraOP Medical Inc, Sunnyvale, CA USA). Both Novac7® and Liac® have been used in a phase-III trial, the ELIOT trial. The irradiation procedure is easily completed in 2 min, and the delivered dose is 21 Gy with the depth of 90% isodose ranging from 13 (3 MeV) to 24 mm (9 MeV). The breast tissue is mobilized over a lead/aluminum shield placed posteriorly to protect the chest wall and viscera. By means of these systems are delivering electrons, non-shielded operating rooms can be used but the team has to leave the operation room while the radiation is delivered.

High dose rate (HDR) afterloader (Mick Radio-Nuclear Instruments, Inc., Mount Vernon, NY, USA) within a dedicated shielded operating facility (Brachytherapy Unit) was assessed by Memorial Sloan—Kettering Cancer Centre. Treatment is delivered with HDR to the tumor bed using an iridium 192 (192Ir) source connected to a quadrangular silastic template applicator named Harrison-Anderson-Mick (H.A.M.®). A dose of 18 Gy was used as a standard approach. At 5 years (median follow-up 68 months), local recurrence of 7% reported by this techniques but has a limited use due to the high cost and the need of special shielded operating room.

Several single institution studies have been present in the literature on the feasibility and effectiveness of IORT, but only two phase-III trials have been published, the targeted intraoperative radiotherapy-alone (TARGIT-A) trial and the electron intraoperative treatment (ELIOT) trial with results at a medium follow-up of 2.4 and 5.8 years, respectively. TARGIT-A is an international cohort of 3451 patients who were randomized to either whole breast radiotherapy (40 to 56 Gy ± 10 to 16 Gy boost) or Intrabeam®, with a single 20 Gy fraction prescribed to the surface of the applicator. All clinical T1–T2 ≤3.5 cm, N0–1 invasive breast cancer patients were eligible if they were aged 45 years or older and suitable for wide local excision for invasive ductal carcinoma that was unifocal on conventional examination and imaging [105]. After the pathological evaluation, if the patients had adverse pathologic features including LCIS, lymphovascular space invasion, positive nodal status or other parameters defined at each center, postoperative WBI was added, and the APBI was counted as the boost. At a median follow-up of 2 years and 5 months, local recurrence rate was 3.3% in the APBI group and 1.3% in the WBI group (p = 0.04). Interestingly, even though cases were selected carefully, local recurrence in patients treated with TARGIT as a second invasive procedure by reopening the wound (n = 1143) was 5.4% and higher than with EBRT (1.7%). The difference was explained as a possibility of a delay in wound fluid suppression of tumor cells, a delay of radiation or a geometric miss when inserting the applicator postsurgery by authors [106], and "postpathology" TARGIT by reopening the wound was not recommended. Furthermore, OS or distant metastases, the rates were similar with low skin toxicity profile. There was no difference in hematomas needing surgical aspiration, seromas needing greater than three aspirations, infections requiring intravenous antibiotics or surgical intervention or skin breakdown or delayed healing rates between APBI and WBRT [105].

The ELIOT trial also uses intraoperative electrons as a single dose of 21 Gy prescribed to the 90% depth compared 50 Gy of external beam radiation therapy in which 1305 patients presented with tumors 2.5 cm or smaller and 48 years or older. After tumor excision, the breast tissue was mobilized and a lead/aluminum shield was placed to protect chest wall and underlying structures. The breast tissue as a target was rearranged over the shield. An appropriately sized collimator (4–8 cm) was inserted. At a median follow-up of 5.8 years, the 5-year recurrence rate was 4.4% for ELIOT versus 0.4% for the EBRT. For low risk women the 5-year IBTR was 1.7%. For patients with one or more high risk features (tumor size, receptor status, nodal positivity and grade), the 5-year IBTR was 11.8% for the 178 women (30.4%) with 1 or more risk factors versus 1.7% for the 407 ELIOT low risk women (69.6%) [107]. The rate of ELIOT patients who could be defined as ASTRO suitable subgroup was 23%, and ipsilateral breast recurrences ratio for them was 1.5% at 5 years and alike to whole breast group. ELIOT study results revealed low rates of skin and pulmonary damage [108]. There was no difference in terms of pain, retraction or fibrosis. Overall survival was the same between the two arms. The applicator sizes used in the ELIOT trial are not specified, but it has been advised that to guarantee uniform coverage of microscopic residual disease, the IOERT applicator dimension size has to be chosen at least 1.5 to 2 cm larger than the maximum tumor dimension [109]. Although the above IO-APBI trials show some promising early results, the follow-up for ELIOT is short especially given that breast cancer can recur many years later.

Cochrane meta-analysis including all types of APBI has been published in 2016 consisting seven randomized trials studying 7586 women of the 8955 enrolled [110]. Local recurrence-free survival decreased from HR-1.62 to HR-1.11 for women receiving PBI/APBI compared to WBRT, in addition to poorer physician-reported cosmesis with PBI/APBI. Oncological outcomes as cause-specific, distant metastasis-free, relapse-free survival or mastectomy rates were not affected by this small local recurrence difference, besides no difference in overall survival with PBI/APBI. As acute toxicities seem to be reduced by partial irradiation, this effect did not lead into an advantage for late term subcutaneous fibrosis. 'Elsewhere primaries' (new primaries in the ipsilateral breast) found to be more frequent with PBI/APBI. This meta-analysis cannot help to determine which technique increased the local recurrence or elsewhere primary detection. Ongoing trial will address the questions in future [110]. Despite small differences in local control, the advantages of the patients with APBI such as short treatment duration or easy application during surgery can increase patient treatment compliance. IO-APBI could be a reasonable option for highly selected subpopulation of early-stage breast cancer patients out of a clinical trial.

3.7. Breath hold-cardiac sparing methods

Breast cancer radiotherapy reduces the risk of cancer recurrence and death demonstrated by randomized trials, but as radiation delivery requires tangential and selectively mammaria interna fields, meta-analyses also have found an increase in cardiac deaths following breast cancer radiotherapy associated with the volume of the heart receiving 5 Gy or more [111]. Decreased myocardial function or coronary artery diseases are the most common cardiotoxicity besides less common toxicities of myocardial infarction, congestive heart failure, pericarditis, arrhythmias, angina or valve dysfunction [112]. Darby et al. steered a population-based case-control study of major coronary events in 2168 women who underwent radiotherapy for breast cancer between 1958 and 2001 in Sweden and Denmark. The overall average of the mean doses to the whole heart was 4.9 Gy (range 0.03–27.72), and the rates of major coronary events were associated with a 7% increase in risk of ischemic events per gray increase in mean heart dose with no apparent threshold. This effect of radiation on heart was increasing within the first 5 years after radiotherapy and found to be unrelated to the presence of cardiac risk factors at the time of radiotherapy.

Due to the interplay between respiratory motion and MLC motion during IMRT delivery, the planned and expected doses could be different. Respiratory motion is a well-known factor during treatment planning for breast IMRT, dosimetric studies presented that PTV dose heterogeneity increases as respiratory motion grows. The lung and heart doses also change with respiratory motion. As a result, a larger margin is proposed from CTV to PTV margin [113]. The breath-hold technique could help to minimize the effect of potential negative dosimetric impact arising from interplay effect of multileaf collimator and breathing motion during delivery of IMRT [114, 115].

In clinical practice, there are two commercially available devices: active breathing coordinator™ (ABC_DIBH) (Elekta, Crawley, UK) and Varian RPM system guiding patients to hold their breath while radiotherapy is delivered, which pushes the heart down and away from the radiotherapy field. Even the benefits of these systems were proved by dosimetric studies, they are not used more widespread as it was used in only 19% of EORTC centers in 2010 and just 4% of UK centers [116, 117]. This could be due to additional cost, education of staff and time-consuming procedure depending on patient's capacity and therapist's experience.

In the early 2000s, the Real-time Position Management (RPM) system from Varian Medical System (Palo Alto, USA) consisting of two reflectors attached to an external marker-cube placed on the patient's abdomen was released. The motion of the cube marker, reflecting the breathing pattern of the patient, is evaluated by software that controls the scanner, based on predefined criteria [118]. The advantage of this RPM system is the constant monitorization of patient respiration, and a beam-hold condition automatically occurs if the breath-hold level departs from the planned one [119]. The patient can easily track their performance on screen, also reproducibility is the other important advantage of this system.

The ABC method was established at William Beaumont Hospital and is currently commercialized by Elekta, Inc. as the active breathing coordinator. Also the VMAX Spectra 20C (VIASYS Healthcare Inc, Yorba Linda, CA, USA) and the SpiroDyn'RX (Dyn'R, Muret, France) which are working in the similar principles [120]. The ABC apparatus can be used to suspend breathing at any predetermined position along the normal breathing cycle, or at active inspiration. A digital spirometer is used measure the respiratory cycle, which is connected to a balloon valve. In an ABC procedure, the patient breathes normally through the apparatus. When an operator "activates" the system, the lung volume and the phase (i.e., inhalation or exhalation) at which the balloon value will be closed are specified. The patient is then instructed to proceed to reach the specified lung volume, typically after taking two preparatory breaths. At this point, the valve is inflated with an air compressor for a predefine duration of time, thereby "holding" the patient's breath [120].

There is solid evidence from retrospective and dosimetric planning studies, demonstrating reduction in dose to the heart and coronary arteries with deep inspiration breath-hold treatment of left-sided breast cancers for both early and locally advanced breast cancer therapy with regional irradiation. In a dosimetric analysis, free and breath-hold technique were planned with both forward and inverse IMRT showing a significant reduction in radiation exposure to the contralateral breast, left and right ventricles, as well as proximal and especially distal LAD by breath hold with forward IMRT, as inverse IMRT provided no additional advantage [121]. For whole breast radiotherapy, Wang et al. reported a reduction in mean heart dose from 3.2 Gy forward-planned IMRT in free-breathing to 1.3 Gy for forward-planned IMRT in breath hold. Another confirming study, recruiting 319 breast cancer patients revealed that deep inspiration breath-hold plans expressed large reductions in dose to the heart compared with left-sided FB plans; V20Gy of the heart is reduced from 7.8 to 2.3%, V40Gy from 3.4 to 0.3% and mean dose from 5.2 to 2.7 Gy (−48%, $p < 0.0001$) while median target coverage is slightly improved [122].

In William Beaumont Hospital experience revealed that moderate deep inspiration breath hold achieved using an active breathing control (ABC) device, compared with free breathing (FB) during treatment with deep tangents fields (DT) for locoregional (LR) irradiation of 15 breast cancer patients, reduced the heart V30 for 6 of the 9 left breasted patients, entirely avoiding heart irradiation in 2 of these 6 patients and the mean percentage of both lungs receiving more than 20 Gy from 20.4 to 15.2% [123]. Twenty centers in order to compare clinical aspects of respiratory-gated conformal radiotherapy during breast cancer irradiation versus conventional conformal radiotherapy and reassured the feasibility and good reproducibility of the respiratory gating systems with the reduction in the dose delivered to the

http://dx.doi.org/10.5772/66906

heart during irradiation of the left breast [119]. Even locoregional irradiation is considered, breath-hold technique still added benefit with breath-hold technique significantly by reducing Dmean Heart and Dmean LAD compared to free breathing for both the whole breast and chest wall and regional irradiation groups. When Dmean Heart of <4 Gy had been set as a criteria for planning, all the plans in whole breast radiotherapy has been met this apart from breathing pattern, but only five of nine patients (56%) in the comprehensive breast irradiation group were able to meet this constraint with free breathing, compared to all patients with deep breath hold was in compliance with the criteria of Dmean Heart <4 Gy [124]. Addition to the routine use of deep breath old techniques for left breast cancer patients, Essen et al. recommend it to use for right breast also. The gain for locoregional breast treatment without IMN, the average mean lung dose reduced from 6.5 to 5.4 Gy for the total lung and from 11.2 to 9.7 Gy for the ipsilateral lung while if internal mammaria lymph node irradiation is added significant gain will continue for lung doses, which can translate into a lower risk of pneumonitis and secondary lung cancer rates in future [125]. As a summary of the published literature, deep breath hold reduced the mean heart dose by up to 3.4 Gy when compared to a free breathing approach. Also deep breath-hold technique was announced as stable and reproducible on a daily basis [126].

Breath-hold technique's dosimetric benefits have been clearly in the literature, but these techniques are not yet in widespread use. The reasons for this could be explained by this technique needs commercially available solutions necessitate specialist equipment. Another breath-hold technique described as 'voluntary breath-hold technique' described. This breath-holding technique monitories breath-hold consistency using the distance moved by the anterior and lateral reference marks away from the treatment room lasers in breath hold to monitor constancy at CT-planning and treatment setup. Light fields are then visually checked breath-hold consistency before and during treatment. This technique is announced as simple and inexpensive, but still there is concerns about the reproducibility and consistency [127]. A randomized study conducted at the Royal Marsden Hospital (Sutton, UK), The UK HeartSpare Study, has confirmed that interfraction reproducibility with the voluntary breath-hold technique is analogous to the performed with the spirometry-based device. Addition to this, voluntary technique offers a time advantage at planning-CT and treatment setup and is preferred by patients and radiographers alike compared to using the spirometry-based device [128]. In HeartSpare II study, the VBH technique is currently being ongoing at 10 UK radiotherapy centers to confirm that the technique is applicable in a multicenter setting where presented preliminary data suggest multicenter application of VBH is found to be both actual and practicable at heart-sparing [129].

According to Royal Marsden Hospital protocol firstly patient's asked to practice at home holding their breath, while lying down, initially for 5 s, and building up in 5 s intervals to 20 s. During the standard CT simulation procedure, position of crosses in free breathing and while taking a deep breath in marked on the patient. The duration of the breath hold has to be noted. All the details and a video related to this technique has been published by Barnett et al. [127]. Systematic and random error range for each beam and in each plane reported as 1.5–1.8 mm and 1.7–2.5 mm, respectively [127].

As a conclusion, to date, there is only retrospective or dosimetric studies were presented and no data studying the clinical benefits and oncological outcomes for patients treated with this technique. Especially, the cardiac data will be presented in 15–20 years. Under these circumstances, the clinical application of deep breath-hold technique is important and advisable. In our clinic, we routinely train all our left breast cancer patients and use RPM system during the simulation and treatment to provide the consistency and reproducibility of breath-holding period. After forward IMRT planning, DVH are evaluated according to criteria's as follows: Spinal cord Max <45 Gy or Max <36 Gy (if >2.5 Gy/Fx), heart V20 <4%, V10 <15%, total lung V20 <35%. Our aim is to reduce mean heart dose as low as possible. Average mean heart doses were usually under 4–5 Gy and 2.5 Gy for left-sided RT and right-sided RT including IM nodes. After adding segments, the 105% isodose line cloud should not been seen except in the corners due to lung transmission.

4. Conclusion

Modern radiotherapy techniques have been evolving in the last two decades. Supine positioning will be continued to be used for breast cancer simulation for several decades over the world as it provides patient comfort and position reproducibility for the whole treatment period, while in rare indications such as a very large pendulous breast or depending on institution choice lateral decubitus or prone position can help. The reflection of modern techniques such as three-dimensional (3D), intensity-modulated radiotherapy (IMRT), volumetric modulated arc therapy (VMAT) has been evolving in breast therapy. Even dosimetric studies has demonstrated more homogenous dose distribution and normal organ sparing, still survival data, and the long-term effects of normal tissue sparing on survival will be answered in future. Especially, forward IMRT, using tangential bream angels and creating multiple segment, can be used in clinical practice taking into the considerations of acute toxicity but using tangential radiotherapy field design is still acceptable. There is an increasing attention to hypofractionation in the treatment of breast cancer, while there are still unanswered questions in regional lymph node and expander irradiation. Another attractive approach—APBI could be a reasonable option for highly selected subpopulation of early-stage breast cancer patients out of a clinical trial. Results of ongoing trial comparing APBI techniques to external radiotherapy will address the future of APBI techniques as a routine clinical approach. The most important advance could be named as cardiac sparing-deep breath-hold approach in all the modern technique improvement. Retrospective or dosimetric studies were presented the benefit of using commercially available techniques or voluntary performance, while clinical outcomes could be presented in 15–20 years. Under these circumstances, the clinical application of deep breath-hold technique is important and advisable.

Although most advanced techniques in management of breast cancer have not been proved to increase survival, we suggest recommending resource stratified advanced techniques to be decided institutionally in order to provide best technical and clinical care in this long-term survivor candidates.

http://dx.doi.org/10.5772/66906

Abbreviations

RT	Radiation therapy
2D	Two-dimensional
3D	Three-dimensional
IMRT	Intensity-modulated radiotherapy
VMAT	Volumetric modulated arc therapy
4D	Four-dimensional
CT	Computed tomography
CBCT	Cone-beam computed tomography
3DCRT	Three-dimensional conformal radiotherapy
ICRU	International Commission on Radiation Units and Measurements
IGRT	Image-guided RT
RTOG	Radiation Therapy Oncology Group
EORTC	European Organisation for Research and Treatment of Cancer
OAR	Organ-at-risk
DVH	Dose volume histograms
IMLNs	Internal mammary lymph nodes
ASTRO	American Society for Radiation Oncology
LDR	Low dose rate
PDR	Pulsed dose rate
HDR	High dose rate
APBI	Accelerated partial breast irradiation
DCIS	Ductal carcinoma in situ
PBI	Partial breast irradiation
Dmean	Mean dose

Author details

Yasemin Bolukbasi[1,2] and Ugur Selek[1,2]*

*Address all correspondence to: uselek@mdanderson.org

1 Department of Radiation Oncology, School of Medicine, Koc University, Istanbul, Turkey

2 Department of Radiation Oncology, MD Anderson Cancer Center, The University of Texas, Houston, TX, USA

References

[1] Buchholz TA, Haffty BG, Breast cancer: locally advanced and recurrent disease, post-mastectomy radiation, systemic therapies. In: Halperin CE, Perez CA, Brady LW (eds) Principles and practice of radiation oncology. Philadelphia: Lippincott Willians & Wilkins. 2013. pp. 1140–1163.

[2] Batumalai V, Holloway L, Delaney GP, A review of setup error in supine breast radio-therapy using cone-beam computed tomography. Med Dosim 2016 ;41(3):225-9.

[3] Sethi RA et al., Comparison of three-dimensional versus intensity-modulated radiother-apy techniques to treat breast and axillary level III and supraclavicular nodes in a prone versus supine position. Radiother Oncol 2012;**102**(1):74–81.

[4] Griem KL et al., Three-dimensional photon dosimetry: a comparison of treatment of the intact breast in the supine and prone position. Int J Radiat Oncol Biol Phys 2003;**57**(3):891–899.

[5] Cross MA, Elson HR, Aron BS, Breast conservation radiation therapy technique for women with large breasts. Int J Radiat Oncol Biol Phys 1989;**17**(1):199–203.

[6] Wurschmidt F et al., Incidental dose to coronary arteries is higher in prone than in supine whole breast irradiation. A dosimetric comparison in adjuvant radiotherapy of early stage breast cancer. Strahlenther Onkol 2014;**190**(6):563–568.

[7] Kirby AM et al., Prone versus supine positioning for whole and partial-breast radiotherapy: a comparison of non-target tissue dosimetry. Radiother Oncol 2010;**96**(2):178–184.

[8] Varga Z et al., Individual positioning: a comparative study of adjuvant breast radiother-apy in the prone versus supine position. Int J Radiat Oncol Biol Phys 2009;**75**(1):94–100.

[9] Mahe MA et al., Preliminary results for prone-position breast irradiation. Int J Radiat Oncol Biol Phys 2002;**52**(1):156–160.

[10] Algan O et al., Use of the prone position in radiation treatment for women with early stage breast cancer. Int J Radiat Oncol Biol Phys 1998;**40**(5):1137–1140.

[11] Kirby AM et al., A randomised trial of supine versus prone breast radiotherapy (SuPr study): comparing set-up errors and respiratory motion. Radiother Oncol 2011;**100**(2):221–226.

[12] Campana F et al., Breast radiotherapy in the lateral decubitus position: a technique to prevent lung and heart irradiation. Int J Radiat Oncol Biol Phys 2005;**61**(5):1348–1354.

[13] Piroth MD et al., Usefulness of a thermoplastic breast bra for breast cancer radiotherapy:a prospective analysis. Strahlenther Onkol 2016; 192(9):609-16

[14] Purdy JA, Current ICRU definitions of volumes: limitations and future directions. Semin Radiat Oncol 2004;**14**(1):27–40.

http://dx.doi.org/10.5772/66906

[15] Cheung KY, Intensity modulated radiotherapy: advantages, limitations and future developments. Biomed Imaging Interv J 2006;**2**(1):e19.

[16] Offersen BV et al., ESTRO consensus guideline on target volume delineation for elective radiation therapy of early stage breast cancer. Radiother Oncol 2015;**114**(1):3–10.

[17] Gentile MS et al., Contouring guidelines for the axillary lymph nodes for the delivery of radiation therapy in breast cancer: evaluation of the RTOG breast cancer atlas. Int J Radiat Oncol Biol Phys 2015;**93**(2):257–265.

[18] Li XA et al., Variability of target and normal structure delineation for breast cancer radiotherapy: an RTOG Multi-Institutional and Multiobserver Study. Int J Radiat Oncol Biol Phys 2009;**73**(3):944–951.

[19] Feng M et al., Development and validation of a heart atlas to study cardiac exposure to radiation following treatment for breast cancer. Int J Radiat Oncol Biol Phys 2011;**79**(1):10–18.

[20] Van de Velde J et al., An anatomically validated brachial plexus contouring method for intensity modulated radiation therapy planning. Int J Radiat Oncol Biol Phys 2013;**87**(4):802–808.

[21] Min M et al., External evaluation of the Radiation Therapy Oncology Group brachial plexus contouring protocol: several issues identified. J Med Imaging Radiat Oncol 2014;**58**(3):360–368.

[22] Chen GP et al., A planning comparison of 7 irradiation options allowed in RTOG 1005 for early-stage breast cancer. Med Dosim 2015;**40**(1):21–25.

[23] Guilbert P et al., Conventional 2D and monoisocentric 3D techniques in breast and lymphatic irradiation: a dosimetric comparison. Cancer Radiother 2012;**16**(5–6):473–478.

[24] Leite ET et al., Incidental irradiation of internal mammary lymph nodes in breast cancer: conventional two-dimensional radiotherapy versus conformal three-dimensional radiotherapy. Radiol Bras 2016;**49**(3):170–175.

[25] Nakamura K et al., Recent advances in radiation oncology: intensity-modulated radiotherapy, a clinical perspective. Int J Clin Oncol 2014;**19**(4):564–569

[26] McDonald MW et al., Long-term outcomes of IMRT for breast cancer: a single-institution cohort analysis. Int J Radiat Oncol Biol Phys 2008;**72**(4):1031–1040.

[27] McCormick B, Hunt M, Intensity-modulated radiation therapy for breast: is it for everyone? Semin Radiat Oncol 2011;**21**(1):51–54.

[28] Donovan E et al., Randomised trial of standard 2D radiotherapy (RT) versus intensity modulated radiotherapy (IMRT) in patients prescribed breast radiotherapy. Radiother Oncol 2007;**82**(3):254–264.

[29] Barnett GC et al., A randomised controlled trial of forward-planned radiotherapy (IMRT) for early breast cancer: baseline characteristics and dosimetry results. Radiother Oncol 2009;**92**(1):34–41.

[30] Pignol JP et al., A multicenter randomized trial of breast intensity-modulated radiation therapy to reduce acute radiation dermatitis. J Clin Oncol 2008;**26**(13):2085–2092.

[31] Harsolia A et al., Intensity-modulated radiotherapy results in significant decrease in clinical toxicities compared with conventional wedge-based breast radiotherapy. Int J Radiat Oncol Biol Phys 2007;**68**(5):1375–1380.

[32] Keller LM et al., Five-year results of whole breast intensity modulated radiation therapy for the treatment of early stage breast cancer: the Fox Chase Cancer Center experience. Int J Radiat Oncol Biol Phys 2012;**84**(4):881–887.

[33] Yang JF et al., Long-term breast cancer patient outcomes after adjuvant radiotherapy using intensity-modulated radiotherapy or conventional tangential radiotherapy. Medicine (Baltimore) 2016;**95**(11):e3113.

[34] Hardee ME et al., Prone hypofractionated whole-breast radiotherapy without a boost to the tumor bed: comparable toxicity of IMRT versus a 3D conformal technique. Int J Radiat Oncol Biol Phys 2012;**82**(3):e415–e423.

[35] Lohr F et al., Potential effect of robust and simple IMRT approach for left-sided breast cancer on cardiac mortality. Int J Radiation Oncol Biol Phys 2009;**74**(1):73–80.

[36] Rabinovitch R et al., Evaluation of breast sentinel lymph node coverage by standard radiation therapy fields. Int J Radiation Oncol Biol Phys 2008;**70**(5):1468–1471.

[37] Ma C, Zhang W, Lu J, Wu L, Wu F, Huang B, Dosimetric comparison and evaluation of three radiotherapy techniques for use after modified radical mastectomy for locally advanced left-sided breast cancer. Sci Rep 2015:**21**(5):12274.

[38] Tyran M et al., Volumetric-modulated arc therapy for left-sided breast cancer and all regional nodes improves target volumes coverage and reduces treatment time and doses to the heart and left coronary artery, compared with a field-in-field technique. J Radiation Res 2015: **56**(6):927-37.

[39] Popescu CC et al., Volumetric modulated arc therapy improves dosimetry and reduces treatment time compared to conventional intensity-modulated radiotherapy for locoregional radiotherapy of left-sided breast cancer and internal mammary nodes. Int J Radiat Oncol Biol Phys 2010;**76**(1):287–295.

[40] Marta G, Hanna S, Gadia R, Treatment with intensity-modulated radiation therapy (IMRT) for breast cancer. Rev Assoc Méd Brasil 2014;**60**:508–511.

[41] Rudat V et al., Tangential beam IMRT versus tangential beam 3D-CRT of the chest wall in postmastectomy breast cancer patients: a dosimetric comparison. Radiat Oncol 2011;**6**:26.

[42] Dayes I et al., Intensity-modulated radiotherapy in the treatment of breast cancer. Clin Oncol 2012;**24**(7):488–498.

[43] Yong JH et al., Estimating the costs of intensity-modulated and 3-dimensional conformal radiotherapy in Ontario. Curr Oncol 2016;**23**(3):e228–e238.

[44] Mackie TR, History of tomotherapy. Phys Med Biol 2006;**51**(13):R427–R453.

[45] Mackie TR et al., Tomotherapy: a new concept for the delivery of dynamic conformal radiotherapy. Med Phys 1993;**20**(6):1709–1719.

[46] Kaidar-Person O, Kostich M, Zagar TM, Jones E, Gupta G, Mavroidis P, Das SK, Marks LB, Helical tomotherapy for bilateral breast cancer: clinical experience. Breast 2016;**28**:4.

[47] Goddu SM et al., Helical tomotherapy planning for left-sided breast cancer patients with positive lymph nodes: comparison to conventional multiport breast technique. Int J Radiat Oncol Biol Phys 2009;**73**(4):1243–1251.

[48] Jacob J, Campana F, Chira C, Peurien D, Daveau C, Can helical tomotherapy be used as a safe treatment alternative for breast cancer patients? J Nucl Med Radiat Ther 2012; S6:002.

[49] O'Donnell H et al., Early experience of tomotherapy-based intensity-modulated radiotherapy for breast cancer treatment. Clin Oncol 2009;**21**(4):294–301.

[50] Boram L et al., Radiotherapy-induced secondary cancer risk for breast cancer: 3D conformal therapy versus IMRT versus VMAT. J Radiol Prot 2014;**34**(2):325.

[51] Abo-Madyan Y et al., Second cancer risk after 3D-CRT, IMRT and VMAT for breast cancer. Radiother Oncol 2014;**110**(3):471–476.

[52] Han EY et al., Estimation of the risk of secondary malignancy arising from whole-breast irradiation: comparison of five radiotherapy modalities, including TomoHDA. Oncotarget 2016;**7**(16):22960–22969.

[53] Verma V, Shah C, Mehta MP, Clinical outcomes and toxicity of proton radiotherapy for breast cancer. Clin Breast Cancer 2016;**16**(3):145–154.

[54] Group, P.T.C.-O. http://www.ptcog.ch/index.php/facilities-in-planning-stage. Accessed 7/27/2016.

[55] Galland-Girodet S et al., Long-term cosmetic outcomes and toxicities of proton beam therapy compared with photon-based 3-dimensional conformal accelerated partial-breast irradiation: a phase 1 trial. Int J Radiat Oncol Biol Phys 2014;**90**(3):493–500.

[56] Bush DA et al., Partial breast radiation therapy with proton beam: 5-year results with cosmetic outcomes. Int J Radiat Oncol Biol Phys 2014;**90**(3):501–505.

[57] Xu N et al., Can proton therapy improve the therapeutic ratio in breast cancer patients at risk for nodal disease? Am J Clin Oncol 2014;**37**(6):568–574.

[58] MacDonald SM et al., Proton radiotherapy for chest wall and regional lymphatic radiation; dose comparisons and treatment delivery. Radiat Oncol 2013;**8**:71.

[59] Cuaron JJ et al., Early toxicity in patients treated with postoperative proton therapy for locally advanced breast cancer. Int J Radiat Oncol Biol Phys 2015;**92**(2):284–291.

[60] Bradley JA et al., Initial report of a prospective dosimetric and clinical feasibility trial demonstrates the potential of protons to increase the therapeutic ratio in breast cancer compared with photons. Int J Radiat Oncol Biol Phys 2016;**95**(1):411–421.

[61] Lundkvist J et al., Economic evaluation of proton radiation therapy in the treatment of breast cancer. Radiother Oncol 2005;**75**(2):179–185.

[62] Bhattacharyya T et al., Hypofractionated radiotherapy in carcinoma breast: what we have achieved? J Cancer Res Ther 2015;**11**(2):259–263.

[63] Overgaard M et al., The value of the NSD formula in equation of acute and late radiation complications in normal tissue following 2 and 5 fractions per week in breast cancer patients treated with postmastectomy irradiation. Radiother Oncol 1987;**9**(1):1–11.

[64] Owen JR et al., Effect of radiotherapy fraction size on tumour control in patients with early-stage breast cancer after local tumour excision: long-term results of a randomised trial. Lancet Oncol 2006;**7**(6):467–471.

[65] Whelan TJ et al., Long-term results of hypofractionated radiation therapy for breast cancer. N Engl J Med 2010;**362**(6):513–520.

[66] Bentzen SM et al., The UK Standardisation of Breast Radiotherapy (START) Trial A of radiotherapy hypofractionation for treatment of early breast cancer: a randomised trial. Lancet Oncol 2008;**9**(4):331–341.

[67] Haviland JS et al., The UK Standardisation of Breast Radiotherapy (START) trials of radiotherapy hypofractionation for treatment of early breast cancer: 10-year follow-up results of two randomised controlled trials. Lancet Oncol 2013;**14**(11):1086–1094.

[68] Bentzen SM et al., The UK Standardisation of Breast Radiotherapy (START) Trial B of radiotherapy hypofractionation for treatment of early breast cancer: a randomised trial. Lancet 2008;**371**(9618):1098–1107.

[69] Smith BD et al., Fractionation for whole breast irradiation: an American Society for Radiation Oncology (ASTRO) evidence-based guideline. Int J Radiat Oncol Biol Phys 2011;**81**(1):59–68.

[70] Bane AL et al., Tumor factors predictive of response to hypofractionated radiotherapy in a randomized trial following breast conserving therapy. Ann Oncol 2014;**25**(5):992–998.

[71] Agrawal RK et al., First results of the randomised UK FAST Trial of radiotherapy hypofractionation for treatment of early breast cancer (CRUKE/04/015). Radiother Oncol 2011;**100**(1):93–100.

[72] Wallner P et al., Workshop on Partial Breast Irradiation: State of the Art and the Science, Bethesda, MD, December 8–10, 2002. J Natl Cancer Inst 2004;**96**(3):175–184.

[73] The American Society of Breast Surgeons. Consensus statement for accelerated partial breast irradiation, statements/PDF_Statements/APBI.pdf: https://www.breastsurgeons.org/.

[74] Shah C et al., The American Brachytherapy Society consensus statement for accelerated partial breast irradiation. Brachytherapy 2013;**12**(4):267–277.

[75] Wobb JL et al., Nomogram for predicting the risk of locoregional recurrence in patients treated with accelerated partial-breast irradiation. Int J Radiat Oncol Biol Phys 2015;**91**(2):312–318.

[76] Wazer DE, Kramer B, Schmid C, Ruthazer R, Ulin K, Schmidt-Ulrich R, Factors determining outcome in patients treated with interstitial implantation as a radiation boost for breast conservation therapy. Int J Radiat Oncol Biol Phys. 1997;**39**(2):12.

[77] Polgar C et al., Accelerated partial-breast irradiation using high-dose-rate interstitial brachytherapy: 12-year update of a prospective clinical study. Radiother Oncol 2010;**94**(3):274–279.

[78] Ott OJ et al., Accelerated partial breast irradiation with interstitial implants: risk factors associated with increased local recurrence. Int J Radiat Oncol Biol Phys 2011;**80**(5):1458–1463.

[79] Strnad V et al., Accelerated partial breast irradiation: 5-year results of the German-Austrian multicenter phase II trial using interstitial multicatheter brachytherapy alone after breast-conserving surgery. Int J Radiat Oncol Biol Phys 2011;**80**(1):17–24.

[80] Arthur DW et al., Partial breast brachytherapy after lumpectomy: low-dose-rate and high-dose-rate experience. Int J Radiat Oncol Biol Phys 2003;**56**(3):681–689.

[81] Wazer DE et al., Preliminary results of a phase I/II study of HDR brachytherapy alone for T1/T2 breast cancer. Int J Radiat Oncol Biol Phys 2002;**53**(4):889–897.

[82] Fentiman IS et al., Caesium(137) implant as sole radiation therapy for operable breast cancer: a phase II trial. Radiother Oncol 2004;**71**(3):281–285.

[83] Ott OJ et al., GEC-ESTRO multicenter phase 3-trial: accelerated partial breast irradiation with interstitial multicatheter brachytherapy versus external beam whole breast irradiation: early toxicity and patient compliance. Radiother Oncol 2016: 120(1):119-23.

[84] White J et al., Long-Term Cancer Outcomes From Study NRG Oncology/RTOG 9517: a Phase 2 study of accelerated partial breast irradiation with multicatheter brachytherapy after lumpectomy for early-stage breast cancer. Int J Radiat Oncol Biol Phys 2016;**95**(5):1460–1465.

[85] Rodríguez N et al., Five-year outcomes, cosmesis, and toxicity with 3-dimensional conformal external beam radiation therapy to deliver accelerated partial breast irradiation. Int J Radiat Oncol Biol Phys 2013;**87**(5):1051–1057.

[86] Olivotto IA et al., Interim cosmetic and toxicity results from RAPID: a randomized trial of accelerated partial breast irradiation using three-dimensional conformal external beam radiation therapy. J Clin Oncol 2013;**31**(32):4038–4045.

[87] Hepel JT, Tokita M, MacAusland SG, Evans SB, Hiatt JR, Price LL, Toxicity of three-dimensional conformal radiotherapy for accelerated partial breast irradiation. Int J Radiat Oncol Biol Phys 2009;**75**(5):6.

[88] Jagsi R, Ben David M, Moran JM, Marsh RB, Griffith KA, Hayman JA, Unacceptable cosmesis in a protocol investigating intensity-modulated radiotherapy with active breathing control for accelerated partial-breast irradiation. Int J Radiat Oncol Biol Phys 2010;**76**(1):7.

[89] Vicini F, Winter K, Wong J, Pass H, Rabinovitch R, Chafe S, Initial efficacy results of RTOG 0319: three-dimensional conformal radiation therapy (3D-CRT) confined to the region of the lumpectomy cavity for stage I/II breast carcinoma. Int J Radiat Oncol Biol Phys 2010;**77**(4):7.

[90] Lei RY, Lenoard C, Howell KT, Henkenberns PL, Johnson TK, Hobart TL, Four-year clinical update from a prospective trial of accelerated partial breast intensity-modulated radiotherapy (APBIMRT). Breast Cancer Res Treat 2013;**140**(1):14.

[91] Group, R.T.O., NSABP Protocol B-39/RTOG Protocol 0413: a randomized phase III study of conventional whole breast irradiation (WBI) versus partial breast irradiation (PBI) for women with stage 0, I, or II breast cancer. Clin Adv Hematol Oncol 2004;**4**:3.

[92] Dickler A, Xoft Axxent electronic brachytherapy: a new device for delivering brachytherapy to the breast. Nat Clin Pract Oncol 2009;**6**(3):138–142.

[93] Dooley WC et al., Electronic brachytherapy as adjuvant therapy for early stage breast cancer: a retrospective analysis. Onco Targets Ther 2011;**4**:13–20.

[94] Beitsch PD et al., Post-surgical treatment of early-stage breast cancer with electronic brachytherapy: an intersociety, multicenter brachytherapy trial. Onco Targets Ther 2010;**3**:211–218.

[95] Mann JM et al., Excellent long-term breast preservation rate after accelerated partial breast irradiation using a balloon device. Clin Breast Cancer 2016;**16**(3):217–222.

[96] Small W Jr. et al., Clinical outcomes with the MammoSite radiation therapy system: results of a prospective trial. J Radiat Oncol 2015;**4**(4):395–400.

[97] Gitt A et al., Treatment results of mammosite catheter in combination with whole-breast irradiation. Anticancer Res 2016;**36**(1):355–360.

[98] Vargo JA et al., Extended (5-year) outcomes of accelerated partial breast irradiation using MammoSite balloon brachytherapy: patterns of failure, patient selection, and dosimetric correlates for late toxicity. Int J Radiat Oncol Biol Phys 2014;**88**(2):285–291.

[99] Hieken TJ et al., A novel treatment schedule for rapid completion of surgery and radiation in early-stage breast cancer. Ann Surg Oncol 2016 ;23(10):3297-303.

[100] Rehman S et al., Prospective analysis of toxicity in patients treated with strut-adjusted volume implant for early-stage breast cancer. Brachytherapy 2016;**15**(5):625-30.

[101] Wobb JL et al., Comparison of chronic toxicities between brachytherapy-based accelerated partial breast irradiation and whole breast irradiation using intensity modulated radiotherapy. Breast 2015;**24**(6):739–744.

[102] Abbott AM et al., Prospective multicenter trial evaluating balloon-catheter partial-breast irradiation for ductal carcinoma in situ. Int J Radiat Oncol Biol Phys 2013;**87**(3):494–498.

[103] Vaidya JS et al., Reduced mortality with partial-breast irradiation for early breast cancer: a meta-analysis of randomized trials. Int J Radiat Oncol Biol Phys 2016;**96**(2):259-65.

[104] Smith GL et al., Association between treatment with brachytherapy vs whole-breast irradiation and subsequent mastectomy, complications, and survival among older women with invasive breast cancer. JAMA 2012;**307**(17):1827–1837.

[105] Vaidya JS et al., Risk-adapted targeted intraoperative radiotherapy versus whole-breast radiotherapy for breast cancer: 5-year results for local control and overall survival from the TARGIT—a randomised trial. Lancet 2014;**383**(9917):603–613.

[106] Silverstein MJ et al., Intraoperative radiation therapy: a critical analysis of the ELIOT and TARGIT Trials. Part 2—TARGIT. Ann Surg Oncol 2014;**21**(12):3793–3799.

[107] Veronesi U et al., Intraoperative radiotherapy versus external radiotherapy for early breast cancer (ELIOT): a randomised controlled equivalence trial. Lancet Oncol 2013;**14**(13):1269–1277.

[108] Maluta S et al., Intraoperative electron radiotherapy (IOERT) as an alternative to standard whole breast irradiation: only for low-risk subgroups? Breast Care (Basel) 2014;**9**(2):102–106.

[109] Leonardi MC et al., Accelerated partial breast irradiation with intraoperative electrons: using GEC-ESTRO recommendations as guidance for patient selection. Radiother Oncol 2013;**106**(1):21–27.

[110] Hickey BE, Lehman M, Francis DP, See AM, Partial breast irradiation for early breast cancer. Cochrane Database of Systematic Reviews 2016, 7:Cd007077.

[111] Clarke M et al., Effects of radiotherapy and of differences in the extent of surgery for early breast cancer on local recurrence and 15-year survival: an overview of the randomised trials. Lancet 2005;**366**(9503):2087–2106.

[112] Gramatyka M, Cardiotoxicity as undesired side effect in the treatment of breast cancer. Postepy Hig Med Dosw (Online) 2014;**68**:483–497.

[113] George R et al., Quantifying the effect of intrafraction motion during breast IMRT planning and dose delivery. Med Phys 2003;**30**(4):552–562.

[114] Vedam S et al., Dosimetric impact of geometric errors due to respiratory motion prediction on dynamic multileaf collimator-based four-dimensional radiation delivery. Med Phys 2005;**32**(6):1607–1620.

[115] Duan J et al., Dosimetric and radiobiological impact of dose fractionation on respiratory motion induced IMRT delivery errors: a volumetric dose measurement study. Med Phys 2006;**33**(5):1380–1387.

[116] van der Laan HP et al., Current technological clinical practice in breast radiotherapy; results of a survey in EORTC-Radiation Oncology Group affiliated institutions. Radiother Oncol 2010;**94**(3):280–285.

[117] Bartlett FR et al., The UK HeartSpare Study (Stage IB): randomised comparison of a voluntary breath-hold technique and prone radiotherapy after breast conserving surgery. Radiother Oncol 2015;**114**(1):66–72.

[118] Giraud P, Simon L, Saliou M, Respiratory gated radiotherapy: the 4D radiotherapy. Bulletin du Cancer 2005;**92**(1):6.

[119] Giraud P et al., Dosimetric and clinical benefits of respiratory-gated radiotherapy for lung and breast cancers: results of the STIC 2003. Cancer Radiother 2012;**16**(4):272–281.

[120] Keall PJ et al., The management of respiratory motion in radiation oncology report of AAPM Task Group 76. Med Phys 2006;**33**(10):3874–3900.

[121] Bolukbasi Y et al., Reproducible deep-inspiration breath-hold irradiation with forward intensity-modulated radiotherapy for left-sided breast cancer significantly reduces cardiac radiation exposure compared to inverse intensity-modulated radiotherapy. Tumori 2014;**100**(2):169–178.

[122] Nissen HD, Appelt AL, Improved heart, lung and target dose with deep inspiration breath hold in a large clinical series of breast cancer patients. Radiother Oncol 2013;**106**(1):28–32.

[123] Remouchamps VM et al., Significant reductions in heart and lung doses using deep inspiration breath hold with active breathing control and intensity-modulated radiation therapy for patients treated with locoregional breast irradiation. Int J Radiat Oncol Biol Phys 2003;**55**(2):392–406.

[124] Yeung R et al., Cardiac dose reduction with deep inspiration breath hold for left-sided breast cancer radiotherapy patients with and without regional nodal irradiation. Radiat Oncol 2015;**10**:200.

[125] Essers M et al., Should breathing adapted radiotherapy also be applied for right-sided breast irradiation? Acta Oncol 2016;**55**(4):460–465.

[126] Smyth LM et al., The cardiac dose-sparing benefits of deep inspiration breath-hold in left breast irradiation: a systematic review. J Med Radiat Sci 2015;**62**(1):66–73.

[127] Bartlett FR et al., Voluntary breath-hold technique for reducing heart dose in left breast radiotherapy. Journal of visualized experiments : JoVE 2014(89).

[128] Bartlett FR et al., The UK HeartSpare Study: randomised evaluation of voluntary deep-inspiratory breath-hold in women undergoing breast radiotherapy. Radiother Oncol 2013;**108**(2):242–247.

[129] Bartlett FR et al., OC-0387: The UK HeartSpare Study (Stage II): multicentre evaluation of a voluntary breath-hold technique. Radiother Oncol 2015;**115**:S186.

Chapter 15

Breast Cancer and Flavonoids as Treatment Strategy

Pinar Obakan-Yerlikaya, Elif Damla Arisan,

Ajda Coker-Gurkan and Narcin Palavan-Unsal

Additional information is available at the end of the chapter

http://dx.doi.org/10.5772/66169

Abstract

Breast cancer is the most prevalent cancer type among women. Despite recent progress in early detection and therapeutic strategies, the rate of mortality is increasing. Anti-estrogens or aromatase inhibitors are preferred to treat the women diagnosed with estrogen-receptor (ER) positive tumors. However, breast tumors usually show intra-tumoral heterogeneity with ER-positive and -negative cells. The advanced breast cancer cells lose the estrogen responsiveness and become aggressive by developing new strategies for rapid proliferation such as mutations in cell cycle machinery. New promising drugs are still being investigating against these types of tumors especially to overcome acquired resistance against chemotherapeutic drugs; however, a successful treatment for metastatic tumors is still unclear. Flavonoids, with various pharmacological activities, are plant or fungus secondary metabolites present in human diet. In plants, beside their role in pigmentation, they may also act as messengers, regulators and cell cycle inhibitors. Therefore, they are being tested in ovarian, cervical as well as breast cancer. Due to the positive correlation between flavonoids-rich diet and lower risk of cancer, flavonoids are referred as chemopreventive agents. The current chapter emphasizes the therapeutic potential of flavonoids and their synthetic analogues as anti-cancer agents in breast cancer providing new insights into the molecular mechanisms.

Keywords: breast cancer, chemoprevention, flavonoids

1. Introduction

The use of natural and dietary agents for cancer chemoprevention and therapy received attention for their health benefits. As consumption of fruits or vegetables has been associated with a reduced risk of human cancers especially breast cancer [1], dietary flavonoids, found particularly in these alimentary groups with more than 5000 polyphenolic compounds, have been identified as potential cancer-preventive components [2, 3]. Polyphenols can be divided into ten different classes based on their chemical structure [4]. Flavonoids, phenolic acids, stilbenes, and lignans are the most abundant polyphenols in plants. Polyphenols, mainly flavonoids, possess a number of functions including pollination, pollen tube growth, resorption of minerals, and tolerance to abiotic stress [5]. Flavonoids represented greater attention with the decreased incidence of cancer and cardiovascular diseases in Mediterranean population, which was associated with vegetables, fruits, and red wine consumption. Therefore, they have been under investigation for their therapeutic significance in the protection of human health for decades. Flavonoids are one of the common components in the human diet and generally are present as O-glycosides with sugars bound at C3 position [6].

Breast cancer is the leading cause of cancer death among women worldwide. Despite the presence of new promising advances in therapeutics, the breast cancer mortality rate is still increasing. Recent reports suggest that breast cancer prognosis is lower in countries consuming a healthy, plant-based diet [7]. The possible cause to this scenario has been suggested as flavonoids in fruits and vegetables. Epidemiologic investigations showed that flavonoids exhibit important effects on cancer chemoprevention and chemotherapy. They have been shown to interact with different genes and enzymes including those playing role in antiproliferation, cell cycle arrest, apoptosis, angiogenesis, and multidrug resistance. Therefore, this chapter focuses on the chemopreventive and chemotherapeutical roles of flavonoids in the treatment of breast cancer [6].

2. Structure, classification and metabolism in humans

The chemical structure of flavonoids is based on a C15 skeleton with a chromane ring bearing a second aromatic ring B in position 2, 3, or 4 (**Figure 1**).

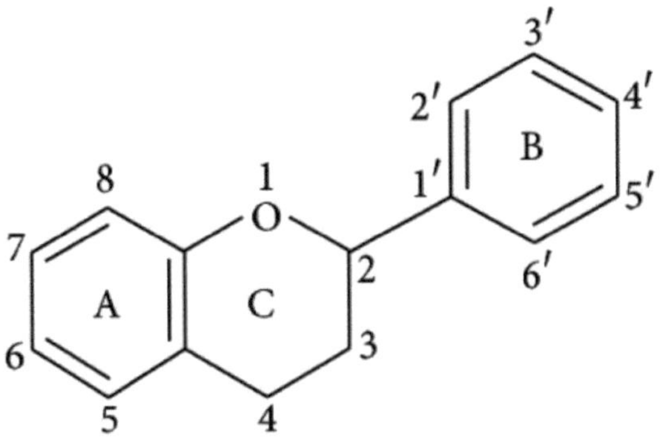

Figure 1. Basic flavonoid structure [8].

http://dx.doi.org/10.5772/66169

Flavonoids are subdivided into different groups based on the nature of C3 element: flavones, flavonols, flavanones, flavanols, anthocyanins, and isoflavones (**Figure 2**).

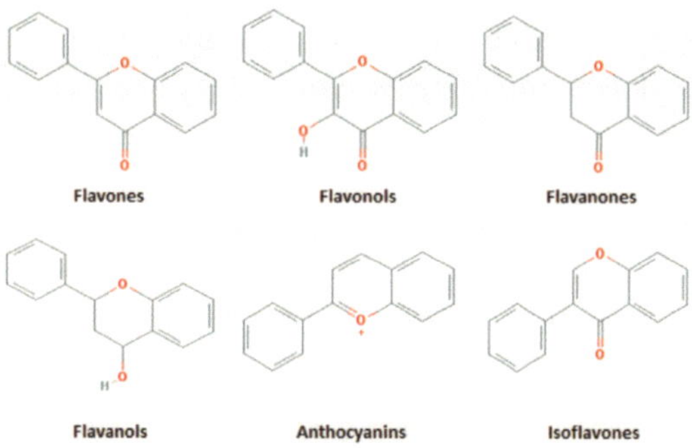

Figure 2. Subclasses of flavonoids (PubChem).

Flavonoids participate light-dependent phase of photosynthesis [9], and they catalyze electron transport. They have been shown to be synthesized from phenylalanine and tyrosine, the aromatic amino acids, with acetates [10]. First, aromatic amino acids are converted to cinnamic acid and parahydroxycinnamic acid, respectively, by phenylalanine and tyrosine ammonia lyase enzymes [11]. Then, parahydroxycinnamic acid accumulates with acetate units to give rise to cinnamoyl, which is the derivative of caffeic acid and chlorogenic acid. Cinnamoyl, then, is converted to ortho-hydroxyacetophenone with a benzaldehyde derivative generating flavonones. If ortho-hydroxyacetophenone condenses with a benzoic acid derivative, flavones are formed. Anthocyanins are naturally occurring glycosides of flavylium (2-phenyl-1-benzopyrylium) ions substituted by hydroxyl and methoxyl groups. Biotransformation of flavonoids occurs in the gut and various secondary metabolites are produced as well such as phenolic acids, lignins, lignans, and stilbenes [11].

Flavonoids, mainly flavanols and quercetin glucosides, are absorbed from the small intestine, while quercetin, quercetin galactoside, and many others are not [12]. Those absorbed by the intestine have been shown to be transported through membrane and use both ATP-dependent pumps and ATP-independent transporters [13]. Following absorption, they are metabolized *via* microbial catabolism and conjugated in the liver and enterocytes [14]. Depending on the subclass, only 5–10% of the amount consumed was shown to be absorbed in the intestine; the rest excreted through the colon where they are further metabolized. The absorbed part in the duodenum is found as methylated, sulfate-conjugated, glucuronide-conjugated, or glycine-conjugated forms [15]. Firstly, in 1992, Hertog et al. measured the content of flavonoids in different fruits, vegetables, and wine. Their findings indicated that mostly quercetin, kaempferol, myricetin, apigenin, and luteolin are found as flavonoid subclasses in the diet. They also suggested that the mean daily intake of flavonoids was higher than the antioxidants β-carotene, vitamin E, and vitamin C [16]. However, the measurement of daily flavonoid intake is difficult to estimate since a standardized method is lacking [17]. Flavonoids, except catechins, exist in nature as glycosides. Following flavonoid intake, the glucosides are cleaved and glucuronated. Glucuronides can be metabolized, released, or stored as aglycones by glucuronidases in a tissue-specific manner [18]. Although the glycosylation of flavonoids has been suggested important for their absorption, the non-glycosylated form of catechin intake has been shown relatively efficient [19]. Flavonoids, especially flavanols, flavonols, and anthocyanins, are relatively abundant in human diet and are shown to play role in cancer, cardiovascular, and neurodegenerative disease disorder prevention [20].

3. Flavonoid-rich food and medicinal plants

The plant extracts have been used as folk remedies against various health problems, including metabolic diseases, cancer, and neurodegenerative disorders. According to in vitro and in vivo studies, a number of plant species have antiproliferative and antitumoral role in breast cancer pathogenesis. In addition, plants which have higher amount of flavonoids are accepted as chemopreventive agents. According to the United States Department of Agriculture (USDA) database, the six subclasses of flavonoids are listed for 506 food items. According to the database, flavonols (quercetin, kaempferol, myricetin, isorhamnetin), flavones (luteolin, apigenin), flavanones (hesperetin, naringenin, eriodictyol), flavan-3-ols ((+)-catechin, (+)-gallocatechin (GC), (−)-epicatechin (EC), (−)-epigallocatechin (EGC), (−)-epicatechin 3-gallate, (−)-epigallocatechin 3-gallate, theaflavin, theaflavin 3-gallate, theaflavin 3′-gallate, theaflavin 3,3′ digallate, thearubigins), anthocyanidins (cyanidin, delphinidin, malvidin, pelargonidin, peonidin, petunidin), and isoflavones (genistein, daidzein, glycitein) are listed.

Generally, these dietary compounds are known with their antioxidant, anti-inflammatory, and anticarcinogenic effects. According to the Seven Countries Study report, the average consumption of quercetin, kaempferol, myricetin, luteolin, and apigenin in composite food samples have ranged from 6 mg/day in Finland to 64 mg/day in Japan, with intermediate intakes in the United States (13 mg/day), Italy (27 mg/day), and the Netherlands (33 mg/day). In a similar study report, average flavonoid intake in Hungarian population was lower compared to Dutch, Danish, and Finnish citizens. The intake of five flavonoids in 17 different diets was estimated. When diet types were compared to each other according to flavonoid consumption ratio, it was shown that South African diet is the lowest flavonoid consumed diet type as 1–9 mg/day consumption. In contrary, Scandinavian diet in correlation with population-based study outcomes was the higher flavonoid intake diet type (75–81 mg/day).

In addition dietary origin of the flavonoids varied between countries. While tea is the main dietary source of flavanoids in Japan by 95% and the Netherlands by 64%, alcoholic beverages such as famous resveratrol based popularity of red wine and beer in Italy by 46%. The vegetables and fruits are the most common dietary sources of Scandinavian countries such as Finland by 100%. Similar ratio was also observed in the United States by 80%. In Australia, tea is the major source of flavonoid, and flavan-3-ols are 75% of whole intake. Therefore, it is important to evaluate the chemopreventive and chemotherapeutic potential of flavonoids in breast cancer disease.

In this section, it is aimed to discuss potential molecular mechanism of above-listed flavanoids in breast cancer studies.

3.1. Flavanols

3.1.1. Quercetin

Quercetin is a natural dietary flavonoid which exerts antioxidant, anti-inflammatory and anticancer properties. Quercetin is found in barks of many plants, fruits, and vegetables. It is one of the well-established grape polyphenols like other members, resveratrol, naringenin, and catechin, can exert antitumoral, antioxidant, anti-angiogenic properties and modify selectively estrogen-receptor (ER). According to a recent study, it is found that quercetin at IC50 value (37 μM) modulated Twist and p38 MAPK signaling, which lead to apoptosis in MCF-7 and MDA-MB-231 breast cancer cells [21]. In addition it is well documented that quercetin exerts its therapeutic effect through modulating different cellular targets. According to the previous study, it was shown that quercetin induced p21 CDK inhibitor with a concomitant decrease of phosphorylation of retinoblastoma (Rb), which inhibits the G1/S cell cycle progression by trapping E2F1. A low dose of quercetin induced mild DNA damage and Chk2 activation, which is the main regulator of p21 expression by quercetin. In addition, quercetin downregulated the cyclin B1 and CDK1, essential components of G2/M cell cycle progression. Inhibition of the recruitment of key transcription factor NF-Y to cyclin B1 gene promoter by quercetin led to transcriptional inhibition SKBR3, MDA-MB-453, and MDA-MB-231 cells [22, 23].

Similar to previous findings, MCF-7 breast cancer cells were exposed to the increasing concentrations of quercetin; consequently, cell viability ratios were decreased, and apoptosis was triggered. Following exposure of cells to moderate cytotoxic dose of quercetin for 48 h, cells undergo apoptosis due to activation of caspases. In addition, quercetin mediates the disruption of Bcl-2/Bax ratio in MCF-7 cells [24].

3.1.2. Kaempferol

A dietary flavonoid, kaempferol (3,5,7-trihydroxy-2-(4-hydroxyphenyl)-4H-1-benzopyran-4-one), is found in edible plants such as kale, beans, endive, tea, broccoli, cabbage, tomato, and grapes, is commonly used in traditional medicine (e.g., *Ginkgo biloba*, *Tilia* spp., *Equisetum* spp., *Moringa oleifera*, *Sophora japonica*, and propolis) has been reported as antimicrobial, anticancer, antioxidant, neuroprotective, cardioprotective, and antiallergic activity [25]. Kaempferol leads to anti-angiogenic effect via reducing vascular endothelial growth factor (VEGF) expression in ovarian cancer cells [26]. Moreover, it enhanced the effect of cisplatin in ovarian cancer and induced cell cycle arrest and apoptosis by modulating Bcl-2-Bax expression. In vitro studies about kaempferol on breast cancer cases, time-dependent exposure of cells to flavonoid (50 μM) induced G2/M arrest *via* inhibiting CDK1; cyclin A, and cyclin B and induced apoptosis by p53 phosphorylation in MDA-MB-453 breast cancer cell [27]. Although kaempferol treatment significantly induced cell viability loss in MCF-7 cells, no significant effect has been reported in MDA-MB-231 breast cancer cells or HC-11 mammary epithelial cells. Kaempferol-induced ERK activated apoptotic cell death and reactive oxygen species (ROS) generation and N-acetyl cysteine (NAC) co-treatment prevented kaempferol-mediated poly (ADP-ribose) polymerase (PARP) cleavage in MCF-7 breast cancer cells [28]. Kaempferol could be extracted from *Murraya koenigii* leaf, which was reported to induce caspase-3-dependent apoptotic cell death and inhibited endogenous 26S proteasomal enzyme activity in MDA-MB-231 breast cancer cells. Moreover, dose-dependent kaempferol treatment reduced the tumor growth through inhibiting the expression of angiogenic and antiapoptotic genes in breast cancer xenografts [29]. In vivo breast cancer xenograft mice models, kaempferol-mediated anticancer effect reported *via* downregulation of IRS-1, pAkt, pMEK1/2, and ERK gene expression and decreased the tumor growth and volume. In addition, kaempferol treatment prevents breast cancer invasion and metastasis in MDA-MB-231 breast cancer cells due to reduction in MMP-2 and MMP-9 expressions, suppression of transcription factor activator protein-1 (AP-1) and MAPK signaling [30]. Lymphangiogenesis, a new lymphatic vessels formation process, is a major step in spreading of tumor cells. Lymphangiogenesis inhibitors might be focused as an important drug target strategy in breast cancer cells. A VEGFR2/3 kinase inhibitor, kaempferol, inhibited mammalian lymphangiogenesis in metastatic breast cancer xenograft models [31].

3.1.3. Myricetin

The use of plant derivatives, which exert biological functions, has gained importance in recent years. Myricetin (3,5,7,3′,4′,5′-hexahydroxyflavone cannabiscetin) is a natural flavonol, which has a unique hydrophobic chemical structure found in different varieties of fruits, vegetables, tea, berries, etc. [32]. The dietary intake of myricetin from our foods is about 0.98–1.1 mg per day, which is quite higher than some other flavonols [33]. Recent studies showed that myricetin is an antioxidant and it possesses cytoprotective, anticarcinogenic, antiviral, and antimicrobial effects [34].

3.1.4. Isorhamnetin

Isorhamnetin is one of the important flavanols found in *G. biloba* leaf extracts. Isorhamnetin is also found in parsley, and thereby it is a common dietary flavonoid as the metabolite of quercetin. Generally, it is well known as antagonist of peroxisome proliferator-activated receptor γ (PPARγ), which inhibits adipocyte differentiation induced by the PPARγ agonist rosiglitazone [35]. Isorhamnetin is a naturally occurring compound in fruits and vegetables; recent study showed that isorhamnetin could significantly inhibit the invasion of MDA-MB-231 cells by downregulating matrix metalloproteinases (MMP-2 and MMP-9) through inhibiting p38 MAPK and STAT3 [36]. Similar results were also obtained in another study, which showed that isorhamnetin inhibited cell proliferation and led to apoptosis. In addition, isorhamnetin was found effective on Akt/mTOR/MAPKs signaling axis. It was established that isorhamnetin-induced autophagy can be reversed by the co-treatment of 3-methyl-adenine in lung cancer cells. The results indicated that isorhamnetin exerts antitumor effect in breast cancer through targeting multiple molecular targets [37].

3.1.5. Silymarin

In recent years, chemopreventive potential of fruits, vegetables, and medicinal herbs such as tea due to ingredients rich in phytochemicals that act as an antioxidant become an important agent. One of the polyphenolic flavonoids silymarin that is isolated from milk thistle (*Silybum marianum* (L.) *Gaertn*) has been shown for its antioxidant action against liver toxicity [38]. Recently, studies reported the anticarcinogenic effect of silymarin in several mouse skin tumorigenic samples and cervical, prostate, liver, and breast cancers. The molecular machinery of silymarin was more frequently shown in the treatment of human umbilical vein endothelial cells (HUVECs), and downregulation of survivin, Akt, and nuclear factor (NF)-κB was observed [39]. Beside cell growth and proliferation inhibition, silymarin was demonstrated as an inhibitor of MMPs and *in vitro* angiogenesis. Silymarin induced liver cancer prevention due to membrane stabilizing antioxidant effect through acting on tumor necrosis factor alpha (TNF-α) expression in hepatocellular carcinoma cells [40]. Moreover, VEGF secretion suppression instead of normal epithelial cells, in prostate and breast cancer epithelial cells, has also been reported in Ref. [41]. In MCF-7 breast cancer cells, silymarin treatment inhibited cell growth *via* upregulating ERB. However, ER alpha (ERα) downregulation is reported to be an important key player in drug-induced autophagy and apoptosis in MCF-7 breast cancer cells *via* Akt/mTOR/ERK signaling pathway [42].

3.2. Flavanes

3.2.1. Luteolin

Luteolin (3′,4′,5,7-tetrahydroxyflavone) which belongs to flavonoids is a heat-stable and non-toxic compound. It is found in vegetables and fruits such as celery, parsley, broccoli, onion leaves, carrots, peppers, cabbages, apple skins, and mignonette and chrysanthemum flowers. As well as other flavanoids, cardiovascular protection, immune system stimulation, antioxidant, anti-inflammatory, and anticarcinogenesis capacities of luteolin have been shown in previous studies [43]. Luteolin exerts its molecular effect *via* inducing different signaling routes in dose-dependent manner. According to previous studies, it is well documented that lutein is both pro- and antioxidant compound. The pro-oxidant activity of flavonoids may be related to their ability to undergo autoxidation catalyzed by transition metals to produce superoxide anions [44]. Due to structural differences including bioactive phenolic ring, prooxidant status of luteolin may increase the cytotoxicity in cells. Luteolin is important in ER-expressing cells. It was shown that luteolin at low concentrations is an antiestrogenic agent and reduces cell proliferation. In addition, luteolin may inhibit aromatase whose function is to catalyze the production of estrogens [44]. A recent study indicated that luteolin downregulates ER and thus caused the degeneration of ER protein. Because the etiology of breast cancer is strongly correlated with nuclear hormone receptor activity, the consumption of luteolin in diet may reduce risk through regulation of estrogen-induced cellular effects. In vitro and in vivo studies showed that luteolin prevented estrogen-induced cell proliferation. It was shown that luteolin impaired estrogen signaling pathway (ESP) in MCF-7 cells by microarray analysis [45]. Luteolin altered cell cycle regulation signaling targets, including CCNA2, PLK1, PCNA, and CDKN1A. This result was considered as the final consequence of ESP modulation, which suppresses cell proliferation in breast cancer cells. A previous study showed that luteolin (5 μM) could be utilized as a chemosensitizing mechanism to target the expression level of cyclin E2 and to overcome tamoxifen resistance in breast cancer patients. In vivo studies also showed that luteolin may exert its effect *via* modulating miRNA expressions such as miR-34a and miR-181a which bidirectionally reduced notch and suppressed invasion mechanism [46].

3.2.2. *Apigenin*

Apigenin is known as the phytoestrogen, used in postmenapausal symptom treatment, and presented in various plant species. Although it is a nontoxic and non-mutagenic plant derivative, it exerts antitumoral activity in different types of cancers and induces oxidative stress in breast cancer cells [47]. However, there are contradictory reports showing that apigenin might stimulate cell proliferation in ERα-positive MCF-7 and T47D cells, but not effective in ERα-negative MDA-MB-435 breast cancer cells [48]. The molecular mechanism of apigenin-induced apoptotic cell death was caspase-dependent, mitochondria [49] and NF-κB, STAT signaling-mediated [50]. Moreover, apigenin inhibited cell growth, metastasis, and invasion in breast cancer cells *via* acting on PI3K/Akt signaling and beta 4 integrin in MDA-MB-231 breast cancer cells [51].

3.3. Flavanones

It was shown that flavanone-rich diet mediated 0.1 –100 μM physiologically achievable concentration in the plasma. One of the mostly known flavanones is naringenin, which is especially abundant in the Mediterranean diet, rich for consumption of grapes, tomato, and citrus. Naringenin was shown with anticancerous effect in various cancer cells. According to in vitro studies, it was shown that naringenin modulated NF-κB to induce apoptosis in the cells. Naringenin was effective in MCF-7 ERα+/ERβ + cell line, but not in ER-independent SKBR-3 (ERα−/ERβ−) cell line [52–55]. *Thymus vulgaris* ethanol extraction originated in naringenin induced cell cycle arrest at S and G2/M phases, which led to apoptotic induction in HTB26 and HTB132 breast cancer cells [52]. The apoptotic efficiency of naringenin was found due to alteration of different cell cycles and apoptosis-related genes such as cyclin-dependent kinases and Bcl-2 family members. Naringenin may activate T cells to induce antitumoral activity in mice and lead to increased interferon (IFN)-γ and interleukin (IL)-2 expressing T cell population [54, 56]. Naringenin promotes the therapeutic effect of tamoxifen in breast cancer cells [57, 58]. Thus, naringenin might promote the potential therapy outcomes and good prognosis in breast cancer cases.

Similar to naringenin, eriodictyol has promising therapeutic effects in cancer cells. Eriodictyol, a flavanone, activated Nrf2 and induced phase II proteins to exert its antioxidant effects [59, 60]. However, there are less studies to evaluate the molecular mechanism of eriodictyol compared to naringenin.

Hesperetin is also a promising flavanone and induced cell cycle arrest at G1 phase. According to the previous study, hesperetin regulated CDK4 and p21 (Cip1) in MCF-7 cells and led to block of cell cycle. Hesperetin is also known with its apoptotic effect in breast cancer cells without effecting normal mammary epithelial cells. It was shown that hesperetin induced apoptosis in dose- and time-dependent manner in MCF-7 cells through triggering ROS generation. Pretreatment of NAC prevented hesperetin-induced apoptosis, which is under control of ASK1/JNK pathway. In addition, hesperetin also induced apoptosis in triple-negative breast cancer MDA-MB-231 cells *via* intrinsic apoptotic pathway [53, 61–64]. In the light of previous findings, both naringenin and hesperetin are known as promising therapeutic candidates in breast cancer due to their sensitizing effect of HER2-positive breast cancer cells.

3.4. Flavan-3-ols

The most important member of flavan-3-ols (catechins) is abundantly present in green and black tea, red wine and chocolate. Catechins, which are generally found in green tea, comprise epigallocatechin gallate (EGCG), epicatechin (EC), gallocatechin (GC), epigallocatechin (EGC), catechin gallate (CG), epicatechin gallate (ECG), gallocatechin gallate (GCG), and catechin (C). Although green tea is a favorable catechin source, it is required to design more bioavailable structures to treat various cancer types, including breast cancer. The detailed investigation for EGCG was established in different studies. According to xenograft model studies, EGCG with tamoxifen has potential in ER-negative breast cancer models. The MDA-MB-231-mediated tumor volume was decreased following 25 mg/kg treatment of EGCG and/or EGCG + tamoxifen in athymic nude female mice model [65–68]. The potentiation of green tea catechins is generally acted on mTOR and EGFR pathways. Similar to these findings, studies indicated that EGCG produces anticancer effect by modulating the activity of MAPKs, IGF/IGF-1 receptor, Akt, NF-κB, and HIF-1α [69–73]. Although catechins have multiple molecular targets in the cells, it is required to improve their structural properties to achieve powerful treatment results.

3.5. Anthocyanins

Anthocyanins confer the bright red, blue, and purple colors to plants such as berries, grapes, and apples. Anthocyanidins lack the sugar component of the anthocyanin [74]. Six anthocyanidins occurred most commonly in nature are pelargonidin, cyanidin, peonidin, delphinidin, petunidin, and malvidin. It has been suggested that the consumption of cyanidin lowers the risk of cardiovascular disease, diabetes, and cancer due to the antioxidant and anti-inflammatory activities [75]. The phenolic structure is responsible for the antioxidant activity such as the ability to scavenge superoxide ($O_2^{\cdot-}$), singlet oxygen ($^{\prime}O_2$), peroxide (ROO^-), hydrogen peroxide (H_2O_2), and hydroxyl radical (OH·), members of ROS [76], in in vitro cell lines including colon, liver, and breast cancer cells [77].

3.5.1. Cyanidin

The anticancer effect of cyanidin-rich extracts of different plant has been shown in MCF-7 ERα (+), MDA-MB-231 ER α (−), and MDA-MB-453 ER α (−) breast cancer cell lines. Moreover, apoptotic induction in MDA-MB-453 cells through the intrinsic pathway of apoptosis by activating caspase cascade, cleaving poly (ADP-ribose) polymerase (PARP), depolarizing mitochondrial membrane potential, and releasing cytochrome C has been shown [78]. In addition, in the same study, 100 mg/kg/day oral administration of cyanidin has been shown to reduce tumor growth and angiogenesis by affecting the expression of angiogenic factors MMP-9, MMP-2, and cell/extracellular matrix (ECM) interaction in nude mice bearing MDA-MB-453 cell xenografts [78]. Furthermore, inhibition of proliferation and cell cycle arrest were induced in MCF-7 human breast cancer cells after the treatment of bilberry extract, which contains high amount of cyanidin [79]. The same study also compared the effect of cyanidin with a well-known antioxidant Trolox, a vitamin E analog, and showed that cyaniding induced apoptosis and cell cycle arrest as much as Trolox [80]. In another study, pycnogenol, derived from pine bark, which contains high amounts of procyanidins, has been shown to induce cell death in breast cancer cells (derived from human fibrocystic mammary tissue) but not in normal human mammary MCF-10A cells [81].

Human epidermal growth factor receptor 2 (HER2) is overexpressed in 20% cases of breast cancer. Therefore, HER2-targeted therapies have been evaluated in recent years. In Liu et al.'s [82] study, cyanidin-3-glucoside, extracted from black rice, inhibited phospho-HER2 and phospho-AKT and induced apoptosis both in vitro and in vivo HER2-positive breast cancer cells and tissues. Another study also revealed that anthocyanidin-rich extracts from berries and grapes have been shown to exhibit proapoptotic effects in multiple cell types in vitro [83]. They induce apoptosis through both intrinsic (mitochondrial) and extrinsic (FAS) pathways.

3.5.2. Delphinidin

Delphinidin is a member of anthocyanins mainly found in pomegranate extract and found in many dietary supplements as complementary cancer medicine. A recent study showed that delphinidin treatment inhibited cell proliferation and induced apoptosis in ER-positive, triple-negative, and HER2-overexpressing breast cancer cell lines without any toxic effect in normal breast epithelial cells [84]. In addition, the same study also indicated that MAPK signaling was inhibited in both triple-negative and ER-negative breast cancer cells but not in MCF-10A normal epithelial cells.

Breast cancer cells overexpressing p65, the unit of NF-κB responsible from cell survival and proliferation, underwent apoptosis following delphinidin treatment. The possible explanation to this process was shown as the inhibition of phosphatidylinositol 3,4,5-trisphosphate (PI3K)-dependent phosphorylation of AKT in vitro and inhibition of the activation of NF-κB in vivo [85]. The same study also pointed out that miR-27a and miR-155 were able to inhibit PI3K and NF-κB and responsible from the anti-inflammatory and cytotoxic activity of delphinidin in MDA-MB-231 breast cancer cell line [86]. Delphinidin has been also shown to inhibit hepatocyte growth factor (HGF)-mediated tyrosyl phosphorylation of focal adhesion kinase (FAK), Src, paxillin, Gab-1, and GRB-2, which are inducers of cell proliferation upon phosphorylation by growth factor signaling. Delphinidin, in the same study, was found to repress Ras-ERK MAPKs and PI3K/AKT/mTOR/p70S6K pathways [16]. The compound also has anti-angiogenic and anti-invasive properties by decreasing MMP-9 activity in ER+ MCF-7 cells. Im et al. showed that delphinidin inhibited MMP-9 transcription by blocking NF-κB through MAPK signaling pathways [87].

3.5.3. Pelargonidin

Pelargonidin, a subclass of anthocyanin with estrogenic activity, was tested in MCF-7 breast cancer cells. The cytotoxic dose (5 μg/ml) of strawberry extract containing pelargonidin-3-O-glucoside caused 50% decrease in cell proliferation [88]. A study performed in breast cancer tissue of rats showed that pelargonidin could inhibit the synthesis of cytochrome c p450 family 1 subfamily A member 1 (CYP1A1) enzyme which converts estradiol into 2-hydroxy-estradiol that can cause DNA damage [89]. The inhibition of the estrogenic activity by 55% was also indicated following pelargonidin containing pomegranate seed oil in ER+ MCF-7 cells. On the other hand, pelargonidin treatment induced apoptosis in both MCF-7 and MDA-MB-231 (ER-). Seventy-five percent inhibition of invasion across a Matrigel was also observed in MCF-7 cells at 10 μg/ml pomegranate seed oil concentration. Studies suggest that further investigations on chemopreventive and therapeutic applications of pelargonidin should be performed against human breast cancer [90].

3.6. Isoflavonoids

3.6.1. Daidzein

Daidzein, is one of the isoflavonoid present in various plants and herbs such as soybeans, tofu, kwao krua (*Pueraria mirifica*), kudzu (*Pueraria lobata*), and also isolated from *Maackia amurensis* cultures [91]. Breast tumor growth inhibition by lower concentration of daidzein (10 μM) treatment in *in vitro* and *in vivo* has been reported. Daidzein prevented T47D breast cancer cell proliferation and acted as antiestrogenic agent [92]. Fifty micrometer daidzein concentration decreased the cell viability in MDA-MB-231 and MCF-7 breast cancer cells by 50 and 42%, respectively, for 48 h. Moreover, daidzein inhibited cell migration and invasion in breast cancer cells by using MicroRaman techniques [93]. As a soybean extract, daidzein stabilized proto-oncogene BRF2 mRNA and decreases BRF2 promoter methylation in ERα and ERβ breast cancer cells and female breast cancer mice models [94]. Antiproliferative effect of daidzein on breast cancer cells was reported by acting on TNF-α expression, down-regulating MMP-9 mRNA expression, and suppressing hedgehog signaling through preventing the Gli1 nuclear translocation. In in vivo MCF-7 athymic nude mice breast cancer models, fed daidzein prevented tumor growth through suppressing ATP2A3 and BLNK expression and decreased MYC oncogene expression [95]. However, no significant association between breast cancer risk and plasma equol and/or equol: daidzein concentrations have been reported in the Chinese population [96].

3.6.2. Genistein

Soybean is one of the dietary components, which contains phytoestrogens and genistein acting as a chemopreventive agent against various cancer cells such as prostate and breast cancer. As a predominant isoflavone, genistein inhibits growth and proliferation of ER-positive and ER-negative breast cancer cells by inhibiting receptor-associated tyrosine kinase (RTK) signaling [97]. Genistein inhibited cell proliferation, growth, invasion, and metastasis and acted as anticarcinogenic and anti-angiogenic compound on breast cancer in vitro and in vivo models

[98]. The molecular mechanism of anticarcinogenic effect of genistein on breast cancer cells is due to DNA topoisomerase, 5-reductase enzyme inhibition, suppressing the NF-κB, Akt and MAPK signaling pathways [99]. Genistein is one of the flavonoids that has been shown to effect on chronic diseases such as atherosclerosis and hereditary hemorrhagic telangiectasia. The molecular target of genistein was reported to enhance the action of transforming growth factor-β (TGF-β) [77]. Like other plant secondary metabolites (tocopherols, curcumin), flavonoids reported to regulate VEGF in breast tumors in vivo and in vitro studies. The anti-angiogenic, anticarcinogenic effect of genistein target VEGF receptor-2 (VEGFR-2) mediated PI3K/Akt/mTOR signaling pathway [100]. Angiogenesis is the formation of new blood vessels and sprouting of circulation by activation of VEGF family member, VEGF-A, leading to endothelial cell proliferation, migration, and destruction of matrix metalloproteins. Although the anti-angiogenic effect of isoflavonoids has been reported in various studies, the exact molecular inhibition mechanism has not been clarified yet. One of the anti-angiogenic effects of genistein is the inhibition of VEGF and its receptor secretion. Ten to fifty micrometer genistein prevented basal VEFG expression both in breast cancer and human umbilical vein endothelial cells (HUVECs) [101]. Moreover, under hypoxia conditions genistein has been shown to induce both VEGF downregulation and inhibition of hypoxia-inducible factor 1 (HIF-1) activation. The anti-angiogenic effect of genistein has been accelerated with curcumin-combined treatment in HUVEC cells by VEGFR-1 and VEGFR-2 downregulation [102]. According to in vivo experiments such as xenografts, chick chorioallantoic membrane or zebra fish experimental models showed the reduction of microvessel density due to genistein treatment mediated by plasminogen activator inhibitor-1, endostatin, angiostatin, and thrombospondin-1 activation. Pretreatment with genistein leads to the reduction of MMP-2, MMP-3, MMP-13, and MMP-15 mRNA expression and VEGF-mediated plasminogen activator (PA) and PAI1 expression blockage. However, no significant effect has been determined on MMP-2 and MMP-9 activity. Antiproliferative and anti-angiogenic effect of genistein is also shown by inhibition of cadherin, integrin V, connexin 43 mRNA expression, and genistein (40 mmol/L), or daidzein (110 μm/L) treatment suppresses epidermal growth factor (EGF) and insulin-like growth factor (IGF-I) [103]. NF-κB signaling pathway plays an important role in not only angiogenesis but also cell growth apoptosis, inflammation, and invasion. Thus, genistein treatment inhibited MMP-9 by NF-κB nuclear translocation-induced NF-κB signaling inactivation [104]. In addition, genistein induced cell proliferation suppression by acting on MAPKs such as ERK-1/2, c-Jun N-terminal kinases (JNK), and p38 dephosphorylation. In order to clarify the anti-angiogenic effect of flavonoids, genistein, one of the major catalytic enzymes of prostaglandin production [cyclooxygenase-2 COX-2], associated VEGF production was investigated [105]. COX isoenzyme catalyzes the production of prostaglandins, VEGF production, and angiogenesis induction. In MCF-7 breast cancer cells, genistein alone or combined treatment with capsaicin leads anti-angiogenic and anticarcinogenic effect *via* acting on reduced COX-2 expression. According to in vivo studies, in TPA-treated animals, genistein or daidzein suppresses NF-κB and COX-2 activity [77]. During cancer progression, various molecules have been involved in various steps such as cell proliferation, differentiation, migration, and extracellular matrix formation. Moreover, some tumor microenvironment modulators such as immunosuppressive and/or angiogenic-inducing factors play essential roles. One of the key targets during these hypoxic breast tumors is galectin-3 that

http://dx.doi.org/10.5772/66169

is involved by overexpression in cancer niche. Soy compound isoflavonoid genistein chemopreventive effect has been reported due to potential action on galectin-3 expression inhibition in breast cancer. The phytoestrogen genistein, which induced G2/M arrest due to galentin-3 downregulation, has been determined in human breast carcinoma cell lines [106]. As shown in **Figure 3**, analysis of transcriptomic profile of mammary epithelial cells of rat females fed a diet containing the soy isoflavone genistein or soy protein isolate showed that soy consumption is associated with reduced breast cancer risk in women. Results provide insight into the molecular basis of the beneficial effect of soy-rich diets.

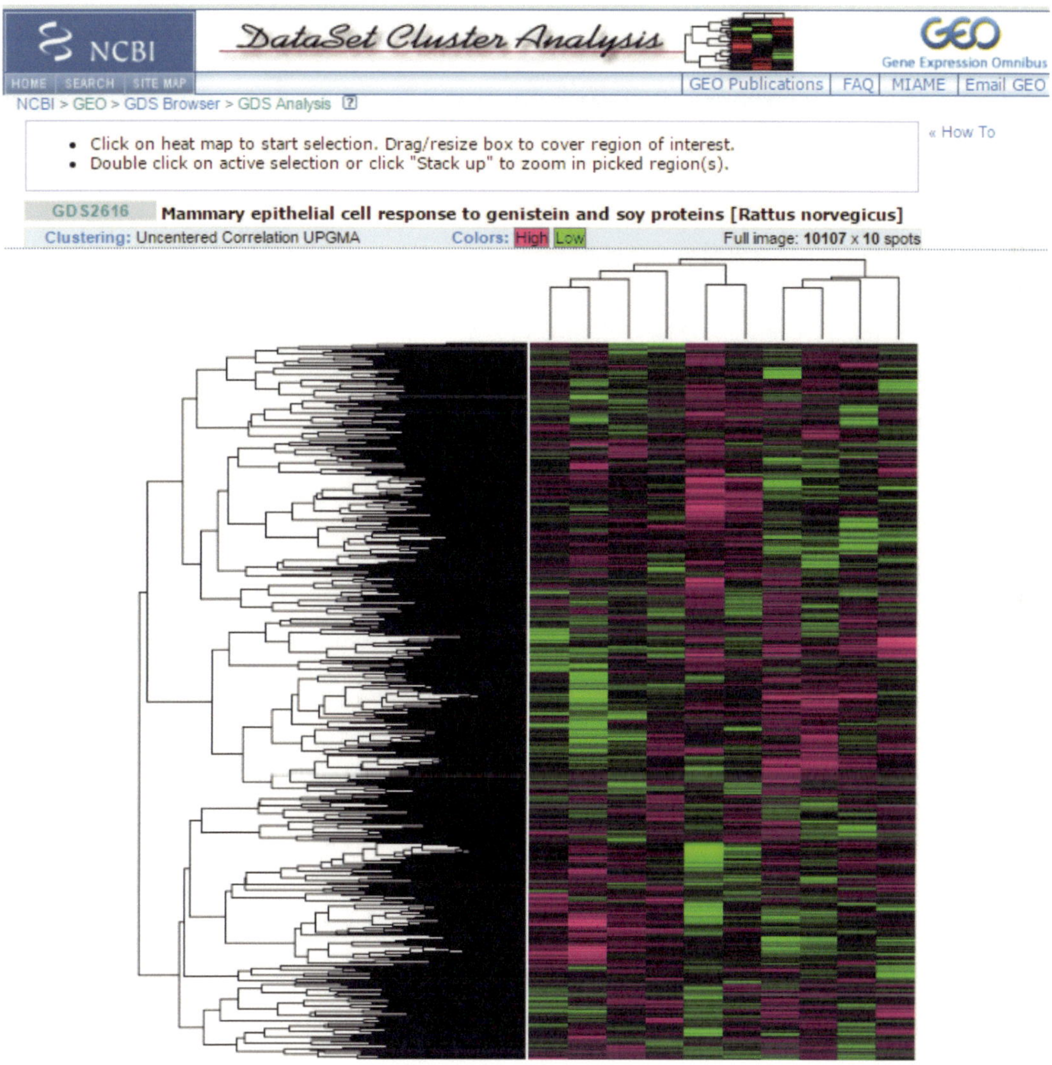

Figure 3. GEO Dataset (GDS2616) demonstration for soy protein genistein protective effect against mammary epithelial cells in *Rattus norvegicus*.

4. Conclusion

In summary, flavonoids can potentially contribute to breast cancer prevention and treatment either by antioxidant or apoptotic activity (**Table 1**). Previous studies highlighted that plant-derived flavonoids are promising when their bioavailability is increased to provide better therapeutic approach in the treatment of disease. However, elucidation of their molecular targets in cell type-specific manner may increase their potential therapeutic effects. Noteworthy that consumption of dietary flavonoids in diet types might be advised to control disease and poor prognosis.

		The effect caused by flavonoid treatment in breast cancer models		
Group of flavonoid	**Subgroup**	**Apoptotic**	**Anti-angiogenic**	**Antioxidant**
Flavanols	Quercetin	+		+
	Kaempferol	+	+	+
	Myricetin			+
	Isorhamnetin	+	+	
	Silymarin	+	+	
Flavanes	Luteolin		+	+
	Apigenin	+	+	
Flavanones	Naringenin	+		
	Eriodictyol			+
	Hesperetin	+		
Flavan-3-ols	Cyanidin	+	+	+
	Delphinidin	+		
	Pelargonidin	+		
Isoflavonoids	Daidzein	+		
	Genistein	+	+	

Table 1. The summary of the effects of flavonoids in breast cancer.

Author details

Pinar Obakan-Yerlikaya*, Elif Damla Arisan, Ajda Coker-Gurkan and Narcin Palavan-Unsal

*Address all correspondence to: p.obakan@iku.edu.tr

Department of Molecular Biology and Genetics, Istanbul Kultur University, Bakirkoy-Istanbul, Turkey

References

[1] Zhang, C.X., et al., Greater vegetable and fruit intake is associated with a lower risk of breast cancer among Chinese women. Int J Cancer, 2009. 125(1): pp. 181-8.

[2] Hui, C., et al., MicroRNA-34a and microRNA-21 play roles in the chemopreventive effects of 3,6-dihydroxyflavone on 1-methyl-1-nitrosourea-induced breast carcinogenesis. Breast Cancer Res, 2012. 14(3): p. R80.

[3] Ni, F., et al., Flavonoid ampelopsin inhibits the growth and metastasis of prostate cancer in vitro and in mice. PLoS One, 2012. 7(6): p. e38802.

[4] Ramos, S., Effects of dietary flavonoids on apoptotic pathways related to cancer chemoprevention. J Nutr Biochem, 2007. 18(7): pp. 427-42.

[5] Aune, D., et al., Fruits, vegetables and breast cancer risk: a systematic review and meta-analysis of prospective studies. Breast Cancer Res Treat, 2012. 134(2): pp. 479-93.

[6] Sak, K., Cytotoxicity of dietary flavonoids on different human cancer types. Pharmacogn Rev, 2014. 8(16): pp. 122-46.

[7] Aune, D., et al., Fruits, vegetables and breast cancer risk: a systematic review and meta-analysis of prospective studies. Breast Cancer Res Treat, 2012. 134(2): pp. 479-93.

[8] Martinez-Perez, C., et al., Novel flavonoids as anti-cancer agents: mechanisms of action and promise for their potential application in breast cancer. Biochem Soc Trans, 2014. 42(4): pp. 1017-23.

[9] Das, D.K., Naturally occurring flavonoids: Structure, chemistry, and high-performance liquid chromatography methods for separation and characterization. Methods Enzymol, 1994. 234: pp. 410-20.

[10] Harborne, J.B., The flavonoids: advances in research since 1980, 2013: Springer, London, UK.

[11] Wagner, H. and L. Farkas, Synthesis of flavonoids, in The Flavonoids, 1975. pp. 127-213: Springer, Dordrecht, Netherlands.

[12] Cermak, R., S. Landgraf, and S. Wolffram, Quercetin glucosides inhibit glucose uptake into brush-border-membrane vesicles of porcine jejunum. Br J Nutr, 2004. 91(6): pp. 849-55.

[13] Gonzales, G.B., et al., Flavonoid interactions during digestion, absorption, distribution and metabolism: a sequential structure-activity/property relationship-based approach in the study of bioavailability and bioactivity. Drug Metab Rev, 2015. 47(2): pp. 175-90.

[14] Passamonti, S., et al., Bioavailability of flavonoids: a review of their membrane transport and the function of bilitranslocase in animal and plant organisms. Curr Drug Metab, 2009. 10(4): pp. 369-94.

[15] Kroon, P.A., et al., How should we assess the effects of exposure to dietary polyphenols in vitro? Am J Clin Nutr, 2004. 80(1): pp. 15-21.

[16] Hertog, M.G., et al., Intake of potentially anticarcinogenic flavonoids and their determinants in adults in The Netherlands. Nutr Cancer, 1993. 20(1): pp. 21-9.

[17] Scalbert, A. and G. Williamson, Dietary intake and bioavailability of polyphenols. J Nutr, 2000. 130(8): pp. 2073S-85S.

[18] Seelinger, G., et al., Anti-carcinogenic effects of the flavonoid luteolin. Molecules, 2008. 13(10): pp. 2628-51.

[19] Okushio, K., et al., Absorption of tea catechins into rat portal vein. Biol Pharm Bull, 1996. 19(2): pp. 326-9.

[20] Stoclet, J.C. and V. Schini-Kerth, Dietary flavonoids and human health. Ann Pharm Fr, 2011. 69(2): pp. 78-90.

[21] Ranganathan, S., D. Halagowder, and N.D. Sivasithambaram, Quercetin suppresses twist to induce apoptosis in MCF-7 breast cancer cells. PLoS One, 2015. 10(10): p. e0141370.

[22] Deng, X.H., et al., Effects of quercetin on the proliferation of breast cancer cells and expression of survivin in vitro. Exp Ther Med, 2013. 6(5): pp. 1155-58.

[23] Dechsupa, S., et al., Quercetin, Siamois 1 and Siamois 2 induce apoptosis in human breast cancer MDA-mB-435 cells xenograft in vivo. Cancer Biol Ther, 2007. 6(1): pp. 56-61.

[24] Duo, J., et al., Quercetin inhibits human breast cancer cell proliferation and induces apoptosis via Bcl-2 and Bax regulation. Mol Med Rep, 2012. 5(6): pp. 1453-6.

[25] Kim, S.H. and K.C. Choi, Anti-cancer effect and underlying mechanism(s) of kaempferol, a phytoestrogen, on the regulation of apoptosis in diverse cancer cell models. Toxicol Res, 2013. 29(4): pp. 229-34.

[26] Luo, H., et al., Kaempferol inhibits VEGF expression and in vitro angiogenesis through a novel ERK-NFkappaB-cMyc-p21 pathway. Food Chem, 2012. 130(2): pp. 321-328.

[27] Choi, E.J. and W.S. Ahn, Kaempferol induced the apoptosis via cell cycle arrest in human breast cancer MDA-MB-453 cells. Nutr Res Pract, 2008. 2(4): pp. 322-5.

[28] Kim, B.W., et al., Sustained ERK activation is involved in the kaempferol-induced apoptosis of breast cancer cells and is more evident under 3-D culture condition. Cancer Biol Ther, 2008. 7(7): pp. 1080-9.

[29] Noolu, B., et al., In Vivo Inhibition of Proteasome Activity and Tumour Growth by Murraya koenigii Leaf Extract in Breast Cancer Xenografts and by its active flavonoids in breast cancer cells. Anticancer Agents Med Chem, 2016. 16:12 (1605-1614).

[30] Kim, S.H., K.A. Hwang, and K.C. Choi, Treatment with kaempferol suppresses breast cancer cell growth caused by estrogen and triclosan in cellular and xenograft breast cancer models. J Nutr Biochem, 2016. 28: pp. 70-82.

[31] Astin, J.W., et al., An in vivo antilymphatic screen in zebrafish identifies novel inhibitors of mammalian lymphangiogenesis and lymphatic-mediated metastasis. Mol Cancer Ther, 2014. 13(10): pp. 2450-62.

[32] Rodgers, E.H. and M.H. Grant, The effect of the flavonoids, quercetin, myricetin and epicatechin on the growth and enzyme activities of MCF7 human breast cancer cells. Chem Biol Interact, 1998. 116(3): pp. 213-28.

[33] Jayakumar, J.K., et al., Evaluation of protective effect of myricetin, a bioflavonoid in dimethyl benzanthracene-induced breast cancer in female Wistar rats. South Asian J Cancer, 2014. 3(2): pp. 107-11.

[34] Maggiolini, M., et al., The red wine phenolics piceatannol and myricetin act as agonists for estrogen receptor alpha in human breast cancer cells. J Mol Endocrinol, 2005. 35(2): pp. 269-81.

[35] Kim, B., Y.E. Choi, and H.S. Kim, Eruca sativa and its flavonoid components, quercetin and isorhamnetin, improve skin barrier function by activation of peroxisome proliferator-activated receptor (PPAR)-alpha and suppression of inflammatory cytokines. Phytother Res, 2014. 28(9): pp. 1359-66.

[36] Li, C., et al., Inhibitory effects of isorhamnetin on the invasion of human breast carcinoma cells by downregulating the expression and activity of matrix metalloproteinase-2/9. Nutr Cancer, 2015. 67(7): pp. 1191-200.

[37] Bruning, A., Inhibition of mTOR signaling by quercetin in cancer treatment and prevention. Anticancer Agents Med Chem, 2013. 13(7): pp. 1025-31.

[38] Zhu, X.X., et al., Silibinin: a potential old drug for cancer therapy. Expert Rev Clin Pharmacol, 2016: 18: 1-8.

[39] Singh, R.P., et al., Silibinin strongly inhibits growth and survival of human endothelial cells via cell cycle arrest and downregulation of survivin, Akt and NF-kappaB: implications for angioprevention and antiangiogenic therapy. Oncogene, 2005. 24(7): pp. 1188-202.

[40] Manna, S.K., et al., Silymarin suppresses TNF-induced activation of NF-kappa B, c-Jun N-terminal kinase, and apoptosis. J Immunol, 1999. 163(12): pp. 6800-9.

[41] Deep, G., et al., Angiopreventive efficacy of pure flavonolignans from milk thistle extract against prostate cancer: targeting VEGF-VEGFR signaling. PLoS One, 2012. 7(4): p. e34630.

[42] Zheng, N., et al., ER beta up-regulation was involved in silibinin-induced growth inhibition of human breast cancer MCF-7 cells. Arch Biochem Biophys, 2016. 591: pp. 141-9.

[43] Birt, D.F., S. Hendrich, and W. Wang, Dietary agents in cancer prevention: flavonoids and isoflavonoids. Pharmacol Ther, 2001. 90(2-3): pp. 157-77.

[44] Lien, E.J., et al., Quantitative structure-activity relationship analysis of phenolic antioxidants. Free Radic Biol Med, 1999. 26(3-4): pp. 285-94.

[45] Markaverich, B.M., K. Shoulars, and M.A. Rodriguez, Luteolin regulation of estrogen signaling and cell cycle pathway genes in MCF-7 human breast cancer cells. Int J Biomed Sci, 2011. 7(2): pp. 101-11.

[46] Chen, P.Y., et al., Up-Regulation of miR-34a Expression in Response to the Luteolin-Induced Neurite Outgrowth of PC12 Cells. J Agric Food Chem, 2015. 63(16): pp. 4148-59.

[47] Harrison, M.E., et al., Exposure of breast cancer cells to a subcytotoxic dose of apigenin causes growth inhibition, oxidative stress, and hypophosphorylation of Akt. Exp Mol Pathol, 2014. 97(2): pp. 211-7.

[48] Scherbakov, A.M. and O.E. Andreeva, Apigenin inhibits growth of breast cancer cells: the role of ERalpha and HER2/neu. Acta Naturae, 2015. 7(3): pp. 133-9.

[49] Choi, E.J. and G.H. Kim, Apigenin induces apoptosis through a mitochondria/caspase-pathway in human breast cancer MDA-MB-453 cells. J Clin Biochem Nutr, 2009. 44(3): pp. 260-5.

[50] Seo, H.S., et al., Apigenin induces apoptosis via extrinsic pathway, inducing p53 and inhibiting STAT3 and NFkappaB signaling in HER2-overexpressing breast cancer cells. Mol Cell Biochem, 2012. 366(1-2): pp. 319-34.

[51] Lee, W.J., et al., Apigenin inhibits HGF-promoted invasive growth and metastasis involving blocking PI3K/Akt pathway and beta 4 integrin function in MDA-MB-231 breast cancer cells. Toxicol Appl Pharmacol, 2008. 226(2): pp. 178-91.

[52] Abaza, M.S., et al., Growth inhibitory and chemo-sensitization effects of naringenin, a natural flavanone purified from Thymus vulgaris, on human breast and colorectal cancer. Cancer Cell Int, 2015. 15: p. 46.

[53] Chandrika, B.B., et al., Hesperetin and naringenin sensitize HER2 positive cancer cells to death by serving as HER2 tyrosine kinase inhibitors. Life Sci, 2016.

[54] Zhang, F., et al., Naringenin prevents TGF-beta1 secretion from breast cancer and suppresses pulmonary metastasis by inhibiting PKC activation. Breast Cancer Res, 2016. 18(1): p. 38.

[55] Zierau, O., et al., Naringenin-type flavonoids show different estrogenic effects in mammalian and teleost test systems. Biochem Biophys Res Commun, 2005. 326(4): pp. 909-16.

[56] Chung, S.Y., et al., Inhibition of P-glycoprotein by natural products in human breast cancer cells. Arch Pharm Res, 2005. 28(7): pp. 823-8.

[57] Hatkevich, T., et al., A naringenin-tamoxifen combination impairs cell proliferation and survival of MCF-7 breast cancer cells. Exp Cell Res, 2014. 327(2): pp. 331-9.

[58] Meiyanto, E., A. Hermawan, and Anindyajati, Natural products for cancer-targeted therapy: citrus flavonoids as potent chemopreventive agents. Asian Pac J Cancer Prev, 2012. 13(2): pp. 427-36.

[59] Jing, X., et al., Eriodictyol-7-O- glucoside activates Nrf2 and protects against cerebral ischemic injury. Toxicol Appl Pharmacol, 2013.

[60] Lou, H., et al., Eriodictyol protects against H(2)O(2)-induced neuron-like PC12 cell death through activation of Nrf2/ARE signaling pathway. Neurochem Int, 2012. 61(2): pp. 251-7.

[61] Guthrie, N. and K.K. Carroll, Inhibition of mammary cancer by citrus flavonoids. Adv Exp Med Biol, 1998. 439: pp. 227-36.

[62] Palit, S., et al., Hesperetin induces apoptosis in breast carcinoma by triggering accumulation of ROS and activation of ASK1/JNK pathway. J Cell Physiol, 2015. 230(8): pp. 1729-39.

[63] So, F.V., et al., Inhibition of proliferation of estrogen receptor-positive MCF-7 human breast cancer cells by flavonoids in the presence and absence of excess estrogen. Cancer Lett, 1997. 112(2): pp. 127-33.

[64] So, F.V., et al., Inhibition of human breast cancer cell proliferation and delay of mammary tumorigenesis by flavonoids and citrus juices. Nutr Cancer, 1996. 26(2): pp. 167-81.

[65] Farabegoli, F., A. Papi, and M. Orlandi, (−)-Epigallocatechin-3-gallate down-regulates EGFR, MMP-2, MMP-9 and EMMPRIN and inhibits the invasion of MCF-7 tamoxifen-resistant cells. Biosci Rep, 2011. 31(2): pp. 99-108.

[66] Parvez, S., et al., Catechin prevents tamoxifen-induced oxidative stress and biochemical perturbations in mice. Toxicology, 2006. 225(2-3): pp. 109-18.

[67] Scandlyn, M.J., et al., A new role for tamoxifen in oestrogen receptor-negative breast cancer when it is combined with epigallocatechin gallate. Br J Cancer, 2008. 99(7): pp. 1056-63.

[68] Stuart, E.C., R.M. Jarvis, and R.J. Rosengren, In vitro mechanism of action for the cytotoxicity elicited by the combination of epigallocatechin gallate and raloxifene in MDA-MB-231 cells. Oncol Rep, 2010. 24(3): pp. 779-85.

[69] Butt, M.S., et al., Green tea and anticancer perspectives: updates from last decade. Crit Rev Food Sci Nutr, 2015. 55(6): pp. 792-805.

[70] Delgado, L., et al., Anti-proliferative effects of quercetin and catechin metabolites. Food Funct, 2014. 5(4): pp. 797-803.

[71] Rathore, K., et al., Green tea catechin intervention of reactive oxygen species-mediated ERK pathway activation and chronically induced breast cell carcinogenesis. Carcinogenesis, 2012. 33(1): pp. 174-83.

[72] Rathore, K. and H.C. Wang, Green tea catechin extract in intervention of chronic breast cell carcinogenesis induced by environmental carcinogens. Mol Carcinog, 2012. 51(3): pp. 280-9.

[73] Sen, T. and A. Chatterjee, Epigallocatechin-3-gallate (EGCG) downregulates EGF-induced MMP-9 in breast cancer cells: involvement of integrin receptor alpha5beta1 in the process. Eur J Nutr, 2011. 50(6): pp. 465-78.

[74] Singletary, K.W., K.J. Jung, and M. Giusti, Anthocyanin-rich grape extract blocks breast cell DNA damage. J Med Food, 2007. 10(2): pp. 244-51.

[75] Prior, R.L. and X. Wu, Anthocyanins: structural characteristics that result in unique metabolic patterns and biological activities. Free Radic Res, 2006. 40(10): pp. 1014-28.

[76] Wang, S.Y. and H. Jiao, Scavenging capacity of berry crops on superoxide radicals, hydrogen peroxide, hydroxyl radicals, and singlet oxygen. J Agric Food Chem, 2000. 48(11): pp. 5677-84.

[77] Kim, H., T.G. Peterson, and S. Barnes, Mechanisms of action of the soy isoflavone genistein: emerging role for its effects via transforming growth factor beta signaling pathways. Am J Clin Nutr, 1998. 68(6 Suppl): pp. 1418S-1425S.

[78] Hui, C., et al., Anticancer activities of an anthocyanin-rich extract from black rice against breast cancer cells in vitro and in vivo. Nutr Cancer, 2010. 62(8): pp. 1128-36.

[79] Tang, J., et al., Delphinidin and cyanidin exhibit antiproliferative and apoptotic effects in MCF7 human breast cancer cells. Integr Cancer Sci Ther, 2015. 2: pp. 82-86.

[80] Rimm, E.B., et al., Relation between intake of flavonoids and risk for coronary heart disease in male health professionals. Ann Intern Med, 1996. 125(5): pp. 384-9.

[81] Yao, L.H., et al., Flavonoids in food and their health benefits. Plant foods for human nutrition, 2004. 59(3): pp. 113-122.

[82] Liu, W., et al., Selective anti-proliferation of HER2-positive breast cancer cells by anthocyanins identified by high-throughput screening. PLoS One, 2013. 8(12): p. e81586.

[83] Bunea, A., et al., Anthocyanin determination in blueberry extracts from various cultivars and their antiproliferative and apoptotic properties in B16-F10 metastatic murine melanoma cells. Phytochemistry, 2013. 95: pp. 436-44.

[84] Ozbay, T. and R. Nahta, Delphinidin inhibits HER2 and Erk1/2 signaling and suppresses growth of HER2-overexpressing and triple negative breast cancer cell lines. Breast Cancer (Auckl), 2011. 5: pp. 143-54.

[85] Martin, S., et al., Delphinidin inhibits endothelial cell proliferation and cell cycle progression through a transient activation of ERK-1/-2. Biochem Pharmacol, 2003. 65(4): pp. 669-75.

[86] Syed, D.N., et al., Delphinidin inhibits cell proliferation and invasion via modulation of Met receptor phosphorylation. Toxicol Appl Pharmacol, 2008. 231(1): pp. 52-60.

[87] Im, N.K., et al., Delphinidin suppresses PMA-induced MMP-9 expression by blocking the NF-kappaB activation through MAPK signaling pathways in MCF-7 human breast carcinoma cells. J Med Food, 2014. 17(8): pp. 855-61.

[88] Weaver, J., et al., Strawberry polyphenols are equally cytotoxic to tumourigenic and normal human breast and prostate cell lines. Int J Oncol, 2009. 34(3): pp. 777-86.

[89] Jeyabalan, J., et al., Chemopreventive and therapeutic activity of dietary blueberry against estrogen-mediated breast cancer. J Agric Food Chem, 2014. 62(18): pp. 3963-71.

[90] Kim, N.D., et al., Chemopreventive and adjuvant therapeutic potential of pomegranate (*Punica granatum*) for human breast cancer. Breast Cancer Res Treat, 2002. 71(3): pp. 203-17.

[91] Fedoreyev, S.A., et al., Isoflavonoid production by callus cultures of *Maackia amurensis*. Fitoterapia, 2000. 71(4): pp. 365-72.

[92] de Lemos, M.L., Effects of soy phytoestrogens genistein and daidzein on breast cancer growth. Ann Pharmacother, 2001. 35(9): pp. 1118-21.

[93] Medeiros, P.S., et al., Raman microspectroscopy for probing the impact of a dietary antioxidant on human breast cancer cells. Food Funct, 2016. 7(6): pp. 2800-10.

[94] Koo, J., et al., Induction of proto-oncogene BRF2 in breast cancer cells by the dietary soybean isoflavone daidzein. BMC Cancer, 2015. 15: pp. 905.

[95] Bao, C., et al., Daidzein suppresses tumor necrosis factor-alpha induced migration and invasion by inhibiting hedgehog/Gli1 signaling in human breast cancer cells. J Agric Food Chem, 2014. 62(17): pp. 3759-67.

[96] Atkinson, C., et al., Plasma equol concentration is not associated with breast cancer and fibrocystic breast conditions among women in Shanghai, China. Nutr Res, 2016. 36(8): pp. 863-71.

[97] Akiyama, T., et al., Genistein, a specific inhibitor of tyrosine-specific protein kinases. J Biol Chem, 1987. 262(12): pp. 5592-5.

[98] Hsieh, C.Y., et al., Estrogenic effects of genistein on the growth of estrogen receptor-positive human breast cancer (MCF-7) cells in vitro and in vivo. Cancer Res, 1998. 58(17): pp. 3833-8.

[99] Li, Z., et al., Genistein induces cell apoptosis in MDA-MB-231 breast cancer cells via the mitogen-activated protein kinase pathway. Toxicol In Vitro, 2008. 22(7): pp. 1749-53.

[100] Morgan, T.M., T.D. Koreckij, and E. Corey, Targeted therapy for advanced prostate cancer: inhibition of the PI3K/Akt/mTOR pathway. Curr Cancer Drug Targets, 2009. 9(2): pp. 237-49.

[101] Yu, X., et al., Anti-angiogenic genistein inhibits VEGF-induced endothelial cell activation by decreasing PTK activity and MAPK activation. Med Oncol, 2012. 29(1): pp. 349-57.

[102] Buchler, P., et al., Antiangiogenic activity of genistein in pancreatic carcinoma cells is mediated by the inhibition of hypoxia-inducible factor-1 and the down-regulation of VEGF gene expression. Cancer, 2004. 100(1): pp. 201-10.

[103] Sounni, N.E., et al., Up-regulation of vascular endothelial growth factor-A by active membrane-type 1 matrix metalloproteinase through activation of Src-tyrosine kinases. J Biol Chem, 2004. 279(14): pp. 13564-74.

[104] Gupta, S.C., et al., Regulation of survival, proliferation, invasion, angiogenesis, and metastasis of tumor cells through modulation of inflammatory pathways by nutraceuticals. Cancer Metastasis Rev, 2010. 29(3): pp. 405-34.

[105] Chung, M.H., et al., Genistein inhibits phorbol ester-induced NF-kappaB transcriptional activity and COX-2 expression by blocking the phosphorylation of p65/RelA in human mammary epithelial cells. Mutat Res, 2014. 768: pp. 74-83.

[106] Lin, H.M., et al., Galectin-3 mediates genistein-induced G(2)/M arrest and inhibits apoptosis. Carcinogenesis, 2000. 21(11): pp. 1941-5.

Chapter 16

Translational Challenges and Therapeutic Opportunities in BRCA1-Related Breast Cancer

Jeffrey Johnson, William Audeh, Hisashi Tanaka,
Farin Amersi, Armando E. Giuliano and
Xiaojiang Cui

Additional information is available at the end of the chapter

http://dx.doi.org/10.5772/66168

Abstract

Although significant progress has been made in the management of the hereditary cancer syndrome related to mutations of BRCA1, two fundamental and clinically relevant questions regarding BRCA1-related cancer syndrome remain unresolved: (1) What factors account for the tissue specificity of the BRCA1-related cancer risk? (2) How does a mutation or loss of BRCA1 lead to the basal-like phenotype of breast cancer? This review focuses on recent studies in BRCA1-related pathways that lead to specific characteristics of the hereditary cancer syndrome and discusses the current translational evidence for exploiting these pathways in new therapeutic strategies. Mounting evidence suggests that estrogen signaling and metabolism, oxidative stress, specific secondary mutations, and regulation of specific progenitor cells and transcriptional programs are critical in BRCA1-associated breast cancer. Strategies geared toward estrogen reduction may play a role in treatment and prevention. Therapies aimed at mitigating oxidative stress may be a strategy for risk reduction, while cancer-cell-specific sensitivity to oxidative stress may also be an opportunity for specific targeting. BRCA1-related transcriptional regulation and signaling provide a number of therapeutic targets, including the PI3-AKT and Notch pathways. Thus, significant opportunities exist in translational and clinical research for developing the treatment strategies for the management of BRCA1-related breast cancer.

Keywords: BRCA1, basal-like breast cancer, DNA repair, estrogen, reactive oxygen species

1. Introduction

In 1866, Pierre Paul Broca described the remarkable pedigree of his wife's family in his treatise *Traité des Tumeurs*: Of 19 women from five generations who lived to the age of 30 years, cancer developed in 14 women, including nine cases of breast cancer [1]. The French physician and surgeon observed: "This deadly predisposition, impossible to foretell, impossible to escape, inaccessible to surgery, and until now even inaccessible to internal or medical treatment, is an indication of a general state which precedes each local manifestation ... in certain cases this predisposition transmits itself by heredity through several generations" [1]. Progress was slow for the next 100 years. Further identification of family pedigrees suggested the hereditary passage of breast cancer, but this remained controversial [2]. With the second half of the twentieth century came the recognition of a familial breast cancer syndrome that in some cases could be associated with an autosomal dominant allele encoding a tumor suppressor gene [3]. In 1990, linkage analysis mapped the putative allele to chromosome 17q21, and the gene, BRCA1, was finally cloned in 1994 [4, 5]. The identification of BRCA2 followed a similar trajectory, with its localization to 13q12-13 in 1994 and cloning the following year [6, 7]. In addition to BRCA1/2, a number of genes have been implicated in familial breast cancer with varying degrees of conferred risk that are generally inversely related to population allele frequency; BRCA1, for example, has rare mutations with high penetrance [8]. Since that time, significant advances have been made in understanding the risks and mechanisms of BRCA1/2-related carcinogenesis. For patients with BRCA1/2 mutations, estimates of lifetime cancer risk widely vary due to different studies of cohorts and varying penetrance attributed to different mutation-related phenotypes, family/genetic history, and environmental exposures. Cumulative risk by 70 years of age for patients with germline BRCA1 mutations ranges between 46% and 87% for breast cancer and between 27% and 63% for ovarian cancer, with the low-risk and general population studies falling in the lower range of the estimate and high-risk families in the upper range. For BRCA2 mutations, the risks are 31–56% and up to 11%, respectively [9]. Beyond female breast and ovarian cancer, BRCA1 mutations may also be associated with the risk for melanoma, whereas BRCA2 is associated with male breast cancer, pancreatic cancer, and prostate cancer [10].

A number of therapeutic strategies have been developed to manage hereditary breast cancer. The National Comprehensive Cancer Network evidence-based guidelines provide an algorithm for the management of hereditary breast cancer, including identification of high-risk individuals and families, genetic testing, cancer screening, risk mitigation through prophylactic salpingo-oophorectomy and possible mastectomy, locoregional and systemic treatment, and ongoing surveillance [11]. Newer therapies and combination strategies are being designed to target more specific features of the cancer genotype and phenotype. The use of PARP inhibitors in the model of synthetic lethality to exploit deficiency in homologous repair in BRCA1/2 deficient cells is one such example [12–15]. This targets one aspect of BRCA1/2 function, but the development of further strategies is desirable, especially as BRCA1-related cancer and cancer risk have a more complicated etiology than defective homologous repair alone. The BRCA1 cancer syndrome may be related to the myriad cellular processes in which BRCA1 is involved, including recognition and repair of genomic damage, regulation of chromosome sorting and mitosis, control of cell-cycle checkpoints, protein ubiquitination, cell signaling, and transcriptional regulation [16–20]. Further, abrogation of BRCA1 function can be the result of a multitude of lesions and processes with variable penetrance and relative hypomorphism, including mutations resulting in a premature stop codon with or without mRNA transcription and expression of a truncated protein, mutations resulting in loss of the function of particular functional domains, intronic mutations resulting in splice variants, large rearrangements, variation in mRNA splicing, methylation and silencing of the gene, and regulation by microRNA [21–23]. Although most BRCA1 mutant mRNAs have shortened half-life, some BRCA1 mutant proteins are translated [24]. However, characterizing cellular localization and function of these proteins is difficult. Staining for intracellular BRCA1 in mutants is inconsistent, as patterns vary with different antibodies, fixation methods, and methods of exposing epitopes, which may lead to a lack of correlation between BRCA1 staining and qPCR levels [25, 26]. Despite nearly two decades of genetic testing, there remain a significant number of variants of uncertain significance. Even when a mutation is established as pathogenic, targeted therapies against DNA repair may not always be effective, as preclinical data suggest in the case of at least one common pathogenic mutation, C61G [27].

Out of this complicated picture, two fundamental questions arise regarding specific characteristics of the BRCA1-related cancer syndrome, both with the potential to guide cancer prevention and therapy: (1) What accounts for the tissue specificity of the BRCA1-related cancer risk? (2) How does mutation or loss of BRCA1 lead to the basal-like phenotype of breast cancer, as opposed to the luminal phenotype of BRCA2 mutations? We searched PubMed for English-language studies and reviews related to BRCA1 function, estrogen metabolism, oxidative stress, basal-like breast cancer, and BRCA1-related therapy. Reference lists of selected articles were searched to track the provenience of key ideas and findings.

2. BRCA1/2 and carcinogenesis

The best known and perhaps dominant roles for the BRCA proteins in tumor suppression lie in the maintenance of chromosomal stability, a role played in nearly all tissues [28]. Both BRCA1 and BRCA2 are essential for homologous repair, a high-fidelity repair mechanism for double-stranded breaks and daughter strand gaps, lesions that can arise from DNA damage and at stalled replication forks [29, 30]. Lack of BRCA proteins results in these lesions being shunted into error-prone repair pathways resulting in chromosomal rearrangements and deletions [30–32]. Both BRCA1/2 have additional roles in chromosomal stability: BRCA1 functions in the recognition of DNA damage and the recruitment and assembly of protein complexes for repair of lesions, and BRCA2 stabilizes stalled replication forks to allow for repair rather than degradation and prevents spontaneous hyperrecombination [28, 33, 34]. BRCA1 also heterodimerizes with BARD1 at the N-terminal ring domain, conferring E3 ubiquitin ligase activity and regulating mitotic spindle assembly; loss of this interaction also results in loss of tumor suppressor activity [27, 35]. Dysregulation of the mitotic spindle assembly as well as centrosome amplification, along with failure of the G2-M checkpoint, leads to defects in chromosome segregation, abnormal division, and aneuploidy [35, 36]. BRCA2 may also have a role in cell-cycle checkpoint control [37].

Maintenance of chromosomal stability alone cannot explain comprehensively the related cancer syndrome beyond an increased risk of carcinogenesis. Other factors are needed to account for the tissue tropism of BRCA1/2-related cancers as well as the particular phenotype of BRCA1-related cancer: basal subtype cancer developing specifically in the epithelium of the breast and papillary serous cancer developing most likely in the fimbria of the fallopian tube —cancers that have similar mutational profiles and likely similar early driving events in carcinogenesis [38]. Several explanations may account for the tissue specificity of the carcinogenic potential. First, breast and fallopian tube cells are subject to a unique exposure resulting in accumulating mutations and genomic damage, possibly related to the genotoxic effects of estrogen metabolism and the generation of reactive oxygen species (ROS), or related to abrogation of normal cell-cycle control in tissues periodically undergoing multiple cycles of rapid proliferation. These tissues may provide an environment that is permissive for, or even driving, cell survival and proliferation despite mounting genomic damage. Further, functions of BRCA1 unrelated to genomic stability may contribute both to the tissue-specific risk as well as the particular phenotype including transcription-related roles in the regulation of mammary progenitor cells and moderation of the proliferative effects of estrogen signaling.

2.1. BRCA1 cancer tissue specificity: estrogen and oxidative stress

Maintenance of the genome alone cannot explain the tissue-specific nature of BRCA1-related cancer risk. It is well documented that cumulative estradiol exposure is linked to lifetime risk of the development of breast cancer [39]. Estrogen-linked carcinogenesis could be related to the transcriptional program of estrogen signaling, which promotes cell proliferation, or to the toxic side effects of estrogen metabolism. BRCA1 interacts with the classical estrogen signaling pathway in combination with BARD1 by repressing ERα-related transcription through ubiquitination, a function lost with deleterious mutations of the BRCA1 RING domain [40, 41]. However, estrogen signaling is not restricted to the nuclear receptors ERα and ERβ and likely plays a role in estrogen receptor negative cancers. Recent studies have shown an alternative mechanism of BRCA1 cell survival based on nonclassical binding of estrogen to cytoplasmic and membrane-associated proteins with downstream effects preventing damage from oxidative stress [42]. Gorrini et al. showed that both oxidative stress and estrogen induced the expression of NRF2, a master regulator of antioxidant capacities, through the PI3K-AKT pathway, and that NRF2 induced by estrogen was crucial for cell survival. They also showed that apoptosis may be prevented in BRCA1 knockdown mammary epithelial cells with exposure to estrogen [43, 44]. This is consistent with clinical observations that reduction in estrogen load reduces risk of cancer in women carrying a BRCA mutation, even if BRCA1-related cells are estrogen receptor negative [45].

BRCA1 mutants may be particularly sensitive to estrogen metabolites, and the early risk of developing cancer reflects the rapid, uncorrected accumulation of genotoxic damage from exposure to both estrogen metabolites and reactive oxygen species produced by oxidative metabolism of estrogen through the catechol pathway, a topic reviewed by Yager and Davidson [39]. Metabolism of estrogen by cytochrome P-450 enzymes, including some tissue-specific enzymes, leads to the formation of estrogen-3,4-quinone, which can form stable DNA adducts and depurinating DNA adducts resulting in mutagenesis. Reduction of oxidized estrogen metabolites leads to reactive oxygen species, which may further damage DNA, proteins, and lipids [39]. Recently, Santen et al. have shown in ER knockout mice the dose-dependent accumulation of toxic estrogen metabolites and concordant rates of tumor formation along with mitigation by estrogen reduction via oophorectomy or aromatase inhibitor treatment [46]. Further, Savage et al. showed that treatment with the estrogen metabolites, 2-hydroxyestradiol and 4-hydroxyestradiol, resulted in double-strand breaks, produced primarily during S-phase, and that BRCA1 deficiency, including both heterozygous and homozygous mutants, led to increased double-strand breaks and loss of efficient repair [47]. Further, wild-type BRCA1 represses the expression of estrogen metabolizing genes, resulting in decreased damage to DNA [47].

Reactive oxygen species (ROS) are produced during normal aerobic metabolism and multiple other cellular processes. ROS and the redox state of a cell are also essential components in cell signaling and homeostasis. Imbalance of pro- and antioxidant factors, whether from endogenous sources or exogenous sources (e.g., UV radiation and tobacco), results in oxidative damage to nucleic acids, amino acids, and fatty acids, and contributes to a number of disease processes. Among the most common DNA lesions resulting from oxidative stress is 8-oxoguanine, which results in a mutagenic template during DNA replication resulting in base pair substitutions and stalling of RNA polymerase II at the site of the lesion with inhibition of nucleotide excision repair [48, 49]. Bae et al. showed that BRCA1 has a role in the response to oxidative stress by upregulating expression of antioxidant genes and enhancing the activity of NRF2 [50]. Further, BRCA1 maintains balance of the cellular redox state, making cells more resistant to exogenous oxidative stress. BRCA1 overexpression and deficiency result in increased and decreased resistance to exogenous oxidative stress, respectively [50]. Besides activating cellular defenses to oxidative stress, BRCA1/2 also mediate repair of DNA damage resulting from oxidative stress. Le Page et al. showed that BRCA1- and BRCA2-deficient cells are unable to repair 8-oxoG lesions and that reconstitution of wild-type BRCA proteins leads to recovery of the transcription-coupled repair mechanism [49]. These studies suggest that BRCA1 tumor suppression involves mitigating the damage of oxidative stress before it is required to repair the resulting DNA lesions.

2.2. BRCA1 cancer phenotype: progenitor cells and transcriptional regulation

Tumors arising in the setting of a germline BRCA1 mutation share common features from the level of genomic alterations, gene expression, histologic phenotype, clinical behavior and prognosis, and response to therapy. Histologically, they are high grade with high mitotic index, pushing tumor margins, central necrosis, and a lymphocytic infiltrate [51]. A subset of sporadic tumors, often demonstrating a relative decrease in BRCA expression through mechanisms other than germline loss, and arising in the same tissues as germline mutants, appears to share this constellation of traits [52]. Turner et al. coined the term BRCAness to identify "the phenotypes that some sporadic tumors share with familial-BRCA cancers" [52]. This is in contrast to BRCA2-related breast cancer, which has a significantly different gene expression profile, and which is more typically lower grade, more differentiated, appearing later in life, and of the luminal/ER-positive subtype [51, 53]. Interestingly, the relative risk profiles for BRCA1 and BRCA2 mutations are also different, further suggesting different etiologic mechanisms. Compared to the aged-matched general population, the relative risk for BRCA1 mutation carriers is greatest in the young population and approaches the population risk in the later decades of life; the relative risk for BRCA2 remains constantly elevated over the population risk throughout the patient's lifetime [54].

BRCAness may be a feature related to the progenitor cell of origin from which these cancers arise. Foulkes hypothesized that BRCA1 acting as a regulator of mammary stem cell function may drive the phenotype of BRCA1-related cancers [55]. In this model, immortal mammary stem cells absent a BRCA1 signal would maintain a relatively undifferentiated, proliferative phenotype that would require very few additional genomic "hits" in order to become malignant; genomic instability conferred by loss of BRCA1-mediated DNA repair functions would account for the proclivity for malignant derangement and the early age of presentation. The general model is appealing, although it appears more likely that BRCA1-associated cancer arises from luminal epithelial progenitors, not mammary stem cells [56].

The mammary epithelium can be sorted into subgroups representing different stages of the differentiation from multipotent mammary stem cell to mature luminal epithelium, which requires BRCA1 for proper development [57]. Depletion of BRCA1 results in failure of mammary cells to differentiate and form acini in culture, but increases cell proliferation [58]. Liu et al. showed that BRCA1 knockdown increases stem/progenitor cell population while preventing mammosphere formation [59]. Furthermore, in human mammary tissue, BRCA1 heterozygotes showed lobules comprised of ALDH1 (stem cell marker) positive cells with minimal ER expression and evidence of BRCA1 loss of heterozygosity. These lobules occurred in normal tissue, showing that mammary progenitor cells can survive without BRCA1 expression and create atypical, nonmalignant lobules. This suggests that the tissue tropism of BRCA1-related tumors is due to a permissive environment, possibly due to release of paracrine factors from luminal epithelium, for the survival of BRCA1 negative cells [60].

Lim et al. [62] demonstrated that normal mammary cells sorted by basal and epithelial markers showed varied potency and clonogenic activity *in vivo* corresponding to bipotent progenitor, committed luminal progenitor, and mature luminal cells. These may represent the cells of origin of the different subtypes of mammary epithelial tumors that can be segregated by gene expression [53, 61]. Comparison of gene expression profiles between normal mammary subpopulations of mammary stem cells, luminal progenitor cells, and mature luminal cells showed significant associations with, respectively, claudin-low, basal, and luminal A and B cancer cell populations [62]. Further analysis of these subtypes reveals few somatic mutations common to all breast cancers, but within the well-defined subtypes, genetic and epigenetic changes give rise to their common phenotypes [38]. These tumor subtypes can also be segregated by clinical behavior, prognosis, and response to treatment [63].

Gene-expression profiles of BRCA1-associated tumors correlated most closely with luminal progenitor cells and loss of BRCA1 in a mouse luminal breast cancer model leads to epithelial-mesenchymal transition (EMT), dedifferentiation, and basal tumor development [62, 64, 65]. BRCA1 transcriptionally regulates a number of genes associated with basal-like breast cancer, including Notch ligands and receptors, with loss of BRCA1 associated with decreased luminal differentiation and ER-α signaling and also with increased basal-like and proliferation markers [66]. Increased Notch signaling due to BRCA1 loss may contribute to the basal-like phenotype as well as suppression of apoptosis [67]. Wild-type BRCA1 represses expression of a number of genes associated with basal-like and BRCA1-related cancers, including FOXC1, *p*-Cadherin, and CK5 and 17 [68, 69]. The luminal progenitor, as the cell of origin for BRCA1-related cancer, is consistent with an important role for ROS as mammary stem cells and multipotent progenitor cells have lower concentrations of ROS than more mature progenitor cells [70].

Around 80–90% of BRCA1 tumors are basal, as opposed to 10–15% of all tumors, although may also sort with the claudin-low subtype [38, 71, 72]. Conversely, around 20% of basal tumors show germline or somatic BRCA1/2 mutation [38]. BRCA1-related cancers exhibit common mutational profiles. A total of 81–89% of BRCA1 tumors, both ER+ and ER−, have a loss of heterozygosity of the wild-type allele, which is correlated with higher grade and increased proliferation [73]. For cells lacking functional BRCA1, cell survival is generally dependent on secondary mutations. BRCA1 tumors commonly show mutations of PTEN and TP53 allowing cell proliferation to continue in spite of mounting genomic irregularities. These mutations appear to follow a general evolutionary pattern preceding the loss of the WT BRCA allele [74]. This is significantly different than tumorigenesis in luminal cancers, with rare PTEN mutations and late loss of TP53. Even without loss of wild-type allele, heterozygotes display altered gene expression, including in genes related to cell differentiation and proliferation [75].

3. Developments in targeted therapy

Therapy for BRCA1/2 related tumors involves surgery, radiation, and systemic chemotherapy and endocrine therapy. Specific treatment for cancer developing in the setting of BRCA1/2 has targeted deficient DNA repair. Platinum-based chemotherapy creates intra- and interstrand DNA crosslinks resulting in double-stranded breaks. In the absence of homologous repair, the accumulation of genomic damage results in cell death. Pegylated liposomal doxorubicin has also been shown to have a survival advantage [76].

PARP inhibitors have been used to exploit the DNA repair defect [13]. PARP-1 binds to DNA strand breaks and signals DNA damage by hydrolyzing NAD+ to form poly(ADP-ribosyl) tails on histones and itself, resulting in the recruitment of the protein machinery for repair [77]. PARP inhibitors include a nicotinamide moiety that competes with NAD+, inhibiting the enzymatic function of PARP, and trapping the PARP enzyme at the site of DNA damage, preventing repair [78]. Loss of PARP-mediated regulation and repair of single strand breaks leads to stalled replication forks, and double strand breaks develop, which leads to cell death in a process referred to as synthetic lethality. Loss of BRCA1 prevents homologous repair from occurring; loss of PARP function results in loss of regulation of nonhomologous end joining, which leads to error-prone repair, genomic instability, and cell death [79]. A number of clinical trials assessing the efficacy of PARP inhibitors in BRCA-mutated breast cancer are currently underway, in metastatic disease as well as in the adjuvant and neoadjuvant setting (http://www.cancer.gov/about-cancer/treatment/clinical-trials).

However, not all BRCA1-related tumors are sensitive to DNA damaging agents and PARP inhibitors. BRCA1 deleterious mutations in the RING finger domain lose tumor suppressor function related to loss of interaction with PALB but retain some homologous repair activity, rendering them less responsive to PARP inhibitors and platinum chemotherapy [27]. There is also evidence that BRCA1/2-associated tumors gain resistance to platinum and PARP inhibitor therapy through mutations resulting in reversion to the wild-type sequence or other restoration of the open reading frame [80]. Lord and Ashworth also review preclinical data suggesting that loss of 53BP1 or the related RAP1-interacting factor 1 (RIF1), proteins involved in nonhomologous end joining, leads to reduced genomic damage from PARPi-induced nonhomologous end joining and at least partial restoration of homologous repair and survival for BRCA1-deficient cells. However, clinical data supporting this mechanism are lacking [80].

Further specific treatment for BRCA1 cancer risk includes targeting estrogen production and signaling and prophylactic surgery to eliminate or reduce the number of potential tumorigenic cells. Bilateral salpingo-oophorectomy has been shown to significantly reduce the risk of breast cancer incidence by about 50% and breast cancer mortality by 90% [45, 81]. The use of tamoxifen, independent of estrogen receptor status, reduced the risk of contralateral breast cancer in BRCA1 mutation carriers with HR 0.38 (95% CI, 0.27–0.55) in a pooled prospective/retrospective cohort [82]. Specific therapy to prevent formation of ROS or toxic estrogen metabolites without endocrine ablation or blockade present a possible target that would modify cancer risk without the possible side effects and complications of surgery and iatrogenic menopause, including loss of fertility. Alternatively, strategies that exploit increased oxidative stress in tumor cells may provide strategy for targeted therapy. In normal cells, ROS are produced at low concentrations and can be effectively neutralized by the antioxidant system of the cells. In contrast, cancer cells produce elevated levels of ROS due to increased metabolic activity, resulting in a state of chronic oxidative stress. As noted above, BRCA1-mutant cells have a dysregulated response and increased sensitivity to oxidative stress as well as a decreased ability to repair DNA lesions resulting from ROS. As such, induction of ROS-mediated damage in cancer cells by proper pharmacological agents that either promote ROS generation beyond the cellular antioxidative capacity or disable the cellular antioxidant system have been considered as a "radical" therapeutic strategy to preferentially kill cancer cells [83]. Elesclomol, a small molecule that increases ROS production in mitochondria and induces apoptosis, has shown *in vitro* potential for treating breast cancer cells with defective DNA repair [84, 85].

The PI3K-AKT pathway is another target for therapy. PI3K is involved in both oxidative stress and escape mechanisms of DNA repair from PARP inhibitors. Combination treatment with PI3K and PARP inhibitors showed significant efficacy in inhibiting tumor cell growth *in vitro* and reducing tumor volume in mouse models [86]. PI3-AKT also functions downstream of Notch, a critical cancer stem cell regulator associated with basal-like breast cancer, in suppression of apoptosis [87, 88]. Although targeting the Notch pathway alone is not sufficient to reduce proliferation or cause cell death, combination with inhibition of the EGFR

http://dx.doi.org/10.5772/66168

pathway or AKT pathway results in enhanced cell death [88]. These results suggest that combination therapies targeting signaling pathways implicated in basal-like breast cancer or BRCA1-regulated cell function would provide new avenues for combating BRCA1-related breast cancer.

4. Conclusion

A great volume of knowledge regarding the molecular functions of BRCA1 and BRCA2 has developed in the last 20 years since the cloning of the genes. Despite some challenging issues in understanding BRCA1-mutant breast cancer development, there is great potential for advances in tying elucidated molecular pathways in cell and animal models to the clinical and epidemiological presentation of BRCA1/2-related breast cancer (**Table 1**). Such translational advances may be exploited not only to advance the treatment of breast cancer but also to diminish the risk described by Pierre Paul Broca—inaccessible to treat, impossible to escape—so long ago.

Challenges in BRCA1-associated breast cancer	Opportunities in BRCA1-associated breast cancer
1. Mechanisms for the tissue specificity of the BRCA1-related cancer risk	1. Development of targeted therapy based on hyperactive signaling pathways in BRCA1-associated breast cancer
2. Mechanisms for the unique BRCA1-related breast cancer phenotype	2. Improvement of synthetic lethal approaches in the treatment of BRCA1-associated breast cancer
3. Differential effects of BRCA1 mutations in different mammary epithelial cell and breast cancer cell populations	3. Prevention strategies based on BRCA1-associated breast cancer biology
4. Individualized breast cancer risk prediction for BRCA1 mutation carriers	

Table 1. Challenges and opportunities in BRCA1-related breast cancer research and treatment.

Acknowledgements

We apologize to many scientists and clinicians whose work was not referenced due to space limitations. This work was supported by National Institutes of Health (CA151610), the Avon Foundation (02-2014-063), Eleanor and Glenn Padnick Discovery Fund in Cellular Therapy, and David Salomon Translational Breast Cancer Research Fund to XC, and the Fashion Footwear Charitable Foundation of New York, Inc., the Entertainment Industry Foundation, Associates for Breast and Prostate Cancer Studies, the Margie and Robert E. Petersen Foundation, Linda and Jim Lippman Research Fund to AG. The funders/sponsors had no role in the design and conduct of the study; collection, management, analysis, and interpretation of the data; preparation, review, or approval of the manuscript; and decision to submit the manuscript for publication. The authors declare no conflicts of interest.

Author details

Jeffrey Johnson[1], William Audeh[2,3], Hisashi Tanaka[1,2], Farin Amersi[1,2], Armando E. Giuliano[1,2] and Xiaojiang Cui[1,2*]

*Address all correspondence to: xiaojiang.cui@cshs.org

1 Department of Surgery, Cedars-Sinai Medical Center, Los Angeles, CA, USA

2 Samuel Oschin Comprehensive Cancer Institute, Cedars-Sinai Medical Center, Los Angeles, CA, USA

3 Division of Hematology/Oncology, Cedars-Sinai Medical Center, Los Angeles, CA, USA

References

[1] Krush A. Contributions of Pierre Paul Broca to cancer genetics. Trans Nebraska Acad Sci Affil Soc. 1979;VII:125–9.

[2] Penrose LS, Mackenzie HJ, Karn MN. A genetical study of human mammary cancer. Br J Cancer. 1948;2(2):168–76.

[3] Go RC, King MC, Bailey-Wilson J, Elston RC, Lynch HT. Genetic epidemiology of breast cancer and associated cancers in high-risk families. I. Segregation analysis. J Natl Cancer Inst. 1983;71(3):455–61.

[4] Hall JM, Lee MK, Newman B, Morrow JE, Anderson LA, Huey B, et al. Linkage of early-onset familial breast cancer to chromosome 17q21. Science. 1990;250(4988):1684–9.

[5] Miki Y, Swensen J, Shattuck-Eidens D, Futreal PA, Harshman K, Tavtigian S, et al. A strong candidate for the breast and ovarian cancer susceptibility gene BRCA1. Science. 1994;266(5182):66–71.

[6] Wooster R, Neuhausen SL, Mangion J, Quirk Y, Ford D, Collins N, et al. Localization of a breast cancer susceptibility gene, BRCA2, to chromosome 13q12-13. Science. 1994;265(5181):2088–90.

[7] Wooster R, Bignell G, Lancaster J, Swift S, Seal S, Mangion J, et al. Identification of the breast cancer susceptibility gene BRCA2. Nature. 1995;378(6559):789–92.

[8] Gracia-Aznarez FJ, Fernandez V, Pita G, Peterlongo P, Dominguez O, de la Hoya M, et al. Whole exome sequencing suggests much of non-BRCA1/BRCA2 familial breast cancer is due to moderate and low penetrance susceptibility alleles. PLoS One. 2013;8(2):e55681.

[9] Fackenthal JD, Olopade OI. Breast cancer risk associated with BRCA1 and BRCA2 in diverse populations. Nat Rev Cancer. 2007;7(12):937–48.

[10] Mersch J, Jackson MA, Park M, Nebgen D, Peterson SK, Singletary C, et al. Cancers associated with BRCA1 and BRCA2 mutations other than breast and ovarian. Cancer. 2015;121(2):269–75.

[11] NCC N. Breast Cancer 2014. 3: Available from: www.nccn.org/professionals/physician_gls/f_guidelines.asp.

[12] Bryant HE, Schultz N, Thomas HD, Parker KM, Flower D, Lopez E, et al. Specific killing of BRCA2-deficient tumours with inhibitors of poly(ADP-ribose) polymerase. Nature. 2005;434(7035):913–7.

[13] Farmer H, McCabe N, Lord CJ, Tutt AN, Johnson DA, Richardson TB, et al. Targeting the DNA repair defect in BRCA mutant cells as a therapeutic strategy. Nature. 2005;434(7035):917–21.

[14] Garber K. PARP inhibitors bounce back. Nat Rev Drug Discov. 2013;12(10):725–7.

[15] Maxwell KN, Domchek SM. Cancer treatment according to BRCA1 and BRCA2 mutations. Nat Rev Clin Oncol. 2012;9(9):520–8.

[16] Welcsh PL, King MC. BRCA1 and BRCA2 and the genetics of breast and ovarian cancer. Hum Mol Genet. 2001;10(7):705–13.

[17] Mullan PB, Quinn JE, Harkin DP. The role of BRCA1 in transcriptional regulation and cell cycle control. Oncogene. 2006;25(43):5854–63.

[18] Gunsalus GL, Musto NA, Bardin CW, Kunz HW, Gill TJ, 3rd. Rats homozygous for the grc complex have defective transport of androgen-binding protein to the epididymis, but normal secretion into the blood. Biol Reprod. 1985;33(5):1057–63.

[19] Di LJ, Fernandez AG, De Siervi A, Longo DL, Gardner K. Transcriptional regulation of BRCA1 expression by a metabolic switch. Nat Struct Mol Biol. 2010;17(12):1406–13.

[20] Koutedakis Y, Sharp NC. Lactic acid removal and heart rate frequencies during recovery after strenuous rowing exercise. Br J Sports Med. 1985;19(4):199–202.

[21] Sanz DJ, Acedo A, Infante M, Duran M, Perez-Cabornero L, Esteban-Cardenosa E, et al. A high proportion of DNA variants of BRCA1 and BRCA2 are associated with aberrant splicing in breast/ovarian cancer patients. Clin Cancer Res. 2010;16(6): 1957–67.

[22] Arnold AG, Otegbeye E, Fleischut MH, Glogowski EA, Siegel B, Boyar SR, et al. Assessment of individuals with BRCA1 and BRCA2 large rearrangements in high-risk breast and ovarian cancer families. Breast Cancer Res Treat. 2014;145(3):625–34.

[23] Chang S, Sharan SK. BRCA1 and microRNAs: emerging networks and potential therapeutic targets. Mol Cells. 2012;34(5):425–32.

[24] Perrin-Vidoz L, Sinilnikova OM, Stoppa-Lyonnet D, Lenoir GM, Mazoyer S. The nonsense-mediated mRNA decay pathway triggers degradation of most BRCA1 mRNAs bearing premature termination codons. Hum Mol Genet. 2002;11(23):2805–14.

[25] Perez-Valles A, Martorell-Cebollada M, Nogueira-Vazquez E, Garcia-Garcia JA, Fuster-Diana E. The usefulness of antibodies to the BRCA1 protein in detecting the mutated BRCA1 gene. An immunohistochemical study. J Clin Pathol. 2001;54(6):476–80.

[26] Turner NC, Reis-Filho JS, Russell AM, Springall RJ, Ryder K, Steele D, et al. BRCA1 dysfunction in sporadic basal-like breast cancer. Oncogene. 2007;26(14):2126–32.

[27] Drost R, Bouwman P, Rottenberg S, Boon U, Schut E, Klarenbeek S, et al. BRCA1 RING function is essential for tumor suppression but dispensable for therapy resistance. Cancer Cell. 2011;20(6):797–809.

[28] Venkitaraman AR. Cancer suppression by the chromosome custodians, BRCA1 and BRCA2. Science. 2014;343(6178):1470–5.

[29] Moynahan ME, Chiu JW, Koller BH, Jasin M. Brca1 controls homology-directed DNA repair. Mol Cell. 1999;4(4):511–8.

[30] Moynahan ME, Pierce AJ, Jasin M. BRCA2 is required for homology-directed repair of chromosomal breaks. Mol Cell. 2001;7(2):263–72.

[31] Snouwaert JN, Gowen LC, Latour AM, Mohn AR, Xiao A, DiBiase L, et al. BRCA1 deficient embryonic stem cells display a decreased homologous recombination frequency and an increased frequency of non-homologous recombination that is corrected by expression of a brca1 transgene. Oncogene. 1999;18(55):7900–7.

[32] Tutt A, Bertwistle D, Valentine J, Gabriel A, Swift S, Ross G, et al. Mutation in Brca2 stimulates error-prone homology-directed repair of DNA double-strand breaks occurring between repeated sequences. EMBO J. 2001;20(17):4704–16.

[33] Cousineau I, Abaji C, Belmaaza A. BRCA1 regulates RAD51 function in response to DNA damage and suppresses spontaneous sister chromatid replication slippage: implications for sister chromatid cohesion, genome stability, and carcinogenesis. Cancer Res. 2005;65(24):11384–91.

[34] Schlacher K, Christ N, Siaud N, Egashira A, Wu H, Jasin M. Double-strand break repair-independent role for BRCA2 in blocking stalled replication fork degradation by MRE11. Cell. 2011;145(4):529–42.

[35] Joukov V, Groen AC, Prokhorova T, Gerson R, White E, Rodriguez A, et al. The BRCA1/BARD1 heterodimer modulates ran-dependent mitotic spindle assembly. Cell. 2006;127(3):539–52.

[36] Xu X, Weaver Z, Linke SP, Li C, Gotay J, Wang XW, et al. Centrosome amplification and a defective G2-M cell cycle checkpoint induce genetic instability in BRCA1 exon 11 isoform-deficient cells. Mol Cell. 1999;3(3):389–95.

[37] Lee H, Trainer AH, Friedman LS, Thistlethwaite FC, Evans MJ, Ponder BA, et al. Mitotic checkpoint inactivation fosters transformation in cells lacking the breast cancer susceptibility gene, Brca2. Mol Cell. 1999;4(1):1–10.

[38] Cancer Genome Atlas N. Comprehensive molecular portraits of human breast tumours. Nature. 2012;490(7418):61–70.

[39] Yager JD, Davidson NE. Estrogen carcinogenesis in breast cancer. N Engl J Med. 2006;354(3):270–82.

[40] Eakin CM, Maccoss MJ, Finney GL, Klevit RE. Estrogen receptor alpha is a putative substrate for the BRCA1 ubiquitin ligase. Proc Natl Acad Sci U S A. 2007;104(14):5794–9.

[41] Fan S, Ma YX, Wang C, Yuan RQ, Meng Q, Wang JA, et al. Role of direct interaction in BRCA1 inhibition of estrogen receptor activity. Oncogene. 2001;20(1):77–87.

[42] Renoir JM, Marsaud V, Lazennec G. Estrogen receptor signaling as a target for novel breast cancer therapeutics. Biochem Pharmacol. 2013;85(4):449–65.

[43] Gorrini C, Baniasadi PS, Harris IS, Silvester J, Inoue S, Snow B, et al. BRCA1 interacts with Nrf2 to regulate antioxidant signaling and cell survival. J Exp Med. 2013;210(8):1529–44.

[44] Gorrini C, Gang BP, Bassi C, Wakeham A, Baniasadi SP, Hao Z, et al. Estrogen controls the survival of BRCA1-deficient cells via a PI3K-NRF2-regulated pathway. Proc Natl Acad Sci U S A. 2014;111(12):4472–7.

[45] Rebbeck TR, Kauff ND, Domchek SM. Meta-analysis of risk reduction estimates associated with risk-reducing salpingo oophorectomy in BRCA1 or BRCA2 mutation carriers. J Natl Cancer Inst. 2009;101(2):80–7.

[46] Santen RJ, Yue W, Wang JP. Estrogen metabolites and breast cancer. Steroids. 2015;99(Pt A):61–6.

[47] Savage KI, Matchett KB, Barros EM, Cooper KM, Irwin GW, Gorski JJ, et al. BRCA1 deficiency exacerbates estrogen-induced DNA damage and genomic instability. Cancer Res. 2014;74(10):2773–84.

[48] Cheng KC, Cahill DS, Kasai H, Nishimura S, Loeb LA. 8-Hydroxyguanine, an abundant form of oxidative DNA damage, causes G-T and A-C substitutions. J Biol Chem. 1992;267(1):166–72.

[49] Le Page F, Randrianarison V, Marot D, Cabannes J, Perricaudet M, Feunteun J, et al. BRCA1 and BRCA2 are necessary for the transcription-coupled repair of the oxidative 8-oxoguanine lesion in human cells. Cancer Res. 2000;60(19):5548–52.

[50] Bae I, Fan S, Meng Q, Rih JK, Kim HJ, Kang HJ, et al. BRCA1 induces antioxidant gene expression and resistance to oxidative stress. Cancer Res. 2004;64(21):7893–909.

[51] Hedenfalk I, Duggan D, Chen Y, Radmacher M, Bittner M, Simon R, et al. Gene-expression profiles in hereditary breast cancer. N Engl J Med. 2001;344(8):539–48.

[52] Turner N, Tutt A, Ashworth A. Hallmarks of 'BRCAness' in sporadic cancers. Nat Rev Cancer. 2004;4(10):814–9.

[53] Sorlie T, Tibshirani R, Parker J, Hastie T, Marron JS, Nobel A, et al. Repeated observation of breast tumor subtypes in independent gene expression data sets. Proc Natl Acad Sci U S A. 2003;100(14):8418–23.

[54] Antoniou A, Pharoah PD, Narod S, Risch HA, Eyfjord JE, Hopper JL, et al. Average risks of breast and ovarian cancer associated with BRCA1 or BRCA2 mutations detected in case Series unselected for family history: a combined analysis of 22 studies. Am J Hum Genet. 2003;72(5):1117–30.

[55] Foulkes WD. BRCA1 functions as a breast stem cell regulator. J Med Genet. 2004;41(1): 1–5.

[56] Molyneux G, Geyer FC, Magnay FA, McCarthy A, Kendrick H, Natrajan R, et al. BRCA1 basal-like breast cancers originate from luminal epithelial progenitors and not from basal stem cells. Cell Stem Cell. 2010;7(3):403–17.

[57] Kubista M, Rosner M, Kubista E, Bernaschek G, Hengstschlager M. Brca1 regulates in vitro differentiation of mammary epithelial cells. Oncogene. 2002;21(31):4747–56.

[58] Furuta S, Jiang X, Gu B, Cheng E, Chen PL, Lee WH. Depletion of BRCA1 impairs differentiation but enhances proliferation of mammary epithelial cells. Proc Natl Acad Sci U S A. 2005;102(26):9176–81.

[59] Liu S, Ginestier C, Charafe-Jauffret E, Foco H, Kleer CG, Merajver SD, et al. BRCA1 regulates human mammary stem/progenitor cell fate. Proc Natl Acad Sci U S A. 2008;105(5):1680–5.

[60] Elledge SJ, Amon A. The BRCA1 suppressor hypothesis: an explanation for the tissue-specific tumor development in BRCA1 patients. Cancer Cell. 2002;1(2):129–32.

[61] Perou CM, Sorlie T, Eisen MB, van de Rijn M, Jeffrey SS, Rees CA, et al. Molecular portraits of human breast tumours. Nature. 2000;406(6797):747–52.

[62] Lim E, Vaillant F, Wu D, Forrest NC, Pal B, Hart AH, et al. Aberrant luminal progenitors as the candidate target population for basal tumor development in BRCA1 mutation carriers. Nat Med. 2009;15(8):907–13.

[63] van 't Veer LJ, Dai H, van de Vijver MJ, He YD, Hart AA, Mao M, et al. Gene expression profiling predicts clinical outcome of breast cancer. Nature. 2002;415(6871):530–6.

[64] Bai F, Smith MD, Chan HL, Pei XH. Germline mutation of Brca1 alters the fate of mammary luminal cells and causes luminal-to-basal mammary tumor transformation. Oncogene. 2013;32(22):2715–25.

[65] Bai F, Chan HL, Scott A, Smith MD, Fan C, Herschkowitz JI, et al. BRCA1 suppresses epithelial-to-mesenchymal transition and stem cell dedifferentiation during mammary and tumor development. Cancer Res. 2014;74(21):6161–72.

[66] Bouras T, Pal B, Vaillant F, Harburg G, Asselin-Labat ML, Oakes SR, et al. Notch signaling regulates mammary stem cell function and luminal cell-fate commitment. Cell Stem Cell. 2008;3(4):429–41.

[67] Lee CW, Raskett CM, Prudovsky I, Altieri DC. Molecular dependence of estrogen receptor-negative breast cancer on a notch-survivin signaling axis. Cancer Res. 2008;68(13):5273–81.

[68] Gorski JJ, James CR, Quinn JE, Stewart GE, Staunton KC, Buckley NE, et al. BRCA1 transcriptionally regulates genes associated with the basal-like phenotype in breast cancer. Breast Cancer Res Treat. 2010;122(3):721–31.

[69] Ray PS, Wang J, Qu Y, Sim MS, Shamonki J, Bagaria SP, et al. FOXC1 is a potential prognostic biomarker with functional significance in basal-like breast cancer. Cancer Res. 2010;70(10):3870–6.

[70] Diehn M, Cho RW, Lobo NA, Kalisky T, Dorie MJ, Kulp AN, et al. Association of reactive oxygen species levels and radioresistance in cancer stem cells. Nature. 2009;458(7239): 780–3.

[71] Foulkes WD, Stefansson IM, Chappuis PO, Begin LR, Goffin JR, Wong N, et al. Germline BRCA1 mutations and a basal epithelial phenotype in breast cancer. J Natl Cancer Inst. 2003;95(19):1482–5.

[72] Prat A, Parker JS, Karginova O, Fan C, Livasy C, Herschkowitz JI, et al. Phenotypic and molecular characterization of the claudin-low intrinsic subtype of breast cancer. Breast Cancer Res. 2010;12(5):R68.

[73] Tung N, Miron A, Schnitt SJ, Gautam S, Fetten K, Kaplan J, et al. Prevalence and predictors of loss of wild type BRCA1 in estrogen receptor positive and negative BRCA1-associated breast cancers. Breast Cancer Res. 2010;12(6):R95.

[74] Martins FC, De S, Almendro V, Gonen M, Park SY, Blum JL, et al. Evolutionary pathways in BRCA1-associated breast tumors. Cancer Discov. 2012;2(6):503–11.

[75] Feilotter HE, Michel C, Uy P, Bathurst L, Davey S. BRCA1 haploinsufficiency leads to altered expression of genes involved in cellular proliferation and development. PLoS One. 2014;9(6):e100068.

[76] Lee JM, Ledermann JA, Kohn EC. PARP Inhibitors for BRCA1/2 mutation-associated and BRCA-like malignancies. Ann Oncol. 2014;25(1):32–40.

[77] Rouleau M, Patel A, Hendzel MJ, Kaufmann SH, Poirier GG. PARP inhibition: PARP1 and beyond. Nat Rev Cancer. 2010;10(4):293–301.

[78] Murai J, Huang SY, Das BB, Renaud A, Zhang Y, Doroshow JH, et al. Trapping of PARP1 and PARP2 by Clinical PARP Inhibitors. Cancer Res. 2012;72(21):5588–99.

[79] Patel AG, Sarkaria JN, Kaufmann SH. Nonhomologous end joining drives poly(ADP-ribose) polymerase (PARP) inhibitor lethality in homologous recombination-deficient cells. Proc Natl Acad Sci U S A. 2011;108(8):3406–11.

[80] Lord CJ, Ashworth A. Mechanisms of resistance to therapies targeting BRCA-mutant cancers. Nat Med. 2013;19(11):1381–8.

[81] Domchek SM, Friebel TM, Neuhausen SL, Wagner T, Evans G, Isaacs C, et al. Mortality after bilateral salpingo-oophorectomy in BRCA1 and BRCA2 mutation carriers: a prospective cohort study. Lancet Oncol. 2006;7(3):223–9.

[82] Phillips KA, Milne RL, Rookus MA, Daly MB, Antoniou AC, Peock S, et al. Tamoxifen and risk of contralateral breast cancer for BRCA1 and BRCA2 mutation carriers. J Clin Oncol. 2013;31(25):3091–9.

[83] Trachootham D, Alexandre J, Huang P. Targeting cancer cells by ROS-mediated mechanisms: a radical therapeutic approach? Nat Rev Drug Discov. 2009;8(7):579–91.

[84] Kirshner JR, He S, Balasubramanyam V, Kepros J, Yang CY, Zhang M, et al. Elesclomol induces cancer cell apoptosis through oxidative stress. Mol Cancer Ther. 2008;7(8): 2319–27.

[85] Qu Y, Wang J, Sim MS, Liu B, Giuliano A, Barsoum J, et al. Elesclomol, counteracted by Akt survival signaling, enhances the apoptotic effect of chemotherapy drugs in breast cancer cells. Breast Cancer Res Treat. 2010;121(2):311–21.

[86] Juvekar A, Burga LN, Hu H, Lunsford EP, Ibrahim YH, Balmana J, et al. Combining a PI3K inhibitor with a PARP inhibitor provides an effective therapy for BRCA1-related breast cancer. Cancer Discov. 2012;2(11):1048–63.

[87] Lee CW, Simin K, Liu Q, Plescia J, Guha M, Khan A, et al. A functional Notch-survivin gene signature in basal breast cancer. Breast Cancer Res. 2008;10(6):R97.

[88] Dong Y, Li A, Wang J, Weber JD, Michel LS. Synthetic lethality through combined Notch-epidermal growth factor receptor pathway inhibition in basal-like breast cancer. Cancer Res. 2010;70(13):5465–74.

Chapter 17

Molecular Fingerprints and Biomarkers of Breast Cancer

Hala Fawzy Mohamed Kamel,
Hiba Saeed Bagader Al-Amodi and
Hanan Mohamed AbdElmoneim

Additional information is available at the end of the chapter

http://dx.doi.org/10.5772/66899

Abstract

Substantial progress has been made over the past three decades in understanding breast cancer (BC) molecular biology, genomics, and targeted therapy. The recent comprehensive molecular and pathological diversity observed in BC patients indicates that BC is not a homogeneous disease; It may be appropriately defined as a myriad of diseases. The explosion of molecular information in the past 10 years has led to a better understanding of the biologic diversity of breast cancers (BCs), and clues to the different etiologic pathways to BC development. It will be useful to study the epigenetics of BC cells and define the mechanisms of both genetic and epigenetic driving alterations beside the mutations. Identifying the oncogenes and tumor suppressor genes is the purpose cancer diagnostics and therapeutics. Oncogenes as well as novel ones involved in the significantly altered regions would enable researchers to identify new causes and molecular pathways that may be targeted at BC treatment. Our main goal is to provide comprehensive understanding of underlying molecular mechanisms and hallmarks of BC, focusing on the identification of fingerprints and novel molecular targets that will greatly improve the cancer predictive, prognostic, and diagnostic biomarkers and, in addition, the possible targets for novel therapies.

Keywords: breast cancer, carcinogenesis, molecular markers, omics, personalized medicine

1. Introduction

Cancers, including breast cancer, are generally thought to develop from a single cell in which mutations and/or epigenetic events have modified the function of genes responsible for cellular growth regulation. These events establish the malignant phenotype, and subsequent molecular events may lead to the emergence of malignant subclones with enhanced growth and metastatic potential [1]. Cancer cells, replicating inappropriately, eventually interfere with normal tissue and organism functions, cause morbidity and may ultimately prove fatal in the absence of effective therapy. The rate of growth of tumours including, breast tumours, is determined by a balance between cell proliferation and cell death; if the rate of proliferation exceeds that of death, tumour growth will occur. Not surprisingly, many of the genes involved in neoplasia turn out to be concerned with control of cell death, as well as with control of cell proliferation [2].

The genes involved in neoplasia are usually classified as oncogenes or tumour suppressor genes, depending on whether the affected gene has gained or lost function in its mutated form. In keeping with this model, breast cancer is the result of imbalance in complex regulatory controls of cellular development and growth. Genetic abnormalities detected in breast carcinomas include mutation and amplification of oncogenes, mutation of tumour suppressor genes, and loss of heterozygosity at certain chromosomal loci. Sex hormones, growth factors, oncogenes, and tumour suppressor genes all regulate gene expression and thereby influence growth and function of breast epithelial cells. Influences favouring cell proliferation or inhibiting cell death may promote tumour progression [3].

Breast carcinoma is phenotypically complex: carcinoma in situ and invasive carcinoma may coexist, as mixed histological types of invasive carcinoma, and infiltrating ductal carcinomas often contain areas with different grades of disease. This morphological heterogeneity mirrors molecular heterogeneity, as well as morphologically similar tumours may differ in genetic and metabolic processes, and specific genetic abnormalities may influence clinical outcome [4, 5].

Prognosis and likely responses to therapy are clinically important in breast cancer and many variables have been evaluated. Classical morphological variables including histological type, tumour size, grade, lymph node status, and whether or not there is blood or lymphatic vascular invasion remain the strongest predictors of tumour behaviour. Attempts to evaluate breast tumour prognosis from individual or combined expression of variables such as oestrogen and progesterone receptor, cell proliferation index, S-phase fraction, DNA ploidy, growth factors and their receptors, oncogenes, tumour suppressor genes, proteases, components of the plasminogen system, and cell cycle regulators have yet to match the clinical utility of the classical morphological factors [6].

The chief forms of carcinoma of the breast are breast cancers that are classified into those that have not penetrated the limiting basement membrane (noninvasive) and those that have (invasive). The WHO current classification [7] is illustrated in **Figure 1**.

Breast cancer is the most commonly diagnosed cancer in women with an increased incidence of 14.1 million new cases in year 2012 and high mortality rate about 8.2 million deaths all over the world [8]. The incidence rate is expected to increase by year 2020 to reach about double the rate in 2012 [9]. Young women aged 20–59 years are expected to suffer from breast cancer with increased rate of death from cancer among their age group [10].

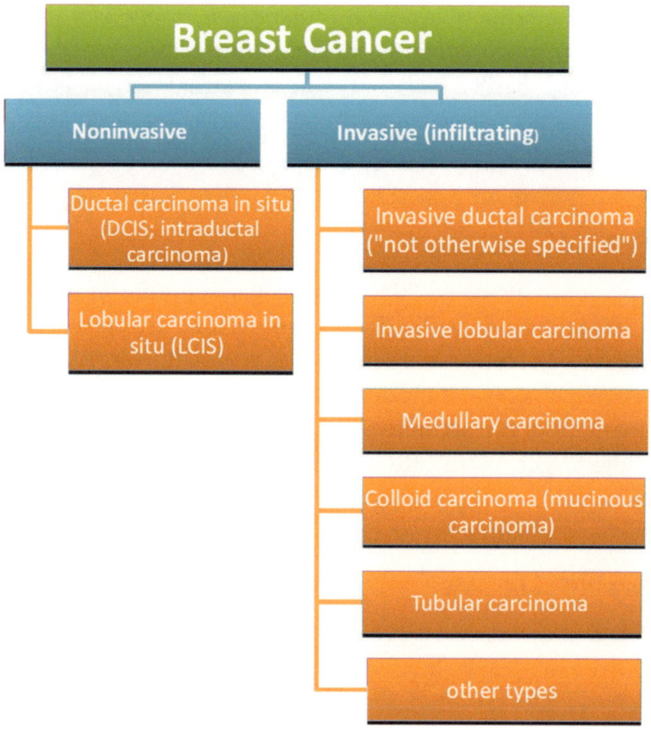

Figure 1. Classification of cancer breast.

2. Breast cancer risk factors

The transformation of the normal epithelium into carcinoma is a multistep process. Genetic background and environmental and dietary factors have a role in breast cancer development. In the normal breast tissue, there is a balance between negative and positive growth factors, so to develop, breast cancer requires loss or gain in some functions [5]. The following factors are thought to be related to breast cancer development:

2.1. Age

The increased incidence of breast cancer with age may reflect the accumulation of somatic mutation. Early menarche and late menopause prolong the exposure to ovarian hormones and are associated with a higher incidence of breast cancer. There is some evidence that breast cancer in younger women is more aggressive than in older women, consistent with a more rapidly evolving disease declaring itself sooner clinically [11].

2.2. Genetic factors

Complex acquired genetic alterations are considered to cause breast cancer, and genetic abnormalities in the premalignant and malignant breast epithelium are likely to have a causal role [12].

That most breast cancers are due to acquired mutations is implied by the fact that only 5% of breast cancer patients have a strong family history indicating inheritance of tumour-promoting mutations in the germ line. Inherited early-onset breast cancer is largely attributable to two genes, BRCA1 and BRCA2. Li-Fraumeni syndrome, ataxia telangiectasia, and Cowden's disease are also associated with increased risk of breast cancer [13].

2.3. Hormonal status

Breast cancer risk appears to increase with exposure to mammotropic hormones, mainly oestrogen, progesterone, prolactin, and insulin-like growth factor 1 during adolescence and adult life. This may be explained by an increased epithelial cell population at risk during the preinitiation stage, affecting clonal expansion and modulating growth enhancement in subclinical tumours. Estrogen is a dominant influence on breast growth, but its role depends on oestrogen receptor (ER) expression in the target tissues. Recently, it has been suggested that overexpression of oestrogen receptors in the normal breast epithelium increases breast cancer risk in women [5].

2.4. Previous benign breast disease

Clear evidence exists that certain subtypes of benign breast disease are associated with breast cancer. In benign breast neoplasia, inactivation of tumour suppressor genes may occur and loss of heterozygosity is also reported. Ductal and lobular carcinomas in situ have a partly malignant morphological phenotype, lacking the ability to invade and metastasize, but are associated with elevated invasive cancer risk. Other lesions associated with abnormal cell proliferation are also associated with more modestly elevated cancer risk, notably the atypical hyperplasia (ductal and lobular) and florid hyperplasia of usual type (that is, without atypia). Frequent coexistence of premalignant lesions with invasive breast cancer is consistent with progression from these lesions to cancer, but there are many controversies in this area, and clonal relationships are not always clear [4].

3. Carcinogenesis and pathogenesis of breast cancer

The prognosis of breast cancer is variable and affected by the heterogeneity of breast cancer, different pattern of breast subtypes, and aggressive genetic behaviour. All these factors may be associated with worsen patient outcome if accumulated with effect of hormonal status, and bilateral oophorectomy may improve prognosis in breast cancer. Depending upon these data, reduced breast cancer mortality is achieved, but still breast cancer is the most prevalent cancer in young women [14]. Aggressive behaviour of breast cancer is due to collision of biologically active tumour and genetic abnormalities, but targeted interventions may improve the survival rate and patient outcome [3].

Estrogen has a crucial role in many tumours including ovaries, endometrium, and mammary gland cancers and also prostate cancer. Estrogen is linked to enhanced proliferation, decreased apoptosis, and DNA damage in breast cancer. Several experiments on animals have demonstrated that estradiol administration increased the risk of breast cancer, while antioestrogen agents had an opposite effect. Response of breast cancer to antioestrogen therapy after the confirmed presence of high percentage of hormonal receptors is defined as hormonal-dependent breast cancer [15].

The presented framework of circulating tumour cell (CTC) biology and classification of CTC assays might help to structure this dynamic field of translational cancer research. Better insights into the biology of CTCs will further improve CTC assay development [1, 16]. Based on the theories proposed that tumour cells are heterogeneous and breast cancer is the most famous heterogeneous tumour. Therefore, CTC belonging to breast cancer requires special detection approach. Specific profile for CTCs could be targeted for successful detection of complex aggressive breast cancer [17].

Tumorigeneses are postulated by many research works due to multiple steps and may start as chronic disease and processed to cancer. Intervention and prevention of these steps before cancer emerge is a good chance for reducing breast cancer risk. Adjuvant therapies as tamoxifen are effective and safe in significantly reducing and preventing molecular changes that lead to cancer. Those targeted hormonal therapies are very important to stop invasion and metastasis of tumour cells. Blocking DNA mutation is also initiated by using micronutrients and gene therapy to target abnormal pathways that claimed to had a role in carcinogenesis [5].

4. Gene expression profiling of breast cancer

Management of breast cancer depends on clinicopathologic parameters including age, stage, hormonal status, and Ki67 status. Alteration of molecular genetic character including alterations at DNA, RNA, and the protein functional changes contributes to oncogenesis. However, epigenetic changes and regulatory or transcriptional molecules as snRNA, siRNA, and miRNA may be other significantly contributing molecules as well. Successful therapy depends on hormone receptor and human epidermal growth factor receptor 2 (Her2) pathway by analysing their immunohistochemical expression. Failure to respond to the traditional treatment increases morbidity and mortality, and so further discovery of molecular variation in individuals could help in classifying breast cancer subtypes. Clonal analysis of different breast cancer types to understand molecular modifications and genetic expression help in producing full accurate histopathological diagnosis [18].

In the past decade, where breast cancer is clustered in families due to a common genetic factor BRCA1 or BRCA2 mutation, environmental factors shared between relatives may also be relevant. There has been progress in development of new therapeutic approaches that target these BRCA1 and BRCA2 cancer susceptibility genes, which led to loss of functional mutations in either BRCA1 or BRCA2 [19].

Recent delivery of nucleic acid mimics and therapeutic-based miRNA could be used for nano-delivery of target therapy to specific site. In addition, miRNA were recently studied as biological biomarkers in breast cancer, specifically for diagnosis, predicting cancer behavior and outcome [20].

5. Hormone receptors

The breast epithelium undergoes hyperplasia or involution in response to hormone supplementation or withdrawal, and oestrogen and progesterone receptors in the breast tissue mediate proliferative effects. Certain genetic alterations (alteration to the DNA-binding domain) are associated with high overall tumour grade and lack of steroid hormone receptors; an inverse correlation between both receptor expression and nuclear anaplasia also indicates a relation with cellular differentiation. Steroid hormone receptor expression in breast neoplasia has prognostic value. Moreover, there is an independent correlation between oestrogen and progesterone receptor status in breast cancer and tumour progression [21, 22].

5.1. Oestrogen receptors (ER) and progesterone receptors (PR)

Estrogen and progesterone receptors are unique signature to define personalized therapy of breast cancer, and their genetic expression may contribute to breast cancer management through using antioestrogen-targeted therapy. If mutated DNA is spilled from dying cancerous cells into the blood stream, it will become habitant into lymphatic or blood channels and so-called circulating tumor cells. Circulating tumour cells are capable of stimulating other tissues towards continuous proliferation and could be a tool to measure tumour power and ability to enhance metastases [18]. Further research is mandatory to identify those patients at high risk of breast cancer and to understand method of optimization of circulating tumour cell measurement. In addition, there is progressive need for clinical evolution of new agents and targeted therapy, especially to whom with BRCA positive and triple-negative breast cancer patients [23].

5.2. HER2

The HER2/neu oncogene is located on chromosome 17 at band q 21. It is related to the cerbB-1 (EGFR, HER1) gene which encodes the epidermal growth factor receptor. In addition to its function as a growth factor receptor, it is involved in the regulation of cellular differentiation, adhesion, and motility. When HER2/neu gene is amplified and as a result HER2/neu protein is substantially overexpressed, it is very likely that this plays a role in tumour development and progression [3]. HER2 amplification and overexpression may provide prognostic and therapeutic information in breast cancer and predict resistance to adjuvant therapy. Amplification of this gene is associated with rapid proliferation, shorter disease-free survival, and poorer prognosis in both node-negative and node-positive ductal breast carcinomas and a risk factor for the development of distant metastases. It has true independent prognostic significance but is associated with hormone-independent tumours. Progress of personalized medicine does well for patients to depend on Herceptin treatment. The ultimate goal is to understand cancer behaviour and improve patient survival rate and treatment outcome [6]. Some of the currently utilized cancer biomarkers for breast cancer and their clinical significance are illustrated in **Table 1**.

Biomarker	Clinical utility	References
ER	ER positivity indicates better prognosis in breast cancer patients who have better survival than ER-negative breast cancer patients	[55, 56]
	Predict responsiveness to tamoxifen as when highly expressed, it predicts better response to tamoxifen therapy particularly in node-negative patients	[56]
PR	Prognostic marker indicating better survival when positively expressed (PR +ve)	[55]
	High expression of PR predicts beneficial response to tamoxifen chemotherapy	[57]
HER2/neu	Prognostic marker for worse prognosis in patients with HER2/neu-positive tumours as they have more aggressive breast cancers	[58]
	Predictor marker for the response to therapy with trastuzumab	[59]
BRCA1	Prognostic marker for poor prognosis. High expression of BRCA1 indicates worse prognosis	[60]
	If highly expressed, BRCA1 can predict response to chemotherapy in breast cancer patients	[61]
MammaPrint	Prognosticator in a heterogeneous population for stratification of breast cancer patients into good or poor prognosis, it is a 70-gene assay	[38]
Oncotype DX	A 21-gene multiplex prognostic assay used for determination of recurrence score.	[62, 63]
Isoforms Akt kinase	Akt kinase isoforms and activity are predictive markers to suggest the most likely response to trastuzumab therapy in HER2-neu-positive patients of breast cancer	[64]

Table 1. Currently utilized cancer biomarkers for breast cancer and their clinical significance.

6. Molecular targeting therapy and personalized medicine in breast cancer

Breast cancer is a heterogeneous disease that encompasses subtypes characterized by specific molecular biomarkers: oestrogen receptor (ER) positive, human epidermal growth factor receptor 2 (HER2) positive, and triple-negative (TNBC) which are ER, progesterone receptor (PR), and HER2 negative breast cancers [5]. Perfect diagnosis and detection of molecular abnormalities help in improvement of personalized therapies to block these mutations by targeted therapy. The best example is using HER2 expression by immunohistochemistry or gene amplification to develop accurate therapy with trastuzumab [24]. Trastuzumab is targeted against domain IV of HER2 [25], while pertuzumab (Perjeta) is targeted monoclonal antibody against the ligand domain II of HER2. Lapatinib is dual targeting therapy for both HER2 and epidermal growth factor receptor (EGFR 1), specifically against its intracellular domain; it acts as tyrosine kinase inhibitor (TKI) as well [26]. Patients on combined lapatinib and trastuzumab have better outcome and survival; such therapy could be assessed with HER2 expression [27]. In fact, combining the HER2 targeting therapies as a neoadjuvant or for metastatic late stage, as trastuzumab and lapatinib or pertuzumab, will significantly improve patient's outcome in comparison with single anti-HER2 therapy [28–30]. Using combined and synergistically acting therapy on the same target (HER2) would achieve better response because of the concomitant action on same receptor against two different epitopes, in addition to the likely deaddiction effect of target that may involve stimulation of the immune system [31].

6.1. mechanistic target of rapamycin (mTOR)/PI3K/Akt-pathway inhibitors

Preclinical studies of the effects of AZD2014 in breast cancer are promising steps to confirm anti-proliferative role of mTOR signalling. Targeting mTOR pathway could suppress the development and progression of cancer, specifically gastrointestinal malignancies and breast cancer. The functions of mTOR pathway are mainly targeted for growth signaling, nutrient status, and metabolism with recent undiscovered impact in obesity development [23].

6.2. Therapeutic cancer vaccine

The monoclonal antibody drugs encourage T cells to detect and destroy cancer and increase the ability of the immune system to respond to tumours. Application of therapeutic cancer vaccine stimulates tumour antigen aiming at activation of tumour-specific T cells [32]. Therapeutic cancer vaccines require the selection of appropriate antigens that are not prone to central immunological tolerance induction in the thymus. Each type of cancer has its own particular immune-suppressive mechanisms guided by information of the immune memory. Selection of the best vaccine and its antigen delivery points should take place and be applied in treatment properly [33]. Breast cancer has the advantage of being based on huge antigen pool for an individual tumour, thus using tumor based-vaccines in breast cancer stimulate the activation of polyclonal immune responses. However, tolerance could occur to the immune system for expression of these antibodies. Co-stimulation and sensitization of the immune molecules will deliver all signals needed for activating T cells under the effect of antigen-specific immune response. Cytokines in breast cancer could be an ideal example of the immune costimulatory molecules [34].

7. "Omics" and promising biomarkers in breast cancer

Recently, with the merging of "omic" technologies such as genomics, proteomics, metabolomics, transcriptomics, etc., a great advancement has been achieved in the field of cancer biology with better understanding of carcinogenesis, cancer progression, metastasis, and target therapy [35]. Microarray, mass spectrometry, and sequencing techniques provide evolutionary era for promising cancer biomarkers [36]. Transcriptional profiling has been reported as a valuable tool for classification and determination of prognosis in patients of breast cancer [37, 38]. Apart from diagnosis, prediction of response to therapy, and prediction of breast cancer patients' outcomes, biomarkers may estimate risk assessment of getting cancer [39]. Genetic alterations in breast cancer or methylation of promoters of cancer-specific or associated genes will definitely linked to altered expression of certain proteins and may be used as emerging cancer biomarkers [40].

7.1. Genomic biomarkers: MammaPrint and Oncotype DX

MammaPrint is one of the emerging genomic assays that have been reported as prognostic biomarker, MammaPrint assay analyses 70 genes' expression signatures, and it is used to stratify patients into good or poor risk groups for recurrence [41]. Another example of promising genomic markers is the 21-gene signature assessing test, Oncotype DX. It is a quantitative real-time qRT-PCR-based assay, and both assays may provide physicians with very effective prognostic information and consequently would help in selecting early-stage hormone responsive breast cancer patients who will have a likelihood of disease recurrence [38]. Signatures for both assays include genes as ER, HER2, PR-regulated transcripts and proliferation-linked genes that mainly have been utilized as a very effective tool for assessing the probability of recurrence as well as for classifying patients accordingly into high-, intermediate- or low-risk groups for recurrence. In addition, Oncotype DX assay may be used for assessing response to tamoxifen therapy [42].

7.2. Proteomics

Proteomic approach has been investigated through mass spectrometry, two-dimensional gel electrophoresis, and other strategies and successfully has identified promising markers for early diagnosis of ovarian cancer [43, 44]. In spite of being invalidated, their results have paved the path for applying the proteomic approach, via mass spectrometry, for identification of other biomarkers in serum in breast cancer [45] and nipple aspirate as well [46]. Moreover, a panel of proteins has also been identified by high-throughput antibody arrays' technique, and their levels were significantly increasing in malignant breast tissue when compared to normal tissue. Such panel included p53, MAP kinase 7, and casein kinase Ie and annexin [47]. In fact, recent proteomics techniques such as nano-techniques are evolutionally emerging and promising to overcome few limitations of the conventional techniques for identification of potential biomarkers for early detection of cancer; thus, these techniques have to be applied on larger scale of cancer patients and, more importantly, with standardized protocols in order to validate the potentially valuable biomarkers [48].

7.3. DNA methylation

DNA methylation is an example of DNA modification that could be detected and linked with the unique identity of that gene; thus, DNA methylation patterns differ between normal and tumour tissues, and hence, targeting candidate genes could be used to identify and detect cancer cells in the blood or body fluid [49]. Identification of DNA methylation mapping and assays has been applied to nipple aspirate as well for detection of cancer cells at early stage of breast cancer [50]. DNA methylation assessment has been investigated as a prognostic marker for breast cancer in serum, and it was reported that methylation of adenomatous polyposis coli (APC) gene and Ras association domain family 1 isoform A was significantly linked and independently associated with poor outcome in breast cancer patients [51].

7.4. Circulating tumour cells (CTCs)

Circulating tumour cells (CTCs) are detached or disseminated cells from solid tumours or their metastasis into circulation. It has been firstly detected in the bone marrow, called disseminated tumour cell (DTC) patients with early-stage breast cancer [52]. Once CTCs dislodged from cancerous tissues into circulation, they retain the proliferating capacity and ability to settle in other tissues. CTCs have the capability to proliferate and eventually forming metastasis.

Hence, CTC could be a predictor marker for invasion and metastases [18]. Recently, CTCs were considered a dynamic prognostic marker whether in early- or late-metastasizing breast cancer cases [53]. Evaluation of CTCs might contribute for efficient therapy monitoring; in addition, expression profiles of CTCs may predict the likely responses to treatment. As well, assessment of the molecular features of them may be a pivotal step for the optimization of therapy [54].

8. Conclusion and prospective

Breast cancer with its heterogeneous nature and complex behaviour in great needs requires potential biomarkers to improve screening, diagnosis, classification, prognosis, and prediction to therapies. Understanding biology of breast tumour cell, host immune defences, and the tumour microenvironment may allow early detection and recurrence in breast cancer patients.

Breast cancer patients, clinician, pharmaceutical companies, and targeted therapy developer in great needs for flexible, simple, and inexpensive tests with sharp accurate comprehensive diagnosis. The identified molecular aberrations could be arrested and held up by the corresponding targeted compounds, which are best exemplified by detection of HER2neu expression in breast cancer by immunohistochemistry and gene amplification tests for accurate treatment with trastuzumab. Molecular fingerprint for breast cancer generated to help medical practitioner and healthcare providers to focus on patient's prognosis and adopted the preferred best therapeutic option. Designation of distinctive incompatible genetic markers enhances shrinkage of toxic side effect from overuse of therapies and exaggerated gains to patients.

Author details

Hala Fawzy Mohamed Kamel[1,2]*, Hiba Saeed Bagader Al-Amodi[1] and Hanan Mohamed AbdElmoneim[3,4]

*Address all correspondence to: kamelhala@msn.com; dr.halakamel@gmail.com

1 Biochemistry Department, Faculty of Medicine, Umm AL Qura University, Makhha, Saudi Arabia

2 Medical Biochemistry Department, Faculty of Medicine, Ain Shams University, Cairo, Egypt

3 Pathology Department, Faculty of Medicine, Umm AL Qura University, Makhha, Saudi Arabia

4 Pathology Department, Faculty of Medicine, El-Minia University, El-Minia, Egypt

References

[1] Allison, K.H., *Molecular pathology of breast cancer: what a pathologist needs to know*. Am J Clin Pathol, 2012. **138**(6): p. 770–80.

[2] Davies, E.L., *Breast cancer*. Medicine, 2016. **44**(1): p. 42–46.

[3] Daly, B. and Olopade, O.I., *A perfect storm: how tumor biology, genomics, and health care delivery patterns collide to create a racial survival disparity in breast cancer and proposed interventions for change*. CA Cancer J Clin, 2015. **65**(3): p. 221–238.

[4] Petridis, C., et al., *Genetic predisposition to ductal carcinoma in situ of the breast*. Breast Cancer Res, 2016. **18**(1): p. 22.

[5] Maresso, K.C., et al., *Molecular cancer prevention: current status and future directions*. CA Cancer J Clin, 2015. **65**(5): p. 345–383.

[6] Anaya, J., et al., *A pan-cancer analysis of prognostic genes*. PeerJ, 2015. **3**: p. e1499.

[7] Lebeau, A., et al., *Invasive breast cancer: the current WHO classification*. Pathologe, 2014. **35**(1): p. 7–17.

[8] Ferlay, J., et al., *Cancer incidence and mortality worldwide: sources, methods and major patterns in GLOBOCAN 2012*. Int J Cancer, 2015. **136**(5): p. E359–E386.

[9] Cho, W.C., *Contribution of oncoproteomics to cancer biomarker discovery*. Mol Cancer, 2007. **6**: p. 25.

[10] Goossens, N., et al., *Cancer biomarker discovery and validation*. Transl Cancer Res, 2015. **4**(3): p. 256–269.

[11] Brenner, D.R., et al., *Breast cancer survival among young women: a review of the role of modifiable lifestyle factors*. Cancer Causes Control, 2016. **27**(4): p. 459–472.

[12] Tian, F., et al., *Functional characterization of breast cancer using pathway profiles*. BMC Med Genom, 2014. **7**: p. 45.

[13] Aloraifi, F., et al., *Gene analysis techniques and susceptibility gene discovery in non-BRCA1/BRCA2 familial breast cancer*. Surg Oncol, 2015. **24**(2): p. 100–109.

[14] Rakha, E.A., Reis-Filho, J.S., and Ellis, I.O., *Combinatorial biomarker expression in breast cancer*. Breast Cancer Res Treat, 2010. **120**(2): p. 293–308.

[15] Wysokinski, D., Blasiak, J., and Pawlowska, E., *Role of RUNX2 in breast carcinogenesis*. Int J Mol Sci, 2015. **16**(9): p. 20969–20993.

[16] Hanash, S.M., Baik, C.S., and Kallioniemi, O., *Emerging molecular biomarkers–blood-based strategies to detect and monitor cancer*. Nat Rev Clin Oncol, 2011. **8**(3): p. 142–150.

[17] Alix-Panabières, C. and Pantel, K., *Challenges in circulating tumor cell research*. Nat Rev Cancer, 2014. **14**(9): p. 623–631.

[18] Naik, R., Veldore, V.H., and Gopinath, K.S., *Genetics and breast cancer–oncologists perspectives*. Indian J Surg Oncol, 2015. **6**(4): p. 415–419.

[19] Lord, C.J. and Ashworth, A., *BRCAness revisited*. Nat Rev Cancer, 2016. **16**(2): p. 110–120.

[20] Kaboli, P.J., et al., *MicroRNA-based therapy and breast cancer: a comprehensive review of novel therapeutic strategies from diagnosis to treatment*. Pharmacol Res, 2015. **97**: p. 104–121.

[21] Deblois, G. and Giguere, V., *Oestrogen-related receptors in breast cancer: control of cellular metabolism and beyond*. Nat Rev Cancer, 2013. **13**(1): p. 27–36.

[22] Yager, J.D. and Davidson, N.E., *Estrogen carcinogenesis in breast cancer*. N Engl J Med, 2006. **354**(3): p. 270–282.

[23] Torres, S., et al., *Patterns in target-directed breast cancer research*. Springerplus, 2016. **5**: p. 109.

[24] Pugliano, L., Zardavas, D., and Piccart, M., *Personalized medicine for breast cancer: dream or reality?* memo–Mag Eur Med Oncol, 2013. **6**(3): p. 158–166.

[25] Hurvitz, S.A., et al., *Current approaches and future directions in the treatment of HER2-positive breast cancer*. Cancer Treat Rev, 2013. **39**(3): p. 219–229.

[26] Badache, A. and Hynes, N.E., *A new therapeutic antibody masks ErbB2 to its partners*. Cancer Cell, 2004. **5**(4): p. 299–301.

[27] Konecny, G.E., et al., *Activity of the dual kinase inhibitor lapatinib (GW572016) against HER-2-overexpressing and trastuzumab-treated breast cancer cells*. Cancer Res, 2006. **66**(3): p. 1630–1639.

[28] Baselga, J., et al., *Lapatinib with trastuzumab for HER2-positive early breast cancer (NeoALTTO): a randomised, open-label, multicentre, phase 3 trial*. Lancet, 2012. **379**(9816): p. 633–640.

[29] de Azambuja, E., et al., *Lapatinib with trastuzumab for HER2-positive early breast cancer (NeoALTTO): survival outcomes of a randomised, open-label, multicentre, phase 3 trial and their association with pathological complete response*. Lancet Oncol, 2014. **15**(10): p. 1137–1146.

[30] Hicks, M., et al., *Neoadjuvant dual HER2-targeted therapy with lapatinib and trastuzumab improves pathologic complete response in patients with early stage HER2-positive breast cancer: a meta-analysis of randomized prospective clinical trials*. Oncologist, 2015. **20**(4): p. 337–343.

[31] Arnedos, M., et al., *Personalized treatments of cancer patients: a reality in daily practice, a costly dream or a shared vision of the future from the oncology community?* Cancer Treat Rev, 2014. **40**(10): p. 1192–1198.

[32] Dragani, T.A., et al., *Major milestones in translational oncology*. BMC Med, 2016. **14**(1): p. 110.

[33] van der Burg, S.H., et al., *Vaccines for established cancer: overcoming the challenges posed by immune evasion*. Nat Rev Cancer, 2016. **16**(4): p. 219–233.

[34] Curigliano, G., et al., *Breast cancer vaccines: a clinical reality or fairy tale?* Ann Oncol, 2006. **17**(5): p. 750–762.

[35] Liotta, L.A. and Petricoin, E.F. 3rd, *-Omics and cancer biomarkers: link to the biological truth or bear the consequences*. Cancer Epidemiol Biomarkers Prev, 2012. **21**(8): p. 1229–1235.

[36] Diamandis, E.P., *Present and future of cancer biomarkers*. Clin Chem Lab Med, 2014. **52**(6): pp. 791–794.

[37] Bertucci, F., et al., *Gene expression profiling of primary breast carcinomas using arrays of candidate genes*. Hum Mol Genet, 2000. **9**(20): pp. 2981–2991.

[38] van't Veer, L.J., et al., *Gene expression profiling predicts clinical outcome of breast cancer*. Nature, 2002. **415**(6871): pp. 530–536.

[39] Ross, J.S., et al., *Breast cancer biomarkers*. Adv Clin Chem, 2005. **40**: pp. 99–125.

[40] Sotiriou, C. and Pusztai, L., *Gene-expression signatures in breast cancer*. N Engl J Med, 2009. **360**(8): pp. 790–800.

[41] Tian, S., et al., *Biological functions of the genes in the mammaprint breast cancer profile reflect the hallmarks of cancer*. Biomark Insights, 2010. **5**: pp. 129–138.

[42] Habel, L.A., et al., *A population-based study of tumor gene expression and risk of breast cancer death among lymph node-negative patients*. Breast Cancer Res, 2006. **8**(3): p. R25.

[43] Jones, M.B., et al., *Proteomic analysis and identification of new biomarkers and therapeutic targets for invasive ovarian cancer*. Proteomics, 2002. **2**(1): pp. 76–84.

[44] Petricoin, E.F., et al., *Use of proteomic patterns in serum to identify ovarian cancer*. Lancet, 2002. **359**(9306): pp. 572–577.

[45] Li, J., et al., *Proteomics and bioinformatics approaches for identification of serum biomarkers to detect breast cancer*. Clin Chem, 2002. **48**(8): pp. 1296–1304.

[46] Paweletz, C.P., et al., *Proteomic patterns of nipple aspirate fluids obtained by SELDI-TOF: potential for new biomarkers to aid in the diagnosis of breast cancer*. Dis Markers, 2001. **17**(4): pp. 301–307.

[47] Hudelist, G., et al., *Use of high-throughput protein array for profiling of differentially expressed proteins in normal and malignant breast tissue*. Breast Cancer Res Treat, 2004. **86**(3): pp. 281–291.

[48] Ray, S., et al., *Proteomic technologies for the identification of disease biomarkers in serum: advances and challenges ahead*. Proteomics, 2011. **11**(11): pp. 2139–2161.

[49] Costanzo, M., et al., *Charting the genetic interaction map of a cell*. Curr Opin Biotechnol, 2011. **22**(1): pp. 66–74.

[50] Szyf, M., Pakneshan, P., and Rabbani, S.A., *DNA methylation and breast cancer*. Biochem Pharmacol, 2004. **68**(6): pp. 1187–1197.

[51] Muller, H.M., et al., *DNA methylation in serum of breast cancer patients: an independent prognostic marker*. Cancer Res, 2003. **63**(22): pp. 7641–7645.

[52] Vincent-Salomon, A., Bidard, F.C., and Pierga, J.Y., *Bone marrow micrometastasis in breast cancer: review of detection methods, prognostic impact and biological issues*. J Clin Pathol, 2008. **61**(5): p. 570–576.

[53] Bidard, F.C., Proudhon, C., and Pierga, J.Y., *Circulating tumor cells in breast cancer*. Mol Oncol, 2016. **10**(3): p. 418–430.

[54] Banys-Paluchowski, M., et al., *Circulating tumor cells in breast cancer–current status and perspectives*. Crit Rev Oncol Hematol, 2016. **97**: p. 22–29.

[55] Dowsett, M., et al., *Benefit from adjuvant tamoxifen therapy in primary breast cancer patients according oestrogen receptor, progesterone receptor, EGF receptor and HER2 status*. Ann Oncol, 2006. **17**(5): p. 818–826.

[56] Morgan, D.A., Refalo, N.A., and Cheung, K.L., *Strength of ER-positivity in relation to survival in ER-positive breast cancer treated by adjuvant tamoxifen as sole systemic therapy*. Breast, 2011. **20**(3): p. 215–219.

[57] Oldenhuis, C.N., et al., *Prognostic versus predictive value of biomarkers in oncology*. Eur J Cancer, 2008. **44**(7): p. 946–953.

[58] Mass, R.D., et al., *Evaluation of clinical outcomes according to HER2 detection by fluorescence in situ hybridization in women with metastatic breast cancer treated with trastuzumab*. Clin Breast Cancer, 2005. **6**(3): p. 240–246.

[59] Ali, S.M., et al., *Value of serum human epidermal growth factor receptor 2 (HER2)/neu testing for early prediction of response to HER2/neu-directed therapies is still an open one and deserves further study in large prospective trials*. J Clin Oncol, 2009. **27**(36): p. e273; author reply e274–e275.

[60] James, C.R., et al., *BRCA1, a potential predictive biomarker in the treatment of breast cancer*. Oncologist, 2007. **12**(2): p. 142–150.

[61] Domagala, P., et al., *Immunophenotypic predictive profiling of BRCA1-associated breast cancer*. Virchows Arch, 2011. **458**(1): p. 55–64.

[62] Goldstein, L.J., et al., *Prognostic utility of the 21-gene assay in hormone receptor-positive operable breast cancer compared with classical clinicopathologic features*. J Clin Oncol, 2008. **26**(25): p. 4063–4071.

[63] Paik, S., et al., *A multigene assay to predict recurrence of tamoxifen-treated, node-negative breast cancer*. N Engl J Med, 2004. **351**(27): p. 2817–2826.

[64] Grell, P., et al., *Akt expression and compartmentalization in prediction of clinical outcome in HER2-positive metastatic breast cancer patients treated with trastuzumab*. Int J Oncol, 2012. **41**(4): p. 1204–1212.

Chapter 18

Cardiac Toxicity of HER2-Directed Therapy in Women with Breast Cancer: Epidemiology, Etiology, Risk Factors, and Management

Shahid Ahmed, Arooba Talat, Nayyer Iqbal,
Mohamed Emara, Duc Le, Amir Sami and Jim Xiang

Additional information is available at the end of the chapter

http://dx.doi.org/10.5772/66437

Abstract

The HER2-targeted therapy have profoundly changed the outcomes of women with HER2-positive breast cancers. Trastuzumab and pertuzumab, HER2-targeting monoclonal antibodies, lapatinib and Neratinib, small molecule inhibitors of HER2 and the epidermal growth factor receptor, and ado-trastuzumab emtansine, a HER2-positive directed antibody drug conjugate, are approved for the treatment of HER2-positive breast cancer.

Cardiac toxicity is a known adverse effects of trastuzumab, and other HER2-directed therapy. In most cases it manifests as mild and reversible left ventricle dysfunction. Nevertheless, symptomatic heart failure is not rare. The incidence and severity of cardiac dysfunction is greatest among women who received HER2-directed therapy in combination with anthracycline-based therapy. In addition, a borderline low normal left ventricle ejection fraction; prior treatment with antihypertensive medication; and older age are other risk factors for trastuzumab-related cardiac dysfunction. HER2 signaling plays an important role in modulating myocardial response to treatment-related injury. Management of trastuzumab and the other HER2 targeted treatment-related cardiac dysfunction has two key components: withdrawal of HER2-directed therapy and treatment of underlying cardiac dysfunction. A multidisciplinary approach is recommended for an optimal outcome. This chapter reviews cardiac toxicity of trastuzumab and other HER2-directed therapy including epidemiology and pathophysiology of cardiac dysfunction, cardiac monitoring, treatment and prevention.

Keywords: breast cancer, HER2-directed therapy, cardiac toxicity, trastuzumab, pertuzumab, lapatinib, T-DM1, Neratinib

1. Introduction

Breast cancer is one of the most common cancers in women worldwide [1]. In 2012, nearly 1.7 million women were diagnosed with breast cancer. This represents about 12% of all new cancer cases and 25% of all cancers in women [2]. Approximately 20–25% of all breast cancers overexpressed the human epidermal growth factor receptor-2 (HER2). This protein is a member of the HER family of transmembrane receptor tyrosine kinases and is located at the cell surface. HER2 is involved in cellular growth and differentiation, and its overexpression has been associated with adverse prognosis. Prior to the development of HER2-targeted therapy, women with HER2-positive breast cancer had poor outcomes. However, access to HER2-directed therapy including monoclonal antibodies, small molecule inhibitors, and antibody-drug conjugates in the management of early and advanced breast cancer has transformed the natural history of HER2-positive breast cancer [3, 4]. HER2-targeted therapy alone or in combination with chemotherapy has been associated with improvements in response rate, disease control rates, and overall survival in HER2-positive metastatic breast cancer [3–5]. Combination of HER2-targeted agents including dual HER2 blockade and selected delivery of potent chemotherapeutic agent along with HER2 inhibition are new therapeutic approaches that in many women have transformed metastatic HER2-positive breast cancer into a chronic disease. More importantly, HER2 blockade in early-stage breast cancer has resulted in lower recurrence and mortality [3, 6].

As the outcomes of women with HER2-positive breast cancer have improved, increasingly attention has been directed toward minimizing both acute and chronic treatment-related toxicities. Cardiac toxicity is a known adverse effect of trastuzumab and other HER2-directed therapy [7, 8]. In most cases, it manifests as mild and reversible left ventricle dysfunction. Nevertheless, overt heart failure is not unusual. Serial monitoring of cardiac function is recommended for women treated with HER2-directed therapy. In women with treatment-related cardiac dysfunction, trastuzumab and other HER2-directed therapy interruptions and treatment of cardiac dysfunction are recommended. This chapter provides a summary of efficacy of HER2-directed therapy in breast cancer and reviews the incidence, pathophysiology, risk factors, monitoring, and management and prevention of HER2-targeted treatment-related cardiac dysfunction.

2. Efficacy of HER2-directed therapy

The current HER2-directed treatments for women with HER2-positive breast cancer include monoclonal antibodies, small molecule inhibitors, and antibody-drug conjugates (**Table 1**). Trastuzumab is the prototype humanized monoclonal antibody directed against the extracellular domain of human epidermal growth factor receptor-2 [9]. It was first evaluated in women with HER2-positive metastatic breast cancer. The combination of trastuzumab and chemotherapy resulted in improvement in progression-free and overall survival compared with chemotherapy alone, in women with HER2-positive metastatic breast cancer [5]. A Cochrane review assessed efficacy and safety of trastuzumab in seven trials, involving 1497 women with advanced breast cancer [10]. The combined hazard ratios (HRs) for overall survival and progression-free survival favored the trastuzumab-containing regimens (HR 0.82, 95% confidence interval (CI) 0.71–0.94, p-value = 0.004; and HR 0.61, 95% CI 0.54–0.70, p-value < 0.00001, respectively).

Class	Comments
Monoclonal antibodies	
Trastuzumab	A humanized monoclonal antibody directed against the extracellular domain of the HER2 receptor that prevents ligand-independent HER2 signaling. It has demonstrated efficacy in both early and advanced stage breast cancer
Pertuzumab	A humanized monoclonal antibody that binds to the extracellular domain II of HER2 and inhibits ligand-dependent HER2-HER3 dimerization. It has been evaluated in combination with trastuzumab in preoperative setting and advanced breast cancer
Antibody-drug conjugates	
Ado-trastuzumab emtansine	An antibody-drug conjugate consisting of the cytotoxic agent DM1 linked to trastuzumab. It has demonstrated efficacy in advanced breast cancer
Small molecules inhibitors	
Lapatinib	An oral dual EGFR/ErbB2 reversible tyrosine kinase inhibitor blocking both HER1 and HER2 that suppresses the downstream pathways. It has been evaluated in both early and advanced breast cancer.
Afatinib, Neratinib	Irreversible tyrosine kinase inhibitor of EGFR/HER2/HER4

Table 1. List of current HER2-directed targeted drugs that are approved for the management of HER2-positive breast cancer.

Later trastuzumab was evaluated in women with early-stage breast cancer, in both adjuvant and neoadjuvant settings, and demonstrated improvement in disease-free and overall survival. A Cochrane review evaluated efficacy and toxicity of trastuzumab in eight studies involving 11,991 women with early-stage breast cancer [11]. The combined HRs for overall survival and disease-free survival significantly favored the trastuzumab-containing regimens (HR 0.66; 95% CI 0.57–0.77, p-value < 0.00001; and HR 0.60; 95% CI 0.50–0.71, p-value < 0.00001, respectively). Based on results from five randomized adjuvant trials in women with node-positive or high-risk node-negative breast cancer, 1 year of adjuvant trastuzumab has become the standard therapy for women with HER2-positive breast cancer [6, 12–14].

Lapatinib is a dual EGFR/HER2 reversible tyrosine kinase inhibitor that suppresses the downstream signaling involving MAPK/Erk1/2 and PI3K/Akt pathways by blocking both HER1 and HER2 [15]. Lapatinib has demonstrated efficacy in HER2-positive advanced breast cancer [16]. In addition, it has been assessed in both adjuvant and neoadjuvant settings in women with early-stage breast cancer. However, overall the data suggest that lapatinib in early-stage breast cancer is inferior compared with trastuzumab [3, 17].

Pertuzumab is a humanized monoclonal antibody that binds to the extracellular domain II of HER2. It inhibits ligand-dependent HER2-HER3 dimerization and reduces signaling via intracellular pathways such as PI3K/Akt [18]. Pertuzumab has limited antitumor clinical activity alone, but it is a very good synergistic drug when combined with trastuzumab and has demonstrated benefit in combination with trastuzumab in the treatment of both early (neoadjuvant setting) and advanced HER2-positive breast cancer [3, 19, 20]. In the neoadjuvant setting, the pooled pathological complete response rate in the dual anti-HER2 therapy group was 54.8% compared with 36% in the monotherapy group when used in combination with chemotherapy (relative risk [RR], 1.56; 95% CI 1.23–1.97; p-value < 0.001). In the metastatic setting, dual anti-HER2 therapy demonstrated significant benefits in both progression-free survival (HR, 0.71; 95% CI 0.62–0.81; p-value < 0.001) and overall survival (HR, 0.68; 95% CI 0.57–0.82; p-value < 0.001) [21].

Ado-trastuzumab emtansine (T-DM1) is an antibody-drug conjugate consisting of an anti-microtubule cytotoxic agent DM1 linked to trastuzumab [22]. In women with HER2-positive advanced breast cancer, who were previously treated with trastuzumab and a taxane, it has shown significant improvement in progression-free and overall survival compared with lapatinib plus capecitabine [23].

Neratinib is an irreversible binder of HER1, HER2, and HER3 receptors [22, 24] It has demonstrated efficacy in HER2-positive breast cancer that progress on trastuzumab [3]. In addition, 1 year of neratinib following adjuvant chemotherapy and trastuzumab in women with HER2-positive breast cancer has been associated with modest improvement in disease-free survival [25].

In summary, over the past 15 years, HER2-directed therapy has revolutionized the management of HER2-positive breast cancer. In women with early-stage cancer, neoadjuvant and adjuvant HER2-directed therapies have substantially improved the disease-free and overall survival. Likewise, for many women, HER2-targeted therapy has transformed HER2-positive advanced breast cancer into a chronic disease. For example, median overall survival of women with HER2-positive advanced cancer has improved from 20.3 months reported by Slamon et al. in the first randomized trial using trastuzumab with chemotherapy to 48 months with the use of triple combination of pertuzumab, trastuzumab, and docetaxel [5, 26].

3. Cardiac safety of HER2-directed therapy

3.1. Trastuzumab

Trastuzumab-related cardiac dysfunction incidence varies according to the underlying treated population and the definition of cardiac toxicity used in the clinical trials. In the pivotal clinical trial that evaluated trastuzumab in combination with chemotherapy (anthracycline or taxane) in women with HER2-positive metastatic breast cancer, a high rate of cardiac dysfunction was noted, especially when trastuzumab was given in combination with an anthracycline-based chemotherapy [5]. In this trial, cardiac dysfunction was observed in

27% of the women who received an anthracycline, cyclophosphamide, and trastuzumab; 8% of the women who received an anthracycline and cyclophosphamide alone; 13% of the women who received paclitaxel and trastuzumab; and only 1% of the women who received paclitaxel alone. Among these women, the incidence of cardiac dysfunction of New York Heart Association class III or IV was 16% among women who were treated with an anthracycline, cyclophosphamide, and trastuzumab; 3% among women who received an anthracycline and cyclophosphamide alone; 2% among women who received paclitaxel and trastuzumab; and 1% among those who were treated with paclitaxel alone (**Table 2**). Given a high risk of symptomatic heart failure with the concomitant use of trastuzumab with anthracycline, in all adjuvant breast cancer trials, trastuzumab was only used after anthracyclines or with anthracycline-free chemotherapy. A Cochrane review assessed efficacy and safety of trastuzumab in seven trials, involving 1497 women with advanced breast cancer [10]. Trastuzumab increased the risk of congestive heart failure (CHF) (RR 3.49, 90% CI 1.88–6.47, p-value = 0.0009) and left ventricular ejection fraction (LVEF) decline (RR 2.65, 90% CI 1.48–4.74, p-value = 0.006).

Class	New York association functional classification	Canadian Cardiovascular Society functional classification
I	Patients with cardiac disease but without resulting limitations of physical activity	Ordinary physical activity, such as walking and climbing stairs, does not cause angina
II	Patients with cardiac disease resulting in slight limitation of physical activity	Slight limitation of ordinary activity
III	Patients with cardiac disease resulting in marked limitation of physical activity	Marked limitation of ordinary physical activity
IV	Patients with cardiac disease resulting in inability to carry on any physical activity without discomfort	Inability to carry on any physical activity without discomfort

Table 2. New York association and Canadian Cardiovascular Society functional classifications.

In the major adjuvant trastuzumab clinical trials, the rates of symptomatic CHF varied from 0.6 to 4.1%, whereas the rates of symptomatic or minimally symptomatic reduction in LVEF ranged from 4 to 34% (**Table 3**). The Herceptin Adjuvant (HERA) trial compared 1 or 2 years of trastuzumab given once every 3 weeks with observation in women with HER2-positive breast cancer. The incidence of trastuzumab discontinuation due to cardiac disorders was 4.3% [8]. The incidence of cardiac end points was higher in the trastuzumab group compared with observation: severe CHF, 0.60% compared with 0.06%; symptomatic CHF, 2.15% compared with 0.12%; and confirmed significant LVEF drops, 3.04% compared with 0.53%. Most women with cardiac dysfunction recovered in fewer than 6 months.

The National Surgical Adjuvant Breast and Bowel Project trial B-31 compared doxorubicin and cyclophosphamide (AC) followed by paclitaxel with AC followed by paclitaxel plus 52 weeks of trastuzumab beginning concurrently with paclitaxel in women with node-positive, HER2-positive breast cancer [27]. Among women with normal post-AC LVEF

Trial	N	Design	Definition of severe cardiotoxicity	Frequency of monitoring	Asymptomatic drop in LVEF (≥10% points to <55%)	Severe CHF/cardiac events (NYHA class III/IV CHF or death)	Discontinued for cardiac reasons
FinHer[12, 29]	232	V or T + H versus V or T[a] ≥FEC × 3	Myocardial infarction; HF; or LVEF decrease >15 points	Echo or MUGA before chemotherapy, after FEC, and 12 and 36 months after chemotherapy	3.5 versus 8.6%	0.9 versus 1.7%	n/a
NSABP B-31[27, 14]	2030	AC + TH + H versus AC + T	Grade III/IV HF or cardiac death; or LVEF decrease >15 points[b]	MUGA 3 weeks, 6, and 9 months after end of initial AC, and 3 months after last trastuzumab dose	34 versus 17%	4.1 versus 0.8%	19%[c]
BCIRG 006[6]	3222	AC + T versus AC + TH + H versus TCaH[d]	Grade III/IV HF; cardiac death; grade 3–4 arrhythmias; grade 3–4 ischemia/infarction; or LVEF decrease >10 points[b]	After AC, after second dose of docetaxel, at end of chemotherapy, and 3, 12, and 36 months after randomization	11 versus 19% versus 9%	0.7 versus 2.0% versus 0.4%	n/a
NCCTG N9831[28, 14]	3505	AC + TH + H versus AC + T + H versus AC + T	Grade III/IV HF or cardiac death; or LVEF decrease >15 points[b]	MUGA or echo at entry, after AC, and 6, 9, 18, and 21 months after entry	5.8–10.4 versus 4.0–7.8% versus 4.0–5.1%	3.3 versus 2.8% versus 0.3%	n/a[b]
HERA[8, 13]	5090	Adj chemoc[e] ≥H versus Adj chemo alone	Severe HF; symptomatic HF; or LVEF decrease >10 points	LVEF (echo or MUGA) at baseline, 3, 6, 12, 18, 24, 30, 36, and 60 months	7.1 versus 2.2%	0.6 versus 0.06%	4.3%

A: anthracycline; C: cyclophosphamide; T: taxane; H: trastuzumab; Ca: carboplatin; V: vinorelbine; F: 5-flourouracil; E: epirubicin; n/a: information not available; HF: heart failure; LV0EF: left ventricular heart failure; MUGA: multi-gated acquisition scan.

[a] No prior anthracycline before H exposure; H exposure limited to 9 weeks.

[b] Measured from baseline.

[c] 6.7% did not receive H after A due to unacceptable drops in LVEF.

[d] Included a nonanthracycline arm.

[e] 96% of chemotherapy was A containing.

Table 3. Rates of asymptomatic and symptomatic cardiac dysfunction in various adjuvant trastuzumab phase 3 clinical trials.

who began post-AC treatment, 5 of 814 (0.006%) women in the control group developed a cardiac event compared with 31 of 850 (0.036%) women treated with trastuzumab. The difference in cumulative incidence at 3 years was 3.3% (4.1% for trastuzumab-treated women minus 0.8% for control patients; 95% CI 1.7–4.9%). Twenty-seven of the 31 patients in the trastuzumab arm have been followed for ≥6 months after diagnosis of a CE; 26 were asymptomatic at last assessment; and 18 remained on cardiac medication. Fourteen percent of patients discontinued trastuzumab because of asymptomatic decreases in LVEF; 4% discontinued trastuzumab because of symptomatic cardiotoxicity.

In the North Central Cancer Treatment Group N9831 adjuvant breast cancer trial, women with HER2-positive operable breast cancer were randomly assigned to AC followed by either weekly paclitaxel (arm A); paclitaxel then trastuzumab (arm B); or paclitaxel plus trastuzumab then trastuzumab alone (arm C) [28]. There were 1944 women with satisfactory or no LVEF evaluation who proceeded to post-AC therapy. Cardiac events (CHF or cardiac death) were as followed: arm A, n = 3; arm B, n = 19; and arm C, n = 19 with 3-year cumulative incidences of 0.3, 2.8, and 3.3%, respectively. Incidence of asymptomatic LVEF decreases requiring holding trastuzumab was 8–10%; LVEF recovered and trastuzumab were restarted in approximately 50%.

The Breast Cancer International Research Group randomly assigned 3222 women with HER2-positive early-stage breast cancer to receive doxorubicin and cyclophosphamide followed by docetaxel every 3 weeks (AC-T), the same regimen plus 52 weeks of trastuzumab (AC-T plus trastuzumab), or docetaxel and carboplatin plus 52 weeks of trastuzumab (TCH) [6]. The incidence of congestive heart failure in the two trastuzumab-containing regimens was higher in the group receiving AC-T plus trastuzumab (2.0%) than in the AC-T group (0.7%) or the TCH group (0.4%); the incidence with AC-T plus trastuzumab as compared with TCH was increased by a factor of five. In addition, a significant difference in sustained, subclinical loss of mean LVEF (defined as >10% relative loss), was observed in the group receiving AC-T plus trastuzumab, as compared with the TCH group (18.6 versus 9.4%, p-value < 0.001), with a rate of 11.2% in the AC-T group. Of 194 of the 1042 patients (19%) who had a relative reduction in LVEF of more than 10% in the group receiving AC-T plus trastuzumab, the decrease persisted for at least 4 years after randomization in 33% of the women.

The FinHer investigators randomly assigned 1010 women to receive three cycles of docetaxel or vinorelbine, followed by three cycles of fluorouracil, epirubicin, and cyclophosphamide (FEC). The 232 women with HER2-positive cancer were further assigned to receive or not to receive nine weekly trastuzumab infusions [12]. The incidence of symptomatic heart failure among the HER2-positive women was 0.9% (one patient) with trastuzumab and 1.7% (two patients) without trastuzumab. The incidence of absolute declines in LVEF >20% points from baseline was 6.8% with trastuzumab and 10.5% without trastuzumab [12, 29].

The Cochrane review evaluated toxicity of trastuzumab in eight studies involving 11,991 women with early-stage breast cancer [11]. Trastuzumab significantly increased the risk of CHF (RR 5.11; 90% CI 3.00–8.72, p-value < 0.00001) and LVEF (RR 1.83; 90% CI 1.36–2.47, p-value = 0.0008).

3.2. Lapatinib and other HER2-directed therapies

In the Adjuvant Lapatinib and/or Trastuzumab Treatment Optimization trial (ALTTO), 8381 women with HER2-positive early breast cancer were randomly assigned to 1 year of adjuvant therapy with trastuzumab, lapatinib, their sequence (T → L), or their combination (L + T). Overall, incidence of primary or secondary cardiac end points was low in all treatment arms; primary cardiac end points occurred in 0.25–0.97% of women. Three fatal cardiac events occurred in the T → L arm and one in each of the other treatment arms [17].

A comprehensive analysis of 49 clinical trials involving 3689 women treated with lapatinib reported a low rated of cardiac events [30]. For example, asymptomatic cardiac events were reported in 53 women (1.4%), and symptomatic grade III and IV systolic dysfunction was observed only in 7 women (0.2%) treated with lapatinib. Cardiac safety of lapatinib in combination with trastuzumab is reviewed in the section of dual HER2-directed therapy.

Cardiotoxicity of pertuzumab was usually reported with the trastuzumab combination, and no additive cardiotoxicity was reported with addition of pertuzumab to trastuzumab. In phase I–III trials of pertuzumab, cardiac dysfunction was seen in 4.5–14.5% of women with pertuzumab treatment and cardiac dysfunction was usually grade I and II [30]. Cardiac safety of pertuzumab is reviewed in more detail in the section of dual HER2-directed therapy.

T-DM1 had a better safety profile compared to trastuzumab, and no significant cardiotoxicity was observed with T-DM1 in heavily pre-treated women. In the EMILIA study, only in 1.7% of women in the T-DM1 group experienced reduction in LVEF and grade III LVEF reduction developed only in one woman (0.2%) in the T-DM1 group compared to the lapatinib plus capacitabine group [23]. In phase I-II trials with neratinib, no cardiotoxicity was reported, whereas cardiotoxicity was seen between 0 and 5.3% with afatinib treatment [30].

3.3. Dual HER2-directed therapy

Several trials have evaluated dual HER2-directed therapy using trastuzumab in combination with lapatinib or pertuzumab in the neoadjuvant setting and metastatic breast cancer. These trials reported the risk of heart failure with dual HER2-directed therapy [20, 26, 31–34]. A meta-analysis of randomized clinical trials compared the risk of cardiac adverse events with dual HER2-directed therapy to HER2 monotherapy and reported a comparable cardiac toxicity between combination and mono-HER2-directed therapies [35]. Overall incidence results for CHF in dual HER2-directed and monotherapy were 0.88% (95% CI 0.47–1.64%) and 1.49% (95% CI 0.98–2.23%). The incidence of LVEF decline was 3.1% (95% CI 2.2–4.4%) and 2.9% (95% CI 2.1–4.1%), respectively. When stratified by each treatment combination, the incidence of CHF was 0.96% (95% CI 0.40–2.31%) for the trastuzumab plus lapatinib combination and 0.80% (95% CI 0.33–1.93%) for the trastuzumab plus pertuzumab combination, while the LVEF decline was 3.2% (95% CI 1.8–5.7%) and 3.1% (95% CI 1.9–4.8%), respectively. The odd ratio of CHF between dual and monotherapy was 0.58 (95% CI 0.26–1.27, p-value = 0.17), while the odd ratio of LVEF decline was 0.88 (95% CI 0.53–1.48, p-value = 0.64). Among the two trials in the metastatic setting [19, 31], there was no association between dual anti-HER2 therapy and either CHF (OR: 0.85, 95% CI 0.31–2.37, *p*-value = 0.76) or LVEF decline (OR: 1.11, 95% CI 0.24–5.02, *p*-value = 0.90). Among the four trials in the neoadjuvant setting, there was also no evidence of an association between dual anti-HER2 therapy and CHF (OR: 0.74, 95% CI 0.02–29.54, *p*-value = 0.87) or LVEF decline (OR: 1.52, 95% CI 0.44–5.32, *p*-value = 0.51) [20, 32–34]. For CHF, the pooled ORs for the comparison trastuzumab plus lapatinib versus trastuzumab and trastuzumab plus lapatinib versus lapatinib were 0.33 (95% CI 0.08–1.41, *p*-value = 0.13), and 0.64 (95% CI 0.22–1.88, *p*-value = 0.42), respectively. For LVEF decline, the pooled ORs for the trastuzumab plus lapatinib versus trastuzumab, trastuzumab plus lapatinib versus lapatinib, and trastuzumab plus pertuzumab versus trastuzumab were 0.53 (95% CI 0.07–3.98, *p*-value = 0.54), 2.27 (95% CI 0.69–7.49, *p*-value = 0.18), and 0.66 (95% CI 0.36–1.23, *p*-value = 0.19), respectively. Another systematic review and meta-analysis compared treatment outcomes for women who received single or combined anti-HER2 therapies [21]. Overall, no statistically significant difference in the risk of heart failure between dual anti-HER2 therapy and monotherapy was noted (RR, 0.79; 95% CI 0.23–2.68; *p*-value = 0.71). Likewise, no statistically significant difference in risk of left ventricular ejection fraction decline was noted single versus dual HER2-directed therapy (RR, 1.12; 95% CI 0.51–2.44; *p*-value = 0.77).

Overall, cardiac toxicity is more often noted with the regimens employing sequential anthracycline and taxanes. Nonetheless, the majority of women who received the therapy displayed neither acute nor delayed cardiac toxicity [29]. The rates of cardiac dysfunction with the novel HER2-targeted therapies are significantly lower than the trastuzumab. Furthermore, the combination of anti-HER2 treatment does not increase the cardiac toxicity compared to trastuzumab alone. Longer-term follow-up is required to determine the full effect of adverse cardiac events.

4. Pathophysiology of cardiac dysfunction

Cardiac dysfunction is a potential short- or long-term complication of several anticancer therapies. Although the underlying pathophysiology of trastuzumab and other novel HER2-directed therapy-induced cardiac toxicity is not fully understood, it is different from that of anthracycline-related or type I cardiac dysfunction and has been classified as type II cardiac dysfunction [36]. Whereas anthracycline-associated or type I cardiac dysfunction is dose dependent, cumulative, and potentially irreversible and has been associated with structural myocardial abnormalities, such as vacuolization, myofibrillar disarray and drop-out, and myocyte necrosis, trastuzumab-related or type II cardiac dysfunction is not dose related, does not appear to occur in all individuals, is expressed in a broad range of severity, is not related to identifiable structural changes, and, more importantly, appears to be reversible (**Table 4**) [36, 37].

Trastuzumab-induced cardiac dysfunction is considered to be the result of attenuated HER2-mediated signaling in the heart, culminating in decreased functionality of cardiac myocytes. HER

	Type I cardiac dysfunction (myocardial damage)	Type II cardiac dysfunction (myocardial dysfunction)
Prototype drug	• Doxorubicin	• Trastuzumab
Natural history	• typically permanent and irreversible • recurrence in months or years may be related to sequential cardiac stress	• reversible with high likelihood of recovery to baseline heart function in 2–4 months
Dose relationship	• dose-dependent • cumulative	• dose independent
Pathophysiology	• oxidative stress/damage • free radical formation	• blockade of HER2 signaling in myocardium
Electron microscopic findings	• vacuoles • myofibrillar disarray and dropout • necrosis • changes resolve over time	• no characteristic structural abnormalities
Noninvasive cardiac testing Findings	• decreased ejection fraction • global decrease in wall motion	• decreasedejection fraction • global decrease in wall motion
Effect of rechallenge	• high risk of progressive recurrent dysfunction • may result in intractable heart failure and death	• may be safe and appropriate for some individuals
Effect of late sequential stress	• High likelihood of sequential stress-related cardiac dysfunction	• Low likelihood of sequential stress-related cardiac dysfunction

Table 4. Cancer treatment-related cardiac dysfunction.

signaling plays an important role in modulating myocardial response to chemotherapy-induced injury and inhibition of the HER-2/erbB2 receptor worsens anthracycline-associated cardiotoxicity [38]. HER or ErbB receptors are family of transmembrane tyrosine kinase receptors that bind extracellular ligands and regulate cell growth, differentiation, and survival [39]. HER2 appears to function as a compensatory mechanism acting against cardiac stress, such as anthracycline-induced cardiotoxicity. Subsequent administration of trastuzumab may then lead to an inhibition of this compensation, resulting in heart failure [40]. Trastuzumab induces down-regulation of HER2 receptors which leads to apoptosis by disrupting downstream cytoprotective signaling pathways and by decreasing expression of Bcl-2 anti-apoptotic protein [41]. Discontinuation or trastuzumab withdrawal allows recovery of signaling pathway and reversal of LVEF decline, in contrast to the permanent myocyte dysfunction and damage caused by anthracyclines.

Trastuzumab-induced cardiotoxicity is demonstrated by inhibiting ErbB2 signaling in rat cardiac myocytes with a suitable antibody. This process promotes intrinsic (mitochondrial) apoptotic pathway that involves an increase in Bcl-XS/Bcl-XL ratio [42, 43]. Some studies showed that trastuzumab down-regulates neuregulin-1 (NRG-1), which is released in endocardium and activates MAPK and the PI3K/AKT cell survival pathways as well as focal adhesion kinases (FAK) in cardiomyocytes which are all important for the function and structure of cardiomyocytes [44].

In general, women who develop cardiotoxicity while receiving trastuzumab therapy improve upon withdrawal of the drug. Evidence suggests that reintroducing trastuzumab may be appropriate for some individuals who previously have experienced trastuzumab-related cardiac dysfunction.

5. Risk factors

The following are the risk factors for trastuzumab-associated cardiotoxicity identified in the adjuvant clinical trials: prior treatment with anthracycline-based chemotherapy; a borderline low normal left ventricle ejection fraction; prior treatment with antihypertensive medication; older age; and a body mass index >25 kg/m^2 [7, 29]. In the HERA trial, the women who had a cardiac end point received a significantly higher dose of epirubicin and doxorubicin than the women without [8]. Furthermore, women with a screening LVEF of <60% had a significantly higher incidence of cardiac end points than women with a higher screening LVEF ≥60% (6.90% versus 2.72%; 95% CI 1.33–7.02%). Women with a risk factor of hypertension, current smoker, diabetes, hypothyroidism, or age ≥60 showed a trend to a higher incidence of cardiac end points that was not significant.

In NSABP B-31 trial, CHFs were more frequent in older women and women with marginal post-AC LVEF [27]. LVEF, assessed either at baseline or after AC, was strongly associated with subsequent CHF ($P < 0.0001$), and age at entry was also predictive ($P = 0.03$). Hypertension was marginally significant ($P = 0.07$). In a multivariate analysis, age and post-AC LVEF remained statistically significant.

The NSABP B31 data about risk factors for a cardiac event are supported by NCCTG N9831 trial [28, 29]. For example, women ≥60 years had a risk of 6.6%, women aged 50–59 years had a 2.8% risk, and women <50 years had a 2.1% risk ($P = 0.003$). Previous or current use of antihypertensive agents increased the risk to 6.0% ($P = 0.005$). Baseline LVEF above the lower limit of normal but <55% increased the risk to 5.6% ($P = 0.033$). BMI ($P = 0.161$) and post-AC LVEF level ($P = 0.134$) were not significantly correlated with LV dysfunction.

6. Monitoring

Women treated with adjuvant trastuzumab and other HER2-directed treatment require appropriate monitoring of LV function. LVEF measurement, obtained by echocardiogram or radionuclide ventriculography (multiple-gated acquisition [MUGA] scans), is currently the generally accepted diagnostic tool to detect cardiotoxicity of antineoplastic agents. It is important to note that the LVEF reflects the functional status of the left ventricle, and until functional impairment occurs, myocardial injury will not be detected by LVEF measurement [40].

With about a decade of follow-up involving women treated in the adjuvant setting with trastuzumab-containing regimens, the optimal surveillance for trastuzumab-related cardiotoxicity is not known. The available evidence does not definitively support a specific schedule of screening or demonstrates improved outcomes for the screened patients [45]. In the adjuvant setting, a baseline evaluation for cardiac function is performed with a repeat testing at 3, 6, 9, and 12 months [46]. In metastatic disease, HER2-directed therapy is continued until disease progression. LVEF is typically monitored at baseline, during the first 3–12 months of therapy and then as clinically indicated such as the presence of symptoms suggestive of cardiac dysfunction.

The optimal cardiac monitoring of women who are receiving novel HER2-directed therapy is not known. The United States Food and Drug Administration (US FDA) prescribing information recommends that all women who are treated with pertuzumab or lapatinib or TDM1 have LVEF assessed at the treatment initiation and subsequently at regular intervals (i.e., every 3 months in the metastatic setting and every 6 weeks in the neoadjuvant setting) [47–49]. Given that cardiac dysfunction rates of novel HER2-targeted therapies are not high and the combination of anti-HER2 treatment does not increase the cardiac toxicity compared with trastuzumab, periodic monitoring of cardiac function in otherwise asymptomatic women with metastatic breast cancer may not be cost effective.

The early detection of injured myocardial cells is required more sensitive diagnostic tools than the use of conventional methods for LVEF measurement. For example, several small studies have evaluated tissue Doppler and strain rate imaging to detect early subclinical changes in cardiac function during and after cancer treatment that preceded a decrease in LVEF [50, 51]. Contrast ECG and real-time 3D ECG are under investigation that may allow improvement in the accuracy of calculating LVEF. In addition, early identification of women at high risk of cardiotoxicity by cardiac biomarkers, in particular, troponin can be more effective for targeted preventive strategies [50].

7. Treatment of cardiac dysfunction

A multidisciplinary approach for the management of treatment-related cardiotoxicity is important for optimal outcomes. Cardio-oncology is a new interdisciplinary field of growing interest focusing on management and prevention of therapy-related cardiac dysfunction in cancer patients [52].

Management of trastuzumab and other HER2-directed treatment-related cardiac dysfunction has two key components: withdrawal of trastuzumab and other HER2-directed therapy and treatment of underlying cardiac dysfunction. Although in the adjuvant clinical trials, various "stopping and restarting" criteria were used for asymptomatic declined in LVEF, the optimal withdrawal and continuation schedule for asymptomatic decline in LVEF in general population are not known.

The NSABP B-31 and the NCCTG N9831 trials used the following dosing guidelines.

- If there is 16% or greater decline in LVEF from the baseline value or 10–15% declined in ejection fraction to below the lower limit of normal of LVEF, trastuzumab is withheld for

4 weeks and reassessment of LVEF at week four. Discontinue trastuzumab if at 4 weeks LVEF remains below that levels.

- Discontinue trastuzumab if a person develop symptomatic heart failure during treatment with trastuzumb, it is discontinued.

Symptomatic heart failure is defined as the presence of:

- dyspnea, pedal edema, and orthopnea;
- the presence of sinus tachycardia, raised jugular venous pressure, tachypnea, crackles, and S3 heart sound;
- radiographic evidence of pulmonary congestion or edema.

One of the algorithms for monitoring of cardiac function for women on adjuvant trastuzumab is described in **Figure 1**.

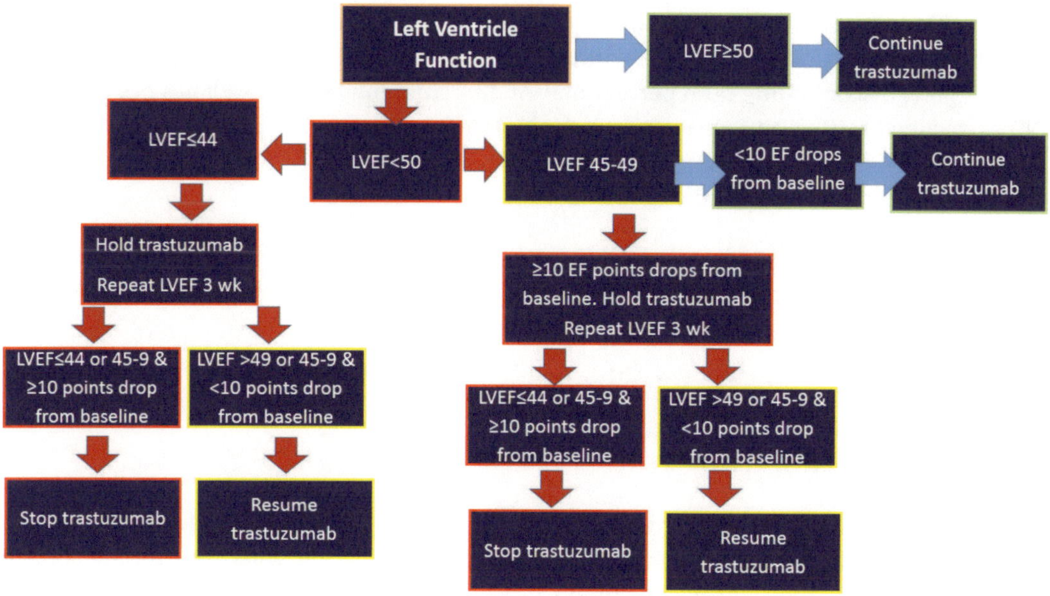

Figure 1. Algorithm for stop and restarting trastuzumab based on LVEF assessments.

Unlike early-stage breast cancer, the dosing criteria for women with metastatic breast cancer are not well defined. In clinical practice, left ventricle function monitoring is infrequently performed in otherwise asymptomatic women with metastatic breast cancer.

Angiotensin-converting enzyme (ACE) inhibitors and beta-blockers have been proven to delay or reverse LV dilation and improve ejection fraction [53–55]. All women with symptomatic heart failure should be treated with an ACE inhibitor in combination with a beta-blocker unless a specific contraindication exists. HER2-directed therapy should be permanently discontinued in such women. ACE inhibitors in combination with a beta-blocker should be used in all asymptomatic women with LV dysfunction and an ejection fraction below 40% unless a specific contraindication exists. Women with LVEF >40% may also get benefit from pharmacological intervention [56, 57]. The optimal duration of therapy is not known and is determined by several factors such as the degree of LV dysfunction, recovery of LV function, patient symptoms, and preference.

7.1. Lapatinib

The US FDA prescribing information recommends discontinuation of lapatinib for a decline in the LVEF to <50%, for those whose LVEF drops below the institution's lower limit of normal and for any women who develop symptomatic heart failure during therapy [49]. Dose reduction is recommended if the LVEF recovers to normal after a minimum of 2 weeks in otherwise asymptomatic patients.

7.2. Pertuzumab

The US FDA prescribing information recommends to withhold both pertuzumab and trastuzumab if LVEF is <45% or is 45–49% with a ≥10% absolute decrease below the baseline value and suggests discontinuing both pertuzumab and trastuzumab if the LVEF has not improved or has declined further on repeat assessment in 3 weeks [47].

7.3. Ado-trastuzumab emtansine (T-DM1)

For women who are treated with T-DM1, at least temporary discontinuation of therapy is recommended if the LVEF falls to <40% or is 40–45% with a ≥10% absolute decrease below the pretreatment value [48].

8. Preventive strategies

The presence of underlying cardiovascular risk factors can increase the risk of treatment-related cardiac dysfunction. Cardiovascular risk reduction with appropriate control of blood pressure, cholesterol, and blood glucose, as well as positive health-promoting behavior, including healthy diet, smoking cessation, regular exercise, and weight control, is recommended for women with breast cancer to reduce the risk of treatment-related cardiotoxicity [50, 58, 59]. Several strategies have been developed to mitigate the risk of both symptomatic and asymptomatic cardiac dysfunction related to HER2-directed therapy. These interventions include periodic cardiac function monitoring, use of a non-anthracycline-based chemotherapy, stopping and restarting HER2-directed therapy, and early detection of cadiotoxicity by biomarkers, followed by prophylactic intervention in selected high-risk patients.

HER2-directed therapy should be avoided in women with a significant cardiovascular history such as recent myocardial infarction, CHF, unstable angina, significant arrhythmias, uncontrolled hypertension, LV hypertrophy, or significant valvular heart disease. The cardiac toxicity data from the adjuvant trastuzmab trials suggest three approaches which have been associated with a reduced risk of cardiac toxicity. The first approach employed by the HERA investigators, which is the sequential use of trastuzumab after completion of adjuvant chemotherapy. This approach resulted in very low rates of cardiac toxic effects, despite the fact that 94% of women received an anthracycline-based regimen [29]. However, the direct comparison of concurrent versus sequential administration of trastuzumab in the N9831 trial suggests that even though the sequential approach is effective, concurrent administration provides greater benefit with minimal increased risk for cardiac toxicity [3, 29].

A second approach was employed in FinHer trial which used 9-week duration of adjuvant trastuzumab and showed a very low rate of cardiac dysfunction [29]. However, the non-inferiority of shorter duration of trastuzumab is not confirmed in a randomized clinical trial. In the Protocol for Herceptin as Adjuvant therapy with Reduced Exposure (PHARE) trial, 3380 women were randomly assigned 6 versus 12 months of trastuzumab [60]. The overall incidences of CHF were 0.65 and 0.53% in the 12 and 6 months arms, respectively ($p > 0.05$). Cardiac dysfunction occurred in 5.9 and 3.4% of women in the 12 and 6 months arms, respectively ($p = 0.001$) [61]. However, with a median follow-up of 42.5 months, treatment for 6 months resulted in a shorter 2-year DFS rate compared with 12 months of therapy (91 versus 94%, respectively; HR 1.28, 95% CI 1.05–1.56). In addition, treatment for 6 months resulted inferior overall survival (93 versus 66 events; HR 1.46, 95% CI 1.06–2.01) and more frequent distant recurrences (HR 1.33, 95% CI 1.04–1.71). Hence, the approach of 6 months or shorter duration of adjuvant trastuzumab is not recommended.

The third approach is the use of a non-anthracycline-based chemotherapy regimen such as docetaxel and carboplatin plus 1 year of trastuzumab (TCH → H) that was employed in the BCIRG 006 trial. The rate of symptomatic congestive heart failure was only 0.4% with TCH → H compared with a rate of 2.0% with AC → TH → H [6]. A non-anthracycline-based regimen also eliminates the risk of cardiac dysfunction from anthracycline that may preclude the use of adjuvant trastuzumab. The risk for cardiotoxicity with an anthracycline-based regimen can be reduced by identifying women who are at increased risk for cardiac dysfunction and avoiding such regimen in these women.

The primary prevention using a beta-blocker or an ACE inhibitor has been employed as an approach to reduce cancer therapy-related cardiac toxicity [62–64]. The results of the PRADA (prevention of cardiac dysfunction during adjuvant breast cancer therapy) trial have shown that candesartan—but not metoprolol—concomitantly administrated with adjuvant chemotherapy including epirubicin, with or without trastuzumab, can protect against early decline in LVEF, assessed with cardiac magnetic resonance [62]. MANTICORE 101-Breast (Multidisciplinary Approach to Novel Therapies in Cardiology-Oncology Research) is a randomized trial that evaluated if conventional heart failure pharmacotherapy can prevent trastuzumab-mediated left ventricular remodeling, measured with cardiac MRI. The study randomized 99 women with HER2-positve breast cancer in a 1:1:1 ratio to an ACE inhibitor (perindopril), beta-blocker (bisoprolol), or placebo [63, 64]. The study failed to achieve its primary end point and neither a beta-blocker nor an ACE inhibitor, used as prophylaxis against trastuzumab's adverse cardiac effects, and successfully prevented left ventricle remodeling. The post-treatment LVEF for placebo patients was significantly but not clinically worse than in either of the experimental arms—56% versus 59% for perindopril and 61% for bisoprolol (down from 61, 62 and 62%, respectively). Although prophylactic beta-blocker or ACE inhibitor is currently not recommended in women with normal baseline LVEF, it may consider in woman at high risk of cardiac dysfunction.

9. Conclusions

The HER2-directed therapy including monoclonal antibodies such as trastuzumab, small molecule inhibitors, and antibody-drug conjugates has revolutionized the management of women with early and advanced HER2-positive breast cancer. Left ventricle dysfunction is a known adverse effect of trastuzumab and other HER-2 directed therapy. In most cases, it is mild and reversible; however, symptomatic heart failure is not a rare complication. The optimal approach to reduce treatment-related LV dysfunction, the best method for its early detection, and the optimal regimen to prevent it remain unknown. Appropriate patient selection for HER2-directed therapy and cardiac monitoring is essential to prevent and manage potential cardiac adverse events. A monitoring schedule that assesses baseline and on-treatment cardiac function but potentially reduces the overall number of assessments is suggested for women on HER2-directed therapy. Intervention strategies with cardiovascular medication such as treatment with ACE inhibitor and beta-blockers and cardiovascular risk reduction to improve cardiac status before, during and after treatment, are important to reduce incidence of heart failure. Simplified rules for starting, interrupting and discontinuing trastuzumab are important for the management of LVEF reduction in women on HER2-directed therapy. We recommend a multidisciplinary approach for the management and prevention of treatment-related cardiac dysfunction for the optimal outcomes.

Author details

Shahid Ahmed[1,2,3]*, Arooba Talat[4], Nayyer Iqbal[1,2], Mohamed Emara[1], Duc Le[1,2], Amir Sami[1,2] and Jim Xiang[1]

*Address all correspondence to: shahid.ahmed@saskcancer.ca

1 Saskatchewan Cancer Agency, University of Saskatchewan, Saskatoon, SK, Canada

2 Department of Oncology, University of Saskatchewan, Saskatoon, SK, Canada

3 Department of Community Health and Epidemiology, University of Saskatchewan, Saskatoon, SK, Canada

4 Department of Medicine, University of Saskatchewan, Saskatoon, SK, Canada

References

[1] Siegel RL, Miller KD, Jemal A. Cancer statistics, 2016. CA Cancer J Clin. 2016; 66:7.

[2] Ferlay J, Soerjomataram I, Ervik M, et al. GLOBOCAN 2012 v1.1, Cancer Incidence and Mortality Worldwide: IARC Cancer Base No. 11 [Internet]. Lyon, France: International Agency for Research on Cancer; 2014. Available from: http://globocan.iarc.fr, accessed on August, 08 2016.

[3] Ahmed S, Sami A, Xiang J. HER2-directed therapy: current treatment options for HER2-positive breast cancer. Breast Cancer. 2015;22:101–116.

[4] Mendes D, Alves C, Afonso N, et al. The benefit of HER2-targeted therapies on overall survival of patients with metastatic HER2-positive breast cancer—a systematic review. Breast Cancer Res. 2015;17:140.

[5] Slamon DJ, Leyland-Jones B, Shak S, et al. Use of chemotherapy plus a monoclonal antibody against HER2 for metastatic breast cancer that overexpresses HER2. N Engl J Med. 2001;344:783–792.

[6] Slamon D, Eiermann W, Robert N, et al. Adjuvant trastuzumab in HER2-positive breast cancer. N Engl J Med. 2011;365:1273–1283.

[7] Curigliano G, Cardinale D, Suter T, et al. Cardiovascular toxicity induced by chemotherapy, targeted agents and radiotherapy: ESMO Clinical Practice Guidelines. Ann Oncol. 2012;23:vii155–vii166.

[8] Suter TM, Procter M, van Veldhuisen DJ, et al. Trastuzumab-associated cardiac adverse effects in the Herceptin adjuvant trial. J Clin Oncol. 2007;25:3859–3865.

[9] Molina MA, Codony-Servat J, Albanell J, Rojo F, Arribas J, Baselga J. Trastuzumab (herceptin), a humanized anti-HER2 receptor monoclonal antibody, inhibits basal and activated HER2 ectodomain cleavage in breast cancer cells. Cancer Res. 2001;61:4744–4749.

[10] Balduzzi S, Mantarro S, Guarneri V, et al. Trastuzumab-containing regimens for metastatic breast cancer. Cochrane Database Syst Rev. 2014;6:CD006242.

[11] Moja L, Tagliabue L, Balduzzi S, et al. Trastuzumab containing regimens for early breast cancer. Cochrane Database Syst Rev. 2012;4:CD006243.

[12] Joensuu H, Kellokumpu-Lehtinen PL, Bono P, et al. Adjuvant docetaxel or vinorelbine with or without trastuzumab for breast cancer. N Engl J Med. 2006;354:809–820.

[13] Piccart-Gebhart MJ, Procter M, Leyland-Jones B, et al. Trastuzumab after adjuvant chemotherapy in HER2-positive breast cancer. N Engl J Med. 2005;353:659–1672.

[14] Romond EH, Perez EA, Bryant J, et al. Trastuzumab plus adjuvant chemotherapy for operable HER2-positive breast cancer. N Engl J Med. 2005;353:1673–1684.

[15] Montemurro F, Valabrega G, Aglietta M. Lapatinib: a dual inhibitor of EGFR and HER2 tyrosine kinase activity. Expert Opin Biol Ther. 2007;6:257–268.

[16] Cameron D, Casey M, Oliva C, et al. Lapatinib plus capecitabine in women with HER-2-positive advanced breast cancer: final survival analysis of a phase III randomized trial. Oncologist. 2010;15:924.

[17] Piccart-Gebhart M, Holmes E, Baselga J, et al. Adjuvant lapatinib and trastuzumab for early human epidermal growth factor receptor 2-positive breast cancer: results from the randomized phase III adjuvant lapatinib and/or trastuzumab treatment optimization trial. J Clin Oncol. 2016;34:1034–1042.

[18] Capelan M, Pugliano L, De Azambuja E, et al. Pertuzumab: new hope for patients with HER2-positive breast cancer. Ann Oncol. 2013;24:273–282.

[19] Baselga J, Cortés J, Kim SB, et al. Pertuzumab plus trastuzumab plus docetaxel for metastatic breast cancer. N Engl J Med. 2012;366(2):109–119.

[20] Gianni L, Pienkowski T, Im YH, et al. Efficacy and safety of neoadjuvant pertuzumab and trastuzumab in women with locally advanced, inflammatory, or early HER2-positive breast cancer (NeoSphere): a randomised multicentre, open-label, phase 2 trial. Lancet Oncol. 2012;13:25.

[21] Zhang X, Zhang XJ, Zhang TY, et al. Effect and safety of dual anti-human epidermal growth factor receptor 2 therapy compared to monotherapy in patients with human epidermal growth factor receptor 2-positive breast cancer: a systematic review. BMC Cancer. 2014;14:625.

[22] Gradishar WJ. HER2 therapy-an abundance of riches. N Engl J Med. 2012;6:176–178.

[23] Verma S, Miles D, Gianni L, et al. Trastuzumab emtansine for HER2-positive advanced breast cancer. N Engl J Med. 2012;367:1783–1791.

[24] Tiwari SR, Mishra P, Abraham J. Neratinib, a novel HER2-targeted tyrosine kinase inhibitor. Clin Breast Cancer. 2016;16(5):344–348.

[25] Chan A, Delaloge S, Holmes FA, Moy B, et al. Neratinib after trastuzumab-based adjuvant therapy in patients with HER2-positive breast cancer (ExteNET): a multicentre, randomised, double-blind, placebo-controlled, phase 3 trial. Lancet Oncol. 2016;17:367.

[26] Swain SM, Kim SB, Cortes J, et al. Pertuzumab, trastuzumab, and docetaxel for HER2-positive metastatic breast cancer (CLEOPATRA study): overall survival results from a randomised, double-blind, placebo-controlled, phase 3 study. Lancet Oncol. 2013;14:461–471.

[27] Tan-Chiu E, Yothers G, Romond E, et al. Assessment of cardiac dysfunction in a randomized trial comparing doxorubicin and cyclophosphamide followed by paclitaxel, with or without trastuzumab as adjuvant therapy in node-positive, human epidermal growth factor receptor 2-overexpressing breast cancer: NSABP B-31. J Clin Oncol. 2005;23:7811–7819.

[28] Perez EA, Suman VJ, Davidson NE, et al. Cardiac safety analysis of doxorubicin and cyclophosphamide followed by paclitaxel with or without trastuzumab in the North Central Cancer Treatment Group N9831 adjuvant breast cancer trial. J Clin Oncol. 2008;26:1231–1238.

[29] Costa RB, Kurral G, Greenberg L, et al. Efficacy and cardiac safety of adjuvant trastuzumab-based chemotherapy regimens for HER2-positive early breast cancer. Ann Oncol. 2010;21:2153–2160.

[30] Sendur MA, Aksoy S, Altundag K. Cardiotoxicity of novel HER2-targeted therapies. Curr Med Res Opin. 2013;29:1015–1024.

[31] Blackwell KL, Burstein HJ, Storniolo AM, et al. Overall survival benefit with lapatinib in combination with trastuzumab for patients with human epidermal growth factor receptor 2-positive metastatic breast cancer: final results from the EGF104900 Study. J Clin Oncol. 2012;30:2585.

[32] Baselga J, Bradbury I, Eidtmann H, et al. Lapatinib with trastuzumab for HER2-positive early breast cancer (NeoALTTO): a randomised, open-label, multicentre, phase 3 trial. Lancet. 2012;379:633–640.

[33] Robidoux A, Tang G, Rastogi P, et al. Lapatinib as a component of neoadjuvant therapy for HER2-positive operable breast cancer (NSABP protocol B-41): an open-label, randomised phase 3 trial. J Clin Oncol. 2013;14:1183–1192.

[34] Guarneri V, Frassoldati A, Bottini A, et al. Preoperative chemotherapy plus trastuzumab, lapatinib, or both in human epidermal growth factor receptor 2-positive operable breast cancer: results of the randomized phase II CHER-LOB study. J Clin Oncol. 2012;30:1989–1995.

[35] Valachis A, Nearchou A, Polyzos NP, et al. Cardiac toxicity in breast cancer patients treated with dual HER2 blockade. Int J Cancer. 2013;133:2245–2252.

[36] Ewer MS, Lippman SM. Type II chemotherapy-related cardiac dysfunction: time to recognize a new entity. J Clin Oncol. 2005;23:2900–2902.

[37] Ewer MS, Vooletich MT, Durand JB, et al. Reversibility of trastuzumab-related cardiotoxicity: new insights based onw clinical course and response to medical treatment. J Clin Oncol. 2005;23:7820–7826.

[38] Crone SA, Zhao YY, Fan L, et al. ErbB2 is essential in the prevention of dilated cardiomyopathy. Nat Med. 2002;8:459–465.

[39] Yarden Y. The EGFR family and its ligands in human cancer: signalling mechanisms and therapeutic opportunities. Eur J Cancer. 2001;37(Suppl 4):S3–S8.

[40] Perik PJ, de Korte MA, van Veldhuisen DJ, et al. Cardiotoxicity associated with the use of trastuzumab in breast cancer patients. Expert Rev Anticancer Ther. 2007;7:1763–71.

[41] Nagata Y, Lan KH, Zhou X, et al. PTEN activation contributes to tumor inhibition by trastuzumab, and loss of PTEN predicts trastuzumab resistance in patients. Cancer Cell. 2004;6:117–127.

[42] Grazette LP, Boecker W, Matsui T, et al. Inhibition of ErbB2 causes mitochondrial dysfunction in cardiomyocytes: implications for Herceptin-induced cardiomyopathy. J Am Coll Cardiol. 2004;44:2231–2238.

[43] Rohrbach S, Muller U, Werdan K, et al. Apoptosis-modulating interaction of the neuregulin/erbB pathway with anthracyclines in regulating Bcl-xS and Bcl-xL in cardiomyocytes. J Mol Cell Cardiol. 2005;38:485–493.

[44] Zeglinski M, Ludke A, Jassal D, et al. Trastuzumab-induced cardiac dysfunction: a 'dual-hit'. Exp Clin Cardiol. 2011;16:70–74.

[45] Dang CT, Yu AF, Jones LW, et al. Cardiac surveillance guidelines for trastuzumab-containing therapy in early-stage breast cancer: getting to the heart of the matter. J Clin Oncol. 2016;34:1030–1033.

[46] National Comprehensive Cancer Network: NCCN clinical practice guidelines in oncology: Breast cancer, version 3. 2015. http://www.nccn.org.

[47] US Food & Drug Administration (FDA). Pertuzumab (PERJATA) http://www.accessdata.fda.gov/drugsatfda_docs/label/2013/125409s051lbl.pdf (Accessed on September 13, 2016).

[48] US Food & Drug Administration (FDA). Ado-Trastuzumab Emtansine (KADCYLA) http://www.accessdata.fda.gov/drugsatfda_docs/label/2013/125427lbl.pdf (Accessed on September 13, 2016).

[49] US Food & Drug Administration (FDA). Lapatinib (TYKERB) http://www.accessdata.fda.gov/drugsatfda_docs/label/2010/022059s007lbl.pdf (Accessed on September 13, 2016).

[50] Cardinale D, Biasillo G, Cipolla CM. Curing cancer, saving the heart: a challenge that cardioncology should not miss. Curr Cardiol Rep. 2016;18:51.

[51] Thavendiranathan P, Poulin F, Lim KD, Plana JC, Woo A, Marwick TH. Use of myocardial strain imaging by echocardiography for the early detection of cardiotoxicity in patients during and after cancer chemotherapy: a systematic review. J Am Coll Cardiol. 2014;63:2751–2768.

[52] Lenihan DJ, Hartlage G, DeCara J, et al. Cardio-oncology training: a proposal from the International Cardioncology Society and Canadian Cardiac Oncology Network for a new multidisciplinary specialty. J Card Fail. 2016. doi:10.1016/j.cardfail.2016.03.012

[53] Bellenger NG, Rajappan K, Rahman SL, Lahiri A, Raval U, Webster J, Murray GD, Coats AJ, Cleland JG, Pennell DJ. Effects of carvedilol on left ventricular remodelling in chronic stable heart failure: a cardiovascular magnetic resonance study. Heart. 2004;90:760–764.

[54] Kalay N, Basar E, Ozdogru I, et al. Protective effects of carvedilol against anthracycline-induced cardiomyopathy. J Am Coll Cardiol. 2006;48:2258–2262.

[55] Abdulla J, Barlera S, Latini R, et al. A systematic review: effect of angiotensin converting enzyme inhibition on left ventricular volumes and ejection fraction in patients with a myocardial infarction and in patients with left ventricular dysfunction. Eur J Heart Fail. 2007;9:129–135.

[56] Mackey JR, Clemons M, Cote MA, et al. Cardiac management during adjuvant trastuzumab therapy: recommendations of the Canadian Trastuzumab Working Group. Curr Oncol. 2008;15:24–35.

[57] Jones AL, Barlow M, Barrett-Lee PJ, et al. Management of cardiac health in trastuzumab-treated patients with breast cancer: updated United Kingdom National Cancer Research Institute recommendations for monitoring. Br J Cancer. 2009;100:684–692.

[58] Albini A, Pennesi G, Donatelli F, et al. Cardiotoxicity of anticancer drugs: the need for cardio-oncology and cardio-oncological prevention. J Natl Cancer Inst. 2010;102:14–25.

[59] Lenihan DJ, Esteva FJ. Multidisciplinary strategy for managing cardiovascular risks when treating patients with early breast cancer. Oncologist. 2008;13:1224–1234.

[60] Pivot X, Romieu G, Debled M, et al. 6 months versus 12 months of adjuvant trastuzumab for patients with HER2-positive early breast cancer (PHARE): a randomised phase 3 trial. Lancet Oncol. 2013;14:741.

[61] Pivot X, Suter T, Nabholtz JM, et al. Cardiac toxicity events in the PHARE trial, an adjuvant trastuzumab randomised phase III study. Eur J Cancer. 2015;51:1660–1666.

[62] Gulati G, Heck SL, Ree AH, et al.Prevention of cardiac dysfunction during adjuvant breast cancer therapy (PRADA): a 2 × 2 factorial, randomized, placebo-controlled, double-blind clinical trial of candesartan and metoprolol. Eur HeartJ. 2016;37:1671–80.

[63] Pituskin E, Mackey JR, Koshman SR, et al. Prophylactic beta blockade preserves left ventricular ejection fraction in HER2-overexpressing breast cancer patients receiving trastuzumab: Primary results of the MANTICORE randomized controlled trial. Cancer Res 2016;76:S1-5.

[64] Pituskin E, Mackey JR, Koshman SR, et al. Prophylactic beta blockade preserves left ventricular ejection fraction in HER2-overexpressing breast cancer patients receiving trastuzumab: primary results of the MANTICORE randomized controlled trial. SABCS. 2015; Abstract S1-05.

Chapter 19

Aspects of Immediate and Delayed Alloplastic Breast Reconstruction After Mastectomy

Michael Friedrich and Stefan Kraemer

Additional information is available at the end of the chapter

http://dx.doi.org/10.5772/66876

Abstract

Seventy percent of patients with early breast cancer can be treated by breast-conserving surgery, while the remaining 30% are forced to receive mastectomy. Nearly 30% of these patients choose breast reconstruction. In the last decade, new alternative techniques and improved surgical devices have significantly improved techniques for breast reconstruction that especially include immediate or delayed breast reconstruction with silicone implants as an excellent option. In general, implant reconstruction may be single- or two-stage procedures. Single-stage reconstruction is the preferred technique for patients with small breasts and minimal ptosis, while large breasts with ptosis require reduction mastopexy either combined with dermoglandular flap or with titane net for covering the caudal pole of the implant. Thus, excellent cosmetic results can be achieved. Recent studies showed a significant survival benefit for postmastectomy irradiation in nodal-positive patients, so that many candidates for breast reconstruction are irradiated with a higher probability of wound-healing complications after breast reconstruction and increased rates of other complications like capsular fibrosis.

Keywords: immediate reconstruction, delayed reconstruction, mastectomy

1. Introduction

Breast cancer affects many women, but with advances in detection and treatment, survival rates have increased. The reconstruction of partial mastectomy defects during breast-conserving surgery and of the whole female breast after mastectomy is an integral part of the surgical treatment of breast cancer [1, 2]. If it is necessary for oncologic reasons and if there are contraindications for breast-conserving therapy, methods of breast reconstruction can contribute significantly to the restoration of physical integrity, including an improvement of life quality for the affected women. Besides an improvement or restoration of the physical image and of the self-esteem, breast reconstruction leads to a processing of an oncologically necessary mastectomy from a psychooncological and rehabilitative point of view [3].

Thus, it is important to understand that there are many reconstructive options available to help ease the psychological burden of mastectomy. Reconstructive options include tissue expander/implants, biologics, and several autologous tissue options, including pedicled latissimus and Transverse Rectus Abdominis Muscle (TRAM) flaps, free TRAM flaps, and perforator flaps.

Breast reconstruction using prosthetic devices (alloplastic reconstruction) is the most commonly performed procedure in women following mastectomy [2]. The goal is to provide an outcome that is predictable and reproducible while minimizing complications and optimizing esthetics. There are various strategies by which this can be achieved. It begins with proper patient selection because most adverse events occur in high-risk patients. This in turn is related to the timing of the reconstruction that can be performed immediately following the mastectomy (primary) or on a delayed basis (secondary). The radiated patient poses additional challenges and limitations that must be understood to achieve a desired outcome.

2. Development of expander and implant technology

The era of modern breast reconstruction started in the early 1960s of the last century with the introduction of silicone-filled implants. Implants of the old generation have a round shape and a smooth surface. Smooth implants tend to have an increased rate of intense capsular contractions, dislocations, and therefore often a bad, asymmetric overall result with a frequent need of correcting surgery such as capsulotomy, capsulectomy, change of implant, explantation surgery, and autologous conversion. Furthermore, implants with a round shape are suitable only for a small breast up to 300 g without contralateral ptosis and little projection, a type of breast that is found *most often* in Asia [4, 5].

Implants of the new generation reflect the developments of implant technology *during* the last years and lead, provided that the medical indications are respected, to very good symmetric reconstructions with long-term stability of the results. By texturizing the surface of the implant, the rate of capsular contractions and the need for correcting surgery declined significantly.

It can actually not be finally judged whether surfacing the implant with polyurethane leads to the same long- term results. In conditions of thin soft tissue, combining *polyurethane* surfacing and surrounding tissue can cause surgical difficulties in case of a necessary change of implants, or it can be a contraindication for reimplanting [2, 6]. The filling of the implants with cohesive silicone gel in combination with an enforced coat of the implant *leads* to significantly higher safety of the implants. Because of their fluid consistency and instability of their form, implants with sodium chloride filling can only be recommended limitedly in regard of the esthetic overall result. The decisive progress in alloplastic breast reconstruction is based on the development and introduction of anatomically shaped implants. This shape of implants facilitates the reconstruction of a natural, symmetrical breast as it is found in Europe and America [2, 6, 7].

In the 1970s, Radovan introduced the expander technology in breast reconstruction [8]. Various progresses in design and technology of expanders lead to more consistent and better results in expansion and therefore made alloplastic breast reconstruction more predictable and safer [9]. Texturizing of the surface of the expanders simplifies the process of expansion and leads to less capsular contractures (especially in combination with textured implants), dislocation, and deformation of the chest wall. The introduction of anatomically shaped expanders enables the expansion of the lower breast pole, which is preferred in most cases, in order to prepare a *symmetric* reconstruction. By integrating a valve directly *into* the expander, the placement of a distant port for filling is unnecessary and increases the comfort for patients and doctors during the expansion phase.

According to our experience, the best results of alloplastic breast reconstruction are achieved by the use of anatomically shaped, textured implants filled with cohesive gel and, in the case of need of tissue expansion, in combination with anatomically shaped, textured expanders [2, 10] (**Figure 1**).

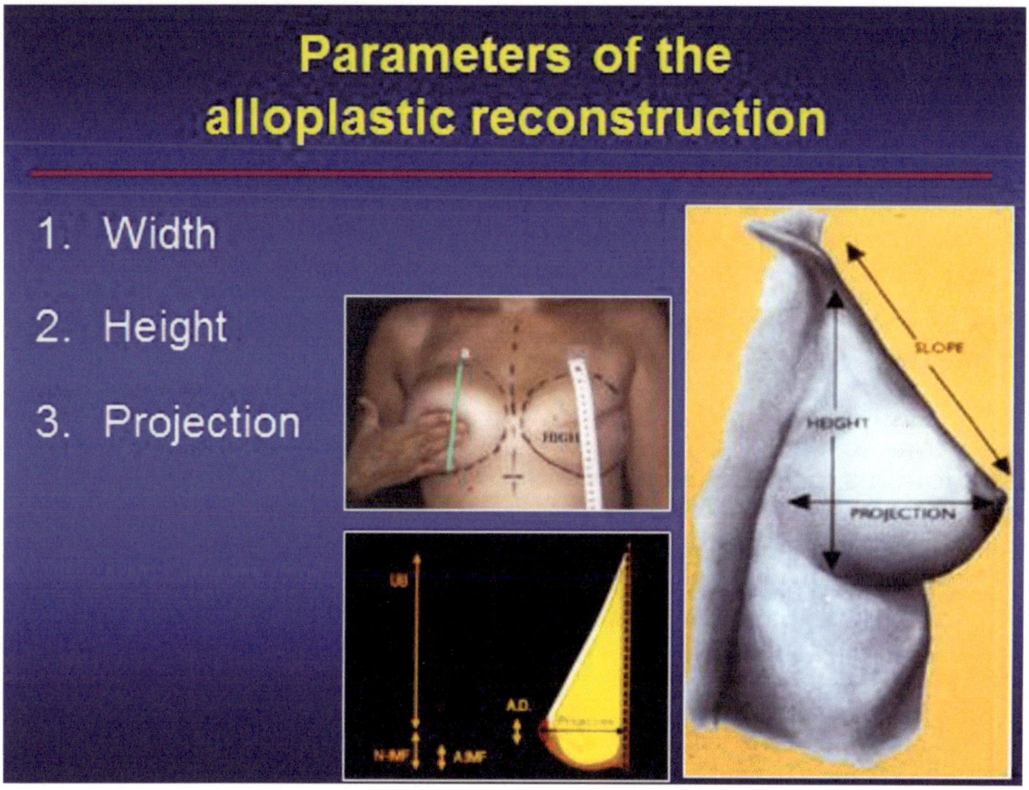

Figure 1. Parameters of alloplastic reconstruction. The preoperative marking of the subpectoral expander-implant loge is performed on the chest wall and can be supported by so-called templates. The lower line of the loge should not be more than 1 cm below the inframammary crease. The submuscular in the caudolateral area subcutaneous loge should have the same extent as the chosen expander and should correspond to the basis and height of the contralateral breast.

3. Basics of alloplastic breast reconstruction

In order to achieve optimal cosmetic results of alloplastic breast reconstruction, these anatomic conditions need to be respected [11, 12]:

1. Conservation of the inframammary crease
2. Integrity of the *pectoralis major muscle*
3. Quality and tautness of the skin

The conservation of the inframammary crease during mastectomy is safe from an oncologic point of view, as only very rarely is there breast parenchyma to be found distal to the inframammary crease. The inframammary crease is formed by fusion of the superficial and the mammary fascia. Its contour is defined by the distribution of fine fibrous retinacula, which connect the dermal as well as the musculofascial layers to a superficial fascia. The mammary fascia represents the natural cover of the mammary gland. The loss of this structural network at the time of mastectomy will lead to an inferior cosmetic result.

Small lesions of the *pectoralis major muscle* present no problem for an alloplastic breast reconstruction. However, larger dehiscences within the muscle should be provided with absorbable sutures. Alloplastic breast reconstruction is planned geometrically according to three parameters: width of the breast (basis of the breast), height of the breast, and projection. The width and the height are defined by the measurements of the contralateral breast. They are then plotted on the side of the chest wall that *has* to be reconstructed precisely to where the planned localization of the expander is.

The projection of the breast can to some extent be predicted by the dimensions of the expander. Depending on the final volume, a permanent *anatomically shaped* implant with corresponding width, height, and projection can be chosen [13].

4. Indications for alloplastic breast reconstruction

Because of a higher overall complication rate in primary expander-implant reconstruction, secondary expander-implant reconstruction should be preferred if alloplastic reconstruction is indicated. For reconstruction of a smaller, non-ptotic breast after mastectomy without radiation of the chest wall, secondary expander-implant reconstruction is suitable to achieve a good cosmetic result, provided that a *subtle* planning and surgical technique are considered [14–16].

Secondary, combined expander-implant reconstruction is the most commonly used method of reconstruction of the female breast after mastectomy in these days. If performed with the most modern expander and implant technologies, this method has various advantages [17]:

1. It is a relatively simple and safe surgical technique, which is easy to be taught, understood, and standardized and thus also suitable for less highly specialized centers.
2. The only tissue of identical texture, color, and sensitivity is used for breast reconstruction.

3. As compared to *autologous* reconstruction with distant *tissue* flaps, there is no morbidity in the area of flap *mobilization and tissue harvest*.

4. Only a small incision with consequently little scarring is necessary.

5. The operation time is significantly reduced as compared to *autologous* reconstruction. The time of postoperative reconvalescence is short.

Generally speaking, a small, not ptotic contralateral breast is suitable for alloplastic breast reconstruction after mastectomy. Patients need to be informed that, in order to adjust symmetry or shape, mastopexy or reduction *mammoplasty* might be necessary. The risk of a secondary, adapting reduction *mammoplasty* increases with size and ptosis of the contralateral breast [2, 9, 16].

Macromastia and extreme ptosis of the contralateral breast are relative contraindications for a reconstruction with expander implant. The most important relative contraindication, however, is radiotherapy of the chest wall [18–21]. Since the indication for radiation of the chest wall has been extended in the last years and primarily depends on histopathologic parameters (tumor size, lymphangiosis, lymph node metastases), the indication for primary reconstruction with implant or expander implant has to be very restricted and well considered. After radiation therapy, fibrosis and interactions with the blood circulation of the skin increase the rate of complications in alloplastic reconstructions such as capsular contractures, necrosis of the skin, or deficient esthetic results. The eschewal of expander reconstruction is very often possible in skin-sparing mastectomy (SSM). Especially in cases of extended ductal carcinoma in situ, SSM is an increasingly common surgical alternative to modified radical mastectomy [22].

It is very important to inform patients about general methods of breast reconstruction. It is necessary to inform about advantages and disadvantages of alloplastic reconstruction as compared to autologous reconstruction including microsurgical *perforator flaps* (e.g., *deep inferior epigastric perforator, DIEP flaps*). When indicating alloplastic reconstruction, the wish of the patient to be intensely informed needs to be respected. Former surgery, age and comorbidity of the patients, previous or postoperative radiation therapy, size of the breast, shape of the breast, symmetry, the personal experience of the surgeon, and, last but not least, the wish of the patients are essential parameters when choosing the optimal method of breast reconstruction [2, 23].

5. Surgical procedure of alloplastic breast reconstruction

When planning the surgical procedure, the incision line and the amount of skin that needs to be removed have to be considered from an oncological as well as a plastic-reconstructive point of view, already at the time of mastectomy. The dimension of the contralateral breast, especially the basis of the breast, defines the size of the expander. The preoperative marking of the subpectoral expander-implant loge is performed on the chest wall and can be supported by so-called templates. The lower line of the loge should not be more than 1 cm below the inframammary crease. The submuscular in the caudolateral area subcutaneous loge should have the same extent as the chosen expander and should correspond to the basis and height of the contralateral breast. During the preparation of the submuscular loge, a consistent dissection is performed visually in cranial, caudal, and medial direction. The caudal and medial insertions of the *pectoralis major muscle* are cut through visually, coming from the subpectoral direction (**Figure 2**). The expander loge in the caudolateral area of the chest wall lies subcutaneously. This is especially important for secondary expander-implant reconstruction. When implanted in the loge, the expander is filled to 50% with a sodium chloride solution. Afterwards, the wound is closed layer by layer. The closing of the major pectoral muscle is especially important in order to achieve a sufficient coverage of the expander with soft tissue (**Figure 3**).

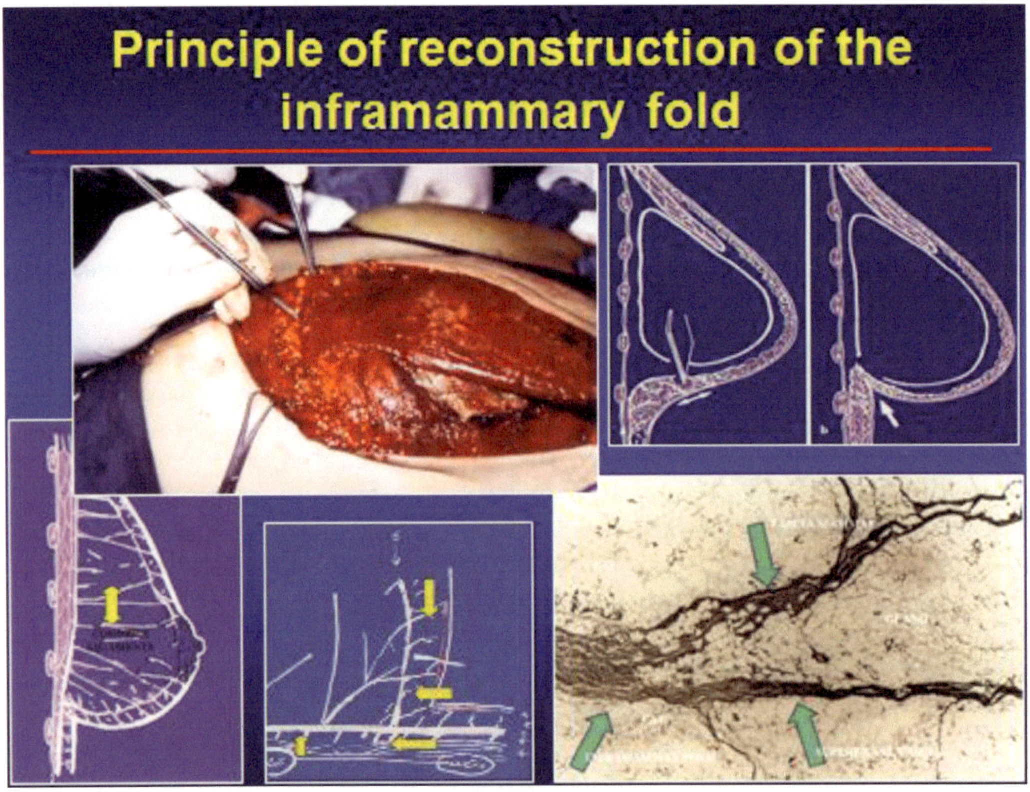

Figure 2. Principle of reconstruction of the inframammary fold. During the preparation of the submuscular loge, a consistent dissection is performed visually in cranial, caudal, and medial direction. The caudal and medial insertions of the *pectoralis major muscle* are cut through visually, coming from the subpectoral direction. The expander loge in the caudolateral area of the chest wall lies subcutaneously. This is especially important for secondary expander-implant reconstruction. When implanted in the loge, the expander is filled to 50% with a sodium chloride solution. Afterward, the wound is closed layer by layer. The closing of the major pectoral muscle is especially important in order to achieve a sufficient coverage of the expander with soft tissue.

http://dx.doi.org/10.5772/66876

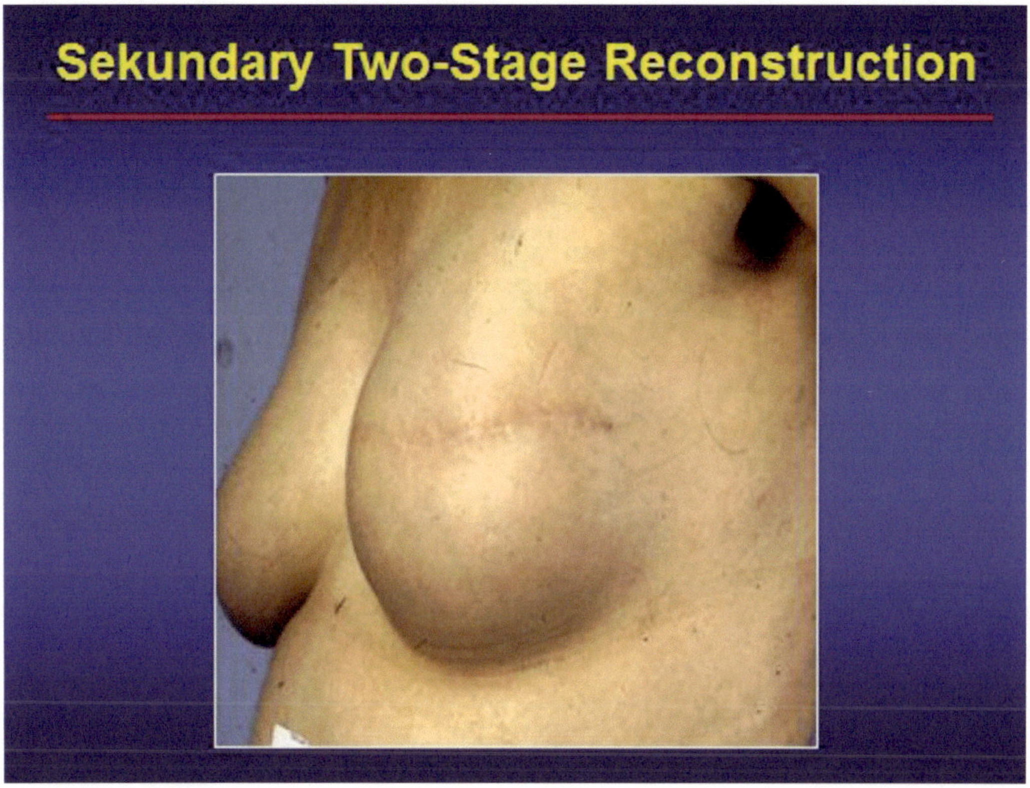

Figure 3. Postoperative result of secondary two-stage reconstruction. This figure demonstrates the postoperative result of a secondary two-stage reconstruction with a very nice shape of the reconstructed breast.

The further expansion starts 1 week after implantation in intervals of 3 days, in steps of 50–100 ml. Rapid expansion is necessary to avoid early development of a *fibrous capsule*.

The filling volume should be at least 70–80% of the possible expander volume. After another 3–6 months, the expander can be replaced by a suitably planned and chosen implant. The form and size of the chosen implant determine the quality of the result of the reconstruction. The implant loge can be optimized by targeted capsulotomy. If the inframammary crease is too high, it can be lowered by caudal capsulotomy. If the inframammary crease is to low, it can be reshaped and relocated by caudal capsulotomy, ellipsoid capsulectomy, and adaptation of the anterior to the posterior capsula with non-resorbable sutures [24, 25]. After insertion of a drain, the final anatomic implant is put in and the wound is closed in multiple layers. The positioning of the implant over the first two postoperative weeks is ensured by a special tape bandage.

An example for the surgical planning of secondary expander-implant reconstruction and the cosmetic result after nipple-areola reconstruction is demonstrated (**Figure 4**).

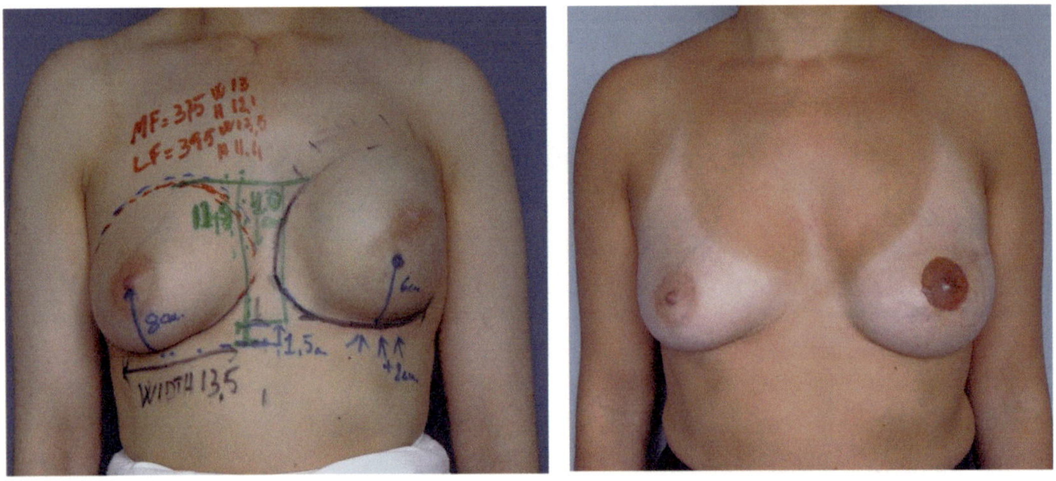

Figure 4. Secondary expander-implant reconstruction: surgical planning with markings and cosmetic result after nipple-areola reconstruction. The drawings show the measurements for the width, the height, and the projection and the markings of the inframammary fold.

6. Complications

The incidence of local complications is lower in primary implant and secondary expander-implant reconstruction than in autologous secondary reconstructions if the medical indications are respected [26, 27]. Early complications include hematoma, necrosis of the skin, infections, and pain. Adjuvant treatments including chemotherapy and radiation therapy can cause delayed wound healing. Delayed complications are infection, implant extrusion, and capsular contracture. Generally speaking, complications are more common after immediate reconstruction than after secondary reconstruction. This can be explained by the application of adjuvant therapies at the time of immediate reconstruction. Chemotherapy affects the immune system and therefore influences processes of regeneration and wound healing. Radiation therapy deteriorates the capacity of skin stretching and leads to excessive fibrosis. Furthermore, it reduces oxygenation of the tissue, which leads to excessive capsular reactions. Persistent infections often lead to removal of the implants. In this case, further reconstructive procedures can only be performed after the final healing of the infections [28].

7. Conclusions

Alloplastic methods of breast reconstruction are the most common methods of reconstructing the female breast after mastectomy. In order to obtain optimal results *for* reconstruction, the use of textured, anatomically shaped expander-implant systems is recommended. If adjuvant therapy is necessary, especially in the case of radiation therapy, an implant or expander-implant reconstruction is relatively contraindicated because of an insufficiently high rate of complication.

http://dx.doi.org/10.5772/66876

The patients need to be informed about the necessity of adapting mastopexy or reduction *mammoplasty* of the contralateral breast and about possible autologous methods *for* reconstruction. In our opinion, adjuvant postmastectomy radiation therapy is *the most important relative* contraindication for alloplastic reconstruction because of an inacceptable complication rate, especially if compared to *secondary* autologous reconstruction.

Author details

Michael Friedrich[1]* and Stefan Kraemer[1, 2]

*Address all correspondence to: friedrichmichael@hotmail.com

1 Department of Obstetrics and Gynecology, HELIOS Medical Center, Krefeld, Germany

2 Department of Obstetrics and Gynecology, Breast Center, University Medical Center, Cologne, Germany

References

[1] Krämer S., Darsow M., Kümmel S., Kimmig R., Rezai M.: "Breast conserving treatment of breast cancer – oncological and reconstructive aspects". *Gynakol. Geburtshilfliche Rundsch.*, 2008, *48*, 56.

[2] Rezai M., Darsow M., Kümmel S., Krämer S.: "Autologous and alloplastic breast reconstruction – overview of techniques, indications and results". *Gynakol. Geburtshilfliche Rundsch.*, 2008, *48*, 68.

[3] Franchelli S., Leone M.S., Berrino P., Passarelli B., Capelli M., Baracco G., et al.: "Psychological evaluation of patients undergoing breast reconstruction using two different methods: autologous tissues versus prostheses". *Plast. Reconstr. Surg.*, 1995, *95*, 1213.

[4] Gabriel S.E., O'Faflon W.M., Kurland L.T., Beard C.M., Woods J.E., Melton L.J. 3rd.: "Risk of connective tissue diseases and other disorders after breast implantation". *N. Engl. J. Med.*, 1994, *330*, 1697.

[5] Jarrett J.R., Cutler R.G., Teal D.F.: "Subcutaneous mastectomy in small, large, or ptotic breasts with immediate submuscular placement of implants". *Plast. Reconstr. Surg.*, 1978, *62*, 702.

[6] Barone F.E., Perry L., Keller T., Maxwell G.P.: "The biomechanical and histopathologic effects of surface texturing with silicone and polyurethane in tissue implantation and expansion". *Plast. Reconstr. Surg.*, 1992, *90*, 77.

[7] Hakelius L., Ohlsen L.: "A clinical comparison of the tendency to capsular contracture between smooth and textured gel-filled silicone mammary implants". *Plast. Reconstr. Surg.*, 1992, *90*, 247.

[8] Radovan C.: "Breast reconstruction after mastectomy using the temporary expander". *Plast. Reconstr. Surg.*, 1982, *70*, 153.

[9] Becker H.: "Breast augmentation using the expander mammary prosthesis". *Plast. Reconstr. Surg.*, 1987, *79*, 192.

[10] Maxwell G.P., Falcone P.A.: "Eighty-four consecutive breast reconstruction using a textured silicone tissue expander". *Plast. Reconstr. Surg.*, 1992, *89*, 1022.

[11] Maillard G.F., Garey L.J.: "An improved technique for immediate retropectoral reconstruction after subcutaneous mastectomy". *Plast. Reconstr. Surg.*, 1987, *80*, 396.

[12] van Straalen W.H., Hage J.J., Bloemena E.: "The inframammary ligament: myth or reality?" *Ann. Plast. Surg.*, 1995, *35*, 237.

[13] Georgiade G.S., Riefkohl R., Cox E., McCarty K.S., Seigler H.F., Georgiade N.G., et al.: "Long-term clinical outcome of immediate reconstruction after mastectomy". *Plast. Reconstr. Surg.*, 1985, *76*, 415.

[14] Beasley M.E.: "Eighty-four consecutive breast reconstructions using a textured silicone tissue expander". *Plast. Reconstr. Surg.*, 1992, *89*, 1035.

[15] Pollock M.: "Capsular contracture: a retrospective study of the effects of textured silicone implants". *Plast. Surg. Forum*, 1991, *14*, 250.

[16] Spear S.L., Spittler C.J. "Breast reconstruction with implants and expanders". *Plast. Reconstr. Surg.*, 2001, *107*, 177.

[17] Beasley M.E.: "Two stage expander/implant reconstruction: delayed reconstruction". In: Spear S.L. (ed) Surgery of the breast: Principles and art. 1st edn. 1998, Lippincott-Raven, Philadelphia

[18] Chawla A.K., Kachnic L.A., Taghian A.G., Niemierko A., Zapton D.T., Powell S.N.: "Radiotherapy and breast reconstruction: complications and cosmesis with TRAM versus tissue expander/implant". *Int. J. Radiat. Oncol. Biol. Phys.*, 2002, *54*, 520.

[19] Rosato R.M., Dowden R.V.: "Radiating as a cause of capsular contracture". *Ann. Plast. Surg.*, 1994, *32*, 342.

[20] Schuster R.H., Kuske R.R., Young V.L., Fineberg B.: "Breast reconstruction in women treated with radiation therapy for breast cancer: cosmesis, complications, and tumor control". *Plast. Reconstr. Surg.*, 1992, *90*, 445.

[21] Victor S.J., Brown D.M., Horwith E.M., Martinez A.A., Kini V.R., Pettinga J.E., et al.: "Treatment outcome with radiation therapy after breast augmentation or reconstruction in patients with primary breast carcinoma." *Cancer*, 1998, *82*, 1303.

[22] Kroll S.S., Ames F., Singletary S.E., Schustermann M.A.: "The oncologic risks of skin preservation at mastectomy when combined with immediate reconstruction of the breast". *Surg. Gynecol. Obstet.*, 1991, *172*, 1.

[23] Audretsch W., Rezai M., Kolotas C., Zamboglou N., Schnabel T., Bojar H.: "Tumor-specific immediate reconstruction (TSIR) in breast cancer patients". *Perspect. Plast. Surg.*, 1998, *11*, 71.

[24] Dowden R.V.: "Achieving a natural inframammary fold and ptotic effect in the reconstructed breast". *Ann. Plast. Surg.*, 1987, *19*, 524.

[25] Handel N., Jensen J.A.: "An improved technique for creation of the inframammary fold in silicone implant breast reconstruction". *Plast. Reconstr. Surg.*, 1992, *89*, 558.

[26] Evans G.R., Schustermann M.A., Kroll S.S., Miller M.J., Reece G.P., Robb G.L., et al.: "Reconstruction and the radiated breast: is there a role for implants?" *Plast. Reconstr. Surg.*, 1995, *96*, 1111.

[27] Kroll S.S., Schustermann M.A., Reece G.P., Miller M.J., Smith B.: "Breast reconstruction with myocutaneous flaps in previously irradiated patients". *Plast. Reconstr. Surg.*, 1994, *93*, 460.

[28] Spear S.L., Maxwell G.P.: "Invited discussion of reconstruction and the radiated breast: is there a role for implants?" *Plast. Reconstr. Surg.*, 1995, *96*, 1116.

Chapter 20

Internal Mammary Sentinel Lymph Node Biopsy

Yong-Sheng Wang, Peng-Fei Qiu and Bin-Bin Cong

Additional information is available at the end of the chapter

http://dx.doi.org/10.5772/66158

Abstract

The conception of internal mammary sentinel lymph node biopsy (IM-SLNB) has been added to the 2009 American Joint Committee on Cancer breast cancer staging manual. However, there has still been slight variation in the surgical treatment model owing to the low visualization rate of internal mammary sentinel lymph nodes (IM-SLN) with the traditional radiotracer injection technique. According to the hypothesis of IM-SLN, a modified injection technique (periareolar intraparenchymal, high volume, and ultrasound guidance) was established, which could significantly improve the IM-SLN visualization rate, and make the IM-SLNB procedure possible in routine practice. IM-SLNB could provide minimally invasive staging, prognosis, and decision-making individually, especially for the patients with clinically positive axilla lymph nodes. Moreover, radiotherapy targeting on internal mammary lymph nodes (IMLN) should be tailored and balanced between the potential benefit and toxicity, and radiotherapy guided by IM-SLNB could achieve this goal. In the era of emphasizing the effective adjuvant therapy, within the changing therapy approach—more systemic treatment, less loco-regional treatment—oncologist should reconsider the application of regional IMLN therapy.

Keywords: breast cancer, internal mammary lymph node, internal mammary sentinel lymph node biopsy, radiotherapy, lymphatic drainage

1. Introduction

Surgical management of the axilla, however, has undergone a paradigm change since the concept of lymphatic mapping in breast was introduced at the John Wayne Cancer Institute in 1991, and sentinel lymph node biopsy (SLNB) has replaced axillary lymph node dissection (ALND) for axillary staging in clinically node-negative early breast cancer. There is a large body of evidence showing that SLNB is an accurate staging procedure in expert hands, and it is now the standard of care for staging clinically node-negative invasive breast cancer.

Furthermore, the results of the ACOSOG Z0011 trial indicated that the patients with a positive axillary sentinel lymph node (ASLN) that may avoid ALND include those with clinical T1–2, N0 breast cancer with one or two positive ASLN who plan to undergo lumpectomy with whole breast radiation and systemic therapy. However, the internal mammary sentinel lymph node biopsy (IM-SLNB) is far behind that of the axilla for the low visualization rate of internal mammary sentinel lymph node (IM-SLN) with the traditional radiotracer injection technique. Based on the hypothesis that the IM-SLN receives the lymphatic drainage from not only the primary tumor area, but also the entire breast organ. The Modified radiotracer injection technique significantly improved the IM-SLN visualization rate, making the routine IM-SLNB possible in daily practice, and further offer individual management for IMLN. In this article, the technical matter, indication and clinical significance of IM-SLNB were discussed, and we would like to identify the breast cancer patients who may benefit from this minimally invasive diagnostic technique.

2. The significant of internal mammary lymph node in breast cancer

In addition to the axillary lymph nodes (ALN), the internal mammary lymph nodes (IMLN) drainage is another first-echelon nodal drainage site in breast cancer [1]. The status of IMLN also provides important regional staging and treatment choice information for breast cancer patients [1, 2]. As reported in the previous studies of extended radical mastectomy, patients with no ALN/IMLN metastases had a 10-year overall survival (OS) rate of 82% compared with 54% for only ALN metastases patients, 38% for only IMLN metastases patients, and 17% for patients with involvement of both nodal, suggesting that regional disease in either nodal chain has the same prognostic relevance [3–5]. The National Comprehensive Cancer Network (NCCN) Clinical Practice Guidelines recommend to strongly consider radiotherapy to IMLN for patients with positive ALN or tumor >5 cm (category 2B), noting "radiotherapy should be given to the IMLN that are clinically or pathologically positive; otherwise, the treatment to the IMLN is at the discretion of the treating radiation oncologist" on this topic.

The nodal status of axillary has been well-established with SLNB and/or ALND in breast cancer patients. However, regional staging and treatment choice could not be achieved just with the ALN status, which might cause under-stage and under-/over-treatment. Handley and Thackray reported that 33% patients had IMLN involvement during survey biopsy, and a back-up IMLN dissection was frequently added to the radical mastectomy starting in the 1950s [6–9]. However, this radical surgical procedure was abandoned due to its extra complications, longer operation time, and lack of survival benefit [10]. Imaging techniques, such as ultrasound, MRI, and PET/CT, could usually detect metastases lesions larger than 5 mm, but due to the deep anatomical location and small size of IMLN, the sensitivity of current imaging techniques cannot satisfy the clinical practice. Therefore, a minimally invasive method is still lacked to evaluate the status of IMLN, and individual IMLN radiotherapy could not be performed.

http://dx.doi.org/10.5772/66158

3. Modified injection technique with high visualization rate

The IM-SLNB provided a less invasive method for assessing IMLN than surgical dissection (**Figure 1**) and may affect decision-making for regional and systemic therapy [11, 12]. Although the 2009 American Joint Committee on Cancer (AJCC) staging incorporated the IM-SLNB concept, there has been little change in surgical practice patterns due to the low visualization rate of IM-SLN with the traditional radiotracer injection technique [13, 14]. Several studies have discovered that superficial injection (intradermal, subdermal, periareolar, and subareolar) of radiotracer was hard to identify IM-SLN, while intraparenchymal injection (peritumoral, intratumoral, or subtumoral) was more reliable [15–18]. These results suggest that the dermal and subdermal lymphatic flow is rarely directed to the internal mammary region, while some intraparenchymal lymphatic flow is directed to the internal mammary region. Unfortunately, with the traditional intraparenchymal injection technique, the internal mammary hotspots were only seen in a small proportion of patients (average 13%, range 0–37%), which has restricted the clinical studies and daily practice of IM-SLNB to date (**Table 4**) [15–20].

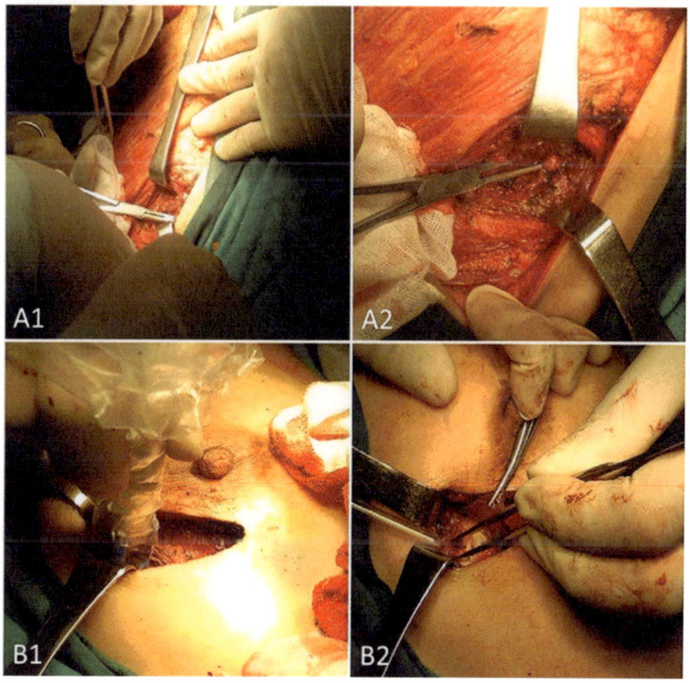

Figure 1. Internal mammary sentinel lymph node biopsy. (A1 & A2 is mastectomy, B1 & B2 is lumpectomy.)

Qiu et al. tried injecting radiotracer with a modified technique (periareolar intraparenchymal, high volume, and ultrasound guidance) and got a high lymphoscintigraphy visualization rate of IM-SLN (71.1%, 248/349) (**Figure 2**) [21, 22]. This might provide a technical feasibility of IM-SLNB, therefore, IM-SLNB could be performed routinely in clinical studies and daily practice and might potentially impact treatment decision-making. However, the basic problem in Qiu's study is the same as all the previous research, because a back up IMLN dissection have not been performed following the IM-SLNB, the accuracy of this minimally invasive technique have not been verified directly. During the IM-SLNB studies, the IM-SLN were concentrated in the 2nd and 3rd intercostal space, which were consistent with the sites of IMLN metastasis in the previous studies of IMLN dissection [6, 10]. These results indirectly confirmed accuracy of IM-SLNB. However, a backup IMLN dissection should be required to validate accuracy of IM-SLNB before its clinical application.

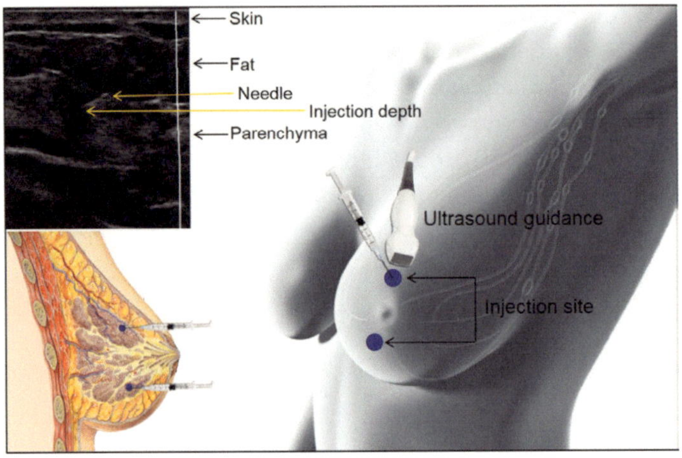

Figure 2. Schematic model of the modified injection techniques.

Additionally, the IM-SLNB is more difficult than axillary SLNB, with success rates of 70–100%. Pleural breach and internal mammary vessel bleeding are the most commonly reported complications from IM-SLNB, occurring in approximately 5% of patients, although pneumothorax and significant postoperative morbidity are rare. Several studies reported the change in clinical management caused by the additional information provided by IM-SLNB [23–28]. IM-SLNB leads to more complete regional staging.

4. Validation study for the hypothesis of internal mammary sentinel lymph node lymphatic drainage in breast cancer

It is generally known that the hypothesis of ASLN lymphatic drainage pattern was proved with subsequent ALND in the breast cancer [29–31]. However, the hypothesis of IM-SLN lymphatic drainage has not been confirmed. As the extended radical mastectomy (included complete internal mammary chain dissection) has been abandoned since 1960s [4, 32, 33], the hypothesis of IM-SLN lymphatic drainage pattern cannot be validated by this way. Now, another method was used to validate the IM-SLN lymphatic drainage hypothesis in our

http://dx.doi.org/10.5772/66158

study. Two different tracers (fluorescence tracer [ICG] and radiotracer [^{99m}Tc-labeled sulfur colloid]) were injected in different sites of the intra-parenchyma to observe whether they could reach to the same IM-SLN in the breast cancer patient. In the clinical practice, the ICG fluorescence tracer is a safe and effective method for sentinel lymph node biopsy (SLNB) in the breast cancer with acceptable sensitivity and specificity comparable to conventional methods (blue dye and radioisotope) [34–36]. In our breast cancer center, it has been compared with the combined method (blue dye with radiotracer [^{99m}Tc-labeled sulfur colloid]) in identifying ASLN. The results showed that all ASLN identified by the combined method also were the ICG fluorescence positive and the non-sentinel lymph nodes were the ICG negative after ALND (n = 69, P < 0.05). The anatomy study of the lymphatics in the breast found that IMLN commonly receive less than 25% of the total lymphatic drainage from the breast [37]. Due to little volume of ICG tracer is difficult to detect by the fluorescence imaging system, it is hard to find IM-SLN by this tracer in the internal mammary lymph chain. But IM-SLN can be detected by radiotracer with the modified radiotracer injection technique and can be performed biopsy in the internal mammary lymph chain guided by this technique. In the validation study of the IM-SLN lymphatic drainage hypothesis, the ICG fluorescence tracer was injected intraparenchymally guided by breast ultrasound at the peritumoral, the radiotracer was injected intraparenchymally with the modified radiotracer injection technique. This method is used to identify different tracers injected in different sites that could reach to the same IM-SLN. The radioactive IM-SLNs were detected by preoperative lymphoscintigraphy (**Figure 3**) 30 min before the surgery and gamma probe during the surgery. IM-SLNB was performed for patients with the radioactive IM-SLNs. After IM-SLN removed, the status of IM-SLN was identified by intraoperative gamma probe and fluorescence imaging system (**Figure 4**). The correlations between the radiotracer and the fluorescence tracer in the same IM-SLN were calculated using the Spearman rank correlation coefficient. The criteria for judging the size of the correlation coefficient were applied: correlations <0.30 are considered minor, correlations between 0.3 and 0.49 are considered medium, and ≥0.5 are considered strong. Cohen's kappa statistic was used to determine inter-examiner agreement. According to Altman's guidelines, it is poor when kappa scores ≤0.20, fair when kappa between 0 and 0.40, moderate when kappa between 0.41 and 0.60, good when kappa 0.61–0.80, and very good when kappa ≥0.80. The results showed that 145 patients underwent IM-SLNB successfully and 127 cases of them identified the radiotracer and the fluorescence tracer reached to the same IM-SLN, 18 cases were detected only the radiotracer positive IM-SLN (**Table 1**). Accordingly, the radiotracer and the fluorescence tracer in the same IM-SLN showed a strong correlation coefficient at 0.836 (*Case-base*, rs >0.5, $P < 0.05$). The degree of agreement between the radiotracer and the fluorescence tracer was *Kappa* = 0.823 (very good), showing high degree of agreement between the two tracers (*Kappa* > 0.8, $P < 0.05$). The results showed that the lymphatic drainage from different location of the breast (the primary tumor, the subareolar plexus) reached to the same IM-SLN, which means that IM-SLN receives lymphatic drainage from not only the primary tumor area but also the entire breast parenchyma. By this method, the hypothesis of IM-SLN lymphatic drainage pattern was demonstrated [38].

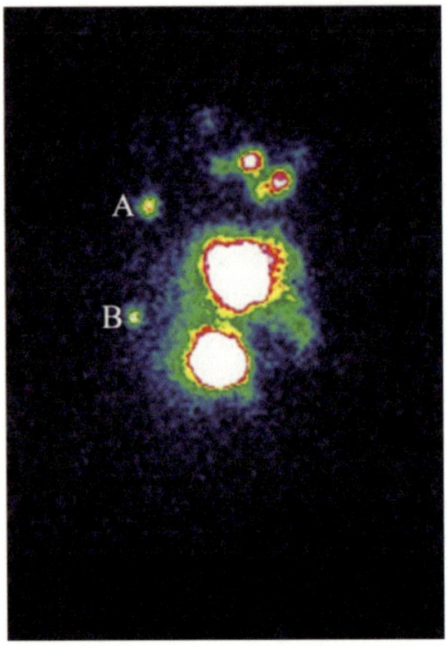

Figure 3. Preoperation lymphoscintigram with radiotracer. Hotspots are evidently shown in both the second intercostal space (A) and the fourth intercostal space (B) in patient with left-sided breast cancer.

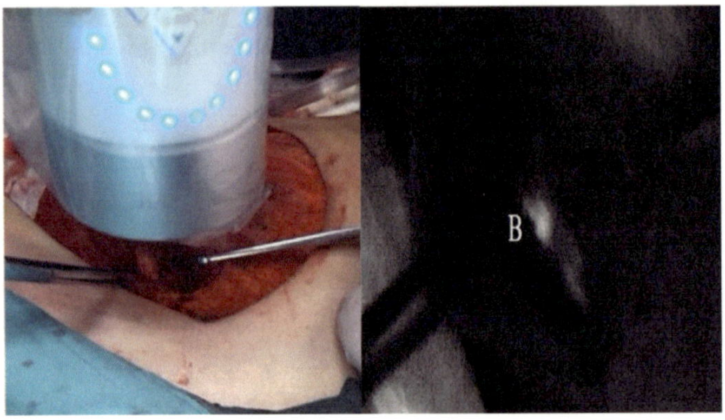

Figure 4. Intraoperative IM-SLNB identified the location of IM-SLN in the fourth intercostal space. The fluorescence imaging system showed the IM-SLN fluorescence tracer positive (B).

Tracers map	Radiotracer+	Radiotracer-	Total
Fluorescence tracer+	127	0	127
Fluorescence tracer-	18	71	89
Total	145	71	216

Table 1. Different tracers identified in IM-SLN.

Furthermore, the radiotracer was not injected in peritumoral intra-parenchyma but in periareolar intra-parenchyma with the modified technique based on the hypothesis. The question arises as to whether all nodes detected by the modified technique should be considered as "true" IM-SLN or whether some of them are actually "second-tier" IMLN. The accuracy of the modified radiotracer injection technique has been confirmed by our team at the previous study [39]. The results showed that IM-SLN detected by the modified technique could reflect the real lymphatic drainage of the whole breast parenchyma. In other words, the modified technique can detect the "true" sentinel node in the internal mammary chain. Also, the results of the metastases site and the number of IM-SLNs were in accordance with the past study of extended radical mastectomy, which could reflect the accuracy of IM-SLNB indirectly [2, 40, 41]. There were no serious adverse events or reactions after the radiotracer injected guiding by the modified injection technique.

5. IM-SLNB should be performed in clinically ALN-positive patients

Several studies indicated that IM-SLNB have little clinical relevance because tumor-positive IM-SLN rarely influence adjuvant treatment strategy and did not affect overall survival [11, 13]. We agree with these results but it should be interpreted with caution for the limitation of their study population. The study population in all current research relate to SLNB (both axilla and internal mammary) was the patients with clinically negative ALN. Because the IMLN involvement is mostly found concomitantly with ALN involvement [10], more attention should be focused on the IM-SLNB in clinically positive ALN patients. Huang et al. [42] retrospectively analyzed 2269 Chinese patients who received extended radical mastectomy and showed that the probability of IMLN metastases was 4.4% for patients with negative ALN, 18.8% for 1–3 positive ALN, 28.1% for 4–6 positive ALN and 41.5% for more than 6 positive ALN. Veronesi et al. also indicated that the IMLN positive rate increased significantly from 9.1% in negative ALN to 29.1% in positive ALN patients [6]. Qiu reported that the IM-SLN positive rate was only 8.1% in clinically negative ALN patient, and adjuvant therapy was altered in a small proportion. However, the IM-SLN positive rate was 20.5% in clinically positive ALN, and individual radiotherapy strategy could be tailored with this IM-SLNB result [22]. To summarize, previous IM-SLNB research failed to assess the IMLN status who really were in need, we could found the evidence from the above results that the patients with clinically positive ALN could get more benefit from the IM-SLNB. Therefore, Qiu et al. suggested that the IM-SLNB research should be encouraged in the clinically positive ALN patients [43].

6. Internal mammary lymph node radiotherapy of breast cancer

For many patients, improvement of systemic therapy will decrease the risk of death due to distant metastasis, after which the importance of optimized local therapy—which will already be better after systemic treatment—will, relatively, contribute more to survival [44]. Radiotherapy could reduce local recurrence and improve survival after mastectomy and breast conserving surgery [45, 46].

The results of Early Breast Cancer Trialists' Collaborative Group (EBCTCG) meta-analysis showed that one breast cancer death being avoided in the first 15 years after radiotherapy for every four recurrences of any type (i.e., either loco-regional or distant) avoided in the 10 years after radiotherapy for patients with breast conserving surgery. And about one breast cancer death was avoided in the 20 years after radiotherapy for every 1.5 recurrences of any type (i.e., either loco-regional or distant) avoided during the first 10 years after radiotherapy for patients with positive lymph node [46].

The meta-analysis from EBCTCG involved 8135 patients and randomly assigned them to the chest wall and regional lymph nodes radiotherapy after mastectomy and axillary surgery versus the same surgery but no radiotherapy. For 1314 patients with 1–3 positive ALN after ALND, postmastectomy radiotherapy could reduce loco-regional recurrence (LRR), overall recurrence (OR, rate ratio [RR] 0.68, 95% confidence interval [CI] 0.57–50.82), and breast cancer mortality (BCM, RR 0.80, 95% CI 0.67–60.95, all $P < 0.05$). For patients with systemic therapy (86.2%, 1133/1314), postmastectomy radiotherapy also could reduce LRR, OR (RR 0.67, 95% CI 0.55–50.82), and BCM (RR 0.78, 95% CI 0.64–60·94, all $P < 0.05$). Furthermore, for 1772 patients with ≥4 positive ALN after ALND, radiotherapy also could reduce LRR, OR (RR 0.79, 95% CI 0.69–60.90), and BCM (RR 0.87, 95% CI 0.77–70.99, all $P < 0.05$). However, the benefit of postmastectomy radiotherapy might be greater for patients irradiated today because of radiotherapy planning changing substantially and patients receiving better coverage of target areas. Today, with the rapid development of the radiotherapy techniques, the doses to normal tissues would be lower, the risks of radiotherapy would be lower, and the benefits of postmastectomy radiotherapy would be larger than in these trials. However, due to the improvement of detection and treatment in breast cancer, which makes the absolute risks lower in breast cancer recurrence and mortality, the absolute benefit of postmastectomy radiotherapy today would be smaller than in this study [47].

The MA.20 trial from National Cancer Institute Common Clinical Trials Group found that the addition of regional nodal radiotherapy (including IMLN) to whole-breast radiotherapy reduced the rate of breast cancer recurrence in patients with node-positive or high-risk node-negative breast cancer. A total of 1832 patients were assigned to the nodal-radiotherapy group or the control group (916 patients in each group) in this trial. At the 10-year follow-up, the rates of disease-free survival (DFS) in the nodal-radiotherapy group was better than that in the control group (82.0 vs. 77.0%; [HR] 0.76 [95% CI, 0.61–60.94], $P = 0.01$). But, there was no significant between group difference in OS, with a rate of 82.8% in the nodal-radiotherapy group and 81.8% in the control group (hazard ratio [HR], 0.91; 95% [CI], 0.72 to 1.13; $P = 0.38$) [48].

In the European Organization for Research and Treatment of Cancer (EORTC) 22922/10925 study, a total of 4004 patients were assigned randomly to the regional nodal radiotherapy (included IMLN) group or the control group. At a median follow-up of 10.9 years, the results showed that regional nodal radiotherapy did not change overall survival (OS) (82.3 vs. 80.7%, HR 0.87, 95% CI, 0.76–71.00, $P = 0.06$), but improved DFS (72.1 vs. 69.1%, HR, 0.89, 95% CI,

http://dx.doi.org/10.5772/66158

0.80–81.00, P = 0.04), the distant metastasis-free survival (DMFS) (78.0 vs. 75.0%, HR, 0.86, 95% CI, 0.76–70.98, P = 0.02), and reduced the breast cancer mortality (12.5 vs. 14.4%, HR, 0.82, 95% CI, 0.70–0.97, P = 0.02) [49].

In the French study, all patients received postoperative radiotherapy to the chest wall and supraclavicular nodes and were randomly assigned to receive IMLN radiotherapy or not. A total of 1334 patients were analyzed after a median follow-up of 11.3 years among the survivors. No benefit of IMLN radiotherapy on OS could be demonstrated: the 10-year OS was 59.3% in the IMLN non-irradiated group versus 62.6% in the IMLN irradiated group (P = 0.8). The overestimation of the risk of IMLN involvement (25%) probably decreased the power of the study [50].

Budach et al. did a meta-analysis of the MA. 20, EORTC22922/10925, French trials and the results showed that additional regional radiotherapy to IMLN statistically significantly improves DFS, DMFS, and OS in stage I–III breast cancer. The absolute benefits in 5-year OS were 1.6% in the MA.20 trial, 10-year OS were 1.6% in the EORTC trial, and 10-year OS were 3.3% in the French trial (HR 0.88 [95% CI 0.80–0.97], P = 0.012). Regional nodal (the medial supraclavicular lymph node and IMLN) irradiation (MA.20 and EORTC) was associated with a significant improvement of DFS (HR 0.85 [95% CI 0.77–0.94]) and DMFS (HR 0.82 [95% CI 0.73–0.92]) [51].

The 2016 NCCN Breast Cancer Clinical Practice Guidelines recommend radiotherapy to IMLN for patients with ≥4 positive ALN (category 1), and strongly consider radiotherapy to IMLN for patients with 1–3 positive axillary nodes (category 2A), both after mastectomy and lumpectomy [52].

The DBCG-IMN Study initiated by Danish Breast Cancer Cooperative Group, a prospective population-based cohort study, found that IMLN radiotherapy increased OS in patients with early-stage node-positive breast cancer. A total of 3089 patients were included in the study, 1492 of them received IMLN radiotherapy and others were no IMLN radiotherapy. With a median of 8.9 years of follow-up time, the 8-year OS rates of IMLN radiotherapy group was higher than that in the no radiotherapy group (75.9% [95% CI 73.6–78.0] vs. 72.2% [95% CI 69.9–74.4]; [HR] 0.82 [95% CI 0.72–70.94], P = 0.005). Breast cancer mortality in IMLN radiotherapy group was lower than that in the no radiotherapy group (20.9% [95% CI 18.8–23.0] vs. 23.4% [95% CI 21.3–25.5]; [HR] 0.85 [95% CI 0.73–70.98], P = 0.03) [53].

In sum, IMLN radiotherapy could reduce loco-regional and distant recurrence and improve survival in breast cancer.

7. Internal mammary lymph node radiotherapy guided by internal mammary sentinel lymph node biopsy

Although the 2016 NCCN Breast Cancer Clinical Practice Guidelines recommend radiotherapy to IMLN for patients with ≥4 positive ALN, and strongly consider radiotherapy to IMLN for patients with 1–3 positive axillary nodes, but according to the status of ALN to estimate the metastasis risk in IMLN, low-risk did not mean IMLN negative and high-risk did not mean IMLN metastases [54]. Studies of extended radical mastectomy reported that 38.3% (36.8–46.2%) patients with ≥4 positive ALN, 19.6% (18.8–26.7%) patients with 1–3 positive ALN identified IMLN metastases, and 9.2% (4.4–16.8%) with negative ALN identified IMLN metastases. It is obvious that negative IMLN was found in about 60% patients with ≥4 positive ALN and positive IMLN was found in about 9% patients with negative ALN [33, 42, 55]. Thus, these inclusion criteria of NCCN Guidelines might induce over- and under-treatment. We should use a more accurate technique to evaluate the pathology status of IMLN and to guide IMLN radiotherapy.

The study by Veronesi et al. found that radiotherapy to IMLN will improve the survival obviously after identifying the metastases by IMLN biopsy. In this clinical study of 68 (10.3%, 68/663) patients receiving radiotherapy to IMLN for histologically proven metastases, radiotherapy was highly effective yielded a 5-year OS of 95% [56].

Currently, IM-SLNB via intercostal space could make it possible—tailored IMLN radiotherapy and minimally invasive staging. Even though breast cancer staging has incorporated IM-SLNB concept since the 6th edition of AJCC, IM-SLNB has not been performed routinely [57]. The studies of IM-SLNB showed that the success rate of IM-SLNB has reached 60–100% with minimal or no changes in operative time, but the visualization rate of IM-SLN was low [12–14, 58], which has been the restriction for both clinical study and daily practice of IM-SLNB.

Now, the modified radiotracer injection technique could improve the IM-SLN detection rate from 15.5 to 71% ($P < 0.001$). Also, the visualization number of IM-SLN was no difference between the modified technique group and the traditional tracer injection technique (peritumoral intraparenchymal injection) group in our pilot study ($P = 0.692$). Up to now, 219 patients with breast cancer received IM-SLNB guided by the modified radiotracer injection technique. The clinically pathological characteristics of the 216 enrolled patients are presented in **Table 2**. The detection rate of ASLN was 98.6% (213/216). The overall visualization rate of IM-SLN detected by preoperative lymphoscintigraphy and gamma probe was 71.8% (155/216). 96.1% (149/155) of them received IM-SLNB. The success rate of IM-SLNB was 97.3% (145/149). The data on clinical outcome of the patients underwent IM-SLNB show in **Table 3**. In 12 patients underwent breast conserving surgery, 5 cases who were identified the location of primary tumor could not reach IM-SLNB had to be made an extra incision in the skin to reach IM-SLNB. In patients who performed IM-SLNB successfully, a total of 279 lymph nodes were removed, the median number of IM-SLNs was 2 (range 1–4 nodes). The IM-SLNs were located in the first (5.4%, 15/279), second (46.2%, 129/279), third (40.5%, 113/279) and forth (7.9%, 22/279) intercostal space. All positive IM-SLNs were in the second (61.1%, 11/18) and the third (38.9%, 7/18) intercostal space. 54.1% (151/279) of IM-SLN was found in the outside of the internal mammary vessels and 45.9% (128/279) was in the inside. Details of IM-SLN mapping and biopsy are shown in **Table 4**. The IM-SLN involvement rate was 8.1% (7/86) in patient with clinically axillary node negative patients and 18.6% (11/59) in positive patients, respectively. All patients with positive IM-SLN received regional nodal radiotherapy to IMLN. The clinical, pathological, and treatment details of these patients were shown in **Table 5**. In patients with ≥4 positive axillary lymph nodes, regional nodal radiotherapy to IMLN had been avoided in

50.0% cases (9/18) with negative IM-SLN. In patients with 1–3 positive axillary lymph nodes, regional nodal radiotherapy to IMLN might be avoided in 91.2% cases (52/57) with negative IM-SLN.

Characteristic	**No.**	**%**
Age (years)		
Median	50	
Range	27–79	
≤50	119	55.1
>50	97	44.9
BMI		
Median	24.1	
Range	17.2–33.5	
Tumor size		
Tis	16	7.4
T1	99	45.8
T2	79	36.6
T3	22	10.2
Tumor location		
UOQ	92	42.6
LOQ	25	11.6
UIQ	48	22.2
LIQ	5	2.3
Central	46	21.3
Tumor type		
Ductal	187	86.6
Lobular	8	3.7
Mixed	5	2.3
Other	16	7.4
Radiotracer intensity (MBq)		
Median	36	
Radiotracer volume (mL/point)		
Median	0.5	
Intervals from injection to SLNB (h)		
2–5	89	41.2
16–22	127	58.8

Abbreviations: BMI, body mass index: UOQ, upper outer quadrant; LOQ, lower outer quadrant: UIQ, upper inner quadrant; LIQ, lower inner quadrant.

Table 2. Descriptive characteristics of eligible patients (N = 216).

Characteristic	No.	%
T stage		
Tis	9	6.2
T1	70	48.3
T2	57	39.3
T3	9	6.2
N stage		
N0	70	48.3
N1	57	39.3
N2	7	4.8
N3	11	7.6
ER		
Positive	101	69.7
Negative	44	30.3
PR		
Positive	98	67.6
Negative	47	32.4
HER-2		
Positive	44	30.3
Negative	101	69.7
Type of surgery		
Lumpectomy + ASLNB	9	6.2
Lumpectomy + ALND	3	2.1
Mastectomy + ASLNB	93	64.1
Mastectomy + ALND	40	27.6
Radiotherapy		
WBI	7	4.8
WBI + RNI	5	3.5
PMRT + RNI	79	54.5
No	54	37.2
Chemotherapy		
Yes	121	83.4
No	24	16.6

Abbreviations: ER, estrogen receptor status; PR, progesterone receptor status; HER-2, human epidermal growth factor receptor-2; WBI, whole breast irradiation; RNI, regional node irradiation; PMRT, postmastectomy radiotherapy.

Table 3. Clinical outcome of patients who underwent IM-SLNB (N = 145).

Characteristic	No.	%
IM-SLN map+	155	71.8 (155/216)
Pt. performed IM-SLNB	149	96.1 (149/155)
Success rate of IM-SLNB	145	97.3 (145/149)
Total no. of IM-SLN	279	
Median	2	
Range	1–4	
IM-SLN metastatic	18	12.4 (18/145)
IM-SLNB time (min)		
Median	10	
Range	3–55	
IM-SLN size (mm)		
Median	5	
Range	3–12	

Table 4. Details of IM-SLN mapping and biopsy.

No.	Tumor location	T stage	No. of positive ALN	N stage without IM-SLN	No. of positive IM-SLN	N stage with IM-SLN	Finally stage	Chemo-therapy	Radio-therapy
1	UOQ	T2	0	pN0	2	pN1b	IIA→IIB	Yes	No→Yes
2	UIQ	T2	2	pN1a	1	pN1c	IIB (no change)	Yes	? →Yes
3	Central	T2	14	pN3a	1	pN3b	IIIC (no change)	Yes	Yes
4	UOQ	T2	9	pN2a	1	pN3b	IIIA→IIIC	Yes	Yes
5	UIQ	T1c	2	pN1a	1	pN1c	IIA (no change)	Yes	? →Yes
6	UOQ	T2	1	pN1a	1	pN1c	IIB (no change)	Yes	? →Yes
7	UIQ	T1a	0	pN0	1	pN1b	IA→IIA	No→Yes	No→Yes
8	UOQ	T2	9	pN2a	2	pN3b	IIIA→IIIC	Yes	Yes
9	LIQ	T2	5	pN2a	1	pN3b	IIIA→IIIC	Yes	Yes
10	UOQ	T1a	3	pN1a	1	pN1c	IIA (no change)	Yes	? →Yes
11	UIQ	T2	0	pN0	1	pN1b	IIA→IIB	Yes	No→Yes
12	UOQ	T3	13	pN3a	1	pN3b	IIIC (no change)	Yes	Yes
13	Central	T1c	1	pN1a	1	pN1c	IIA (no change)	Yes	? →Yes
14	UOQ	T2	13	pN3a	1	pN3b	IIIC (no change)	Yes	Yes
15	Central	T2	11	pN3a	1	pN3b	IIIC (no change)	Yes	Yes
16	UOQ	T2	20	pN3a	1	pN3b	IIIC (no change)	Yes	Yes
17	UOQ	T2	5	pN2a	1	pN3b	IIIA→IIIC	Yes	Yes
18	UIQ	T1c	0	pN0	1	pN1b	IA→IIA	No→Yes	No→Yes

Abbreviations: UOQ, upper outer quadrant; UIQ, upper inner quadrant; LIQ, lower inner quadrant; ?, radiotherapy is controversy.

Table 5. The clinical, pathological, and treatment details of patients with positive IM-SLN.

8. Conclusion

Modified injection technique (two-quadrant, high volume, and ultrasound guidance) could significantly improve the detection rate of IM-SLN and would promote research on IM-SLNB. The hypothesis of IM-SLN lymphatic drainage pattern was demonstrated. As IMLN metastasis is mostly concomitant with ALN metastasis, IM-SLNB should be encouraged in clinically positive ALN patients. IM-SLNB should be performed routinely, for it could lead to accurate IMLN staging and provide IM-SLNB guided IMLN-RT.

Acknowledgements

This work was supported by National Natural Science Foundation of China (81672038), National Natural Science Foundation of China (81502314), Natural Science Foundation of Shandong Province (ZR2014HZ003), and Natural Science Foundation of Shandong Province (ZR2015PH025).

Abbreviations

ALN = axillary lymph nodes

IMLN = internal mammary lymph nodes

SLNB = sentinel lymph node biopsy

IM-SLNB = internal mammary sentinel lymph node biopsy

IM-SLN = internal mammary sentinel lymph nodes

SLN = sentinel lymph nodes

OS = overall survival

DFS = disease-free survival

DMFS = distant metastasis free survival

ALND = axillary lymph node dissection

NCCN = National Comprehensive Cancer Network

EBCTCG = Early Breast Cancer Trialists

Collaborative Group

EORTC = European Organization for Research and Treatment of Cancer

ASLN = axillary sentinel lymph node

ICG = indocyanine green

Author details

Yong-Sheng Wang[1*], Peng-Fei Qiu[1] and Bin-Bin Cong[1,2]

*Address all correspondence to: wangysh2008@aliyun.com

1 Breast Cancer Center, Shandong Cancer Hospital Affiliated to Shandong University, Jinan, China

2 School of Medicine and Life Sciences, University of Jinan and Shandong Academy of Medical Sciences, Jinan, China

References

[1] Chen RC, Lin NU, Golshan M, Harris JR, Bellon JR. Internal mammary nodes in breast cancer: diagnosis and implications for patient management—a systematic review. J Clin Oncol. 2008;26(30):4981–4989.

[2] Livingston SF, Arlen M. The extended extrapleural radical mastectomy: its role in the treatment of carcinoma of the breast. Ann Surg. 1974;179(3):260–265.

[3] Handley RS. Carcinoma of the breast. Ann R Coll Surg Engl. 1975;57(2):59–66.

[4] Dahl-Iversen E, Tobiassen T. Radical mastectomy with parasternal and supraclavicular dissection for mammary carcinoma. Ann Surg. 1969;170(6):889–891.

[5] Urban JA. Management of operable breast cancer: the surgeon's view. Cancer. 1978;42(4):2066–2077.

[6] Veronesi U, Cascinelli N, Greco M, et al. Prognosis of breast cancer patients after mastectomy and dissection of internal mammary nodes. Ann Surg. 1985;202(6):702–707.

[7] Donegan WL. The influence of untreated internal mammary metastases upon the course of mammary cancer. Cancer. 1977;39(2):533–538.

[8] Handley RS, Thackray AC. Invasion of internal mammary lymph nodes in carcinoma of the breast. Br Med J. 1954;1(4853):61–63.

[9] Handley RS, Patey DH, Hand BH. Excision of the internal mammary chain in radical mastectomy: results in 57 cases. Lancet. 1956;270(6921):457–461.

[10] Veronesi U, Marubini E, Mariani L, et al. The dissection of internal mammary nodes does not improve the survival of breast cancer patients. 30-year results of a randomised trial. Eur J Cancer. 1999;35(9):1320–1325.

[11] Madsen EV, Aalders KC, van der Heiden-van der Loo M, et al. Prognostic significance of tumor-positive internal mammary sentinel lymph nodes in breast cancer: a multicenter cohort study. Ann Surg Oncol. 2015;22(13):4254–4262.

[12] Caudle AS, Yi M, Hoffman KE, et al. Impact of identification of internal mammary sentinel lymph node metastasis in breast cancer patients. Ann Surg Oncol. 2014;21(1): 60–65.

[13] Postma EL, van Wieringen S, Hobbelink MG, et al. Sentinel lymph node biopsy of the internal mammary chain in breast cancer. Breast Cancer Res Treat. 2012; 134(2):735–741.

[14] Gnerlich JL, Barreto-Andrade JC, Czechura T, et al. Accurate staging with internal mammary chain sentinel node biopsy for breast cancer. Ann Surg Oncol. 2014;21(2): 368–374.

[15] Shimazu K, Tamaki Y, Taguchi T, et al. Lymphoscintigraphic visualization of internal mammary nodes with subtumoral injection of radiotracer in patients with breast cancer. Ann Surg. 2003;237(3):390–398.

[16] Park C, Seid P, Morita E, et al. Internal mammary sentinel lymph node mapping for invasive breast cancer: implications for staging and treatment. Breast J. 2005;11(1):29–33.

[17] Rodier JF, Velten M, Wilt M, et al. Prospective multicentric randomized study comparing periareolar and peritumoral injection of radiotracer and blue dye for the detection of sentinel lymph node in breast sparing procedures: FRANSENODE trial. J Clin Oncol. 2007;25(24):3664–3669.

[18] Garcia-Manero M, Olartecoechea B, Royo P. Different injection sites of radionuclide for sentinel lymph node detection in breast cancer: single institution experience. Eur J Obstet Gynecol Reprod Biol. 2010;153(2):185–187.

[19] Wang L, Yu JM, Wang YS, et al. Preoperative lymphoscintigraphy predicts the successful identification but is not necessary in sentinel lymph nodes biopsy in breast cancer. Ann Surg Oncol. 2007;14(8):2215–2220.

[20] Sun X, Liu JJ, Wang YS, et al. Roles of preoperative lymphoscintigraphy for sentinel lymph node biopsy in breast cancer patients. Jpn J Clin Oncol. 2010;40(8): 722–725.

[21] Qiu PF, Liu JJ, Liu YB, et al. A modified technology could significantly improve the visualization rate of the internal mammary sentinel lymph nodes in breast cancer patients. Breast Cancer Res Treat. 2012;136(1):319–321.

[22] Qiu PF, Cong BB, Zhao RR, et al. Internal mammary sentinel lymph node biopsy with modified injection technique: high visualization rate and accurate staging. Medicine. 2015;94(41):e1790.

[23] Dupont E, Cox CE, Nguyen K, et al. Utility of internal mammary lymph node removal when noted by intraoperative gamma probe detection. Ann Surg Oncol. 2001;8(10):833–836.

[24] Dupont EL, Salud CJ, Peltz ES, et al. Clinical relevance of internal mammary node mapping as a guide to radiation therapy. Am J Surg. 2001;182(4):321–324.

[25] Galimberti V, Veronesi P, Arnone P, et al. Stage migration after biopsy of internal mammary chain lymph nodes in breast cancer patients. Ann Surg Oncol. 2002;9(9):924–928.

[26] Hong J, Choy E, Soni N, et al. Extra-axillary sentinel node biopsy in the management of early breast cancer. Eur J Surg Oncol. 2005;31(9):942–948.

[27] Jansen L, Doting MH, Rutgers EJ, et al. Clinical relevance of sentinel lymph nodes outside the axilla in patients with breast cancer. Br J Surg. 2000;87(7):920–925.

[28] Johnson N, Soot L, Nelson J, et al. Sentinel node biopsy and internal mammary lymphatic mapping in breast cancer. Am J Surg. 2000;179(5):386–388.

[29] Giuliano AE, Kirgan DM, Guenther JM, Morton DL. Lymphatic mapping and sentinel lymphadenectomy for breast cancer. Ann Surg. 1994;220(3):391–398; discussion 398–401.

[30] Giuliano AE, Dale PS, Turner RR, Morton DL, Evans SW, Krasne DL. Improved axillary staging of breast cancer with sentinel lymphadenectomy. Ann Surg. 1995;222(3):394–399; discussion 399–401.

[31] Turner RR, Ollila DW, Krasne DL, Giuliano AE. Histopathologic validation of the sentinel lymph node hypothesis for breast carcinoma. Ann Surg. 1997;226(3):271–278.

[32] Lacour J, Bucalossi P, Cacers E, Jacobelli G, Koszarowski T, Le M, Rumeau-Rouquette C, Veronesi U. Radical mastectomy versus radical mastectomy plus internal mammary dissection. Five-year results of an international cooperative study. Cancer. 1976;37(1): 206–214.

[33] Veronesi U, Valagussa P. Inefficacy of internal mammary nodes dissection in breast cancer surgery. Cancer. 1981;47(1):170–175.

[34] Wishart GC, Loh SW, Jones L, Benson JR. A feasibility study (ICG-10) of indocyanine green (ICG) fluorescence mapping for sentinel lymph node detection in early breast cancer. Eur J Surg Oncol. 2012;38(8):651–656.

[35] Hirche C, Murawa D, Mohr Z, Kneif S, Hünerbein M. ICG fluorescence-guided sentinel node biopsy for axillary nodal staging in breast cancer. Breast Cancer Res Treat. 2010;121(2):373–378.

[36] Ahmed M, Purushotham AD, Douek M. Novel techniques for sentinel lymph node biopsy in breast cancer: a systematic review. Lancet Oncol. 2014;15(8):e351–362.

[37] Turner-Warwick RT. The lymphatics of the breast. Br J Surg. 1959;46:574–582.

[38] Cong BB, Qiu PF, Liu YB, Zhao T, Chen P, Cao XS, Wang CJ, Zhang ZP, Sun X, Yu JM, Wang YS. Validation study for the hypothesis of internal mammary sentinel lymph node lymphatic drainage in breast cancer. Oncotarget. 2016. doi:10.18632/oncotarget. 9634. [Epub ahead of print]

[39] Cong BB, Cao XS, Qiu PF, Liu YB, Zhao T, Chen P, Wang CJ, Zhang ZP, Sun X, Wang YS. Validation study of the modified injection technique for internal mammary sentinel lymph node biopsy in breast cancer. Onco Targets Ther. 2015;8:2705–2708.

[40] Urban JA, Marjani MA. Significance of internal mammary lymph node metastases in breast cancer. Am J Roentgenol Radium Ther Nucl Med. 1971;111(1):130–136.

[41] Horino T, Fujita M, Ueda N, Ota J, Ryo M, Nakano Y, Taguchi T. Efficacy of internal mammary node dissection in the treatment of breast cancer. Jpn J Clin Oncol. 1991;21(6): 422–427.

[42] Huang O, Wang L, Shen K, et al. Breast cancer subpopulation with high risk of internal mammary lymph nodes metastasis: analysis of 2269 Chinese breast cancer patients treated with extended radical mastectomy. Breast Cancer Res Treat. 2008;107(3):379–387.

[43] Qiu PF, Zhao RR, Liu YB, Wang YS. Internal mammary sentinel lymph node biopsy should still be performed, especially in the patient with clinically positive axillary lymph nodes. Breast. 2013;22(5):999–1000.

[44] Poortmans P. Postmastectomy radiation in breast cancer with one to three involved lymph nodes: ending the debate. Lancet. 2014;383(9935):2104–2106.

[45] Clarke M, Collins R, Darby S, et al. Effects of radiotherapy and of differences in the extent of surgery for early breast cancer on local recurrence and 15-year survival: an overview of the randomised trials. Lancet. 2005;366(9503):2087–2106.

[46] Stemmer SM, Rizel S, Hardan I, et al. The role of radiotherapy of the internal mammary lymph nodes in high-risk stage II to IIIA breast cancer patients after high-dose chemotherapy: a prospective sequential nonrandomized study. J Clin Oncol. 2003;21(14): 2713–2718.

[47] EBCTCG (Early Breast Cancer Trialists' Collaborative Group), McGale P, Taylor C, et al. Effect of radiotherapy after mastectomy and axillary surgery on 10-year recurrence and 20-year breast cancer mortality: meta-analysis of individual patient data for 8135 women in 22 randomised trials. Lancet. 2014;383(9935):2127–2135.

[48] Whelan TJ, Olivotto IA, Parulekar WR, et al. Regional nodal radiotherapy in early-stage breast cancer. N Engl J Med. 2015;373(4):307–316.

[49] Poortmans PM, Collette S, Kirkove C, et al. Internal mammary and medial supraclavicular radiotherapy in breast cancer. N Engl J Med. 2015;373(4):317–327.

[50] Hennequin C, Bossard N, Servagi-Vernat S, et al. Ten-year survival results of a randomized trial of radiotherapy of internal mammary nodes after mastectomy. Int J Radiat Oncol Biol Phys. 2013;86(5):860–866.

[51] Budach W, Kammers K, Boelke E, et al. Adjuvant radiotherapy of regional lymph nodes in breast cancer–a meta-analysis of randomized trials. Radiat Oncol. 2013;8:267.

[52] Gradishar WJ, Anderson BO, Balassanian R, et al. NCCN clinical practice guidelines in oncology: Breast Cancer. Version 1. 2016. NCCN.org.

[53] Thorsen LB, Offersen BV, Danø H, et al. DBCG-IMN: a population-based cohort study on the effect of internal mammary node radiotherapy in early node-positive breast cancer. J Clin Oncol. 2016;34(4):314–320.

[54] Cong BB, Qiu PF, Wang YS. Internal mammary sentinel lymph node biopsy: minimally invasive staging and tailored internal mammary radiotherapy. Ann Surg Oncol. 2014;21(7):2119–2121.

[55] Noguchi M, Ohta N, Thomas M, Kitagawa H, Miyazaki I. Risk of internal mammary lymph node metastases and its prognostic value in breast cancer patients. J Surg Oncol. 1993;52(1):26–30.

[56] Veronesi U, Arnone P, Veronesi P, et al. The value of radiotherapy on metastatic internal mammary nodes in breast cancer. Results on a large series. Ann Oncol. 2008;19(9):1553–1560.

[57] Connolly JL. Changes and problematic areas in interpretation of the AJCC Cancer Staging Manual, 6th edition, for breast cancer. Arch Pathol Lab Med. 2006;130(3):287–291.

[58] Heuts EM, van der Ent FW, von Meyenfeldt MF, Voogd AC. Internal mammary lymph drainage and sentinel node biopsy in breast cancer—a study on 1008 patients. Eur J Surg Oncol. 2009;35(3):252–257.

Chapter 21

Nanobiotechnology for Breast Cancer Treatment

Márcia Rocha, Natalia Chaves and Sônia Báo

Additional information is available at the end of the chapter

http://dx.doi.org/10.5772/66989

Abstract

Despite many technological breakthroughs, even the best breast cancer treatments available today are not 100% effective. Chemotherapy has improved, but many drugs still do not reach the tumor site at effective doses and are often associated with high systemic toxicity and poor pharmacokinetics. Moreover, for many malignancies, diagnosis is obtainable only in metastatic stages of development, reducing the overall effectiveness of treatment. The choice of available treatments depends on tumor characteristics such as biomarkers, tumor size, metastatic disease, ligands, and antigen or endocrine receptor expression. Combined with surgical resection, chemotherapy and radiation remain the first line of treatment for patients with cancer. Even with these treatments, however, cancer continues to have high fatality rates and current therapeutic modalities have yet to significantly improve the often dismal prognosis of this disease. Nanotechnology is a highly focused approach, which may provide more effective and less toxic treatment when compared to chemotherapy. This area of research has emerged as cancer treatment in the form of new drugs and has reached promising results in preclinical and clinical trials proving its value as a potential tumor therapy.

Keywords: breast cancer, therapy, nanomaterials, nano-oncology

1. Introduction

Nanobiotechnology is defined as the biomedical application of nano-sized systems [1]. Nanomaterials, which measure a few nanometers in length, allow for unique interaction with biological systems at the molecular level. They can also facilitate important advances in detection, diagnosis, and treatment of human cancers and this approach is known as nano-oncology. Breast cancer is one of the most common cancers worldwide [2]. The choice of available treatments depends on tumor characteristics such as biomarkers, tumor size, metastatic disease, ligands, and antigens or endocrine receptors expression. Combined with surgical resection, chemotherapy and radiation remain the first line of treatment for patients with cancer [3]. Improvements have been made to chemotherapies, because drugs are still not reaching the tumor site at effective doses, and are often associated with high systemic toxicities and poor pharmacokinetics. The nanotechnology is an approach which allows more effective and less toxic chemotherapy.

For many malignancies, diagnosis is obtainable only during metastatic stages of development, reducing the overall effectiveness of treatment [4]. Multidrug resistance, the principal mechanism by which many cancers develop resistance to drugs, is also a key factor in the failure of many forms of chemotherapy. It affects patients with a variety of blood cancers and solid tumors, including breast cancers [5]. Triple-negative breast cancer (TNBC), with absent or minimal expression of estrogen and progesterone receptors, and human epidermal growth factor receptor 2 are most common in younger women. In later stages, the prognosis is more dire, when compared to that of other breast cancer subtypes, with a higher risk of relapse, often involving other organs [6]. Emerging nanotechnologies have exhibited the possibility of specifically treating or targeting breast cancer. Among nanoparticles, various lipid nanoparticles, namely liposomes, solid lipid nanoparticles, nanostructured lipid carriers, and lipid polymer hybrid nanoparticles, have been developed over the past few years for breast cancer therapy and evidence of this is documented [2].

Nanoparticles are also being actively developed for tumor imaging *in vivo*, biomolecular profiling of cancer biomarkers, and targeted drug delivery. These nanotechnology-based techniques can be widely applied for management of varying malignant diseases [7].

2. Breast cancer

2.1. Incidence and epidemiology

Breast cancer is the most frequent carcinoma in females and the second most common cause of cancer-related mortality in women worldwide. Approximately 61,000 new cases of *in situ* and 246,000 cases of invasive breast carcinoma, respectively, are expected to be diagnosed in the United States in 2016. Within this same period in the United States, breast cancer will account for an estimated 40,500 deaths among women [8]. The decline in cancer-related death rates over the past two decades has been driven by continued decreases in fatalities from breast cancer. Death rates for female breast cancer are down 36% from peak rates, most likely, as a result of improvements in early detection and treatment [9, 10]. By contrast, incidence rates increased in men for cancer of the breast. Some suggestive correlations about the increased cancer rate involve changes in environmental risk factors, such as obesity [8, 11].

2.2. Current breast cancer diagnosis and treatment

Breast cancer diagnosis, according to the European guidelines, is based on clinical examination in combination with imaging and confirmed by pathological assessment [3]. Clinical examination includes manual palpation of the breasts and locoregional lymph nodes, along with assessment for distant metastases (bones, liver, lungs, and neurological examination in the case of symptoms). Other forms of assessment include complete personal and family medical history, including evaluation of menopausal status, physical examination, blood count analysis, liver and renal function tests, and alkaline phosphatase and calcium checks [12].

Pathological diagnosis should be based on core-needle biopsies obtained by manual or preferably by ultrasound or stereotactic guidance. The pathological report should include the histological type, grade, estrogen receptor (ER), and for invasive cancer, progesterone receptor (PgR) along with human growth factor receptor type 2 (HER2) [13]. Routine staging evaluations are directed at locoregional diseases, as asymptomatic distant metastases are very rare and patients do not profit from comprehensive laboratory and radiological staging. Bilateral mammography and ultrasound of the breast and regional lymph nodes are included in imaging [3].

Subsequent to diagnosis, the prognostic and treatment are based on histology and immunohistochemistry (IHC) data. The selection of a treatment strategy is based upon the tumor extent/location (size and location of primary tumor, number of lesions, and number and extent of lymph node involvement) and other factors such as age, lifestyle, and general health status of the patient [14].

Women with a high risk of breast cancer (previous chest wall irradiation for lymphoma or carrying the BRCA1 or BRCA2 gene mutations) may be offered risk-reducing surgery including prophylactic bilateral mastectomy and reconstruction [15].

Ductal carcinoma *in situ* may be treated with breast conservation therapy (BCT), which has replaced radical mastectomy as the treatment of choice for early breast cancer, providing clear resection margins achieve, or with mastectomy, usually followed by radiotherapy and/or chemotherapy [16]. Whole-breast radiotherapy (WBRT) after breast-conserving surgery (BCS) for diagnosis of ductal carcinoma *in situ* (DCIS) decreases the risk of local recurrence [17]. Mastectomy may still be carried out based upon tumor size (relative to breast size), tumor multicentricity, prior radiation of the chest wall or breast, or patient choice [18]. Sentinel lymph node biopsy (SLNB) is now the standard of care. All modalities of chemotherapy, endocrine therapies (ETs), and targeted therapies as adjuvant treatments may be used preoperatively for patients with isolated tumor cells [13].

In HER2-positive breast cancer, trastuzumab therapy should be started in the neoadjuvant setting in association with the taxane part of the chemotherapy regimen. The chemotherapy regimens to be used in the neoadjuvant setting are the same ones used in the adjuvant setting. Unfortunately, there are no validated predictive markers which allow for the tailoring of the regimen to the individual patient. It is therefore recommended that a sequential program of anthracyclines and taxanes is used. ER-positive, HER2-negative carcinomas, especially of the lobular subtype, are generally less responsive to primary chemotherapy than ER-negative and HER2-positive tumors and may benefit more from primary ET. ET is usually given 4–6 months before surgery and continued postoperatively; for post-menopausal patients, aromatase inhibitors (AIs) are more effective than tamoxifen in decreasing tumor size and require less extensive surgery [3, 19].

2.3. Limitations of the current breast cancer treatments

One major challenge to the treatment of cancer is the lack of selective toxicity, which results in a reduced therapeutic index and, as consequence, compromises clinical prognosis. In order to reduce damage to normal tissues, suboptimal doses of anticancer chemotherapeutics are often administered [20].

Furthermore, the high interstitial fluid pressure (IFP) of solid tumors forms a barrier to transcapillary transport and results in poor biodistribution and penetration of drugs [21]. Another determinant of drug distribution within tissues is the half-life of the drugs in circulation; a drug with longer half-life will establish a more uniform distribution in tissues, even if its extravasation and penetration of tissues are relatively slow, whereas a drug that has a short half-life will have nonuniform distribution [22]. Moreover, vessels in tumor sites are heterogenic and may have fenestrations that increase the extravasation of drugs [23].

It has been shown that the amount of drug accumulated in normal viscera is 10- to 20-fold higher than that in a similarly weighted tumor site [24] and that many anticancer drugs are not able to penetrate more than 40–50 mm (equivalent to the combined diameter of three to five cells) from the vasculature [20, 25, 26]. These defects often lead to incomplete tumor response, multiple drug resistance (MDR), and ultimately therapeutic failure [27–29]. MDR, when tumor cells are treated with one anticancer drug and become resistant to a whole spectrum of drugs, is usually based on overexpressed drug efflux proteins and therefore is an important challenge for breast cancer therapy [30–33].

3. Nanobiotechnology-based platforms for breast cancer therapy

3.1. Properties of nanocarriers

The most current anticancer agents do not have an adequate job of differentiating between cancerous and normal cells and can lead to systemic toxicity and severe side effects. To overcome limitations of conventional chemotherapeutics, nanotechnology offers a more targeted approach and could therefore provide significant benefits to cancer patients. The size, shape, and charge are important parameters in nanoparticle systems that indicate the *in vivo* distribution, targeting ability, and biological destination of nanoparticles.

Nanoparticles have many advantages over free drugs. Some of them are listed below:

- Protect the drugs from early degradation.
- Enhance absorption of the drugs into a selected tissue.
- Control the drug tissue distribution and pharmacokinetic.
- Improve intracellular penetration.
- Prevent drugs from premature interaction with the biological environment.
- Reduce systemic toxicity.

Particles with hydrodynamic diameters below 10 nm are subject to rapid kidney clearance. Most of injected nanoparticles end up in the liver and spleen. Resident macrophages will phagocytose nanoparticles, degrade a small part of them, and exocytose both the degraded and intact nanoparticles. To avoid mechanical filtration by the liver and spleen, particles require size limitations above 200 nm [34, 35].

The zeta potential (surface charge) of nanoparticles has been shown to influence the nanoparticles direction within the tumor. It has been described that positively charged nanoparticles show increased cell uptake and binding due to the interaction between cationic nanoparticles and negatively charged cell membranes. Neutral particles have demonstrated lower interaction with the cell membrane than those nanoparticles with the same size and charge, resulting from the lower number of electrostatic interactions between charged cell membranes and nanoparticles surface [36–38]. In addition, studies have shown that systemically administered nanoparticles, with 30–40 nm [39] and 70 nm [40] in size and having a slightly negative surface charge, revealed internalization by tumor cells in mice and movement away from blood vessels [38].

Neutral polymers are used to minimize nanoparticle surface charge. The polymers are generally used to reduce aggregation caused by particle-particle interactions as well as limiting potential electrostatically induced interactions with other components of circulation, such as plasma membranes of cells (negative charge). Supposing the nanoparticle surface charge is increased, both positively and negatively, the probability that the particle will be removed from circulation by macrophage increases [36, 41]. When nanomaterials are administered into the blood, they are taken up within minutes or by the phagocytic cells of mononuclear phagocyte (MPS). The opsonization can be prevented by adding poly (ethylene) glycol (PEG) to the surface of nanomaterials. This addition drastically increases the blood half-life of all nanomaterials regardless of surface charge, improving the circulation time and accumulation in the target tissue. To create long-circulating nanoparticles, a diameter between 30 and 200 nm is desired [42].

The nanoparticle surface is the site that is modified to include targeting ligands. The reason for including a target ligand is that the cell surface of the cognate receptor is elevated in target cancer cells relative to other cells [43]. The advantages of surface coating are that it offers biocompatibilities, biodistribution of the nanoparticles, and modulating interaction between nanoparticles and cells, tissues, and biomolecules [44].

3.2. Nanoparticle drug delivery arsenal

To construct an appropriate nanocarrier for rapid and effective clinical translation, some important characteristics need to be considered. The nanocarriers must be made from a material that is biocompatible and easily functionalized along with being well characterized, soluble, exhibit extended circulation ability, no aggregation, and high uptake efficiency by the target cells.

Nanocarriers can be classified into three categories based upon materials that they are made from: (1) lipid-based, (2) polymeric, and (3) inorganic (**Figure 1**). These nanocarriers have been used for a variety of applications such as drug delivery, imaging, apoptosis detection, radiation sensitizers, and photothermic ablation of tumors [7, 45, 46]. Some of these nanocarriers are described below.

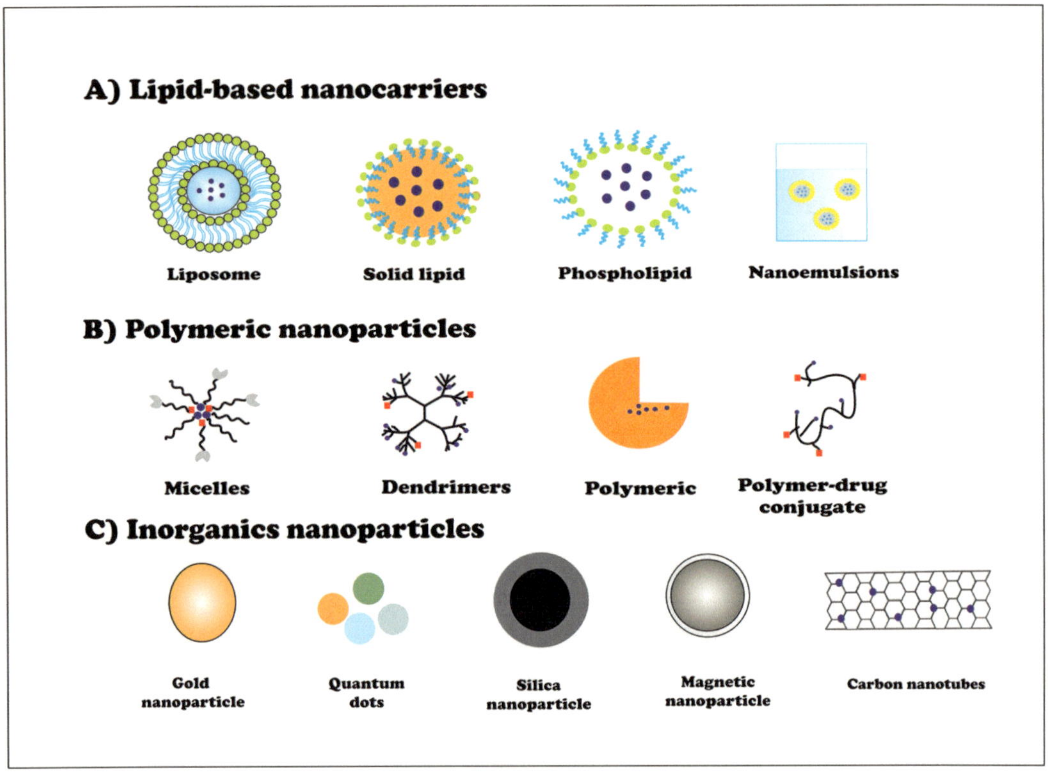

Figure 1. Schematic of different kinds of nanocarriers used for drug delivery. (A) Lipid-based nanocarriers, (B) polymeric nanoparticles, (C) inorganics particles.

3.2.1. Lipid-based nanocarriers

Lipid-based drug delivery systems have attractive properties, as well as biocompatibility, biodegradability, and the ability to entrap both hydrophobic and hydrophilic drugs. Lipid-based nanocarriers include liposomes, nanoemulsion, solid lipid nanoparticles, and phospholipid micelles.

Liposomes were the first nanocarriers, described in 1965 by Bangham [47], and the first that have been clinically approved by the FDA (Food and Drug Administration) to carry chemotherapy drugs (DaunoXome™) (50–80 nm) in 1996 [48]. Liposomes are small vesicles consisting of a bilayer lipid membrane surrounding an aqueous interior compartment [49]. The membranes consist of amphiphilic compounds, such as phospholipids and glycolipids, which make them biodegradable. Hydrophobic molecules are intercalated within the bilayer membrane, and hydrophilic molecules can be entrapped in their aqueous core, making liposomes a good therapeutic carrier [50]. To improve stability and circulation half-life, liposomes can be coated with targeting ligands and polymers such as PEG [51]. For example, a recent study showed that PEG-modified liposomes of ursolic acid enhanced *in vitro* cytotoxicity in gastric cancer cells when compared to standard ursolic acid [38]. Liposomal drug formulation improves the biodistribution and pharmacokinetics of a drug. This means higher drug concentration can be achieved within tumors while reducing drug concentration in normal tissue [51]. Some disadvantages have been identified in the use of liposomes. Studies have shown that 50–80% of liposomes are adsorbed by the reticuloendothelial system (RES) and mainly by liver cells (Kupffer cells) within the first 15–30 min following intravenous administration [52, 53]. Other problems are related to their stability, poor batch-to-batch reproducibility, and difficulty with sterilization [54].

3.2.2. *Polymeric*

Polymeric nanoparticles systems are engineered from biocompatible and biodegradable polymers. Polymeric nanocarriers include micelles, dendrimers, and polymer-drug conjugates.

Many biodegradable polymers have been used to produce polymeric nanoparticles such as poly D L-lactic-co-glycolic acid (PLGA), poly D L-lactic acid (PLA), and poly ethylene glycol (PEG) [55]. Polysaccharides such as chitosan, alginate, and pectin have also been used to encapsulate these nanostructures [56, 57]. These nanoparticles are formulated through a self-assembly process using block copolymers with different hydrophilicity and consisting of two or more polymer chains [58]. Polymeric nanoparticles have been formulated to encapsulate either hydrophilic or hydrophobic drugs. This system facilitates surface modifications, and controlled pH- dependent controlled release [59]. A recent study revealed developed albumin-polymer conjugate nanoparticles of curcumin and demonstrated growth inhibition of three-dimensional LNCaP (epithelial cell line derived from a human prostate carcinoma) multicellular tumor spheroids when compared to native curcumin [60]. This result is an interesting option for controlled and target-based delivery.

Dendrimers are polymeric macromolecules with numerous arms extending from a center, resulting in a well-defined topological structure [61]. They have three main components: (1) a central core with two or more groups and repeated units attached to a central core called generations; (2) peripheral functional groups on the surface which determine the physicochemical properties of a dendrimer; (3) peripheral groups that can be modified to obtain both a charged hydrophilic and lipophilic function [62]. Dendrimers are appealing since they can be synthesized at various sizes, molecular weights, and chemical compositions [62]. With the modification of surface groups, interiors, and core, the properties of dendrimers can be optimized to obtain favorable physical characteristics, biodistribution, and receptor-mediated targeting. Dendrimers have shown promise for biomedical applications because they can be easily conjugated with targeting molecules, are biodegradable, biocompatible, and have high water solubility [63, 64]. A successful study using dendrimers was demonstrated in 2005 when methotrexate conjugated to polyamidoamine (PAMAM) dendrimers resulted in a 10-fold reduction in tumor size compared with that achieved using free systemic methotrexate [60]. In spite of promising results, dendrimers are relatively expensive as compared to other nanoparticles and require many repetitive steps in order to be synthesized, presenting a challenge for large-scale production [65].

3.2.3. *Inorganic*

The iron oxide nanoparticles (IO) are classified based on their sizes as standard superparamagnetic iron oxide (SSPIOs) at 60–150 nm, superparamagnetic iron oxide (USPIO) 5–40 nm, and ultra-small and monocrystalline iron oxide (MION) 10–30 nm. Magnetic nanosystem is attractive due to its ability to become magnetized after exposure to a magnetic field but does not retain permanent magnetization once the field is turned off. These nanoparticles need to be small so that they can be superparamagnetic in order to avoid agglomeration after stoppage of the magnetic field and remain in circulation without being removed by the immune system [36]. The IO can be degraded to Fe+ ions in the body in the acidic compartments of cells, for example, lysosomes, reducing the potential toxicity of nanoparticles (**Figure 2**). The magnetic flux density and permeability of exterior magnetic fields should be optimized to be strong enough to mediate penetration of nanoparticles across the biological barriers, and provide for sufficient accumulation at target sites while reducing risk to normal tissue [66, 67].

Gold nanoparticles have received attention due to their unique properties. These nanoparticles are easily synthesized and size can be readily controlled by turning the synthesis procedure [68]. These nanoparticle conjugates can exhibit increased targeting rapid transport kinetics, long circulatory half-life, size-enhanced tumor uptake, and biocompatibility. These nanoparticles represent one of the most stable and easily surface functionalized for molecular conjugation [69]. Gold is resistant to oxidation under ambient or physiological conditions, which permits interaction in the biological environment. The shape of gold nanoparticles has been demonstrated to penetrate the cell membrane. When functionalized, they can show increased binding affinity and targeting selectivity with multiple targeting groups as well as tumor selective uptake due to their size [69].

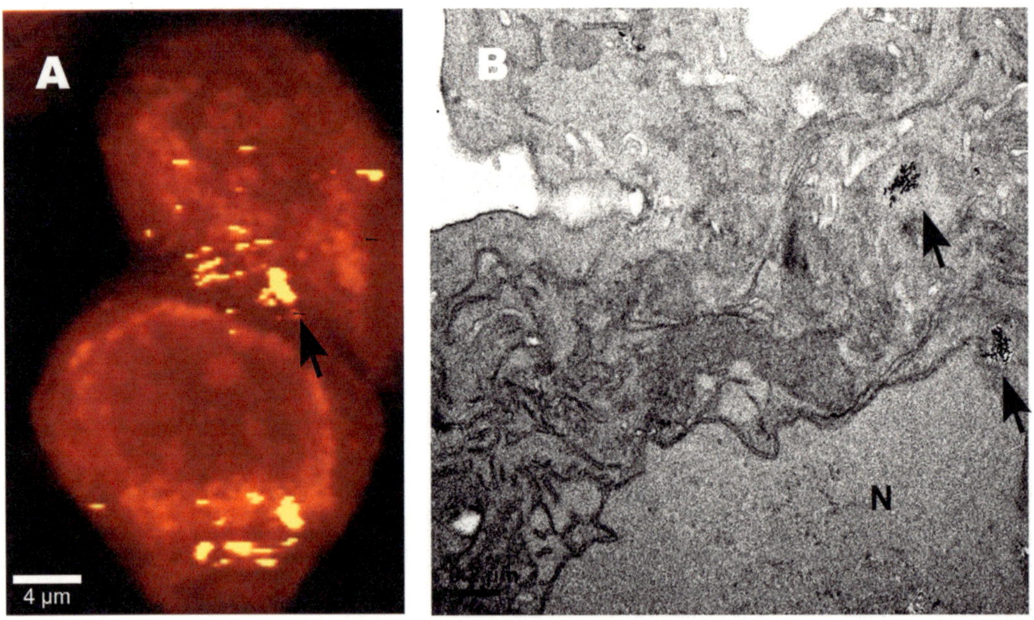

Figure 2. Intracellular occurrence of iron oxide nanoparticles in breast cancer cells analyzed through microscopy. (A) Representative confocal of Raman micrographs after digital contrast enhancement in MDA-MB-231 cells. (B) Ultra-micrographs from transmission electronic microscopic (TEM) in MCF-7 are shown. The cells were treated with 200 μM iron oxide nanoparticles at 37°C for 24 and 6 h, respectively. The black arrow denotes accumulation of particles in the cytoplasm of tumor cells.

Inorganic nanocarriers have been used due to their physiochemical properties, such as chemical composition, size, shape, good stability, ease of functionalization, and higher surface-to-volume ratios. Inorganic nanoparticles include gold nanoparticles, magnetic nanomaterials, carbon nanotubes, silica nanoparticles, and quantum dots [49].

4. Tumor targeting and uptake

4.1. Types of targeting agents

Targeting agents can be broadly classified as proteins (mainly antibodies and their fragments), nucleic acids, peptides, aptamers, vitamins, and carbohydrates, and they may be conjugated to the carriers [70]. The surface marker should be overexpressed on target cells relative to normal cells. When targeting agents are used to deliver nanocarriers to cancer cells, it is essential that the agent binds with high selectivity to molecules that are uniquely expressed on the cell surface. Nanocarriers will recognize and bind to target cells through ligand-receptor interactions. The carriers are then internalized and the drug is released inside the cell [71]. The vitamin folic acid (folate) has also been used because folate receptors (FRs) are overexpressed in many tumor cells including kidney, ovarian, and endometrial cancer. The folate receptor is used to deliver drug conjugates to selectively accumulating drugs into cancer cell-mediated endocytosis [72]. One of the more commonly used ligands for cancer cells is transferrin (Tf) protein. Transferrin interacts with Tf receptors (TfRs), which are overexpressed in a range of tumor cells including lung, colon, pancreatic, and bladder cancers to increased metabolic rates [73]. Tf receptors binding directly to nanoparticles such as liposomes have resulted in improved intracellular delivery and therapeutic outcomes in animal tumor models [65, 74, 75]. Studies show that Tf is also used to facilitate small interfering RNAs (siRNA) delivery through transferrin receptors, allowing for antitumor activity [76]. Targeting receptors whose expression correlates with metabolic rate, such as folate and Tf, are also expressed in fast-growing healthy cells such as endothelial, epithelial, and fibroblasts cells, and this could lead to non-specific targeting and may increase toxicity and decrease drug efficiency [77].

4.2. Passive nanoparticle target

Nanoparticles circulating in the bloodstream can reach the neoplastic tissue by passive drug targeting through the enhanced permeation and retention effect (EPR) (**Figure 3**) [45, 78]. When a solid tumor reaches a certain size, the normal vasculature present in its early stage is not sufficient enough to provide the oxygen required for proliferation [79]. Because of this, the cells start to die and they secrete growth factors, which trigger angiogenesis, where budding of new blood vessels from the surrounding capillaries occurs, increasing their permeability. Angiogenesis in tumors is the process of rapid development of new, irregular blood vessels that present a discontinuous epithelium and lack the basal membrane of normal vascular structures [80, 81]. Fenestrations in the capillaries, depending on the location and tumor type, can reach sizes from 200 to 2000 nm. The fenestrations between endothelial cells facilitate the extravasation of nanocarriers from the surrounding vessels into the tumor [82]. The extracellular fluids are constantly drained into the lymphatic vessels, and this allows for the renewal

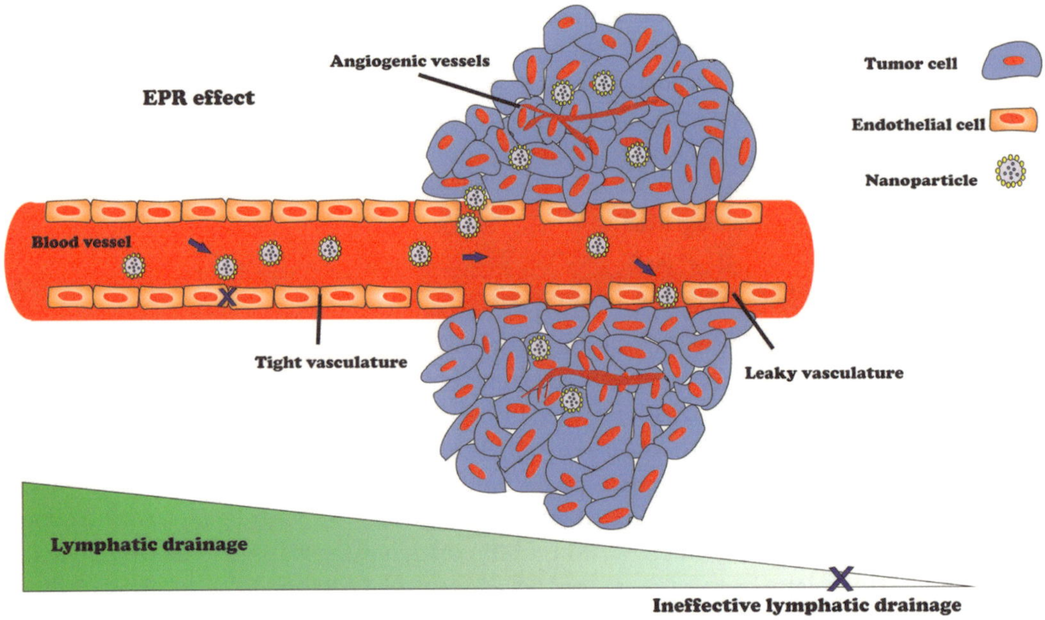

Figure 3. Schematic representation showing enhanced permeability and retention of nanoparticles in tumor.

of interstitial fluid and the recycling of extravagated solutes and colloids back to the circulation [83]. In tumors, the lymphatic function is defective and, consequently, the uptake of the interstitial fluid is minimal [84]. Free drugs may diffuse nonspecifically and a nanocarrier can extravasate into the leaky vessels of tumor tissues through the EPR effect. A study using liposomes of different sizes suggests that particles with a diameter of 200–300 nm are able to extravasate, whereas in another part of the same tumor, molecules only a few nanometers in size may have difficulty entering the interstitium [85]. The success of EPR effect depends on factors such as lymphatic drainage rate, blood flow that is different in various tumor types and degrees of capillary disorder.

4.3. Active nanoparticle target

Passive targeting is available only in certain types of tumors and does not, necessarily, insure internalization of nanocarriers by targeted cells. Nanocarriers can be engineered to attach targeting with selective agents to employ active targeting [86]. As previously described in topic 4.1, some of these agents include peptides [87], proteins [88], antibodies [89], and small organic molecules [90–92]. These agents are complementary to receptors that are overexpressed or present in tumor cells [93]. The objective of passive targeting is to increase interactions between nanoparticles and cells and to enhance internalization of drugs without altering biodistribution [94, 95]. Some physicochemical properties might also affect the efficacy of active targeting *in vitro* and *in vivo*. These properties, such as the size of nanoparticles [96], choice of the targeting ligand [97], and ligand density [98] may affect the efficacy of the active targeting of nanoparticles. The nonspecific biding of proteins during

http://dx.doi.org/10.5772/66989

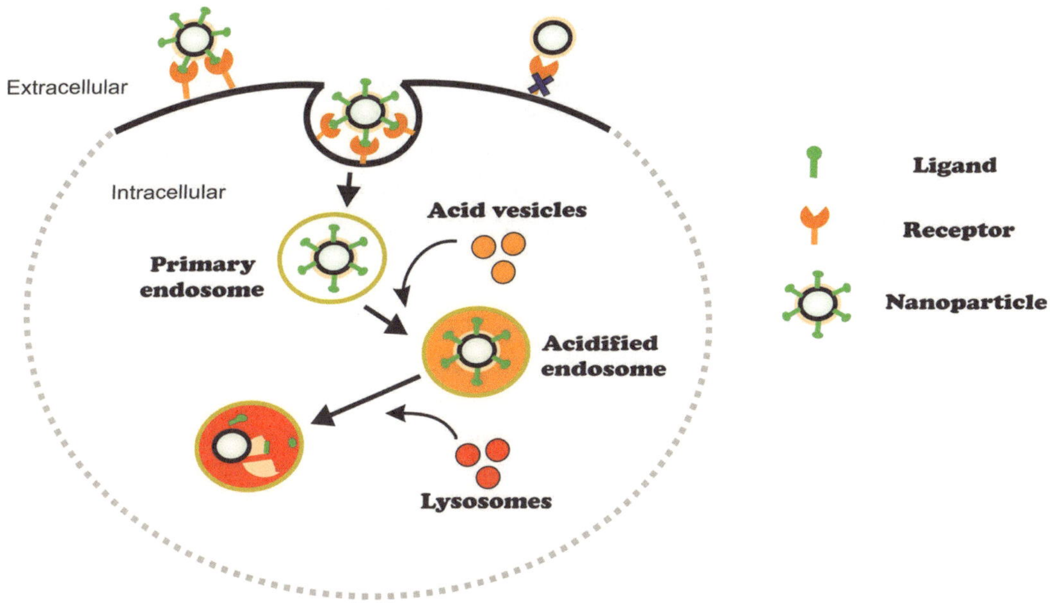

Figure 4. Cellular uptake mechanism. The ligand-coated nanoparticle binds to the membrane receptor, enters the cells by primary endosome, and then forms an acidified endosome. The enzymatic digestion of nanoparticles is done by fusion of lysosomes.

the nanoparticles dislocation through the blood stream and the administration route has been shown to affect the targeting ability of nanocarriers [99]. Active targeting can be used for controlled drug release applications, where the drug is released into the extracellular or intracellular environment. The targeting agents can be used to facilitate nanocarrier internalization into cells, primarily via endocytosis (**Figure 4**) [100].

5. Nanocarriers and multidrug resistance

Multidrug resistance (MDR) limits the potency of many chemotherapeutics can be classified into two types: acquired MDR that can be developed during traditional chemotherapy in common doses and intrinsic MDR that can be developed from preexisting resistance present in tumor cells. MDR is the decreased cell uptake and increased efflux of a drug. MDR transporters carry a variety of anticancer drugs out of cancer cells reducing the intracellular drug doses and produce resistance to chemotherapy [101]. If there is tumor recurrence, chemotherapy may fail because of residual drug-resistant cells dominating the tumor population [5]. Chemotherapy will kill only drug-sensitive cells that do not, or only mildly, express MDR transporters, leaving behind drug-resistant cells that overexpress MDR transporters. The main drug efflux transporters include P-glycoprotein (MDR1 or ABCB1), multidrug resistance-associated proteins (MRP1 or ABCC1), and the breast cancer resistance protein (ABCG2) [102–104]. To combat MDR, stimuli-responsive multifunctional nanoparticle-based drug delivery systems, which can deliver drugs into cells, release the drug in a specific site or at a specific time. To overcome MDR, an optimal drug delivery system has to release drugs into cytoplasm rapidly and completely, leading to sufficiently high intracellular drug concentration to exceed drug efflux and limit concentration, in order to inhibit the proliferation of drug-resistant cancer cells and kill them. A study done using non-ionic copolymer with a hydrophobic core containing doxorubicin, called SP1049C, has been shown to circumvent p-glycoprotein-mediated drug resistance. The study was done on a mouse model of leukemia and it is currently in clinical evaluation. This study demonstrated the possibility of using nanocarriers to bypass MDR transporters [102, 105–107].

6. Preclinical and clinical trials for nanoparticles breast cancer therapy

The nanomedicine industry perspective toward oncology-based nanomedicinal therapeutics is very promising. The aim of these compounds to improve the therapeutic index of anticancer drugs by modifying their pharmacokinetics and tissue distribution to improve delivery to the site of action is well known and has also been demonstrated clinically. The first anticancer nanomedicine approved by the FDA in 1995, Doxil™/Caelyx™ [108], achieves a differential distribution of doxorubicin versus the free drug and is now approved for several applications, including breast cancer, based upon improved safety with equivalent or superior efficacy versus standard therapies.

Nanomedicines for breast cancer therapy or diagnosis in clinical development can be broadly divided into five main types: liposomes, polymeric conjugates, polymeric nanoparticles, polymeric micelles, and others. Examples of marketed anti-breast cancer nanomedicines and those in clinical development are summarized in **Table 1**.

Nanomedicine type	Drug	Product name/company	Indication	Phase
Liposomes	Doxorubicin	Myocet™/Teva UK	Metastatic Breast Cancer	Approved
	Paclitaxel	LEP—ETU/Insys	Breast cancer	Phase II
		EndoTAG-1/MediGene	Breast cancer	Phase II
Polymeric conjugates	Irinotecan	NKTR102 (PEG)/Nektar	Metastatic breast cancer	Phase III
Polymeric micelles	Paclitaxel	Genexol-PM™/Samyang Biopharmaceuticals	Breast cancer	Approved
	Docetaxel	Genexol-PM™/Samyang Biopharmaceuticals	Breast cancer (NSCLC, prostate, ovarian, head and neck, gastric, and esophageal cancer)	Marketed in South Korea
	Paclitaxel	NK105/NanoCarrier™	Breast cancer	Phase III
Other	Paclitaxel	Abraxane ™/Celgene	Advanced breast cancer	Approved
	Phospholipid stabilized microbubble	SonoVue/Bracco Imaging	Ultrasound enhancement for breast and other cancers	Approved

Table 1. Clinically and preclinical nanoparticle for breast cancer therapies and diagnostics, grouped by their trial phases.

7. Conclusions

The choice of appropriate nanocarriers is a difficult one. It is important to understand the key nanoparticle features such as properties, size, targeting ligand, and charge to improve the design for oncology applications. Nanoparticle therapeutics has been used for many treatments of most cancers. Although the field of nanomedicine is developing rapidly, there are still a limited number of nanocarriers approved by the FDA and limited available clinical data. More clinical trials are required to better understand the advantages and disadvantages of nanoparticle therapeutics. Well-designed studies are important for development of these drugs. Further research is needed to develop new nanotherapeutics incorporating a variety of characteristics along with good experimental design in order to achieve improvements in treatments and nanoparticle targeting to overcome current limitations.

Acknowledgements

The authors gratefully acknowledge financial support from the National Council of Technological and Scientific Development (CNPq), Coordination for the Improvement of Higher Education Personnel (CAPES), Financing Agency of Studies and Projects (FINEP), and Foundation for Research Support of the Federal District (FAP-DF).

Author details

Márcia Rocha, Natalia Chaves and Sônia Báo*

*Address all correspondence to: snbao@unb.br

Department of Cell Biology, Institute of Biological Sciences, University of Brasília (UnB), Brasília, Brazil

References

[1] Yezhelyev MV, Gao X, Xing Y, Al-Hajj A, Nie S, O'Regan RM. Emerging use of nanoparticles in diagnosis and treatment of breast cancer. The Lancet Oncology. 2007;**7**(8):657–67. DOI: 10.1016/S1470-2045(06)70793-8

[2] Prabhakar U, Maeda H, Jain RK, Sevick-Muraca EM, Zamboni W, Farokhzad OC, et al. Challenges and key considerations of the enhanced permeability and retention effect for nanomedicine drug delivery in oncology. Cancer Research. 2013;**73**(8):2412–7. DOI: 10.1158/0008-5472.CAN-12-4561

[3] Senkus E, Kyriakides S, Penault-Llorca F, Poortmans P, Thompson A, Zackrisson S, et al. Primary breast cancer: ESMO Clinical Practice Guidelines for diagnosis, treatment and follow-up. In: Annals of Oncology; 2015;26(5)v8-v30 DOI: 10.1093/annonc/mdv298

[4] Morris SA, Farrell D, Grodzinski P. Nanotechnologies in cancer treatment and diagnosis. Journal of the National Comprehensive Cancer Network. 2014;**12**(12):1727–33. DOI: 10.4172/2155-9619.1000195

[5] Koushik O, Rao Y, Kumar P, Karthikeyan R. Nano drug delivery systems to overcome cancer drug resistance-a review. Journal of Nanomedicine and Nanotechnology. 2016;**7**(378):2. DOI: 10.4172/2157-7439.1000378

[6] Johnson R, Sabnis N, McConathy WJ, Lacko AG. The potential role of nanotechnology in therapeutic approaches for triple negative breast cancer. Pharmaceutics. 2013;**5**(2):353–70. DOI: 10.3390/pharmaceutics5020353

[7] Ferrari M. Cancer nanotechnology: opportunities and challenges. Nature Reviews Cancer. 2005;**5**(3):161–71. DOI: 10.1038/nrc1566

[8] Siegel RL, Miller KD, Jemal A. CA: Cancer statistics, 2016. A Cancer Journal for Clinicians. 2016;**77**(1):7–30. DOI: 10.3322/caac.21254

[9] Howlader N, Noone AM, Krapcho M, Garshell J, Miller D, Altekruse SF, Kosary CL, Yu M, Ruhl J, Tatalovich Z,Mariotto A, Lewis DR, Chen HS, Feuer EJ, Cronin KA (eds). SEER Cancer Statistics Review, 1975-2012, SEER [Internet]. April 2015 [Updated: November 2014]. Available from: http://seer.cancer.gov/csr/1975_2012/[Accessed: April 2015]

[10] Berry DA, Cronin KA, Plevritis S, Fryback DG, Clarke L, Zelen M, et al. Effect of screening and adjuvant therapy on mortality from breast cancer. Obstetrical & Gynecological Survey. 2006;**61**(3):179–80. DOI: 10.1056/NEJMoa050518

[11] Schmid D, Ricci C, Behrens G, Leitzmann M. Adiposity and risk of thyroid cancer: a systematic review and meta-analysis. Obesity Reviews. 2015;**16**(12):1042–54. DOI: 10.1111/obr.12321

[12] Chlebowski RT, Rohan TE, Manson JE, Aragaki AK, Kaunitz A, Stefanick ML, et al. Breast cancer after use of estrogen plus progestin and estrogen alone: analyses of data from 2 women's health initiative randomized clinical trials. JAMA Oncology. 2015;**1**(3):296–305. DOI: 10.1001/jamaoncol.2015.0494

[13] van Nijnatten T, Schipper R, Lobbes M, Nelemans P, Beets-Tan R, Smidt M. The diagnostic performance of sentinel lymph node biopsy in pathologically confirmed node positive breast cancer patients after neoadjuvant systemic therapy: A systematic review and meta-analysis. European Journal of Surgical Oncology (EJSO). 2015;**41**(10):1278–87. DOI: 10.1016/j.ejso.2015.07.020

[14] Coates AS, Winer EP, Goldhirsch A, Gelber RD, Gnant M, Piccart-Gebhart M, et al. Tailoring therapies—improving the management of early breast cancer: St Gallen International Expert Consensus on the Primary Therapy of Early Breast Cancer 2015. In: Annals of Oncology; 2015. 2015;26(8)1533-46. DOI: 10.1093/annonc/mdv221

[15] Hartmann LC, Lindor NM. The role of risk-reducing surgery in hereditary breast and ovarian cancer. New England Journal of Medicine. 2016;**374**(5):454–68. DOI: 1056/NEJMra1503523

[16] Curran J. How effective is mammography in detecting breast cancer recurrence in women after Breast Conservation Therapy (BCT)–A systematic literature review. Radiography. 2016; DOI: 10.1016/j.radi.2016.02.001.

[17] Sweldens C, Peeters S, van Limbergen E, Janssen H, Laenen A, Patil S, et al. Local relapse after breast-conserving therapy for ductal carcinoma in situ: a European single-center experience and external validation of the Memorial Sloan-Kettering Cancer Center DCIS nomogram. The Cancer Journal. 2014;**20**(1):1–7. DOI: 10.1097/PPO.0000000000000025

[18] van Dongen JA, Voogd AC, Fentiman IS, Legrand C, Sylvester RJ, Tong D, et al. Long-term results of a randomized trial comparing breast-conserving therapy with mastectomy: European Organization for Research and Treatment of Cancer 10801 trial. Journal of the National Cancer Institute. 2000;**92**(14):1143–50. DOI: 10.1093/jnci/92.14.1143

[19] Guarneri V, Dieci MV, Frassoldati A, Maiorana A, Ficarra G, Bettelli S, et al. Prospective biomarker analysis of the randomized CHER-LOB study evaluating the dual anti-HER2 treatment with trastuzumab and lapatinib plus chemotherapy as neoadjuvant therapy for HER2-positive breast cancer. The Oncologist. 2015;**20**(9):1001–10. DOI: 10.1634/theoncologist.2015-0138

[20] Lu R-M, Chen M-S, Chang D-K, Chiu C-Y, Lin W-C, Yan S-L, et al. Targeted drug delivery systems mediated by a novel peptide in breast cancer therapy and imaging. PLoS One. 2013;**8**(6):e66128. DOI: 10.1371/journal.pone.0066128

[21] Heldin C-H, Rubin K, Pietras K, Östman A. High interstitial fluid pressure—an obstacle in cancer therapy. Nature Reviews Cancer. 2004;**4**(10):806–13. DOI: 10.1038/nrc1456

[22] Trédan O, Galmarini CM, Patel K, Tannock IF. Drug resistance and the solid tumor microenvironment. Journal of the National Cancer Institute. 2007;**99**(19):1441–54. DOI: 10.1093/jnci/djm135

[23] Hida K, Maishi N, Sakurai Y, Hida Y, Harashima H. Heterogeneity of tumor endothelial cells and drug delivery. Advanced Drug Delivery Reviews. 2016;**99**:140–7. DOI: 10.1016/j.addr.2015.11.008

[24] Bosslet K, Straub R, Blumrich M, Czech J, Gerken M, Sperker B, et al. Elucidation of the mechanism enabling tumor selective prodrug monotherapy. Cancer Research. 1998;**58**(6):1195–201. DOI: 10.1128/JB.01028-09 J

[25] Primeau AJ, Rendon A, Hedley D, Lilge L, Tannock IF. The distribution of the anticancer drug Doxorubicin in relation to blood vessels in solid tumors. Clinical Cancer Research. 2005;**11**(24):8782–8. DOI: 10.1158/1078-0432

[26] Minchinton AI, Tannock IF. Drug penetration in solid tumours. Nature Reviews Cancer. 2006;**6**(8):583–92. DOI: 10.1038/nrc1893

[27] Maeda H, Nakamura H, Fang J. The EPR effect for macromolecular drug delivery to solid tumors: Improvement of tumor uptake, lowering of systemic toxicity, and distinct tumor imaging in vivo. Advanced Drug Delivery Reviews. 2013;**65**(1):71–9. DOI: 10.1016/j.addr.2012.10.002

[28] Al-Abd AM, Aljehani ZK, Gazzaz RW, Fakhri SH, Jabbad AH, Alahdal AM, et al. Pharmacokinetic strategies to improve drug penetration and entrapment within solid tumors. Journal of Controlled Release. 2015;**219**:269–77. DOI: 10.1016/j.jconrel.2015.08.055

[29] Khawar IA, Kim JH, Kuh H-J. Improving drug delivery to solid tumors: priming the tumor microenvironment. Journal of Controlled Release. 2015;**201**:78–89. DOI: 10.1016/j.jconrel.2014.12.018

[30] Rebucci M, Michiels C. Molecular aspects of cancer cell resistance to chemotherapy. Biochemical Pharmacology. 2013;**85**(9):1219–26. DOI: 10.1016/j.bcp.2013.02.017

[31] Mimeault M, Mehta PP, Hauke R, Batra SK. Functions of normal and malignant prostatic stem/progenitor cells in tissue regeneration and cancer progression and novel targeting therapies. Endocrine Reviews. 2008;**29**(2):234–52. DOI: 10.1210/er.2007-0040

[32] Shah V, Taratula O, Garbuzenko OB, Taratula OR, Rodriguez-Rodriguez L, Minko T. Targeted nanomedicine for suppression of CD44 and simultaneous cell death induction in ovarian cancer: an optimal delivery of siRNA and anticancer drug. Clinical Cancer Research. 2013;**19**(22):6193–204. DOI: 10.1158/1078-0432

[33] Dreher MR, Liu W, Michelich CR, Dewhirst MW, Yuan F, Chilkoti A. Tumor vascular permeability, accumulation, and penetration of macromolecular drug carriers. Journal of the National Cancer Institute. 2006;**98**(5):335–44. DOI: 10.1093/jnci/djj070

[34] Heidel JD, Mark E. Davis. Clinical developments in nanotechnology for cancer therapy. Pharmaceutical Research. 2011;**28**(2):187–199. DOI: 0.1007/s11095-010-0178-7

[35] Perrault SD, Walkey C, Jennings T, Fischer HC, Chan WC. Mediating tumor targeting efficiency of nanoparticles through design. Nano Letters. 2009;**9**(5):1909–15. DOI: 10.1021/nl900031y

[36] Russ Knapp FF, Ashutosh D. Therapeutic radiopharmaceuticals for cancer therapy. In: Radiopharmaceuticals for Therapy. Springer (India) Pvt. Ltd., New Delhi, India; 2016. p. 167. DOI: 10.1007/978-81-322-2607-9

[37] Barua S, Yoo J-W, Kolhar P, Wakankar A, Gokarn YR, Mitragotri S. Particle shape enhances specificity of antibody-displaying nanoparticles. Proceedings of the National Academy of Sciences. 2013;**110**(9):3270–5. DOI: 10.1073/pnas.1216893110

[38] Zhao T, Liu Y, Gao Z, Gao D, Li N, Bian Y, et al. Self-assembly and cytotoxicity study of PEG-modified ursolic acid liposomes. Materials Science and Engineering: C. 2015;**53**:196–203. DOI: 10.1016/j.msec.2015.04.022

[39] Schluep T, Hwang J, Hildebrandt IJ, Czernin J, Choi CHJ, Alabi CA, et al. Pharmacokinetics and tumor dynamics of the nanoparticle IT-101 from PET imaging and tumor histological measurements. Proceedings of the National Academy of Sciences. 2009;**106**(27):11394–9. DOI: 10.1073/pnas.0905487106

[40] Choi CHJ, Alabi CA, Webster P, Davis ME. Mechanism of active targeting in solid tumors with transferrin-containing gold nanoparticles. Proceedings of the National Academy of Sciences. 2010;**107**(3):1235–40. DOI: 10.1073/pnas.0914140107

[41] Zahr AS, Davis CA, Pishko MV. Macrophage uptake of core-shell nanoparticles surface modified with poly (ethylene glycol). Langmuir. 2006;**22**(19):8178–85. DOI: 10.1021/la060951b

[42] Alexandre Albanese, Peter S. Tang, and Warren C.W. Chan. The Effect of Nanoparticle Size, Shape, and Surface Chemistry on Biological Systems. In: April 18, 2012; Canada: Biomedical Engineering; 2012. p. 1–16. DOI: 10.1146/annurev-bioeng-071811-150124

[43] Tsuchiya K, Nitta N, Sonoda A, Nitta-Seko A, Ohta S, Takahashi M, et al. Evaluation of atherosclerotic lesions using dextran-and mannan–dextran-coated USPIO: MRI analysis and pathological findings. International Journal of Nanomedicine. 2012;**7**:2271. DOI: 10.2147/IJN.S29417

[44] Gregory AE, Williamson D, Titball R. Vaccine delivery using nanoparticles. Frontiers in cellular and infection microbiology. 2013;**3**(13):1–13 10.3389/fcimb.2013.00013. DOI: 10.3389/fcimb

[45] Duncan R. The dawning era of polymer therapeutics. Nature Reviews Drug Discovery. 2003;**2**(5):347–60. DOI: 1038/nrc1958

[46] Lavan DA, McGuire T, Langer R. Small-scale systems for in vivo drug delivery. Nature Biotechnology. 2003;**21**(10):1184–91. DOI: 10.1038/nbt876

[47] Bangham AD, Horne R. Negative staining of phospholipids and their structural modification by surface-active agents as observed in the electron microscope. Journal of Molecular Biology. 1964;**8**(5):660IN2-8IN10. DOI: 10.1016/S0022-2836(64)80115-7

[48] Forssen EA, Ross ME. Daunoxome® treatment of solid tumors: preclinical and clinical investigations. Journal of Liposome Research. 1994;**4**(1):481–512. DOI: 10.3109/08982109409037058

[49] Bangham A. Liposomes: the Babraham connection. Chemistry and Physics of Lipids. 1993;**64**(1):275–85. DOI: 10.1016/0009-3084(93)90071-A

[50] Torchilin VP. Recent advances with liposomes as pharmaceutical carriers. Nature Reviews Drug Discovery. 2005;**4**(2):145–60. DOI: 10.1038/nrd1632

[51] Wang AZ, Langer R, Farokhzad OC. Nanoparticle delivery of cancer drugs. Annual Review of Medicine. 2012;**63**:185–98. DOI: 10.1146/annurev-med-040210-162544

[52] Laverman P, Carstens MG, Boerman OC, Dams ETM, Oyen WJ, van Rooijen N, et al. Factors affecting the accelerated blood clearance of polyethylene glycol-liposomes upon repeated injection. Journal of Pharmacology and Experimental Therapeutics. 2001;**198**(2):607–12.

[53] Litzinger DC, Buiting AM, van Rooijen N, Huang L. Effect of liposome size on the circulation time and intraorgan distribution of amphipathic poly (ethylene glycol)-containing liposomes. Biochimica et Biophysica Acta (BBA)-Biomembranes. 1994;**1190**(1):99–107. DOI: 10.1016/0005-2736(94)90038-8.

[54] Allen T, Hansen C. Pharmacokinetics of stealth versus conventional liposomes: effect of dose. Biochimica et Biophysica Acta (BBA)-Biomembranes. 1991;**1068**(2):133–41. DOI: 10.1016/0005-2736(91)90201-I

[55] Kumari A, Yadav SK, Yadav SC. Biodegradable polymeric nanoparticles based drug delivery systems. Colloids and Surfaces B: Biointerfaces. 2010;**75**(1):1–18. DOI: 10.1016/j.colsurfb.2009.09.001

[56] Arora D, Sharma N, Sharma V, Abrol V, Shankar R, Jaglan S. An update on polysaccharide-based nanomaterials for antimicrobial applications. Applied Microbiology and Biotechnology. 2016;**100**(6):2603–2603. DOI: 10.1007/s00253-016-7315-0

[57] Ankit S, Chetan N, Noor A, Prem NG. Recent advances in chitosan-based nanomedicines for cancer chemotherapy. In: Pradip Kumar Dutta, editor. Chitin and Chitosan for RegenerativeMedicine.India:Springer;2016.p.229–259.DOI:10.1007/978-81-322-2511-9_9

[58] Gu F, Zhang L, Teply BA, Mann N, Wang A, Radovic-Moreno AF, et al. Precise engineering of targeted nanoparticles by using self-assembled biointegrated block copolymers. Proceedings of the National Academy of Sciences. 2008;**105**(7):2586–91. DOI: 10.1073/pnas.0711714105.

[59] Lo Y-L, Sung K-H, Chiu C-C, Wang L-F. Chemically conjugating polyethylenimine with chondroitin sulfate to promote CD44-mediated endocytosis for gene delivery. Molecular pharmaceutics. 2013;**10**(2):664–76. DOI: 10.1021/mp300432s

[60] Jiang Y, Lu H, Dag A, Hart-Smith G, Stenzel MH. Albumin–polymer conjugate nanoparticles and their interactions with prostate cancer cells in 2D and 3D culture: comparison between PMMA and PCL. Journal of Materials Chemistry B. 2016;**4**(11):2017–27. DOI: 10.1039/C5TB02576A

[61] Satija J, Gupta U, Jain NK. Pharmaceutical and biomedical potential of surface engineered dendrimers. Critical Reviews™ in Therapeutic Drug Carrier Systems. 2007;**24**(3):257–306. DOI: 10.1615/CritRevTherDrugCarrierSyst.v24.i3.20

[62] Bai S, Thomas C, Rawat A, Ahsan F. Recent progress in dendrimer-based nanocarriers. Critical Reviews™ in Therapeutic Drug Carrier Systems. 2006;**23**(6):437–495. DOI: 10.1615/CritRevTherDrugCarrierSyst.v23.i6.10

[63] Khandare J, Calderón M. Dendritic polymers for smart drug delivery applications. Nanoscale. 2015;**7**(9):3806–7. DOI: 10.1039/C5NR90030A

[64] Malik N, Wiwattanapatapee R, Klopsch R, Lorenz K, Frey H, Weener J, et al. Dendrimers: Relationship between structure and biocompatibility in vitro, and preliminary studies on the biodistribution of 125I-labelled polyamidoamine dendrimers in vivo. Journal of Controlled Release. 2000;**65**(1):133–48. DOI: 10.1016/S0168-3659(99)00246-1

[65] Kukowska-Latallo JF, Candido KA, Cao Z, Nigavekar SS, Majoros IJ, Thomas TP, et al. Nanoparticle targeting of anticancer drug improves therapeutic response in animal model of human epithelial cancer. Cancer Research. 2005;**65**(12):5317–24. DOI: 10.1158/0008-5472.CAN-04-3921i.

[66] Lee D-E, Koo H, Sun I-C, Ryu JH, Kim K, Kwon IC. Multifunctional nanoparticles for multimodal imaging and theragnosis. Chemical Society Reviews. 2012;**41**(7):2656–72. DOI: 10.1039/c2cs15261d

[67] Thorek DL, Tsourkas A. Size, charge and concentration dependent uptake of iron oxide particles by non-phagocytic cells. Biomaterials. 2008;**29**(29):3583–90. DOI: 10.1016/j.biomaterials.2008.05.015

[68] Das M, Mohanty C, Sahoo SK. Ligand-based targeted therapy for cancer tissue. Expert opinion on drug delivery. 2009;**6**(3):285–304. DOI: 10.1007/s13530-011-0109-y

[69] Ying X, Wen H, Lu W-L, Du J, Guo J, Tian W, et al. Dual-targeting daunorubicin liposomes improve the therapeutic efficacy of brain glioma in animals. Journal of Controlled Release. 2010;**141**(2):183–92. DOI: 10.1016/j.jconrel.2009.09.020.

[70] Shi J, Xiao Z, Kamaly N, Farokhzad OC. Self-assembled targeted nanoparticles: evolution of technologies and bench to bedside translation. Accounts of Chemical Research. 2011;**44**(10):1123–34. DOI: 10.1021/ar200054n

[71] Liang C, Yang Y, Ling Y, Huang Y, Li T, Li X. Improved therapeutic effect of folate-decorated PLGA–PEG nanoparticles for endometrial carcinoma. Bioorganic & Medicinal Chemistry. 2011;**19**(13):4057–66. DOI: 10.1016/j.bmc.2011.05.016

[72] Peer D, et al. Nanocarriers as an emerging platform for cancer therapy. Nature Nanotechnology.2007;**2**(12):751–760. DOI: 10.1038/nnano.2007.387

[73] Vidal J-M, Koulibaly M, Jost J-L, Duron J-J, Chigot J-P, Vayre P, et al. Differential transferrin receptor density in human colorectal cancer: a potential probe for diagnosis and therapy. International Journal of Oncology. 1998;**13**:871–5. DOI: 10.3892/ijo.13.4.871

[74] Iinuma H, Maruyama K, Okinaga K, Sasaki K, Sekine T, Ishida O, et al. Intracellular targeting therapy of cisplatin-encapsulated transferrin polyethylene glycol liposome on peritoneal dissemination of gastric cancer. International Journal of Cancer. 2002;**99**(1):130–7. DOI: 10.1002/ijc.10242.

[75] Ishida O, Maruyama K, Tanahashi H, Iwatsuru M, Sasaki K, Eriguchi M, et al. Liposomes bearing polyethyleneglycol-coupled transferrin with intracellular targeting property to the solid tumors in vivo. Pharmaceutical Research. 2001;**18**(7):1042–8. DOI: 10.1023/A:1010960900254

[76] Cinci M, Mamidi S, Li W, Fehring V, Kirschfink M. Targeted delivery of siRNA using transferrin-coupled lipoplexes specifically sensitizes CD71 high expressing malignant cells to antibody-mediated complement attack. Targeted Oncology. 2015;**10**(3):405–13. DOI: 10.1007/s11523-014-0345-6

[77] Ekblom P, Thesleff I, Lehto VP, Virtanen I. Distribution of the transferrin receptor in normal human fibroblasts and fibrosarcoma cells. International Journal of Cancer. 1983;**31**(1):111–7. DOI: 10.1002/ijc.2910310118

[78] Matsumura Y, Maeda H. A new concept for macromolecular therapeutics in cancer chemotherapy: mechanism of tumoritropic accumulation of proteins and the antitumor agent smancs. Cancer Research. 1986;**46**(12 Part 1):6387–92.

[79] Bates D, Hillman N, Williams B, Neal C, Pocock T. Regulation of microvascular permeability by vascular endothelial growth factors. Journal of Anatomy. 2002;**200**(6):581–97. DOI: 10.1046/j.1469-7580.2002.066.x.

[80] Jain RK. The next frontier of molecular medicine: delivery of therapeutics. Nature Medicine. 1998;**5**(6):655–7. DOI: 10.1038/nm0698-655.

[81] Jain RK, Stylianopoulos T. Delivering nanomedicine to solid tumors. Nature Reviews Clinical Oncology. 2010;**7**(11):653–54. DOI: 10.1038/nrclinonc.2010.139

[82] Hobbs SK, Monsky WL, Yuan F, Roberts WG, Griffith L, Torchilin VP, et al. Regulation of transport pathways in tumor vessels: role of tumor type and microenvironment. Proceedings of the National Academy of Sciences. 1998;**95**(8):4607–12. DOI: 10.1146/annurev-physiol-021909-135833

[83] Swartz MA, Fleury ME. Interstitial flow and its effects in soft tissues. Annual Review of Biomedical Engineering. 2007;**9**:229–56. DOI: 0.1146/annurev.bioeng.9.060906.151850

[84] Padera TP, Stoll BR, Tooredman JB, Capen D, di Tomaso E, Jain RK. Pathology: cancer cells compress intratumour vessels. Nature. 2004;**427**(6976):695. DOI: 10.1038/427695a

[85] Farokhzad OC, Langer R. Impact of nanotechnology on drug delivery. ACS Nano. 2009;**3**(1):16–20. DOI: 10.1021/nn900002m

[86] Lammers T, Kiessling F, Hennink WE, Storm G. Drug targeting to tumors: principles, pitfalls and (pre-) clinical progress. Journal of Controlled Release. 2012;**161**(2):175–87. DOI: 10.1016/j.jconrel.2011.09.063

[87] Gunn J, Wallen H, Veiseh O, Sun C, Fang C, Cao J, et al. A multimodal targeting nanoparticle for selectively labeling T cells. Small. 2008;**4**(6):712–5. DOI: 10.1002/smll.200701103

[88] Jun Y-w, Huh Y-M, Choi J-s, Lee J-H, Song H-T, Kim S, et al. Nanoscale size effect of magnetic nanocrystals and their utilization for cancer diagnosis via magnetic resonance imaging. Journal of the American Chemical Society. 2005;**127**(16):5732–3. DOI: 10.1021/ja0422155

[89] Zhang Y, Kohler N, Zhang M. Surface modification of superparamagnetic magnetite nanoparticles and their intracellular uptake. Biomaterials. 2002;**23**(7):1553–61. DOI: 10.1016/S0142-9612(01)00267-8.

[90] Kohler N, Sun C, Wang J, Zhang M. Methotrexate-modified superparamagnetic nanoparticles and their intracellular uptake into human cancer cells. Langmuir. 2005;**21**(19):8858–64. DOI: 10.1021/la0503451

[91] Sun C, Sze R, Zhang M. Folic acid-PEG conjugated superparamagnetic nanoparticles for targeted cellular uptake and detection by MRI. Journal of Biomedical Materials Research Part A. 2006;**18**(3):550–7. DOI: 10.1002/jbm.a.30781

[92] Kamaly N, Xiao Z, Valencia PM, Radovic-Moreno AF, Farokhzad OC. Targeted polymeric therapeutic nanoparticles: design, development and clinical translation. Chemical Society Reviews. 2012;**41**(7):2971–3010. DOI: 10.1039/c2cs15344k

[93] Byrne JD, Betancourt T, Brannon-Peppas L. Active targeting schemes for nanoparticle systems in cancer therapeutics. Advanced Drug Delivery Reviews. 2008;**60**(15):1615–26. DOI: 10.1016/j.addr.2008.08.005

[94] Alexis F, Pridgen E, Molnar LK, Farokhzad OC. Factors affecting the clearance and biodistribution of polymeric nanoparticles. Molecular Pharmaceutics. 2008;**5**(4):505–15. DOI: 10.1021/mp800051m

[95] Monopoli MP, Åberg C, Salvati A, Dawson KA. Biomolecular coronas provide the biological identity of nanosized materials. Nature Nanotechnology. 2012;**7**(12):779–86. DOI: 1038/nnano.2012.207

[96] Valencia PM, Hanewich-Hollatz MH, Gao W, Karim F, Langer R, Karnik R, et al. Effects of ligands with different water solubilities on self-assembly and properties of targeted nanoparticles. Biomaterials. 2011;**32**(26):6226–33. DOI: 10.1016/j.biomaterials.2011.04.078

[97] Sinha R, Kim GJ, Nie S, Shin DM. Nanotechnology in cancer therapeutics: bioconjugated nanoparticles for drug delivery. Molecular Cancer Therapeutics. 2006;**5**(8):1909–17. DOI: 10.1158/1535-7163.MCT-06-0141

[98] Montet X, Weissleder R, Josephson L. Imaging pancreatic cancer with a peptide-nanoparticle conjugate targeted to normal pancreas. Bioconjugate Chemistry. 2006;**17**(4):905–11. DOI: 10.1021/bc060035

[99] Jiang W, Kim BY, Rutka JT, Chan WC. Nanoparticle-mediated cellular response is size-dependent. Nature Nanotechnology. 2008;**3**(3):145–50. DOI: 10.1038/nnano.2008.30

[100] Veiseh O, Gunn JW, Zhang M. Design and fabrication of magnetic nanoparticles for targeted drug delivery and imaging. Advanced Drug Delivery Reviews. 2010;**62**(3):284–304. DOI. 10.1016/j.addr.2009.11.002

[101] Samaddar JS, Gaddy VT, Duplantier J, Thandavan SP, Shah M, Smith MJ, et al. A role for macroautophagy in protection against 4-hydroxytamoxifen–induced cell death and the development of antiestrogen resistance. Molecular Cancer Therapeutics. 2008;**7**(9):2977–87. DOI: 10.1158/1535-7163.MCT-08-0447

[102] Van Veen HW, Konings WN. The ABC family of multidrug transporters in microorganisms. Biochimica et Biophysica Acta (BBA)-Bioenergetics. 1998;**1965**(1):31–6. DOI: 10.1016/S0005-2728(98)00039-5

[103] Loo TW, Clarke DM. Molecular dissection of the human multidrug resistance P-glycoprotein. Biochemistry and Cell Biology. 1999;**77**(1):11–23. DOI: 10.1139/o99-014

[104] Natarajan K, Xie Y, Baer MR, Ross DD. Role of breast cancer resistance protein (BCRP/ABCG2) in cancer drug resistance. Biochemical Pharmacology. 2012;**83**(8):1084–103. DOI: 10.1016/j.bcp.2012.01.002

[105] Peer D, Margalit R. Fluoxetine and reversal of multidrug resistance. Cancer Letters. 2006;**237**:180–7. DOI: 10.1016/j.canlet.2005.06.003

[106] Haran G, Cohen R, Bar LK, Barenholz Y. Transmembrane ammonium sulfate gradients in liposomes produce efficient and stable entrapment of amphipathic weak bases. Biochimica et Biophysica Acta (BBA)-Biomembranes. 1993;**1151**(2):201–12. DOI: 10.1016/0005-2736(93)90105-9.

[107] Gabizon AA, Shmeeda H, Zalipsky S. Pros and cons of the liposome platform in cancer drug targeting. Journal of Liposome Research. 2006;**16**(3):175–83. DOI: 10.1080/08982100600848769

[108] Barenholz YC. Doxil®—the first FDA-approved nano-drug: lessons learned. Journal of Controlled Release. 2012;**160**(2):117–34. DOI: 10.1016/j.jconrel.2012.03.020

Chapter 22

Immunotherapeutic and Preventive Role of Purified Extract Rich in Beta-Glucans Derived from D-Fraction of *Grifola frondosa* Mushroom in Experimental Mice Biomodel of Mammary Carcinogenesis

Aguilera Braico, Diego Máximo and

Gabriela Andrea Balogh

Additional information is available at the end of the chapter

http://dx.doi.org/10.5772/66890

Abstract

The overall vision of the modern science needs to change to a revalorization of the natural compounds and their beneficial effects on human diseases, such as cancer. Medicinal mushrooms have been used since thousands of years due to its healing properties. Maitake (*Grifola frondosa*) is presented as one of the most interesting medicinal mushrooms that have been studied. Until now, Maitake D-Fraction may have anticarcinogenic activity, preventing oncogenesis and metastasis in certain tumor types. However, the exact molecular mechanism by which D-Fraction acts are yet unknown. The results shown in this chapter suggest that Maitake D-Fraction Pro4X, administered intraperitoneally, prevents significantly the development of mammary tumorigenesis, increases survival, and reduces the process of angiogenesis in BALBc mice. Although yet to determine the active component of the extract and the molecular mechanism by which it operates in the breast carcinogenesis process. The socioeconomic impact of this research project could be important, considering that in Argentina similar studies using natural compounds derived from medicinal mushrooms for cancer therapy have not yet been performed. The beneficial effects of Maitake, if proven, could be useful for the treatment of cancer patients who are undergoing chemotherapy or radiation or for breast cancer prevention in high-risk population.

Keywords: breast cancer, prevention, Maitake D-Fraction

1. Introduction

Breast cancer now represents the second most common type of tumor pathology in the world and the highest incidence representing the leading cause of death in women in the world [1]. During cancer treatment, tumors often develop resistance mechanisms to chemotherapeutics, which occur in about 30% of patients treated with antineoplastic agents. For this reason, and for the many adverse effects of chemotherapy, more effective and less invasive therapeutic alternatives are sought. In the past century, with the development experienced in the chemical-pharmaceutical area, there was an increase in the production of synthetic and semisynthetic chemical drugs. This led to an increase in adverse reactions and negative side effects, in addition to the high cost of acquisition of these compounds. Therefore, there is a widespread tendency to use products derived from natural sources such as plants and edible mushrooms, consumed as dietary supplements in an increasing number of countries in the recent decades [2, 3]. These substances, which exhibit pharmacological properties in a broad spectrum of diseases, have shown their safety compared to drugs with chemical synthetic origin [4, 5].

An approach to the "ideal" anticancer drug could be derived from selective natural agents with low toxicity, such as fungal and extracts of medicinal plants, which possess significant antitumor and anticarcinogenic activities and avoid toxic side effects. Today, there is great interest in the study of natural extracts that meet these characteristics [6]. Plants and medicinal mushrooms are a source of obtaining active ingredients of marked importance in current research. Nature is a rich source of drugs. It is believed, for example, that only about 10% of the estimated 140,000 species of fungi on Earth are known. It is also estimated that only 5% of these species have been known to have pharmacological properties. The international scientific community has focused its efforts on the search for new sources of active ingredients from plants and fungi as potential anticancer drug [7, 8]. From natural products with anticancer activity, the best known are the vinca alkaloids (vincristine and vinblastine) isolated from the Madagascar periwinkle, *Catharanthus roseus, C. roseus* [9]. Probably the most important discovery and development is Paclitaxel (taxol) obtained from *Taxus brevifolia* tree [10, 11]. The new era of anticancer drug has been led by products such as taxol and docetaxol, among others. The discovery of penicillin from Filamentous fungus, *Penicillium notatum* and its therapeutic use, in the 1940s, became a new era of medicine and the "Golden Age" of antibiotics and thus promoted intense research in the nature as a source of new bioactive agents. Plants have a long history in the treatment of cancer, although they have often been observed with some skepticism by the own characteristics of the disease; but now, many people with cancer want to undergo known therapies as alternative products mainly from traditional usage, for example homeopathy and diet, among others, are widely used in oriental medicine. The traditional oriental medicine have been used for thousands of years as a medicinal mushrooms such as *Grifola frondosa* (Maitake) [12], Ganoderma lucidum (Reishi), Inonotus obliquus (Chaga), Lentinus edodes (Shiitake), among others. The production of biologically active fungal metabolites is a very broad field and is a promising study, which until now has been poorly studied [13–15]. Modulation of the immune system through stimulation or suppression of it can contribute to maintaining good health. Numerous immune system stimulating substances have been isolated from higher plants and fungi, and open doors for the development of novel drugs. They are looming, thus, as an effective alternative for the treatment of various health conditions that alter the normal balance of the body's immune response. The use of mushrooms that activate host defense mechanisms (immunostimulatory or immunopotentiating) provides an additional therapeutic tool to conventional chemotherapy. Given the limitations of conventional therapies to reduce cancer mortality rate, many efforts are focused on cancer prevention. Within this context, the use of immunopotentiating and inmunostimulating agents as well as biological response modifiers (BRM), capable of stimulating the immune cells that can identify tumor cells as foreign, eliminate, and prevent carcinogenesis, have gained prominence [16–18]. An immunomodulatory polysaccharide obtained from higher fungi is the grifolano (GRN), derived from *Grifola frondosa*. Several studies suggest that the mechanism of the antitumor activity of GRN is strongly related to immunomodulation [19]. It has been shown that the active grifolano *in vitro* macrophages to produce the tumor necrosis factor-alpha (TNF-α) [20]. The β-glucans are one of the most abundant forms of polysaccharides found in the cell wall of bacteria and fungi, which exert effects on the immune system by stimulating phagocytic activity, activating leukocytes, and inducing the production of various cytokines, which could give them their antitumor activity. It has been shown that oral administration of β-glucans extracts derived from *Grifola frondosa* medicinal mushroom (Maitake) could stimulate hematopoiesis and recovery post-treatment with Paclitaxel in cancer patients [21]. Particularly β-glucans act on a variety of receptors related to immune system, particularly acting on Dectin-1 and CR3 receptors, which trigger a broad spectrum of immune responses [22]. The β-glucans targeting immune cells are macrophages, neutrophils, monocytes, NK cells, and dendrites cells. Immunomodulatory functions induced by β-glucans involve an innate and adaptive immune response. Maitake is an edible and a medicinal mushroom, whose extracts possess β-glucans with different degrees of purification and have antitumor properties [23]. The β-glucans are BRM that, unlike conventional chemotherapeutics, activate or reinforce the host immune system, helping to eliminate or inhibit tumor growth. It has been shown that fractions obtained from Maitake can fight cancer by slowing or stopping tumor growth; and preventing tumor metastasis [23]. On the other hand, could decrease the side effects of chemotherapy such as hair loss, pain, and nausea, and enhance its positive effects [23]. The immunomodulatory functions induced by β-glucans involve an innate response and adaptive immune response. However, the exact mechanisms of immune system activation mediated by β-glucans are still unknown and must be defined.

In this chapter, we present a summary of some experiments done in biomodels of mammary carcinogenesis. So far, we have demonstrated that the treatment with Maitake D-Fraction Pro4X prevents the development of mammary tumorigenesis, blocks tumor invasiveness, reduce tumor angiogenesis, increases overall survival in animals, and exhibits selective cytotoxicity [24–26]. Moreover, we also demonstrated that the use of Maitake D-Fraction Pro4X is safe and nontoxic as well.

2. Direct effect of Maitake D-Fraction compared with Chemotherapy on breast tumour death

2.1. Effect of Maitake vs. chemotherapy on breast tumor death

In order to demonstrate if Maitake D-Fraction is able to kill breast cancer cells in culture, we measured the number of murine breast tumor LM3 cells death after treatment. The effects of increasing concentrations of β-glucans contained in Maitake D-Fraction Pro4X (0.036, 0.091, 0.183, 0.367, and 0.734uM) on cell death were evaluated at 24, 48, and 72 hours of treatment. In parallel, we treated LM3 cells during the same time with chemotherapy drugs using a combination of doxorubicin and cyclophosphamide at increased concentrations from 5 to 40 μM and from 0.5 to 2.5 μM for each drug, respectively. Cell death was determined at 24, 48 and 72 hours of treatment according to the trypan blue exclusion stained method. **Figure 1** shows the cell death values depending on the concentration of the used chemotherapeutic drugs (doxorubicin and cyclophosphamide) for 24, 48, and 72 hours after treatment. In all treatments, cell death was significantly higher (Student's *t*-test, $p \leq 0.05$) relative to untreated controls. It is also observed that the highest percentage of cell death (96.70%) corresponded to the higher concentration of chemotherapy used drugs (40 mM doxorubicin + 2.5 mM cyclophosphamide). The optimal time of the maximal cytolysis was the longest treatment at 72 hours. Cell death values depending on the concentration of Maitake Pro4X Fraction D at 24, 48, and 72 hours of treatment, as shown in **Figure 2**. The percentage of cell death increased depending on both, concentration of Maitake Pro4X used and time of treatment. The highest percentage of cell death (61.52%) corresponded to treatment with the highest dose of Maitake (0.734 μM) for 72 hours, the longest treatment.

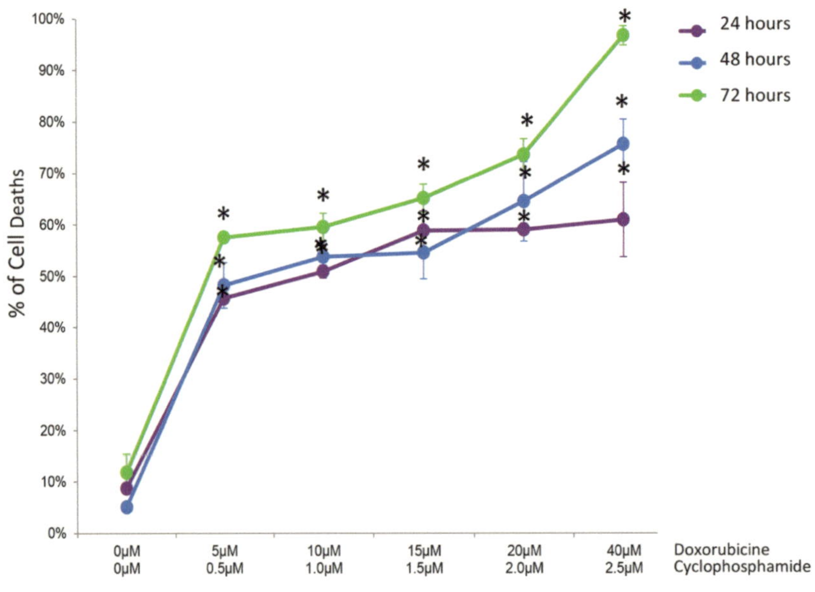

Figure 1. Cell death caused by different concentrations of doxorubicin + cyclophosphamide at 24, 48, and 72 hours of treatment. The values represented the mean ± correspond to SD($N = 2$). *$p < 0.05$ vs. control.

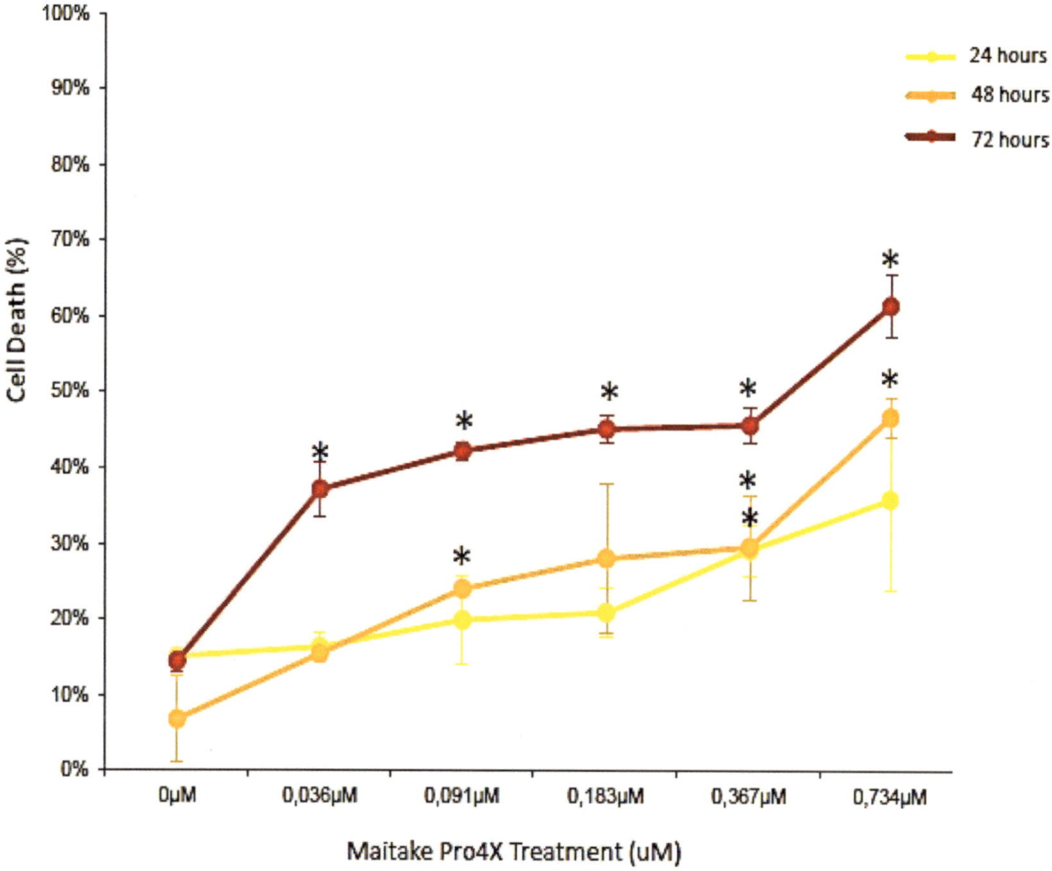

Figure 2. Cell death caused by different concentrations of Maitakeat 24, 48, and 72 hours of treatment. The values represented the mean ± correspond to SD ($n = 2$). *$p < 0.05$ vs. control.

In this work, we observed that both treatments, Maitake or chemotherapy, increased tumor cell death depending on the concentration and time of treatment. These results suggest that Maitake D-Fraction may have a chemotherapeutic effect by inducing a dose-dependent cell death. Here, we observed that the treatment with chemotherapeutic drugs increased mouse tumor cell death in a higher level compared to treatment with Maitake D-Fraction.

2.1.1. *In vitro effect of Maitake on human breast tumour MCF-7 death cells*

By another side, we performed the same experiments measuring the death in tumor human mammary cells (MCF-7). Using the time lapse microscope that takes pictures of the treated MCF-7 cell culture every 10 minutes during 1, 5, 10, and 24 hours (**Figure 3A**), it was found that Maitake D-Fraction increase the number of cell deaths significantly in a dose-dependent form, reaching the maximum deaths at the concentration of 367 μg/ml (equivalent to 0.367 μM) (**Figure 3B**). The treatment of tumoral MCF-7 breast cells at 24 hours with D-Fraction significantly increase ($p < 0.05$) the percentage of cell death in comparison with untreated controls.

2.1.2. Maitake D-fraction decreased MCF7 cell viability and increased apoptosis

These results made us to think about whether Maitake D-Fraction really exerted anticancer effects and induces cell death directly or is toxic for those cells and able to kill any kind of cell. To probe this, we measure the effect of this compound in MCF7 cells viability and examine if the cell death trigger mechanisms are related to apoptosis. The cell deaths were measured by examining using the MTS assay in MCF7 cell cultures incubated with five different concentrations of D-Fraction. A gradual decrease in the number of viable cells was observed with

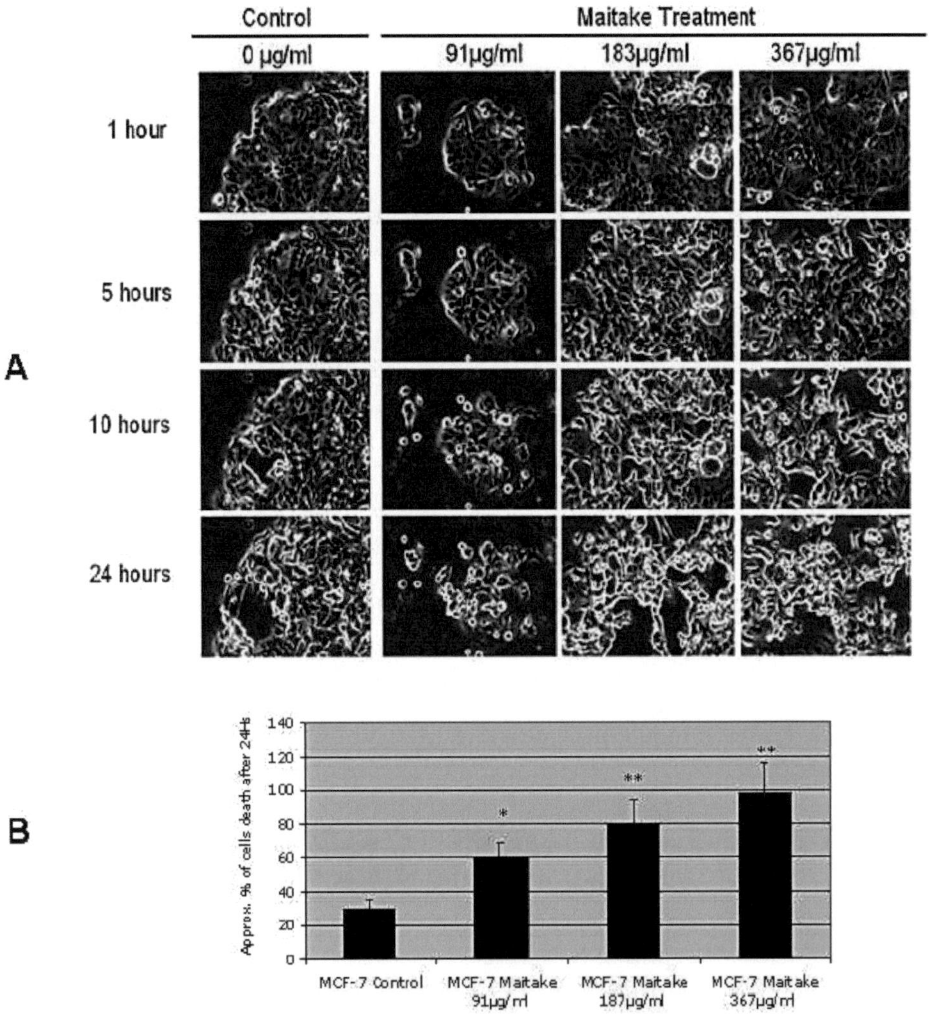

Figure 3. Analysis of cell death induced by Maitake in MCF-7 cells employing the time-lapse microscope. MCF-7 cells at 70% of confluence were treated with and without (control) increased concentrations of Maitake D-Fraction. The experiments were performed by triplicate. Cells were placed in the time-lapse microscope under CO_2 atmosphere, at room temperature during 24 hours. The camera was set up to take pictures every 10 minutes, using the 20× objective. Images and videos were analyzed employing specific software. (A) The representative image corresponding to the cell culture at 1, 5, 10, and 24 hours after Maitake treatment in the conditions indicated in the figure. (B) Corresponding to the approximate percentage of dead cells observed in each movie after 24 hours of Maitake incubation.

http://dx.doi.org/10.5772/66890

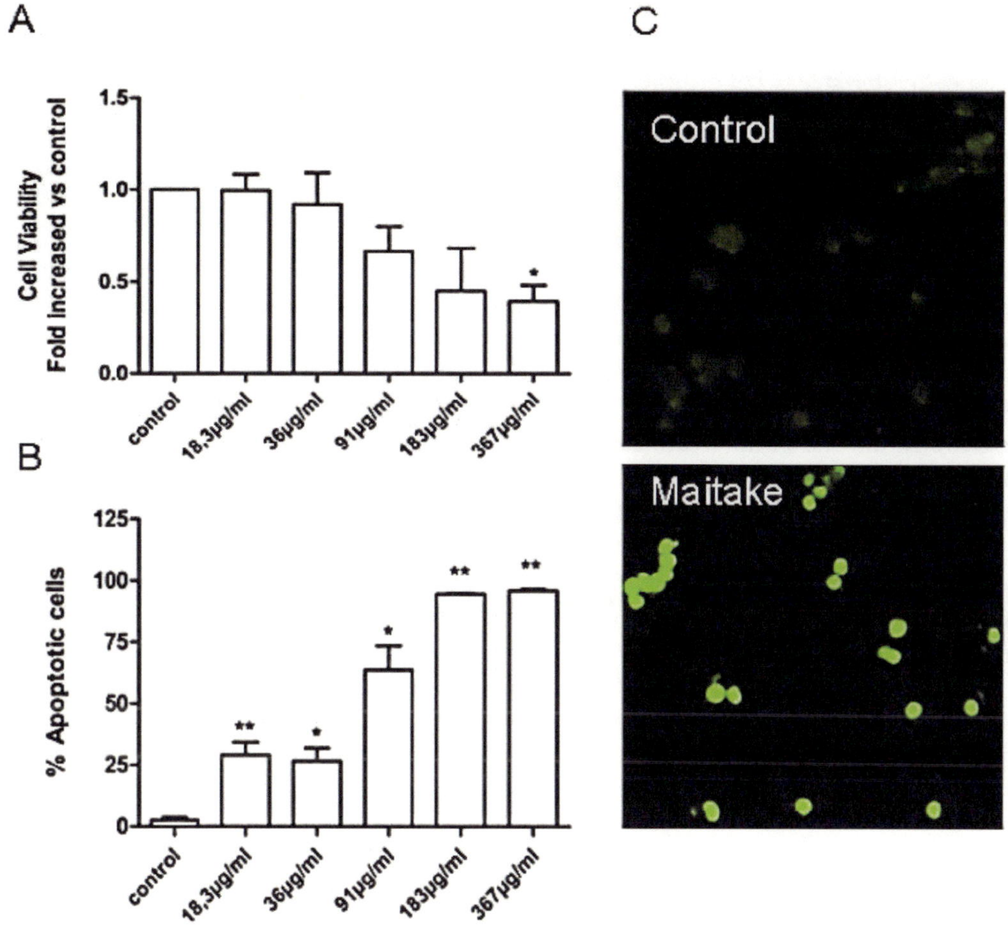

Figure 4. MCF-7 cell viability was evaluated after incubation with five concentrations of Maitake D-Fraction. (A) Cell viability was assessed by MTS assay. The results are expressed in absorbance values at 540 nm and are fold-increase relative to control cell cultures. Three independent experiments were performed in triplicate with identical results. $*p = 0.05$ vs. control ($n = 9$). (B) Apoptosis was increased at every incubation as evaluated by TUNEL assay, reaching statistical significance for every concentration of D-Fraction ($*p < 0.05$ vs. controls; $**p < 0.01$ vs. control). Bars represent the percentage of apoptotic cells evaluated by the ratio between TUNEL-stained cells and DAPI-stained nuclei in every culture. Experiments were repeated three times with identical results ($n = 9$). (C) Immunofluorescence for apoptotic cells (green). Note the increased number of apoptotic cells in 367 µg/ml Maitake-treated cells (Maitake) in comparison to untreated cells (control). Representative images are shown. Magnification ×200.

increasing concentrations of D-Fraction (**Figure 4A**). In fact, we observed that the highest concentration of D-Fraction resulted in a significant decrease in cell viability in comparison to control untreated (**Figure 4A**) ($*p < 0.05$ vs. control). To evaluate whether this decrease in cell viability was due to apoptosis, we employed the TUNEL assay. MCF7 (4×10^4) cells were incubated with increased concentrations of Maitake D-Fraction during 24 hours and the percentage of apoptotic cells was quantified. We observed that the treatment with this fraction, at any concentration, led to a significant increase in the number of apoptotic cells, in a dose-dependent manner (**Figure 4B**). Interestingly, nearly 95% of the cells became apoptotic whenever treated with the highest concentration of Maitake D-Fraction (0.367 μM or 367 μg/ml) (**Figure 4B**). A representative microscope image of these findings is illustrated in **Figure 4C**. As observed, treatment with Maitake D-Fraction led to an effective increase in the number of apoptotic cells (green) as compared to the untreated culture. These findings indicated that Maitake D-Fraction was able to effectively induce apoptosis in human MCF-7 breast cancer cells.

2.2. Effect of Maitake D-Fraction on death of normal human breast cells MCF-10F

To investigate if Maitake D-Fraction is selective to cell death and only induces death on tumor cells not in normal cells, we performed studies using normal human breast cells MCF-10F. We operate at different times and increase concentrations of Maitake D-Fraction using an *in vitro* MCF-10F cell culture and measure cell death after treatment. Cells were incubated by triplicate with D-Fraction at 37°C in controlled atmosphere with 5% CO_2 in a serum-free medium. At the end of the treatment, cell deaths were determined by the technique of trypan blue exclusion assay, counting the percentage of dead and the percentage of live cells in Neubauer chamber. The assay were tested at increased concentrations of Maitake D-Fraction at 91, 183, and 367 μg/ml of culture medium during 24, 48, and 72 hours. All the experiments were performed by triplicate. Surprisingly, treatment of cells, normal mammary MCF-10F cells, with increased concentrations of D-Fraction did not cause significant increases in the percentage of cell death compared to control at the highest dose of 367 μg/ml equivalent to 0.367 μM at any time assayed (**Figure 5**). In conclusion from these experiments, we confirm that Maitake D-Fraction only induced *in vitro* cell death by apoptosis in breast tumor cells without affecting normal breast cells at any concentrations or time of treatment.

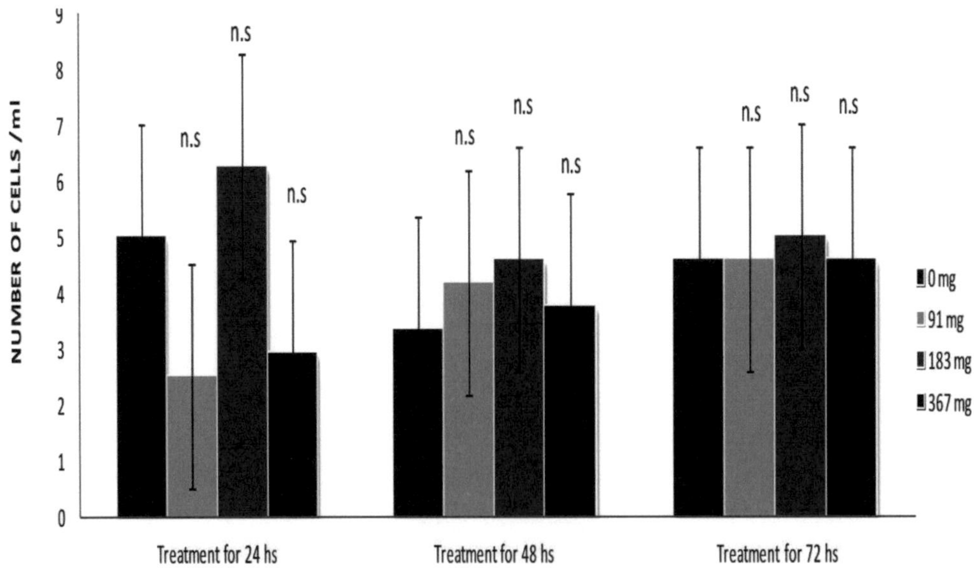

Figure 5. Cell death caused by different concentrations of Maitake D-Fraction on MCF-10F cells at 24, 48, and 72 hours of treatment. The values represented the mean ± correspond to SD ($n = 3$). $*p < 0.05$ vs. control.

3. Breast cancer prevention studies

3.1. Studies of breast tumor prevention by Maitake Pro4X in BALBc mice

3.1.1. Effect of Maitake D-Fraction Pro4X on breast cancer prevention

In order to demonstrate whether the purified extract Maitake D-Fraction Pro4X (from Mushroom Wisdom Inc, NJ, USA) was related to breast cancer prevention or inhibited the mammary tumorigenesis process, three independent experiments were performed employing 20 female nulliparous BALBc mice. Two groups were separated with 10 animals each, control group and Maitake D-Fraction group (5 mg/Kg) that were treated daily during 15 days by intraperitoneal injection. After that, mammary tumorigenesis was induced using implant of 2×10^5 LM3 cells intraperitoneally. All animals were checked weekly for breast tumor development. **Figure 6** shows the picture of mice abdominal area (peritoneal mammary glands) from each condition after 30 days of tumor challenge. From this experiment, we observed that 100% of breast tumorigenesis was developed (10 out 10 animals) in the control group. However, only 3 out 10 animals (30% of tumorigenesis) developed mammary tumors in the condition treated with Maitake D-Fraction Pro4X (Pro4X) (**Figure 6**). The average from all the three independent experiments performed for prevention against breast tumorigenesis development in animals from the control group was 3.333 ± 5.774 (**Figure 7**), which was significantly different from the prevention generated by Maitake Pro4X (64.286 ± 23.862, $p < 0.01$).

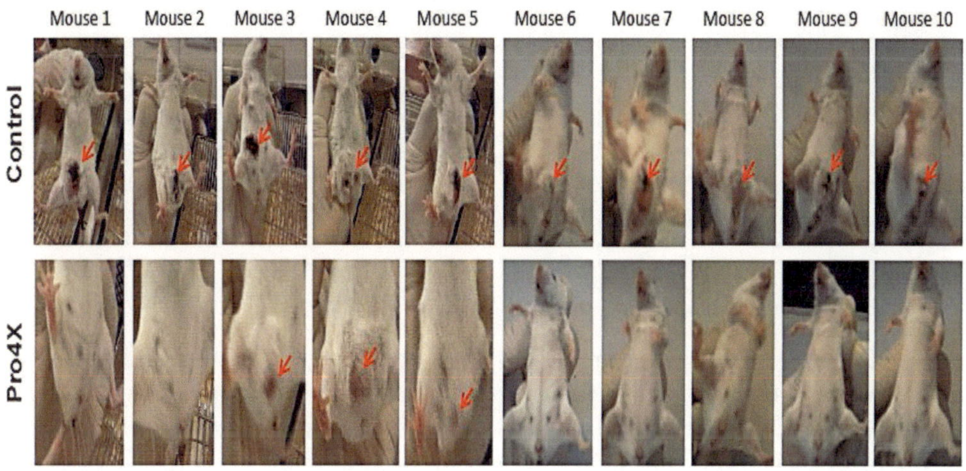

Figure 6. Effect of Maitake D-Fraction on breast cancer prevention in BALBc mice.

3.1.2. Effect of Maitake D-Fraction Pro4X in the tumor grows that escape to treatment

After analyzing the percentage of prevention in each treatment, now is important to study how the tumor grows in the animals that did not respond to the Maitake treatment and escapes its control. From **Figure 6**, 3 of 10 animals escaped the Maitake Pro4X prevention and developed breast tumors. We observed that breast tumor in the control group grew linearly 10–24 days

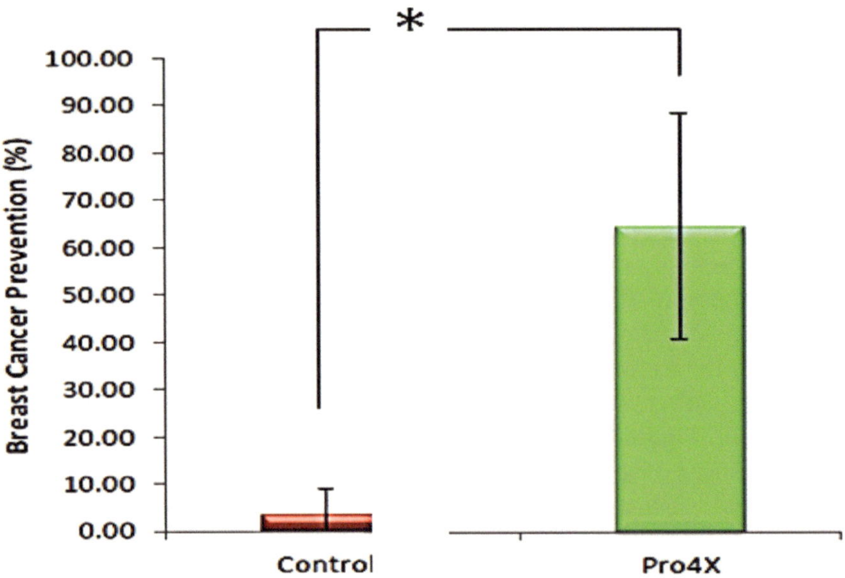

Figure 7. Percentage of breast cancer prevention induced by Maitake D-Fraction Pro4X in BALBc mice.

after tumor challenge; however, in the Maitake group, the breast tumor grew slowly at the same time and at 24 days achieved a similar size to compare the untreated control. At 46 days after Tumorigenesis (the end of experiment), the tumor area (cm^2) did not achieve a significant difference between the groups. The microscopy study of tissue paraffin sections shows that the untreated tumors from the control group were solid and have irregular edges; however, we were surprised to observe that tumors from the Maitake Pro4X group were almost the same size than the controls but full of liquid, not solid, with net tumor round edges, similar to benign tumors.

3.1.3. Effect of Maitake Pro4X on tumor necrosis

From the same experiments, we were interested in analyzing the necrosis area in the breast tumors. **Figure 8** shows the macroscopic aspect of a representative breast tumor at control and Maitake groups at the end of the experiment. After measuring the necrosis area (cm) from breast tumor in each animal group, it can be concluded that Maitake Pro4X reduce significantly ($*p < 0.01$) the area of necrosis in the surface of the breast tumors that escape to its control compared to the untreated group. Maitake D-Fraction Pro4X practically did not develop necrosis in their tumors (**Figure 8**).

3.1.4. Effect of Maitake Pro4X on metastasis in liver and lung tissues

The next question that we made is can Maitake Pro4X avoid the metastasis event in those animals with breast tumors. In order to verify that, lung and liver tissues were isolated from each tumor-bearing mice treated with or without Maitake Pro4X. Weight, macroscopic aspect, and sizes of lung and liver from those mice with breast tumors were checked. The lung and

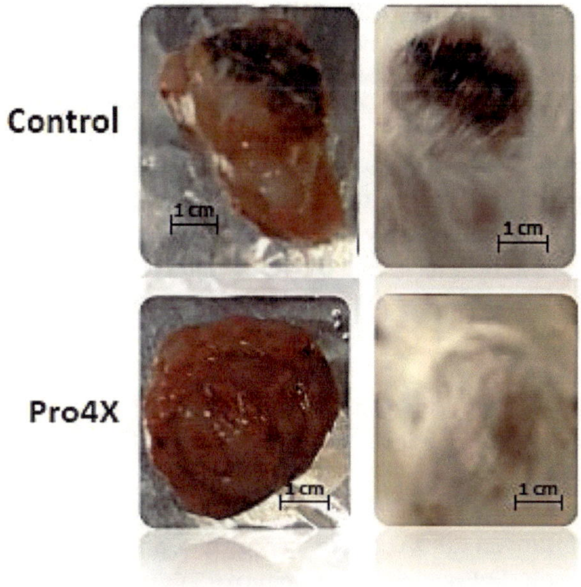

Figure 8. Maitake Pro4X treatment reduces tumor necrosis. The figure represents the pictures of breast tumors isolated (left) and in vivo (right) in both groups.

liver tissues' average area (cm^2) from each experimental group were analyzed. No significant differences in the size of the lung or the liver tissues from those animals in each experimental group were found. But nevertheless, macroscopically, liver tissues from the control group were completely different, colorless, and rigid, compared to those treated with Maitake Pro4X (**Figure 9A**). The histology of control's liver tissue shows and confirms cell proliferation and hyperplasia. However, liver tissues from Maitake Pro4X treated were darker, similar to nor-

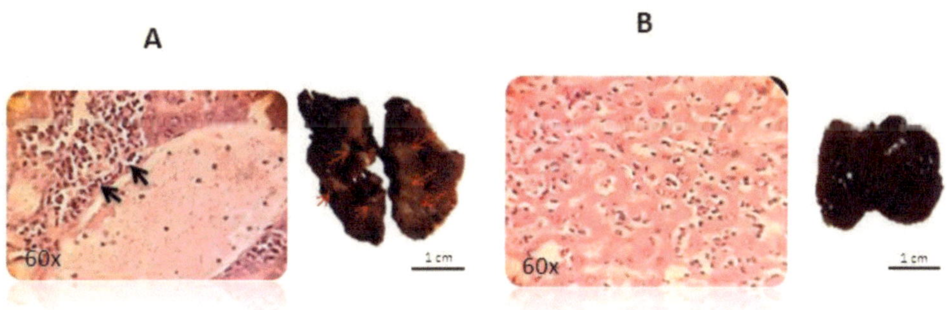

Figure 9. The liver tissues histology (left) of tumor-bearing mice from control (A) and Maitake Pro4X (B). Back arrows represent the cell proliferation area. Right pictures from each histology represent the liver tissue in each condition. Red arrows represent the metastasis area.

mal, with normal texture and aspect (**Figure 9B**). The histology studies from control's liver tissues indicated the presence of bigger blood vessels, with liver structure different than normal and some mitotic changes. Those experiments suggest that the treatment with Maitake Pro4X prevent the liver metastasis development.

The macroscopic study of the lung tissues revealed no morphological differences between tumor-bearing and nontumor-bearing mice. However, surprisingly, were observed higher mitosis percentage in the lung histology sections from control animals (7.50 ± 0.7) compared to Maitake Pro4x treatment (0.1 ± 0.02, $p < 0.001$ in the Pro4X). The percentage of mitosis found in the lung tissues pretreated with Maitake pro4X revealed no differences compared to normal lung tissue.

3.2. Comparison in Breast Tumorigenesis preventive potential: Maitake D-Fraction vs. Tamoxifen in experimental biomodel

In order to study whether Maitake D-Fraction can be adjuvant in breast cancer prevention with tamoxifen, we employed 20 BALBc female mice, 6–8 weeks old, separated into different groups: control group, D-Fraction group, tamoxifen group, and D-Fraction + tamoxifen group. The animals were inbred and kept in the Bioterio from BIOMED-UCA in compliance with National and International Standards of handling of laboratory animals with administration of water and food *ad libitum* kept on a 12-hour light/12-hour dark at room temperature, 22°C. Before performing the experiments, we got the approval of the ethical committee CICUAE from our Institution BIOMED-UCA for the animal use and manipulation in this study. Tumor induction in female mice was performed by exogenous implant of 2×10^5 murine tumor LM3 cells. To study the preventive effects of D-Fraction in mammary tumorigenesis, we have been working with 20 BALBc female mice divided in the following groups: control group treated orally with the dissolution vehicle; Maitake-treated group, with daily administration of 5 mg of β-glucans/kg; tamoxifen-treated group, daily treated with 20 mg of tamoxifen; and combined treatment of tamoxifen and D-Fraction at the indicated doses (tamoxifen + D-Fraction group). The treatments continued for 50 days (equivalent to 5 years in human), after that, mammary tumorigenesis were induced. The animals were observed until day 27 post tumorigenesis (sacrifice day). In this experiment, we observed that Maitake D-Fraction protects mammary tissue against tumor development in about 40% ($^*p < 0.05$) (**Figure 10** shows D-Fraction induce tumorigenesis in about 60%); however, we observed that tamoxifen treatment alone prevent only in about 25% (n.s., *p*-value not significant) against breast carcinogenesis. Surprisingly, the coadministration with tamoxifen + D-Fraction prevented mammary tumorigenesis in about 80% ($^{**}p < 0.01$) (**Figure 10** shows that combined treatment developed only 20% of tumorigenesis). To note, we observed that 100% of control animals developed breast tumor (**Figure 10**).

As for the post-tumorigenesis mortality, 20% of the animals treated with tamoxifen and 25% of control animals died after the tumor induction. Surprisingly, there was no mortality in Maitake and tamoxifen + Fraction D groups, 100% of the animals surviving at the end of the experiment. **Figure 11** show the overall survival rate of the animal from each condition at the end of the treatment.

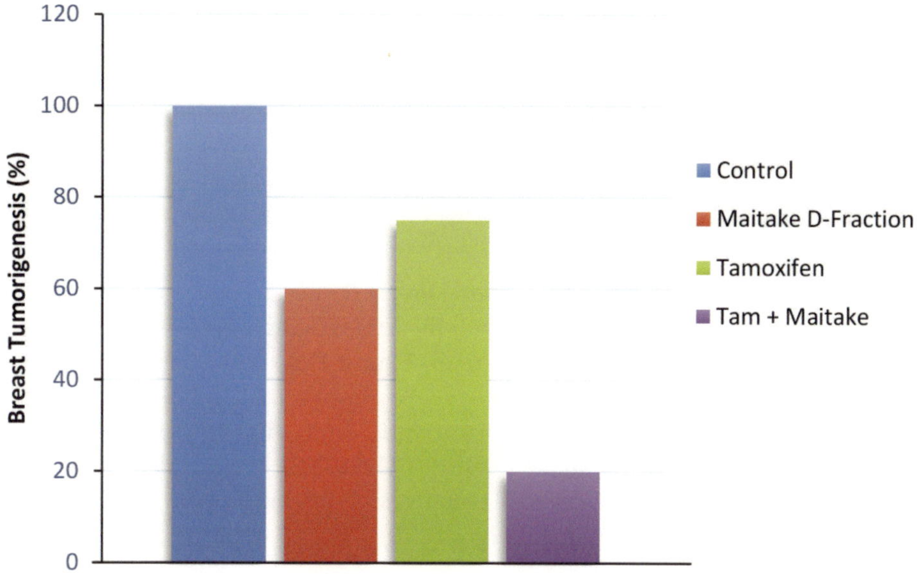

Figure 10. Breast tumorigenesis induced by Maitake or tamoxifen alone or in combination. Maitake D-Fraction was used in a concentration of 5 mg/kg and tamoxifen in concentration of 20 mg/animal. Treatment was performed during 50 days in female BALBc mice.

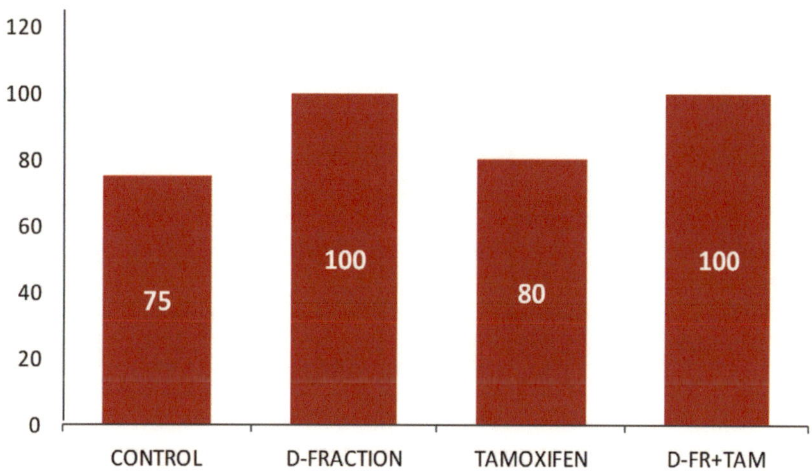

Figure 11. Overall survival rate after treatment with and without Maitake and tamoxifen alone or in combination.

Regarding adverse effects, tamoxifen-treated animals exhibit a remarkable intestinal jaundice, less evident in subjects treated with tamoxifen + Maitake, which was absent in the animals treated only with Maitake. All the treated groups showed significant increase in serum creatinine with $p < 0.05$ compared to control. These results suggest that D-Fraction has a higher preventive potential, compared with tamoxifen, in the development of mammary tumorigenesis.

Moreover, Maitake induce less or no side effects and the maximum overall survival rate in the mice. However, we observed from these experiments that tamoxifen and Maitake D-Fraction are able to achieve the maximal potential in breast cancer prevention when administered in combination.

4. Angiogenesis reduction

We estimate the angiogenic index in the tumoral breast tissues in order to establish if Maitake D-Fraction extracts are able to reduce or avoid the tumoral angiogenesis. **Figure 12A** shows the average blood vessels density in each group. **Figure 12B** shows the microscopy images (25×) of those breast tumors from both groups. We observe that the number of blood vessels/mm^2 in control's breast tumor tissues were significantly higher (0.637 ± 0.182, $p < 0.05$) than breast tumors treated with Maitake Pro4X (0.031 ± 0.028). We can also observe from the microscopy pictures that the area of control blood vessels are bigger compared to those in the breast tissue treated with Maitake Pro4x (**Figure 12B**).

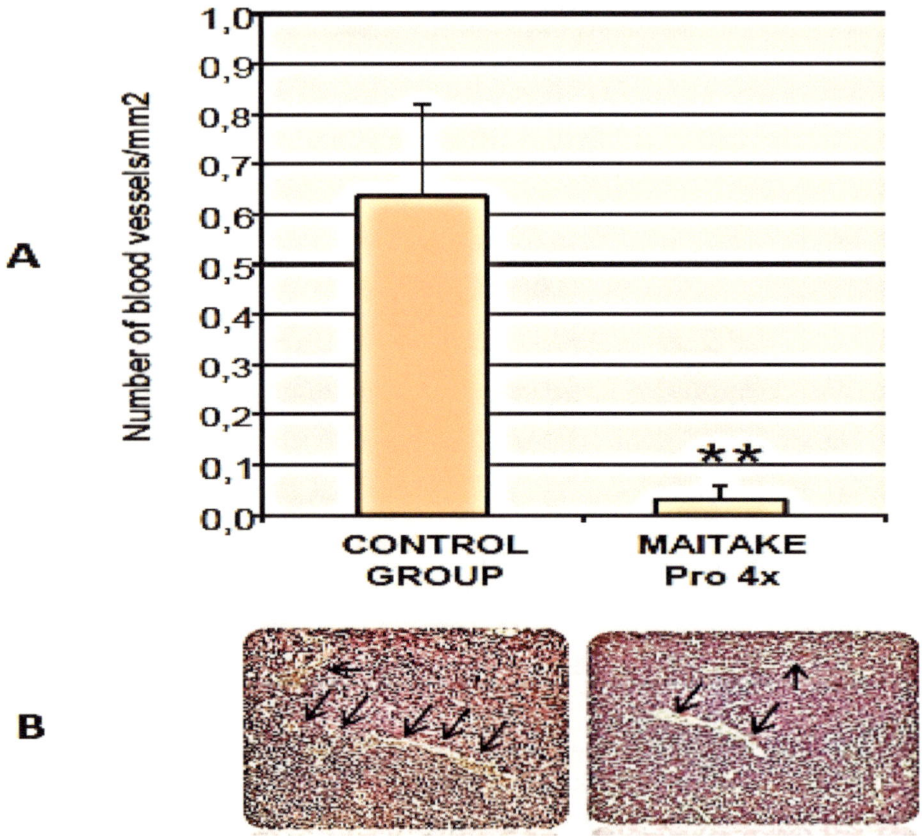

Figure 12. (A) The graphics of average of blood vessels density/mm^2 in each group. (B) The microscopy pictures (25×) of breast tumors analyzed. Black arrows indicated the size of blood vessels in each condition. $^{**}p<0.01$.

http://dx.doi.org/10.5772/66890

5. Survival increase

5.1. Effect of Maitake extract in the relative survival in BALBc mice

Another aspect in which we were interested was the overall survival of mice at the end of the experiment. **Figure 13** shows the percentage of overall relative survival at 46 days after tumorigenesis initiation when the experiment was terminated and the animals were sacrificed to analyze the results. Higher number of animals treated with Maitake D-Fraction lived until the end of the experiment. The overall survival in animals from Maitake Pro4X group at the end was 50% compared to control that was reduced to 10% (**Figure 13**). Here, we also analyzed other Maitake D-Fraction product called Maitake Standard with similar composition of Maitake Pro4X, but less concentrated. Both the Maitake compounds did induce a higher overall survival in BALBc mice at 46 days after tumorigenesis.

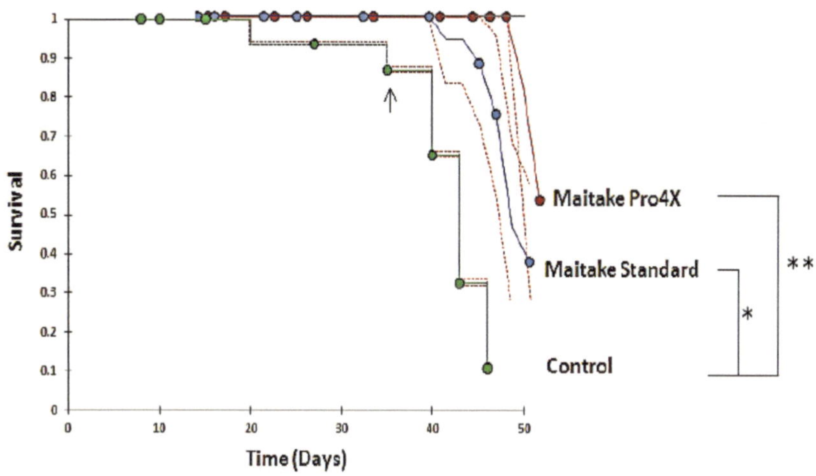

Figure 13. Kaplan-Meier overall survival curves. The graphic represents of overall relative survival from 7 to 50 days after tumorigenesis initiation. A green line represents the control group, a blue line represents the Maitake Standard treatment, and a red line indicates the survival after Maitake Pro4X treatment. *$p<0.05$; **$p<0.01$.

6. Effect of maitake pro4x on specific gene expression related to tumoral phenotype inhibition

With the objective to determine if Maitake D-Fraction PRO4X modifies the genomic expression of tumoral phenotype we isolated total RNA from tumor of all the experimental groups and mammary gland of nontumor-bearing mice. We choose genes such as ABCG2, CUL3, IGFBP5, PTEN, and SPACR, whose expressions were modified after Maitake treatment in MCF-7 cells previously published [25]. For this purpose, total RNA were isolated and after purification RT-PCR were performed in each breast tumor tissue from control, Maitake Standard, and Maitake Pro4X groups. We also isolated total RNA from normal breast tissue treated with Maitake Pro4X resistant to tumorigenesis. In **Figure 14A**, we shown the gene

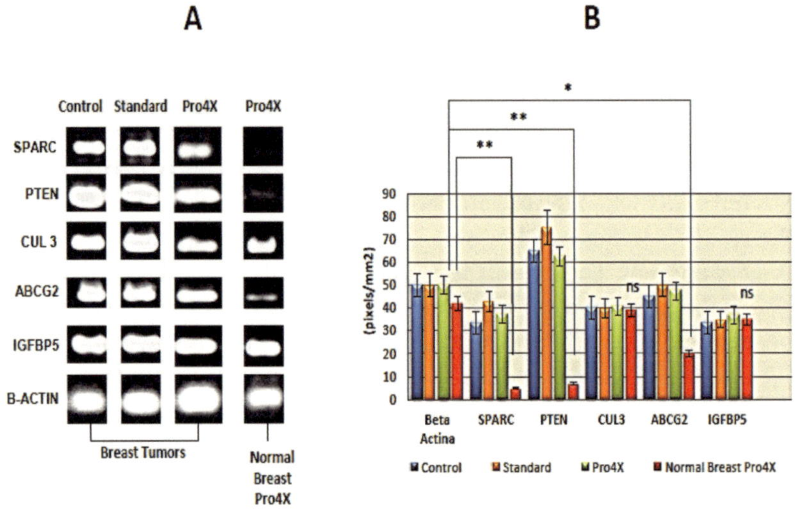

Figure 14. Gene expression analysis. (A) The gene expression at mRNA level in all the conditions. (B) Relative quantification of each RT-PCR reaction. *p<0.05 and **p<0.01.

expression in all the conditions assayed. We observed from this figure that SPARC gene is differentially expressed in all the conditions. SPARC gene expression were upmodulated in the breast tumor tissues treated with Maitake Pro4X (mouse 2 and mouse 3). On the other hand, we observed a downmodulation in the SPACR gene expression corresponding to mouse 4 treated with Maitake Pro4X. We did not observed PCR amplification of SPARC gene in the breast normal tissue without tumor corresponding to a mouse treated with Maitake Pro4X, who was resistant to carcinogenesis. We observed a similar pattern in mouse 2 treated with Maitake Standard. With respect to the gene expression of PTEN, in **Figure 14B**, we observed that are also differentially expressed in the assayed conditions. In the breast tissues of mouse 1 and mouse 4 treated with Maitake Pro4X we observed a downmodulation of this gene; however, we did not observe expression band in the mouse 2 treated with Maitake Standard or in the breast normal tissue resistant to carcinogenesis treated with Maitake Pro4X. ABCGs gene are also expressed differentially in all the conditions. No bands were observed in the tumoral tissue from mouse 2 treated neither with Maitake Standard, nor in the breast normal tissue resistant to carcinogenesis treated with Maitake Pro4X (**Figure 14**). Moreover, CUL3 and IGFBP5 genes were expressed in all conditions (**Figure 14A**). In order to see if there are differences in the level of expression we did quantify the PCR reaction with respect to β-actin amplifying all genes at 10, 20, 35, and 40 cycles. **Figure 14B** shows the quantification of each PCR reaction.

7. Toxicity studies

7.1. Acute Toxicity Studies in BALBc mice as biomodel

To investigate if Maitake D-Fraction Pro4X did not generate acute toxicity, we worked with a really high concentration of Maitake (2000 mg/kg). For this purpose, we employed 10 female and male BALBc mice, 6–8 weeks old. Control group animals received a single oral dose of 514 μl of BD (bi-distilled water) and the treat group animals received one oral dose of 514 μl of D-Fraction (corresponding to 2000 mg/kg of D-Fraction, dose equivalent at approx. 120 times highest compared with the therapeutic dose employed in previous experiments). The animals were observed daily until day 14 after treatment (day of sacrifice). The results show a significant increase in the body weight of the male mice from the control group (24.5 ± 1.49 gs) with respect to males treated with Maitake (22.57 ± 2.19 gs), $p < 0.05$ (**Figure 15**). No significant differences were observed in the body weight of female BALBc mice from both groups. We also observed that the Maitake acute treatment reduce significantly the value of hematocrite percentage from 33.00 ± 1.22 to 28.20 ± 4.44, with $p < 0.05$ in the control group. The percent of hemoglobin were also significantly reduced from 11.18 ± 0.41% to 9.52 ± 1.53%, with $p < 0.05$ in the control group. Toxicity tests revealed that the administration of a single dose of 2000 mg/kg D-Fraction does not cause mortality or any signs of toxicity in any subject. All the individuals survived treatment. Macroscopic examination and histological studies confirmed that breast, liver, lung, and kidney tissues from animals treated with a single dose of 2000 mg/kg of D-Fraction did not reveal histological alterations or significant differences in any tissue compared to controls. We need to study if the slight anemia induced by acute dose of Maitake D-Fraction is due to the reduction of Fe-absorption in duodenum.

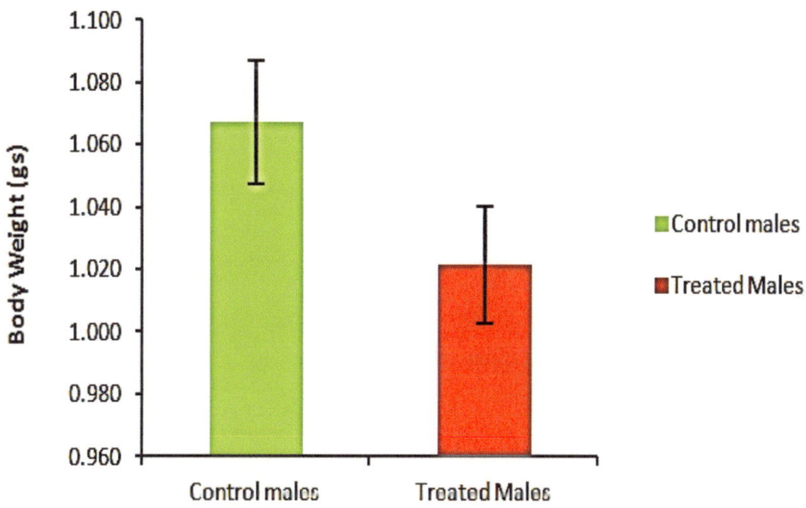

Figure 15. Body weight (grams) of male BALBc mice after treatment in the acute dose of Maitake D-Fraction.

7.2. Sub-Acute Toxicity Studies in biomodels mice BALBc

To determine whether the subacute dose of Maitake D-Fraction induce toxicity in BALBc mice, we worked with 10 female and male mice, 6–8 weeks old, divided into two groups: control group that received a daily volume of BD water and treated group daily treated orally with 5 mg/kg of D-Fraction during 28 days, after that they were proceeded to sacrifice. Toxicity tests revealed that the treatment for 28 days with 5 mg/kg of D-Fraction does not cause mortality or any signs of toxicity in any animal. All the individuals survived treatment. Macroscopic examination and histological studies confirmed that breast, liver, lung, and kidney tissues from animals treated for 28 days with 5 mg/kg of D-Fraction did not reveal histological alterations or significant differences in any tissue compared to controls.

8. Conclusions

Our results demonstrate that Maitake D-Fraction Pro4X prevents mammary tumorigenesis and also increased the overall survival and reduced tumor angiogenesis in BALBc mice. It also protects from the adverse effects of chemotherapy and reduces the toxicity of tamoxifen. The LD50 value is above 2000 mg/kg of D-Fraction, proving to be a nontoxic and safe natural compound for the treatment of animals. It has selective cytotoxicity, causing significant cell deaths in tumor cells without affecting normal cells. Although still we needs to determine which is the active molecule from the Maitake Pro4X extract and which is the exact molecular mechanism utilized to acts as tumor preventive agent. Based upon these results we can postulate that Maitake D-Fraction Pro4X is a good candidate to be used as a preventive agent in breast carcinogenesis in a high-risk population.

All these results suggest that D-Fraction could be applied to the therapy of cancer patients under chemotherapy treatment or as preventive agent in individuals with family history and/or carriers of mutations in BRCA 1 or BRCA2 genes. The beneficial effects of *Grifola frondosa* extract demonstrated in this work could be useful in the near future to reduce the side effects of conventional chemotherapy or to use as a preventive agent against mammary tumorigenesis in high-risk Argentine population.

Author details

Aguilera Braico, Diego Máximo and Gabriela Andrea Balogh*

*Address all correspondence to: gabriela_balogh@uca.edu.ar

Health Department, Medicine Faculty, University of South, Bahia Blanca, Argentina

References

[1] Bray F, McCarron P, Parkin DM. The changing global patterns of female breast cancer incidence and mortality. Breast Cancer Res. 2004; 6(6):229–39.

[2] Chin YW, Balunas MJ, Chai HB, Kinghorn AD. Drug discovery from natural sources. AAPS J. 2006; 8(2):239–53.

[3] Roggo S. Natural products in drug discovery. Chimia. 2007; 61(6):312.

http://dx.doi.org/10.5772/66890

[4] Cragg GM, Nexman DJ. Natural product drug discovery and development. In: Romeo, Ed. Phytochemicals in human health protection, nutrition, and plant defense. New York: Kluwer Academic, Plenum Pub; 1999.

[5] Rodríguez I, Laza D. Scientific information on homeopathy. Resumed 2001; 14(1):105.

[6] Abdullaev FI. Plant-derived agents against cancer. In: Gupta SK, Ed. Pharmacology and Therapeutics in the New Millennium. New Delhi: Narosa Publishing House; 2001. pp. 345–54.

[7] Cragg GM, Nexman DJ. Discovery and development of antineoplastic agents from natural sources. Cancer Investig. 1999; 17(2):153–63.

[8] Popoca Silva J, Villarrel Ortega ML, Aguilar Contreras A. Extracts of some medicinal and antitumoral plants. First National Congress of Medicinal Plants. México, Tlaxcala, 1996. p. 845.

[9] Dowdy SC. Multimodal therapy including neoadjuvant methotrexate, vinblastine, doxorubicin, and cisplatin (MVAC) for stage IIB to IV cervical cancer. Am J Obstet Gynecol. 2002 Jun; 186(6):1167–73.

[10] Kalinowski M, Alfke H, Kleb B, Durfeld F, Joachim Wagner H. Paclitaxol inhibits proliferation of cell lines responsible for metal stent obstruction: possible topical application in malignant bile duct obstructions. Invest Radiol. 2002 Jul; 37(7):399–404.

[11] Hood KA, West LM, Rouwe B, Northcote PT, Berridge MV, Wakefield SJ, et al. A novel antimitotic agent with paclitaxel-like microtubule stabilizing activity. Cancer Res. 2002 Jun 15; 62(12):3356–60.

[12] Cutler RR. The immune system and some natural agents that may help it fight disease. British J Clin Phytomed. 2003; 2:6.

[13] Illana-Esteban C. Maitae mushroom (*Grifola frondosa*) and its therapeutic potentials. Revista Iberoamericana de Micología, 2008; 25(3):141–44.

[14] Moretti A, Susca A, Mule G, Logrieco AF, Proctor RH. Molecular biodiversity of mycotoxigenic fungi that threaten food safety. Int J Food Microbiol. 2013; 167(1):57–66.

[15] Lull C, Wichers HJ, Savelkoul HFJ. Anti-inflammatory and immunomodulating properties of fungal metabolites. Mediat Inflamm. 2005; 2005(2):63–80.

[16] Calvo AM, et al. Relationship between secondary metabolism and fungal development. Microbiol Mol Biol Rev. 2002; 66(3):447–59.

[17] Chan GC, Chan WK, Sze DM. The effects of beta-glucan on human immune and cancer cells. J Hematol Oncol. 2009; 2:25.

[18] Nanba H, Maitake D-Fraction: healing and preventive potential for cancer. J Orthomol Med. 1997; 12:43–49.

[19] Wasser SP, Didukh M, Nevo E. Antitumor and immunomodulatory activities of medicinal mushroom polysaccharide and polysaccharide-protein complexes in animals and humans (Review). Mycol Balcan. 2005; 2:221–50.

[20] Ishibashi K, Miura N, Adachi Y, Ohno N. Relationship between solubility of grifolan, a fungal 1,3 β-D-glucan, and production of tumor necrosis factor by macrophages *in vitro*. Biosci Biotechnol Biochem. 2001; 65(9):1993–2000.

[21] Deng G, et al. A phase I/II trial of a polysaccharide extract from *Grifola frondosa* (Maitake mushroom) in breast cancer patients: immunological effects. J Cancer Res Clin Oncol. 2009; 135(9):1215–21.

[22] Brown GD, et al. Dectin-1 mediates the biological effects of beta-glucans. J Exp Med. 2003; 197(9):1119–24.

[23] Balogh GA, Obiol DJ, Alonso EN. Maitake D-Fraction and its therapeutic effects on breast cancer. Editorial Académica Española. EAE, Ed. AV Akademikerverlag GmbH & Co. KG, Heinrich-Böcking-Str. 6-8 66121, Saarbrücken, Germany. ISBN: 978-3-659-05372-6, August 2012.

[24] Soares R, et al. Maitake (D fraction) mushroom extract induces apoptosis in breast cancer cells by BAK-1 gene activation. J Med Food. 2011; 14(6):563–72.

[25] Alonso E, Orozco M, Nieto A, Balogh GA. Genomic signature induces by Maitake D-Fraction in breast cancer cells. J Med Food. 2013; 16(7):602–17.

[26] Roldan-Deamicis A, Alonso E, Brie B, Aguilera Braico D, Balogh GA. Maitake Pro4X has anti-cancer activity, prevents oncogenesis and reduces metastasis in BALBc mice. Cancer Med. Vol 5 (9):2427–2441, Sept 2016.

Chapter 23

Breast Cancer: From Transcriptional Control to Clinical Outcome

Sudhakar Jha, Deepa Rajagopalan,
Shainan Hora and Shweta Pradip Jadhav

Additional information is available at the end of the chapter

http://dx.doi.org/10.5772/66888

Abstract

Breast cancer is the most common malignancy in women worldwide. The risk of breast cancer in women increases with age, and this is partly attributable to the accumulation of genetic lesions. Growing evidence demonstrates the role played by epigenetic modifiers and the tumor microenvironment in contributing to the increased risk of breast cancer. This chapter provides a comprehensive overview of the epigenetic regulatory signatures that impact the well-studied signaling pathways in breast tissues. Additionally, we will also delve into the therapeutic and diagnostic potential of noncoding RNAs in breast cancer.

Keywords: epigenetic control, noncoding RNA, estrogen receptor α, DNA methylation

1. Introduction

Tumorigenesis is a multistep process that involves accumulation of genetic mutations which confer a selective growth advantage to the cancer cells. However, an emerging area of research suggests that epigenetic changes complement these genetic mutation events and direct the cancer cells towards a full blown malignancy [1–3]. Epigenetic changes refer to the modifications that do not occur on the primary nucleotide sequence of DNA (genetic mutations) but rather affect chromatin structure and function and are reversible in nature. Epigenetic changes involve histone modifications by enzymes that can "write" marks on histone tails such as acetyl and methyl transferases, enzymes that can "erase" these marks such as demethylases and deacetylases and a group of proteins that can "read" the chromatin marks and recruit other proteins to alter gene expression [4].

A recent study in mammary epithelial cells that are on the road to tumorigenic transformation has revealed a coordinated series of events that alter DNA methylation and deregulation of histone marks across large regions of the chromatin [5], thus underlying the need to study these epigenetic modifications to address their diagnostic as well as therapeutic potential in the context of breast cancer. Breast cancer is the most common cause of cancer in women worldwide. It is a complex, heterogeneous disease, thus posing a challenge in the diagnosis and treatment of patients. At the molecular level, based on the gene signature obtained from cDNA microarrays and global mRNA expression studies, breast cancer has been classified into four basic types, namely Luminal A, Luminal B, HER2-enriched, and triple negative/basal-like subtype [6–10]. This classification is based on the molecular characteristics displayed by the tumor, such as hormone receptor status, additional marks such as cytokeratin 5 (CK5) and cell proliferation rate (Ki67 marker[1] status; summarized in **Table 1**). These subtypes, along with displaying unique molecular signatures, also differ in their prognosis and response to treatments. Apart from the aforementioned mRNA markers, recent studies have highlighted the importance of miRNAs in subtyping breast tumors as well as providing directions for diagnosis, prognosis and therapy [11, 12].

However, despite several years of study, a broad-spectrum curative therapy for patients with malignant breast cancer remains elusive. This chapter will focus on key epigenetic regulators including noncoding RNAs identified in breast cancer that affect the hormonal signaling pathways and provide a perspective on combinatorial drug treatments using drugs that target these epigenetic regulators along with tamoxifen, aromatase inhibitors and other conventional therapeutics in specific sub-types of breast cancer.

Breast cancer molecular subtype	Characteristics	Prevalence	Treatment response and clinical outcome
Luminal A	ER positive and/or PR positive HER-2-negative Low Ki67	30–70%	Hormone therapy, chemotherapy; good prognosis and patient survival
Luminal B	ER positive and/or PR positive HER-2 positive (or HER-2 negative with high Ki67)	10–20%	Hormone therapy, chemotherapy; fairly high survival rates, though not as high as Luminal A
HER-2	ER negative PR negative HER-2 positive	10–15%	Trastuzumab and anthracycline-based chemotherapy; generally poor prognosis
Triple negative/basal/ basal-like	ER negative PR negative HER-2 negative	5–15%	Platinum-based chemotherapy and PARP inhibitors; generally poor prognosis

Table 1. Summary of the common molecular subtypes of breast cancer with their characteristics, disease prevalence and treatment response [6].

[1]Ki67 marker: Ki67 is a nuclear protein which is used as a marker for proliferation. It is associated with ribosomal RNA synthesis and thus serves as a proliferation marker. It is present in all cycling cells (G1, S, G2 and M phase) but it is absent in G0 phase cells.

http://dx.doi.org/10.5772/66888

2. Epigenetic alterations in breast cancer

Each cell in our body contains the genetic material in the form of DNA, which is the essential blueprint required for all cellular functions. DNA is packaged into chromatin by wrapping around basic histone proteins to form nucleosomes. These nucleosomes are further condensed into the nucleus to form the chromatin by enzymes that catalyze posttranslational modifications on the histone tails. The chromatin serves to not only condense the DNA within the cellular nucleus but also to control how information in the DNA is retrieved [13]. The histone components of the nucleosomes include a pair of H2A-H2B dimers and a tetramer of H3 and H4 to form the histone octamer around which the DNA is wound. These core histone proteins undergo a wide variety of posttranslational modifications such as acetylation, methylation, ubiquitination, phosphorylation, sumoylation, deamination and ribosylation, to name a few [14]. Since histones regulate accessibility of the DNA to transcription factors and DNA-modifying enzymes, alterations in the structure and posttranslational modifications of histones affects cellular gene expression to a great extent. Enzymes that covalently modify histones, acetyltransferases, methyltransferases and kinases, thus regulate multiple cellular processes that require accessibility to the DNA such as transcription, DNA replication and repair, apoptosis and cell cycle progression [15] (**Figure 1**). It is thus unsurprising that aberrant expression of many epigenetic regulators is prevalent in cancer tissues and contributes to the tumorigenesis process. By altering their epigenetic circuitry, cancer cells overcome the barrier of replicative senescence, accumulate genomic instability and catapult into an organized chaos that is the cancer epigenome (**Figure 2**). This makes it imperative to study the role and activity of proteins involved in epigenetic regulation of gene expression in the context of tumorigenesis. An important attribute of the chromatin-modifying enzymes is that the reactions catalyzed by these molecules such as histone acetylation are easily reversible and thus offer a therapeutic window of opportunity.

Emerging evidence indicates the role played by somatic mutations in the carcinogenesis process. A study by Stephens et al. highlighted the significance of these somatic mutations in the context of breast cancer [16]. Their study which sequenced the genome of 100 tumors for changes in somatic copy numbers and mutations identified point mutations and deletions in known cancer-causing "driver" genes characterized in the context of mammary carcinomas such as *PTEN, BRCA1, TP53, RB1* and *AKT1*. The highlight however was the identification of inactivating somatic mutations in epigenetic regulators such as *ARID1B* and *SMARCD1*, suggesting an altered epigenetic landscape in these tumors [16]. The reversible nature of epigenetic changes and their dynamic role in regulation of cellular gene expression in a tissue specific manner makes them potent tumor stimulating factors and reiterates the need to find suitable "druggable" epigenetic factors to serve both as a biomarker as well as a therapeutic target for the various molecular subtypes of breast cancer [17].

This section will discuss the epigenetic signature, histone posttranslational modifications as well as DNA methylation changes, characterized thus far in the various subtypes of breast cancer and will provide an overview of targeting these chromatin modifiers as a potential combination therapy.

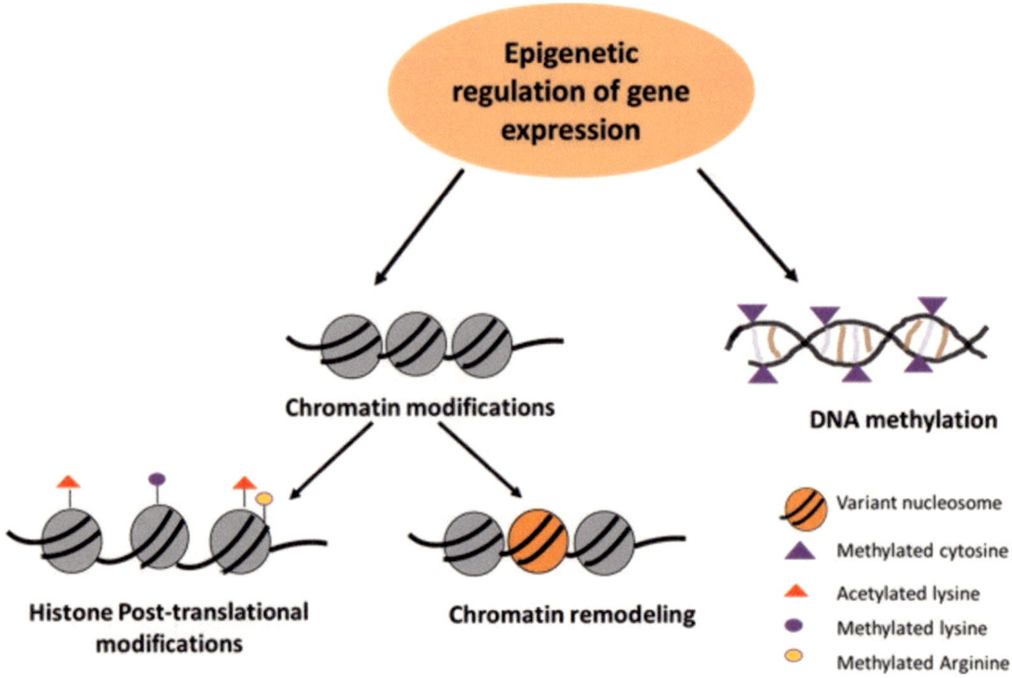

Figure 1. Epigenetic regulatory circuits in cells. A schematic representation of the epigenetic changes which regulate gene expression in normal cells.

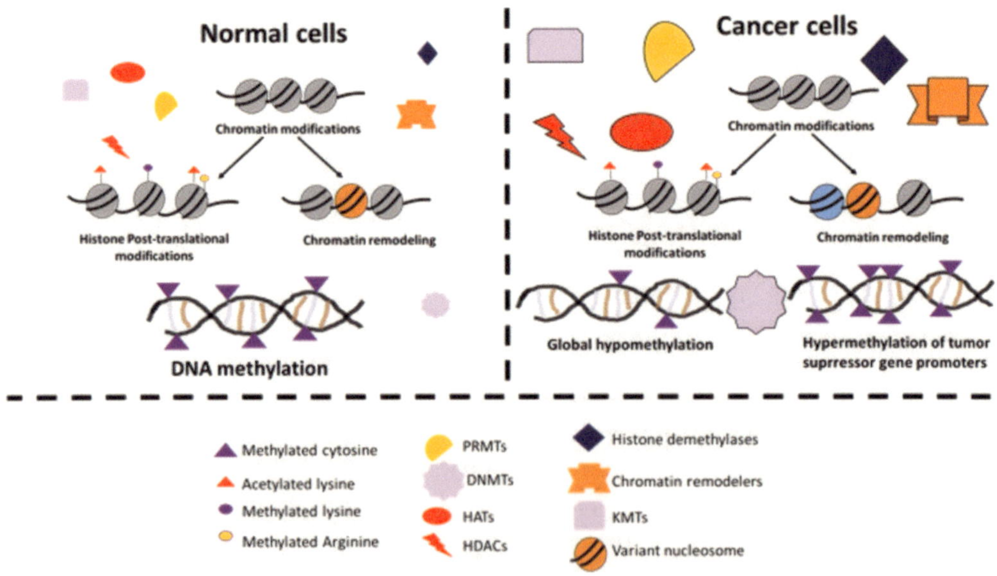

Figure 2. Altered epigenetic pathways in tumorigenic cells. Schematic depiction of the altered epigenetic landscape in cancer cells. Orange nucleosome represents a variant nucleosome which could be introduced as a result of aberrant expression and function of chromatin remodelers. Altered expression and function of HATs, HDACs, DNMTs, KMTs and KDMTs (represented as different sized icons the figure) results in a widespread disarray of the epigenetic marks in cancer cells.

http://dx.doi.org/10.5772/66888

2.1. Histone modifications and histone-modifying enzymes in breast cancer

2.1.1. Aberrant histone acetylation

Histone acetyltransferases (HATs) conventionally play an important role in the activation of gene expression by resulting in an open chromatin structure thus providing access for the transcription machinery to the DNA. There are different families of HATs identified thus far and their role in acetylating histones has been extensively studied. Histone acetylation is regulated by the activity of HATs as well as the histone deacetylases (HDACs), which remove the acetyl moieties from lysine residues. The acetylated lysines are read by reader proteins containing bromodomains (such as BRD2, BRD3 and BRD4) and depending on the complexes recruited by these "readers," gene expression can be switched on or off [4].

In breast cancer, a study by Elsheikh et al. has identified low levels of the histone marks, H3K9Ac, H3K18Ac, H4K12Ac and H4K16Ac, to correlate with poorer prognosis and is associated with basal and HER2-positive tumors. This study has also detailed the status of methylation on H3, which will be discussed in the following sections [18]. This altered epigenetic signature is hypothesized to be due to altered enzymatic activities of the HATs and HDACs, which could be attributed to their dysregulated expression. There are multiple lines of evidence now to support this hypothesis. A ubiquitously expressed acetyltransferase p300/CBP, which is also known to function as transcriptional coactivator, was identified to be overexpressed in breast carcinoma as compared to adjacent normal mammary epithelia. Further, this study also showed that higher expression of p300 as studied by immunohistochemistry from a tissue microarray correlates with poorer prognosis-free survival and increased tumor recurrence [19]. However, it is unclear whether the role of p300 as a histone acetyltransferase or a lysine acetyltransferase (acetylating other non-histone proteins) is involved in this function and remains an interesting avenue for future studies.

Another acetyltransferase, TIP60, belonging to the MYST (MOZ, Ybf1, Sas2, TIP60) family of acetyltransferases is known to undergo mono-allelic losses in breast carcinomas as well as in head and neck tumors [20]. Low nuclear expression of TIP60 as evidenced by IHC correlates with higher tumor grade in breast cancer [20], suggestive of a tumor suppressive role played by this epigenetic regulator. One of the histone targets of TIP60 is the acetylation of Histone H4 at K16. A significant global reduction in histone H4 acetylation and lysine trimethylation has been observed across most cancer types including breast cancer [21]. This loss of mono-acetylation was identified to be due to a reduction in the acetylation status of K16 and not the other putative mono-acetylated lysine on Histone H4 (K5, K8, K12 which are targets of p300/CBP). Other acetyltransferases capable of acetylating K16 on H4 are MOZ (monocytic leukemic zinc finger), MOF (male absent on the first) and MORF (MOZ-related factor). This study also identified the sequence specific loss of recruitment of MOZ, MOF, MORF in cancer cells as compared to the normal cells to the DNA repetitive elements associated with loss of H4K16 acetylation (H4K16Ac) and H4K20 trimethylation (H4K20me3) [21]. In addition, independent studies have identified MOF mRNA and protein expression to be downregulated in breast carcinomas, and this was correlated with the reduced level of H4K16Ac acetylation in these tested primary breast carcinomas [22].

The dysregulated histone acetylation in cancer can also be explained by changes in expression and function of histone deacetylases (HDACs). In breast cancer, HDAC1, HDAC2 and HDAC3 are identified to be differentially expressed as compared to the normal tissue and overexpression of HDAC2 and HDAC3 strongly correlates with a more aggressive tumor type, that is, negative hormone status [23]. This offers the opportunity of treating breast cancers with inhibitors of HDAC to restore acetylation level and suppress the tumorigenesis, and this approach will be detailed in the last part of this section which addresses the therapeutic implication of targeting the epigenetic regulators.

2.1.2. Aberrant histone methylation

Histones can be methylated (mono, di or tri) by enzymes that catalyze the transfer of methyl moiety to the lysine or arginine residues on the histone tails. The enzymes involved are known as histone methyltransferases (HMTs), while another class of enzymes, the histone demethylases (HDMs), is involved in erasing the methyl groups from the histone tails. The dynamic regulation between the HMTs and HDMs regulates the methylation status in the cells, thereby regulating cellular gene expression.

Studies have identified widespread changes in histone methylation in cancer cells as compared to the nontumorigenic counterparts. There is a global reduction in H4K20me3 in multiple cancer types including breast cancer [21]. Global reduction in H4K20me3 was also observed in human breast cancer cell lines compared to the nontumorigenic cells [24]. Further, in an established model of breast cancer in rats, there was a global decrease in H3K9 trimethylation (H3K9me3) and H4K20me3 indicating that these epigenetic dysregulations play an important role in tumorigenesis [25]. In addition, another study has identified low levels of histone methyl marks, H3K4 dimethylation (H3K4me2), H4K20me3 and H4 Arginine dimethylation (H4R3me2) in human tumors, and these were found to correlate with poorer prognosis and more aggressive subtypes of breast cancer such as Luminal and HER2-positive tumors [18]. These global alterations in the level of methylation on histones are suggestive of an imbalance in the expression of methyltransferases as well as the demethylases.

In support of this notion, a variety of histone methyltransferases have been identified to be aberrantly expressed in breast tumors. Frequent overexpression and amplification of the histone methyltransferase NSD3L have been observed in mammary carcinomas, and depletion of this enzyme decreased the invasiveness of breast cancer cells highlighting its potential as an oncogene. However, the targets of NSD3L-affecting tumorigenesis have not been elucidated in detail [26, 27].

Enhancer of zeste 2 (EZH2) a methyltransferase that is a part of the Polycomb Repressive Complex 2 (PRC2) is found to be overexpressed in breast cancer, both at mRNA and protein level. The high expression of EZH2 is correlated with more aggressive cancer and a poor prognosis for patients. Overexpression of EZH2 in normal breast epithelia promotes anchorage independent growth, cell invasion, characteristics of a neoplastic phenotype in these cells, which is dependent on the suppressor of variegation 3-9 (Su(var)3-9), enhancer of zeste (E(z)), and trithorax (Trx) (SET) domain of EZH2 and HDAC activity [28]. This study paved the way

http://dx.doi.org/10.5772/66888

for many other groups to investigate the role of EZH2 enzymatic activity mediated by the SET domain, conventionally known to silence gene expression, in the context of breast carcinomas. H3K27 di and tri methylation are characteristic of Polycomb Group (PcG) target genes and are associated with transcriptional silencing. The PRC2 complex of which EZH2 is the catalytic subunit with the other members being EED and Suz12 is involved in dimethylation and trimethylation of H3K27. The SET domain of EZH2 can function as an N methyltransferase, that is, EZH2 by utilizing S-adenosyl methionine (SAM) as a cofactor can add methyl groups to the lysine residues of substrate proteins. SET domain containing methyltransferases bind SAM and the substrate on opposite sides of the active site of the enzyme, thus SAM can dissociate without interrupting substrate binding to enzyme, resulting in multiple methylations on the lysine residues [29, 30]. In breast cancer cell lines, increased EZH2 expression resulted in the down-regulation of a tumor suppressor, RUNX3. This was identified through chromatin immunoprecipitation to be due to the H3K27me3 at RUNX3 promoter and associated HDAC1, since depletion of EZH2 resulted in the loss of H3K27me3 and HDAC1 from this promoter and increased expression of RUNX3, which was associated with significantly lesser cell growth as compared to the siRNA control [31]. In addition, EZH2 also results in down-regulation of another potential tumor suppressor, FOXC1, a transcription factor that has a role in differentiation and reduces cell migration and invasion. By trimethylating H3K27 at the FOXC1 promoter, EZH2 shuts down the expression of this transcription factor in a highly metastatic breast cancer cell line, MDA-MB-231 [32]. EZH2 is also known to repress RAD51, a protein involved in DNA repair and *CDH1* (E-cadherin), a marker for epithelial cell type, loss of which results in increased invasiveness [33]. However, recent studies have also shown that increased EZH2 expression does not necessarily correlate with the H3K27me3 abundance. In particular, high expression of EZH2 was found in basal-like, HER2-positive and triple-negative tumors, while high H3K27me3 was found in normal-like (ER-negative), HER2-positive and Luminal A type tumors [34]. A possible explanation for this anomaly could be a non-canonical catalytic activity independent function of EZH2. In triple-negative breast cancer (TNBC), it has been reported that EZH2 functions as an activator of NOTCH signaling. EZH2 overexpression could increase *NOTCH1* expression and accelerate mammary tumorigenesis in mice. It can bind to *NOTCH1* promoter, a function that is independent of its ability to methylate histones [35]. This opens new doors to discover other functions of this epigenetic regulator in mediating tumor progression by regulating nonhistone targets or affecting chromatin structure or in a manner independent of its catalytic function.

JARID1C, a histone demethylase, is also known to be upregulated and correlates with increased metastasis in breast cancer lesions compared to the normal counterparts. Mechanistically, JARID1C by modulating H3K4me3 at the promoter of breast cancer metastasis suppressor 1 (*BRMS1*) represses the expression of BRMS1 and depletion of JARID1C results in reduced migration and invasion of breast cancer cells [36]. Enzymes belonging to the demethylase family of KDM4 are seen to be overexpressed in breast cancer and affect cell proliferation and growth of these cells [37]. KDM3A, a histone demethylase, which demethylates H3K9 mono and di-methyl moieties, works as a positive regulator of estrogen receptor (ER) activity. The catalytic activity of this enzyme is essential for ER target gene expression and growth of the cells, highlighting the significance of this methylation status in promoting tumorigenesis [38].

2.1.3. *Other histone modifications*

Phosphorylation of histones is another posttranslational modification, which occurs on histone tails and involves the kinase enzymatic activity. Serine, threonine and tyrosine residues on histone tails are known to be phosphorylated. H3S10 phosphorylation which marks the entry of the cell into mitosis is catalyzed by the enzyme Aurora B Kinase. Elevated expression of this kinase in several cancers is correlated with a poor prognosis for survival; however, it is not determined if this is due to the phosphorylation of H3S10 resulting in increased proliferative ability of cancer cells [39]. Ubiquitination is yet another posttranslational modification found on histones. Mono-ubiquitination of H2B (H2Bub1) is found to be globally reduced, and this is true in the context of breast cancer as well. Proteasome inhibition can reduce ERα-mediated transcription, and this was due to reduction in H2Bub1 levels, which correlated with reduced transcription of ER target genes [40].

2.2. Chromatin remodelers in breast cancer

The chromatin compacts the DNA into the nucleus, and this regulates the accessibility of the wound DNA to transcription and repair machinery. One of the ways through which the chromatin is regulated has been discussed in the preceding section and involves extensive posttranslational modifications on histone tails. Apart from this, the locus-specific DNA methylation status can help in the recruitment of enzymes that alter chromatin structure, and this has also been discussed. Another way to regulate chromatin structure and function is by physically altering the nucleosome location or composition, and this process is known as chromatin remodeling. The groups of enzymes involved in restructuring the chromatin by this mechanism are referred to as chromatin remodelers and are further classified into different families depending on the associated cofactors. All chromatin remodelers utilize the energy of ATP hydrolysis to catalyze the reactions that affect histone-DNA interactions [41].

Remodelers are involved in mobilizing nucleosomes across the genome and regulate chromatin organization. They facilitate proper placement of nucleosomes whenever the DNA is accessed, for instance, before and after replication, repair and transcription. Remodelers also slide or evict nucleosomes and can replace them with a nucleosome that contains a histone variant. A common example is the histone variant H2AZ found flanking the transcription start site [41]. All these functions of remodelers suggest the important underlying role played by this group of epigenetic regulators in controlling basic cellular processes such as transcription, chromatin assembly and DNA repair. Thus, it is not surprising that the altered expression or localization of these chromatin remodelers is correlated with tumorigenesis.

There are several families of chromatin remodelers such as SWI/SNF, INO80 and CHD complexes, all of which are implicated in different cellular processes. Mutations in the SWI/SNF family of chromatin remodelers are found in about 20% of cancers, and some of these mutations could have a gain-of-function phenotype while in the case of breast cancer as well as in leukemia, wild-type SWI/SNF complexes by their diverse protein interactions aid tumor progression [42]. The bipolar function of this important class of chromatin remodelers also implicates the dynamic range of functions of remodelers and the myriad of their cellular interacting

http://dx.doi.org/10.5772/66888

partners, which assist their aberrant functions in cancer cells. In breast cancer, a member of the NuRD complex, a part of the CHD family of remodelers, is known to be aberrantly expressed. Metastasis-associated proteins (MTA-3) are associated with ER-positive breast cancer, and increased expression of these MTA-3 is correlated with increased ER expression as well as invasive behavior. MTA-3 can directly repress *SNAIL* transcription in response to the ER stimulus; therefore, a decrease in either ER expression or MTA-3 expression results in increased metastasis due to aberrant *SNAIL* expression [43].

ARID1A, a member of the human SWI/SNF complex, is known to undergo frequent mutations across many cancer types. In breast cancer, *ARID1A* mRNA expression is seen to be downregulated in tumors as compared to adjacent normal tissues. This decreased expression was correlated with bigger tumor size and with the triple-negative breast cancers. Immunohistochemical staining also revealed a similar correlation between the protein level of ARID1A and tumor stage as well as the triple-negative tumor type [44].

Another member of the SWI/SNF complex, BAF155/SMARCC1 (*BRG1*-associated factor 155/SWI/SNF related, matrix associated, actin dependent regulator of chromatin subfamily C member 1) has been identified to play a critical role in breast cancer tumorigenesis in concert with a protein arginine methyltransferase coactivator-associated arginine methyltransferase 1 (CARM1). CARM1 is highly expressed in many cancers such as breast and prostate with the levels of CARM1 higher in metastatic breast tumors as compared to the primary lesions. CARM1 is also implicated in the growth and proliferation of breast cancers by functioning as a coactivator of the steroid hormone receptors [45]. The arginine methylation of BAF155 at R1064 by CARM1 recruits BAF155 to a unique set of target genes such as genes in the c-MYC pathway. Intriguingly, there was a higher expression of both total and methylated BAF155 as observed by IHC in metastatic tumors, which were also associated with increased expression of CARM1 in these tumor samples. Patients with higher methylated BAF155 had a higher risk of tumor recurrence and poorer prognosis with a hazard ratio[2] very similar to the aggressive triple-negative breast tumors [46]. This and other studies show the significance of chromatin reorganization and altered recruitment/function of chromatin remodelers to be an important hallmark of cancer cells and the need to target these reversible epigenetic changes for development of more specific therapeutics.

Other examples of SWI/SNF family implicated in breast carcinogenesis are the Brahma and Brahma-related gene 1 (*BRM* and *BRG1*) that are overexpressed in breast tumors. Knockdown of either *BRG1* or *BRM* reduced the proliferation of breast cancer cells, whereas a combined knockdown resulted in additive effect, suggesting independent pathways regulated by these chromatin remodelers in breast cancer progression [47].

A genetic mutation in *BRCA1* predisposes women to ovarian cancer and significantly increases the risk for development of breast cancer. *BRCA1* is predominantly found in cells in a complex with members of the SWI/SNF family that is involved in chromatin remodeling. *BRCA1*

[2]Hazard ratio: it is the ratio of the hazard rates of two groups being compared, that is, ratio of how often an event happens in one group compared to the other. In clinical trials, hazard ratios represent survival in a group of patients treated with a drug at any point of time with the other group given a placebo/different treatment. A hazard ratio of 1 indicates no difference in survival while a ratio greater or lesser than 1 indicates one of the groups has a better survival.

directly interacts with BRG1, and this interaction is essential for *BRCA1* transcriptional coactivation function. A dominant negative mutation of *BRG1* or the deletion of exon 11 of *BRCA1* (implicated in cancer) results in abrogation of p53 stimulated *BRCA1* transcriptional activity. This underscores the importance of chromatin organization and remodeling by *BRG1* and *BRCA1* to control *BRCA1* transcriptional activity, loss of which results in increased risk for tumor development [48]. Additionally, interaction of mutant p53 with the SWI/SNF complex leads to open chromatin structure at the Vascular Endothelial Growth Factor Receptor 2 (*VEGFR2*) promoter in breast cancers that leads to the upregulation of VEGF2. This aids the growth of cancer cells in two and three dimensional cultures. Thus, mutant p53 by regulating a major family of chromatin remodelers promotes tumor progression [49].

2.3. Aberrant DNA methylation in breast cancer

DNA methylation is another form of epigenetic regulation that involves the addition of a methyl moiety to the 5′ cytosine of a CG dinucleotide, which are distributed across our genome and are enriched at the gene promoters to form the Cytosine preceding Guanine (CpG) islands. DNA methylation is conventionally associated with gene silencing due to the steric blocking of transcription factors by the methyl moieties, thereby preventing gene expression. In addition, methyl binding proteins such as MeCP2, MBD2 and MBD3 which can physically interact with both DNA methyltransferases as well as histone methyltransferases (Suv39h1 which adds H3K9me3), HDACs and Heterochromatin protein 1 (HP1), recruit this repressive complex to synergistically shut off gene expression of genes with methylated promoters [50, 51]. The enzymes involved in DNA methylation are the *de novo* methyltransferases DNMT3a and DNMT3b which establish new silencing patterns in response to environmental cues and the maintenance methyltransferase DNMT1 which is responsible for maintaining the heritable silencing patterns [50].

Abnormal changes in DNA methylation patterns are widespread across all cancer types including the breast cancer genome. Paradoxically in cancer, there are two distinct aberrations—a global hypomethylation observed as a result of an increased expression of demethylases and gene-specific hypermethylation events possibly due to the inaccessibility of the demethylases to the chromatin structure, both of which could contribute to tumorigenesis [52, 53].

In breast cancer too, a specific cohort of genes is known to be hypermethylated, and therefore, their expression is turned off. This happens at promoters of potential tumor suppressor genes involved in regulation of cellular proliferation, invasion, and metastasis. A few examples of such genes are *CDH1* (E-cadherin), *BRCA1*, *14-3-3σ*, *ERα*, *ERβ*, *RARβ* and *TIMP3* [54].

The importance of methylation in regulating gene expression in a cell- and tissue-specific manner becomes evident on analysis of breast tumor samples for DNA methylation. Different studies by performing methylation specific PCRs have described the concept of methylation index,[3] which is a ratio of genes hypermethylated to the total number of genes studied. It is

[3]Methylation index (MI): It is a reflection of the fraction of genes methylated. It is a ratio of the total number of genes methylated to the total number of genes analyzed. MI can be used to predict the risk of cancer.

http://dx.doi.org/10.5772/66888

observed that a higher methylation index correlates with a poorer prognosis and increased risk of recurrence of breast cancer [55]. Of more clinical significance is the finding that promoter hypermethylation events can be detected from patient serum samples. In a study by Wong et al., the authors, from peripheral blood samples determined that *BRCA1* promoter methylation increases the risk for development of breast cancer by 3.5 fold [56]. Another study has identified genome-wide differential methylation of CpGs in breast tumors compared to normal breast tissues. Interestingly, this study has also identified the differences in methylation between different molecular sub types of breast tumors, highlighting that the altered epigenetic circuitry could result in a different outcome for the disease. While Luminal B, Luminal A and HER2-positive tumors were extensively methylated in the CpGs, the basal-like tumors showed a distinct methylation pattern compared to the other sub types. The DNA methylation in Luminal A and HER2 tumors was more heterogeneous reiterating that breast cancer as a disease is constantly evolving and dynamic. They identified a distinct signature of DNA methylation in Luminal B tumors which are principally associated with CpG methylation at promoters, while, in contrast, basal-like tumors are marked by hypomethylation events in the gene body. This has led to classifying tumors from Luminal A, HER2 subtypes which exhibit signatures of CpG methylation similar to either Luminal B or basal-like as Epi-LumB or Epi-Basal respectively, highlighting the importance of these epigenetic changes in underlying tumor progression. Both Epi-LumB and Epi-Basal types of tumors were significantly correlated with increased tumor size, and Epi-LumB type tumors were found to be associated with shorter patient survival times [57]. This indicates the potential for the use of DNA methylation events in a clinical context for diagnosis and personalized treatment as well as targeting these methylation marks for discovery of therapeutics.

As discussed earlier, hypomethylation events in cancer are also associated with a poorer prognosis. The demethylation of tumor supportive genes that aid proliferation and metastasis such matrix metalloproteases-9 (MMP9) and urokinase plasminogen activator can in part explain this paradox about both hypomethylation and hypermethylation events in breast cancer increasing tumorigenic potential. Treatment of nonmetastatic breast cancer cells with demethylating agents increases their metastatic potential, while, in contrast, treatment with agents that reverse demethylation decreases the invasive capacity of breast cancer cells [58–60].

Apart from 5-methylcytosine, other methylation modifications on DNA include 5-hydroxymethylcytosine (5hmC), 5-formylcytosine (5fC) and 5-carboxylcytosine (5caC), all of which are regulated by Ten-Eleven Translocation (TET) proteins. TET proteins, in an α-Ketoglutarate and Fe(II)-dependent manner, catalyze the oxidation of the methyl groups on DNA, and these modifications could also function as intermediates in the demethylation of DNA [61, 62]. There are three known TET members identified in mammals, which include TET1, TET2 and TET3. They vary in structure and thus catalyze the oxidation reactions with varying efficiencies [63]. Inactivating mutations in *TET2* have been identified in about 15% of myeloid tumors and in patients with myelodysplastic syndromes [64, 65]. Studies by different groups have identified a significant reduction in 5hmC levels in solid tumors including breast, colon, lung, pancreatic, prostate, colon and gastric tumors [66, 67]. Interestingly, these reductions in 5hmC levels were accompanied by a significant decrease in expression of *TET1*, *TET2* and *TET3* in liver and breast carcinomas compared to the adjacent normal epithelia [66].

In the context of breast cancer, 5hmC levels are known to be deregulated. An example is the lower level of 5hmC mark at the promoter of a prominent tumor suppressor, Leucine zipper, putative tumor suppressor 1 (*LZTS1*) in breast cancer patient samples compared to normal breast tissues from healthy individuals. This results in a lower expression of *LZTS1*, and this lower expression as well as reduced *TET1* expression was correlated with 5hmC levels in the tumors. Further, lower levels of 5hmC were also associated with unfavorable prognosis and lymph node involvement [68]. High mobility group AT-hook2 (HMGA2), a chromatin remodeler, which is known to be overexpressed, regulates the expression of *TET* in breast cancers. Knockdown of HMGA2 in both cell lines and mouse breast tumors induces the expression of *TET1*. *TET1* in turn demethylates its own promoter as well as Homeobox A (*HOXA*) genes such as *HOXA7* and *HOXA9*. This induces the expression of *TET1* as well as the *HOXA* genes which together suppress the breast cancer growth and metastasis in mouse xenograft models [69]. This study also uncovers the potential of using the novel *HMGA2/TET1/HOXA9* axis as a prognostic tool for breast cancer patient survival [69]. Further, under hypoxic conditions, which are a characteristic of many solid tumors including breast tumors, studies have shown an increase in expression of *TET1* and *TET3*. The expression of *TET1* and *TET3* correlated with tumor hypoxia in patient samples and poorer prognosis and survival. Under hypoxic conditions, TET1 and TET3 proteins demethylate promoter of TNF-α and thus activate the TNF-α-p38-MAPK signaling pathway and thereby contribute to tumor progression *in vitro* and *in vivo* [70].

The complexity of epigenetic regulation by DNA methylation is evident from these numerous studies. All the studies indicate the possibility of using DNA methylation as well as DNA hydroxymethylation as predictive biomarker for breast cancer especially for early detection of these tumors. Evidence for this is provided by numerous studies which highlight that methylation signatures are more correlated with clinical patterns as compared to the gene expression and suggest a combination of these to expand the current classification and clinical prognosis predictions. Specifically, methylation pattern of promoters of *RASSF1A*, *MAL*, *SFRP1*, *BCAP31*, and *BRCA1* can be used in combination with other gene promoters to increase specificity and statistical power to predict clinical outcome [71, 72].

2.4. Targeting epigenetic regulators in breast cancer

Breast cancer, especially the triple negative subtype, is highly aggressive and needs an exhaustive list of treatment options to be made available for the patients. Understanding the dysregulated epigenetic circuitry has now made it possible to search for cures targeting the reversible marks put by the epigenetic regulators. Furthermore, methylation and acetylation marks as discussed earlier have shown immense potential to serve as candidate biomarkers, highlighting the need to monitor their levels for early diagnosis and treatment. The use of these biomarkers and screening of patients for potential biomarkers also facilitates in improving the individualized therapy and personal medicine, moving away from the conventional "one size fits all" to cater to the needs of the individual patients.

Current treatment strategies for breast cancer include surgery for removal of local tumors, adjuvant therapy in the form of chemotherapy, hormone therapy and targeted therapy.

Treatment of basal-like breast tumors involves treatment with EGFR inhibitors and PARP inhibitors [73]. However, they all suffer from drawbacks mainly due to unprecedented side effects of these drugs. The two most studied therapeutic agents, which regulate epigenetic factors, are DNA methylation inhibitors and histone deacetylase inhibitors and will be detailed in this section. The major challenge for "epi-drugs" is to recapitulate the efficient action from cell-based studies in the clinical context.

The two most used DNA methylation inhibitors are 5′ Azacytidine (5-Aza) and 5-aza-2-deoxycytidine (decitabine). Treatment of ER-negative breast cancer cells with 5-Aza reactivates the expression of ER at both mRNA and protein level. In addition, preclinical evidence suggests a useful role for DNMT inhibitors (DNMTi) in breast cancer treatment. Nanomolar (nM) dose of DNMTi has resulted in reactivation of silenced tumor suppressors such as *ER*, *BRCA1* and *PTEN* in breast cancer cell lines [74]. However, there are no available clinical data for the efficacy of these drugs in breast cancer. These drugs though having improved survival of patients with myelodysplastic syndrome and low blast count AML (lower number of immature blood cells called myeloblasts or blasts for short which are not normally found in the blood) have disappointingly not shown much promise in solid tumors. Other nucleoside analogs like zebularine and antisense oligo to specifically inhibit DNMT1 (MG98) are in clinical development. There have been clinical studies that used a combination of HDAC inhibitors (HDACi) and DNA demethylating agents and have shown promise. A phase I study used a combination of decitabine and vorinostat (HDACi) in cancer patients with advanced disease and showed stabilization of the disease in seven of the 22 evaluable patients of which 2 were patients with breast cancer [75].

HDAC inhibitors function by inhibiting the activity of the enzymes responsible for catalyzing the removal of acetyl moieties from proteins, the HDACs. HDACs are divided into four classes, and current HDACi therapy focuses on inhibitors for Class I and Class II HDACs that include HDACs 1–10. The only HDAC inhibitor that has FDA approval is Vorinostat. HDAC inhibitors result in increased acetylation of histones which is associated with reactivation of tumor suppressor genes such as p21 and p27 which in turn have the potential to inhibit tumor cell growth [76]. Vorinostat can inhibit the proliferation of breast cancer cells irrespective of their ER status. Treatment of vorinostat concomitantly with another HDACi, LAQ824, sensitizes ER positive cells to tamoxifen therapy by downregulating expression of phosphorylated and total Akt (also known as Protein Kinase B [PKB] and originally identified as an oncogene from the AKT-8 retrovirus). HDAC inhibitors such as Vorinostat used in combination can enhance the effect of tamoxifen in the hormonal strategies to treat breast cancer, whereas the mechanistic studies are still exploring the pathways involved in reversal of resistance to hormonal therapy. There are several ongoing phase II trials of combination of HDACs such as vorinostat, entinostat and valproic acid (VA) with tamoxifen, chemotherapeutic agents such as epirubicin and paclitaxel, which show promising results in treatment of the metastatic disease [75].

In a notable exception to the use of HDAC inhibitors, a study found that HDAC inhibitor valproic acid (VA) stimulates the self-renewal and expansion of normal hematopoietic stem cells [77]. In addition to this, VA enables cells to be reprogrammed to induced pluripotent stem cells [81, 82]. VA was found to have a differential effect on breast cancer cells that were differentiated *in vitro* compared to breast cancer cells that had stem cell–like characteristic, in that it radiosensitized the already differentiated cells as compared to radioprotecting the cells that had stem cell–like characteristic [83, 84]. An HDAC inhibitor as such, therefore, can lead to cancer stem cells being formed by dedifferentiating the cells that have non–stem cell–like characteristic to the ones that have the phenotype of stem cells. Chen H. et al. treated the patient-derived breast cancer cells and highly metastatic cell lines with HDAC inhibitors and found that the capacity to initiate tumor formation was high in cell lines that had non–stem cell–like characteristic, and the signaling pathway found to be involved was the WNT/β-catenin [83]. Therefore, in summary, it is extremely important that clinical studies using HDAC inhibitors should be done with extreme caution, and all possible effects should be taken into consideration before combinatorial use in trials.

Intriguingly, these epigenetic regulators and the key aberrantly regulated pathways in breast cancer including ERα signaling share a complex dynamic, which influences the treatment regime and also directs resistance to certain therapeutics. This interplay between epigenetic control and signaling from cell surface receptors has been detailed in the following section.

3. Epigenetic control of signaling pathways in breast cancer

A cell's response to external stimuli requires the activation of a signaling cascade. These signaling cascades can be either linear or multinodal where different signal transduction pathways converge resulting in the translocation and integration of these signals into the activation or repression of gene expression [78]. Signaling pathways crosstalk among each other to regulate the gene expression patterns by modulating downstream effectors such as transcription factors, cofactors and histone modifiers. This coordinated activation of signaling pathways impacts the epigenetic landscape and plays a major role in translating a signaling event into a long-lasting molecular and phenotypic change. Analyzing the relationship between cell signaling and epigenetics is of utmost importance, as it will help us extend our vision on how a cell is able to integrate information from external and/or internal stimuli to gene expression regulation through chromatin modifications.

The combined action of a cell-type–specific transcription factor and signal effectors on regulatory elements of the genome is strongly influenced by the chromatin landscape of a given cell, resulting in the establishment of a dynamic interplay between signaling pathways and the epigenetic machinery leading to the development of different cancer types including breast cancer. Globally, most of the frequently mutated somatic genes are *ER*, *HER2*, *AKT* and *MAPK*, and these are regulated by epigenetic modifications suggesting the interplay of these regulatory networks in breast cancer tumorigenesis [79].

In this section, we will discuss the interplay between signaling pathways and epigenetic regulators with special emphasis on estrogen receptor signaling. We will highlight how chromatin modifications triggered by extrinsic signaling in breast cancer play a critical role in pathological events leading to tumorigenesis.

http://dx.doi.org/10.5772/66888

3.1. Epigenetics of estrogen receptor signaling

Epigenetic changes can be defined as stable molecular alterations of a cellular phenotype that are heritable during somatic cell divisions but do not involve changes in the DNA sequence. Epigenetic regulation is critical in normal growth and development and closely coordinates the transcriptional expression of genes. Estrogen refers to a family of hormones responsible for the development and regulation of the female reproductive system and secondary sexual characteristics. Estrogen is produced by the ovaries and in smaller amounts by the adrenal cortex, testes, and fetoplacental unit [80]. Although estrogen is considered to be a female hormone, it is present in both sexes. Estrogen is found in three naturally occurring forms, such as estrone (E1), estradiol (E2) and estriol (E3). Another type of estrogen called estetrol (E4) is produced only during pregnancy. The steroid 17β-estradiol is the most potent and prevalent estrogen among the group. Estrogen is known to play an important role in a variety of biological processes. It is involved in growth, differentiation, development of brain and has an important role in reproduction [87]. Estrogen plays an important role in controlling hormonal effect; therefore, high levels of estrogen increase the risk of the development of breast cancer as high levels increase the transcription of genes known to be involved in the cell cycle regulation and metabolism pathways [88, 89].

Estrogen diffuses across the cell membrane where it binds and activates its receptor, the estrogen receptor (ER) that plays an important role in the action of estrogen. The biological effects of estrogen are mediated by its binding to the structurally and functionally distinct estrogen receptors (ERα and ERβ) [81]. ERα is a member of the steroid/thyroid hormone and vitamin A/D nuclear receptor super family [82]. ERα plays a role in regulation of genes in a diverse set of target cells that are involved in the estrogen-activated pathway and is therefore also referred to as a nuclear receptor that is activated by ligand. In addition to playing a role in normal development, ERα and its ligand 17β-estradiol have been known to be involved and are implicated in the progression of breast cancer [91]. The function of ERβ has been detailed recently; however, studies to determine its role in breast cancer development and/or prognosis are still ongoing. The role of ERβ in breast cancer remains elusive, but the presence of ERα at the time of diagnosis is used as an indication for endocrine therapy. Pathological estrogens have been associated with a higher risk of breast cancer as estrogen stimulation induces modifications of histones at the promoter region of ERα gene such as phosphorylation, methylation and acetylation by interacting with various enzymes of the epigenetic pathway that induces these histone modifications [88, 92]. These enzymes if deregulated lead to neoplastic transformation driven by ERα [88].

3.1.1. Mechanism of ERα-mediated histone modifications

The transcriptional outcome of ERα is regulated by a dynamic interaction of histone-modifying enzymes and associated coregulators. The multiprotein complexes containing ERα, its coactivators such as p300/CREB-binding protein (p300/CBP), p300/CBP-associated factor (PCAF) [83] and histone-modifying enzymes such as acetylases/deacetylases and methylases/demethylases assemble in response to hormone binding, resulting in transcriptional regulation

[84]. ERα exerts a positive feedback loop on expression of *CYP19A*, which is involved in the synthesis of estrogens in human placenta, thereby promoting induction of its own gene at the transcription level and contributing to local estrogen synthesis by promoting increased acetylation in the *CYP19A* promoter [85]. ERα also enhances the recruitment of metastasis-associated 1 protein (MTA1), a component of the histone deacetylase and nucleosome remodeling complex (NuRD), in a ligand and growth factor signaling dependent manner, resulting in the attenuation of ERα signaling [86]. MTA1 interacts with histone deacetylases directly and hence behaves as a corepressor. Dysregulation of MTA1 leads to cell migration, formation of colonies in semisolid media [97], mammary carcinoma development in transgenic mice [98] and breast cancer cells growth in some experimental observations. In addition, inhibiting the expression of MTA1 protein also led to growth inhibition and reduced invasion of highly metastatic breast cancer cells MDA-MB-231, making it an important molecule in breast tumorigenesis [99].

ERα signaling pathway has traditionally been known to be involved in the activation of genes involved in transcription; however, recent observations using experimental techniques such as microarray and ChIP have found that in transcriptome of more than half of ERα target genes regulated by ERα are repressed [100]. Different chromatin modifications at the ERα target genes as well as recruitment of different regulators of transcription may account for differential regulation by ERα. One of the examples of this regulation is the repressor of estrogen receptor activity (REA) and its binding partner EZH2. EZH2 is an important corepressor that is upregulated during the progression of different cancers, a process accompanied by the silencing of various genes. Interestingly, EZH2-mediated repression of cellular genes was attenuated on inhibition of histone deacetylase activity, implying a dependence of EZH2 targets on acetylation status of histones as well as chromatin remodeling [87]. In another study by Jene-Sanz et al., it was found that EZH2 targets tumor suppressor genes, because EZH2 overexpression not only repressed a significant number of genes but also resulted in increased metastasis [88]. Therefore, the combined interaction of EZH2 with the repressor of estrogen receptor is needed for ERα's recruitment to specific target genes and repression of estrogen-dependent transcription [89]. The inhibition of EZH2 by siRNA was found to be responsible for an increase in estrogen-dependent transcription.

ERα also modifies chromatin organization by affecting the acetylation and deacetylation of conserved lysine residues present in histone tails. Specifically, the coactivators of ERα possess histone acetyl transferase activity and are known to associate with and modulate functions of specific acetyl transferases. In addition, ERα-mediated deacetylation is accomplished by recruitment of histone deacetylases (HDACs), which are recruited indirectly to ERα target genes through multisubunit corepressor complexes. ERα also utilizes corepressor complexes such as nuclear receptor corepressor (NCOR) and silencing mediator of retinoid and thyroid hormone receptors (SMRT) that associate with histone deacetylases [90]. Studies employing siRNA targeting histone deacetylases and corepressors indicated that one such histone deacetylase, HDAC6 functions with a corepressor, ligand-dependent corepressor (LCOR) on some ERα target genes as part of a feedback loop to regulate estrogen-dependent gene regulation in breast cancer cells [91]. The expression levels of HDAC6 correlate with better prognosis and response to endocrine therapy in breast cancer patients. Thus, ERα is known to achieve several histone modifications at target gene promoters using several coregulators.

Studies on ERα target gene regulation have introduced a new degree of complexity, wherein a combination of interactions between ERα and histone acetyltransferases, histone deacetylases, histone methyltransferases, coactivators, corepressors and transcription factors reveals a complex histone code that regulates promoters involved in breast cancer cells proliferation. A dynamic process of DNA methylation is also known to be involved in the control of the cyclic expression of ERα target genes. In a significant fraction of breast cancers, the absence or loss of ER at the time of diagnosis or treatment is due to aberrant methylation of CpG islands, cytosine-guanine-rich areas that are located in the 5′ regulatory regions of the ERα gene [92, 93]. Methylation/demethylation of CpG sites on promoters following estrogen stimulation revealed the importance of DNA methyltransferases control on estrogen-dependent gene expression. Interestingly, ERβ has been found to play a role in the establishment of new and stable methylation. All these results provide strong evidence that estrogen target gene expression is tightly regulated by multiple highly dynamic machinery affecting estrogen receptor in both a transcriptional and an epigenetic manner.

Current endocrine therapy for ERα-positive cancer involves modulating the ERα pathway using antiestrogens (AEs) or aromatase inhibitors (AIs). ERα's ability to modulate epigenetic changes by regulating writers, erasers and readers of epigenetic modifications provides a unique therapeutic opportunity to design novel drugs and small molecular inhibitors for treating ERα-positive cancers [88] (**Figure 3**).

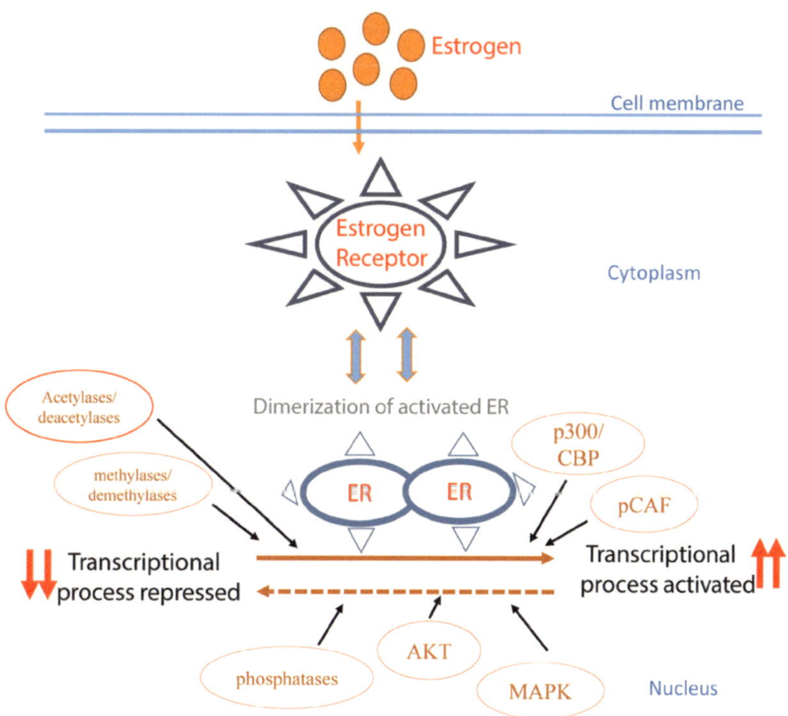

Figure 3. Regulation of epigenetic modifications by ERα. Estrogen signaling activates a set of kinases *via* its extranuclear signaling that modifies histone tails or influences the recruitment and function of histone modifying enzymes. In addition, ERα-driven transcription also involves a coordinated interaction of ERα with acetylases/deacetylases and methylases/demethylases. ERα if deregulated affects tumor progression and its associated therapeutic resistance.

3.2. Linking chromatin to the downstream signaling effectors

Eukaryotes utilize the chromatin landscape as its epigenetic template within the nucleus of living cells to promote gene transcription in response to environmental signals. Different classes of chromatin-associated enzymes or kinases that play important role in modulating chromatin structure within the human genome have been discovered recently. These signal transduction kinases play a pivotal role as chromatin-anchored proteins in eukaryotes, relaying signals from the cytoplasm to the nucleus and direct the association of chromatin-bound transcription complexes at activated targets in the nucleus [94]. These interactions serve to integrate the hormonal signals into a network of coordinated programs, and it is the outcome of this integration that specifies the nature, intensity and duration of the cellular response.

Estrogen and progesterone, two of the hormones known to play a role in breast cancer progression influence a variety of functions *via* their respective signaling cascades. These steroid hormone receptors (SHR) are known to interact with hormone-responsive elements (HREs) in the promoter/enhancer region of target genes, thereby affecting the epigenetic landscape of the cell [95]. SHRs can also activate genes lacking HREs by interacting with other sequence-specific transcription factors bound to their target sequences [96]. In addition to nongenomic interactions that involve the activation of *PI3K/Akt* pathways by the interaction of the ERα with the regulatory subunit of PI3K, SHRs can also induce direct genomic affects by binding to different regulatory elements of the genome and inducing the downstream effector response. Not much has been reported or is known on how progesterone receptor integrates the signaling pathways at the epigenetic level. A study by Ballare et al.using a synthetic progesterone, progestin, found that some of the kinases activated by progestin in the cytoplasm phosphorylate the progesterone receptor (PR) and form a complex with the activated receptor. This complex is recruited to the target sites where the kinases modify the protruding core histone tails and the linker histones. These modifications lead to the displacement of linker histones and a repressive complex, by recruiting specialized ATP-dependent remodelers such as switch/sucrose nonfermentable (SWI/SNF) [97]. In addition, other specialized ATP-dependent remodelers displace histone H2A/H2B dimers from the promoter nucleosome, enabling synergistic access of other transcription factors and additional receptor complexes to previously hidden binding sites on the surface of a histone H3/H4 tetramer particle [95]. It is only after completion of these initial chromatin remodeling steps that complexes containing mediator and RNA polymerase along with associated basal transcription factors are recruited, and further steps in transcription can take place. Thus, these signaling pathways of progestin action converge on the chromatin to enable gene regulation in the case of breast cancer.

3.2.1. Role of kinases in the epigenetic signaling network

Cross talk between signaling kinases and chromatin remodelers are critical for eliciting inducible transcriptional programs that include differentiation of cells, their ability to invade and migrate and to form cancer stem cells. Epigenetic approach targeting breast cancer stem cells (CSCs) may prove to be a good therapeutic option since not much has been known about the cross talk between these signaling kinases and chromatin remodelers. In an exception, one study found the chromatin-associated role of an evolutionarily conserved protein kinase

http://dx.doi.org/10.5772/66888

C (PKC) family protein, PKC-θ. After nuclear translocation to the nucleus, PKC-θ plays a role in generating a T cell–induced immune response by influencing the transcription of genes involved in generating the response that also include some microRNAs [112]. Aberrant expression of this kinase may lead to uncontrolled cell growth leading to tumors, inflammatory disorders or an aggressive form of breast cancer leading to cancer metastasis [113].

PKC-θ is present mainly in ER-negative basal-like breast cancer lines, localized in the nucleus, and an increased nuclear PKC-θ results in epithelial to mesenchymal transition (EMT). Experiments such as ChIP using pan-PKC-θ-specific antibody was performed, and it was found that PKC-θ occupies the proximal promoter region of *CD44* gene in EMT models. Additionally, ChIP analysis demonstrated that RNA polymerase II and PKC-θ coexist on the promoter of CSC-inducible gene suggesting that PKC-θ exists as part of a transcription complex in the mesenchymal state [98]. Thus, active PKC in primary breast cancers tethers the transcription complex to EMT and CSC-inducible genes, and the expression of this complex is found elevated in cancer stem cells leading to breast cancer. The PKC pathway also cooperates with the transforming growth factor β (TGF-β) pathway and collaborates with the NF-κB pathway to promote a distinct transcriptional program of inducible EMT and CSC signature genes [99]. Using the p50 and p65 heterodimer (the subunits of NF-κB pathway), the transcription complex of activated PKC-θ is bound to the chromatin of some inducible genes that are involved in the EMT process. The role of each of the subunit is such that p65 subunit recruits the PKC-θ transcriptional complex to the promoter region of *CD44* and *IL-6* and the p50 subunit is involved in the recruitment of PKC-θ transcriptional complex to only the promoter region of *IL-6* but not to *CD44*. In a cellular system if PKC-θ is knocked out, it is observed that PKC-θ is not only important for maintaining a permissive state for IL-6 and CD44 at the chromatin level but also for the enrichment of certain epigenetic marks such as H3K4me3 and H3K9ac [113]. Using genome-wide analysis, distinct cohorts of inducible PKC-θ sensitive genes in the mesenchymal state that are directly tethered to chromatinized PKC-θ were identified. Some of the genes were found to be EMT regulators and some involved in progression of cancer, suggesting that PKC-θ occupies a position upstream making it a novel regulator of the EMT process and in the progression of cancer. Thus, the chromatin bound PKC-θ engages with factors that play a role in establishing a permissive chromatin state, thereby contributing a new dimension toward the understanding of EMT/CSC process in breast cancer. Targeting CSCs remains an underdeveloped area of cancer therapy; however, a novel epigenetic mechanism using specific inhibitors will pave the way for novel "epitherapeutic" strategies.

Some other examples of signaling pathways influencing the epigenetic circuitry include the NF-κB pathway. Tumor necrosis factor α (TNF-α), an important effector of the NF-κB pathway, is known to induce expression of a lysine demethylase, KDM4D in macrophages and dendritic cells. Enzymes belonging to the demethylase family of KDM4 including KDM4D are overexpressed in breast cancer and affect cell proliferation and growth of these cells [98]. Another lysine demethylase of KDM4 family, KDM4A, has been known to be involved in transcriptional regulation, where it may either stimulate or repress gene transcription [100]. The latter function involves the association with nuclear receptor corepressor complex or association with histone deacetylases. KDM4A is also known to form complexes with ER and to stimulate its activity. Accordingly, depletion of KDM4A in ER-positive breast cancer cells leads to a decrease in the expression of ER targets such as the c-*JUN* and Cyclin D1 oncogenes and reduced cell growth [101]. Similarly, KDM4A knockdown inhibited proliferation of ER-negative MDA-MB-231 and ER-positive MCF7 breast cancer cells [102, 103], suggesting that KDM4A is critical for growth of both ER positive and negative breast cancers. Another example is the progesterone-activated extracellular signal-regulated protein kinase 1/2 (ERK1/2) pathway in breast cancer, which phosphorylates both the progesterone receptor and the downstream kinase, mitogen and stress-activated protein kinase 1(MSK1), forming an active ternary complex that mediates the phosphorylation of histone H3 at serine 10 in breast cancer cells [104]. This initial step triggers the recruitment of histone modifiers and chromatin remodeling complexes, which ultimately leads to displacement of histones H1 and H2A/H2B supporting the role of chromatin remodeling complexes for transcriptional activation of progesterone responsive genes.

In the case of ERα signaling, ER activates a number of kinases in the extranuclear compartment including protein kinase B (AKT) and extracellular signal-regulated protein kinase. In ER-positive breast cancers, mitogen-activated protein kinase (MAPK) pathway exerts an effect at the level of ER-induced transcription as well as at the level of the cell cycle regulation. Estrogen stimulates cell proliferation by activation of MAP kinase, either through rapid, nontranscription effects or by increasing growth factor production and consequently MAP kinase expression. Hormonal stimulation also promotes alterations in the phosphorylation of specific residues in histone tails *via* modulation of these extra-nuclear kinases. Estrogen-ERα signaling activates MAP kinase cascades in breast cancer specifically the one involving ERK-1 and ERK-2 that transmit and amplify signals involved in cellular proliferation [105]. ERα activates ERK2, resulting in its chromatin binding and enabling ERK2 modulation of estrogen-dependent gene expression and proliferation in breast cancers. This convergence of ERK2 and ERα at the chromatin level is also known to activate an oncogenic kinase AuroraA/B to directly affect nuclear receptor activities [106]. The Src-AKTs, which are involved in phosphorylation of Histone H1 and Src-MAPK pathways, are also activated by ERα signaling. Downstream substrates of these kinases such as the ones that phosphorylate histone H1 and core histones are therefore influenced by ERα signaling at the chromatin level [122]. In addition, the expression of several phosphates such as PP1 and PP2A is also regulated by the ERα signaling. In one of the studies, these phosphates were identified as key negative regulators of steroid receptor coactivator 3 (SRC-3). SRC-3 is a coactivator and an oncogene, whose phosphorylation transforms it into a powerful coregulator. It was shown that PDXP and PP2A dephosphorylate SRC-3 and inhibit its ligand-dependent association with estrogen receptor, thus regulating the oncogenic cell proliferation and invasion functions of SRC-3 in breast cancer cells [107]. These observations therefore suggest that ERα-extranuclear signaling has the potential to modulate epigenetic modifications. The direct communication between the extracellular environment and the regulation of gene function may be even more widespread and warrants greater study. It could involve many kinases that are known to regulate gene expression indirectly *via* signaling cascades. In addition, the signaling to chromatin may change the role of these kinases and may rationalize the use of chromatin-modifying enzymes as important cellular targets.

http://dx.doi.org/10.5772/66888

3.3. HDACs and signaling pathways

Sustained and increased hormone and growth factor receptor signaling in breast cancer cells contributes to resistance toward endocrine therapy. It has become important to modulate the signaling pathways so as to design an attractive strategy in overcoming potential resistance to endocrine therapy. In the case of breast cancer, down regulation of ERα expression is one of the mechanisms behind the acquisition of endocrine resistance. Histone deacetylases (HDACs) are important epigenetic regulators and are overexpressed in multiple cancers, including breast cancer. Specifically, histone deacetylase 1 (HDAC1) is an important epigenetic regulator involved in transcriptional regulation through modification of chromatin organization [82]. Although, HDACs are primarily known to repress gene expression as part of corepressor complexes, recent findings by Smith et al. have established a link between HDACs inhibition and repression of gene expression, suggesting that they might also function as coactivators [108]. In some cases, as for the regulation of ERα, HDACs inhibitors (HDACi) can have both positive and negative impact on transcription, depending on the cell context. In breast cancer cells, trichostatin A (TSA), a potent and reversible HDACi, produced a strong decrease in ERα accumulation independent of the presence or absence of ER ligands. The effect was dose dependent and was not restricted to TSA since a similar regulation was obtained with different HDACi, suberoylanilide hydroxamic acid (SAHA), which is structurally similar to TSA [109]. Regulation by TSA takes place at the transcriptional level and therefore the use of different HDACi decreases the expression of *ERα* in ER-positive breast cancer cells. In another study, it was found that the use of HDACi reactivates the expression of the receptor in ER-negative cells and the treatment resulted in dose-dependent and time-dependent re-expression of *ERα* mRNA [110, 111]. This was speculated to be due to the loss of *ERα* expression or that TSA could potentiate the effect of DNA methyltransferase inhibitors such as 5-aza-2-deoxycytidine, treated together on the re-expression of the ERα protein [112]. Activation of the silenced ERα by HDAC1 inhibition and partial re-expression of *ERα* by TSA treatment may provide a possible therapeutic treatment for patients with advanced breast cancer, restoring estrogen-mediated signaling and growth. Thereby, inhibition of HDAC1 expression or activity may provide a new strategy for breast cancer therapy.

The phosphoinositide 3-kinase (PI3K)/mammalian target of rapamycin (mTOR) pathway plays a critical role in multiple cellular functions including metabolism, proliferation, growth, and survival [113]. Studies have found PI3K/mTOR pathway to be a promising target in breast cancer [114]. The p70 S6 kinase (S6K1) is one of the best-characterized downstream targets of mTOR and plays an important role in protein translation and cell proliferation [115]. The mTOR inhibitor rapamycin, tested as an anticancer drug, rapidly dephosphorylates and inactivates S6K1. S6K1 is amplified in 10–30% of breast cancer cell lines, and its overexpression is associated with poor prognosis in breast cancer patients. PI3K inhibitors are able to regulate the expression of ERα through the activity of S6K1, as in cells that have S6K1 overexpression, rapamycin can increase both mRNA and protein levels of ERα, promoting the acetylation of its promoter [114].

In some cases, HDAC1 activity and its binding to the *ERα* promoter is required for the rapamycin-dependent upregulation of ERα expression. Thus, when S6K1 is active and HDAC1 is hyper-phosphorylated, it results in decreased expression of ERα, whereas in the presence of rapamycin or cell starvation, S6K1 activation and mitogen dependent HDAC1 phosphorylation is ablated, increasing the level of ERα in breast cancer cells. Thus, the mitogen-dependent phosphorylation of HDAC1 inhibits the positive transcriptional regulation of the deacetylase on ERα expression [116]. Since both HDACs and mTOR inhibitors are known to have anti-proliferative effect in breast cancer cells, their combinatorial treatment shows promise (**Figure 4**).

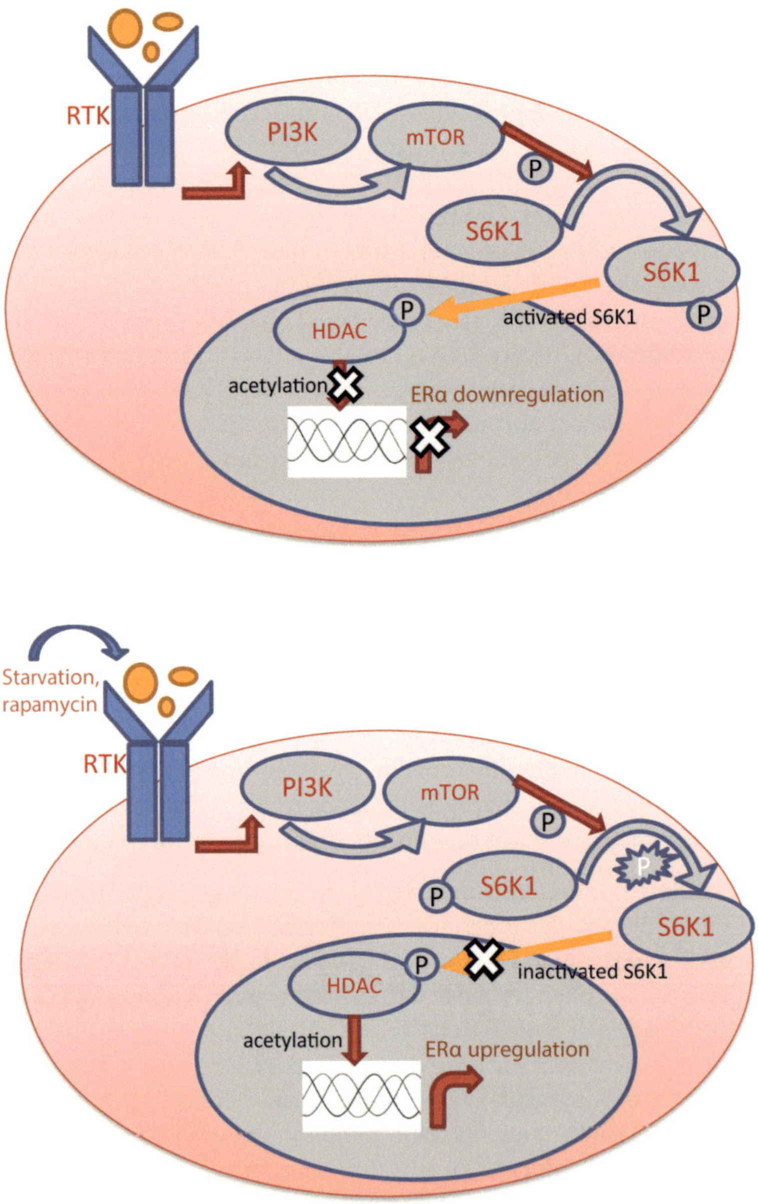

Figure 4. Mitogen-mediated HDAC1 phosphorylation and ERα transcriptional regulation. PI3K/mTOR pathway is activated by the RTK. Subsequently, S6K1 activation controls HDAC1 phosphorylation and thereby reduces acetylation of the ERα promoter and gene expression. In the case of cell starvation or when rapamycin is present, S6K1 is not active and is not able to phosphorylate HDAC1, promoting acetylation of ERα and its gene expression.

http://dx.doi.org/10.5772/66888

3.3.1. The role of antiestrogens in epigenetic silencing

Corepressors are associated with deacetylase activity through the recruitment of HDACs, and these HDACs possess different functional domains responsible for deacetylase activity and interaction with other proteins. The amount of histone acetylation is therefore determined by an equilibrium between acetyltransferases and deacetylases, and that the ratio of corepressors to coactivators is the modulator of transcription in any given context [112]. The ligand-dependant activation of steroid hormones receptor regulates a variety of gene expression. Binding of an agonist leads to the activation of transcription, whereas an antagonist does the opposite, leading to inhibition. ERα bound to an anti-estrogen is unable to activate transcription, and this may be due to the recruitment of a repressor complex with HDAC activity [117] making the use anti-estrogens a feasible treatment option. However, the use of anti-estrogens is limited due to the associated side effects or the development of resistance. Moreover, HDAC activity has also been associated with gene silencing in some eukaryotes [117]. This gene silencing associated with HDAC binding at the *ERα* promoter could be due to the direct targeting of HDAC to estrogen-responsive elements (EREs), thereby mimicking or modulating the effects of the anti-estrogens [118]. The specific sites of the action of HDACs are therefore associated with the binding of corepressors and in-turn lead to the reversible silencing process, thus a potential therapeutic option. An example of this phenomenon was highlighted in one of the studies where treatment of MCF-7 cells with an antiestrogen hydroxytamoxifen (OHT), induced silencing of estrogen-responsive genes [118]. Similarly, the estrogen-dependent expression of the ERα was partially silenced after 3 months of OHT treatment and OHT-resistant cell growth appeared simultaneously. It was found that histone deacetylase activity was involved in the repressive effect by its binding to estrogen-responsive elements (ERE) and the antiestrogen effect might be very similar, if not identical to the ERE-targeted HDAC activity [118].

3.4. Promoter DNA methylation and signaling pathways

DNA methylation profiles of many genes have been linked with cancer initiation and progression [119]. As discussed earlier, in the case of DNA methylation, the most extensively studied mechanism of epigenetic control is global hypomethylation that leads to genome instability. At the same time, hypermethylation of promoter regions has been detected in a vast majority of tumor suppressor genes, which are strongly associated with tumor development. Hypermethylation events can occur early in tumorigenesis, involving the disruption of pathways that may predispose cells to malignant transformation. Gene silencing by hypermethylation of promoter genes is an important mechanism of carcinogenesis and has great potential for cancer prevention and therapy [120].

In the case of breast cancer, the distribution of aberrantly methylated regions in the genome was found to be nonrandom and concentrated in relatively small genomic regions spanning up to several hundred kilobases. DNA hypermethylation also leads to aberrant regulation of the Wnt pathway in breast cancer, and an overstimulated Wnt signaling is a hallmark of different breast cancer tumor subtype [121]. Functional loss of negative Wnt regulators by epigenetic gene silencing, through DNA methylation of the tumor suppressor gene-associated promoters, has been found to contribute to the activation of aberrant WNT/β-catenin signaling [122]. Recent studies have also found impaired regulation of Wnt-antagonists by promoter hypermethylation in breast cancer. The growing list of epigenetically silenced WNT antagonists involved in human cancers indicates an important role for epigenetic inactivation events in tumor initiation and progression [123]. For examples, some Wnt proteins like WNT1, WNT2 and WNT3A are overexpressed in breast cancer, acting as oncogenic activators for canonical Wnt signaling [124]. In contrast, WNT5A acts as a tumor suppressor inhibiting tumor cell proliferation, antagonizing the WNT/β-catenin signaling and is thereby silenced by tumor-specific methylation [125]. In parallel, epigenetic inactivation of Wnt gene family members, *WNT7A* and *WNT9A*, through promoter methylation, has been reported as well [126]. As epigenetic dysregulation of WNT/β-catenin signaling frequently contributes to tumor pathogenesis, identification of aberrant epigenetic events that activate WNT/β-catenin signaling may provide useful biomarkers for cancer detection and prognosis. Some Wnt proteins like Wnt1, Wnt2 and Wnt3A are overexpressed in breast cancer, acting as oncogenic activators for canonical Wnt signaling [124]. In addition, WNT5A acts as a tumor suppressor inhibiting tumor cell proliferation, antagonizing the WNT/β-catenin signaling and is thereby silenced by tumor-specific methylation [125]. In parallel, epigenetic inactivation of Wnt gene family members, *WNT7A* and *WNT9A*, through promoter methylation, has recently been reported [126]. As epigenetic dysregulation of WNT/β-catenin signaling frequently contributes to tumor pathogenesis, identification of aberrant epigenetic events that activate WNT/β-catenin signaling may provide useful biomarkers for cancer detection and prognosis.

In addition, hypermethylation of the gene promoters of Wnt repressors was observed in various cell lines and tissues. The epithelial adhesion molecule E-cadherin (encoded by *CDH1*) also acts as a negative regulator of WNT/β-catenin signaling by affecting the intracellular localization of β-catenin. Epigenetic silencing of *CDH1*, by promoter methylation has been observed in breast cancer, leading to aberrant activation of WNT/β-catenin signaling. The *APC* promoter (adenomatous polyposis coli) of the WNT/β-catenin signaling pathway has also been found to be hypermethylated at the CpG island in ~35–50% of breast cancer tumors and cell lines [127]. The methylation of *APC* gene is a cancer-specific change and may disrupt the regulation in the APC/β-catenin pathway in breast cancers, making it a common mechanism of the inactivation of tumor suppressor gene in primary breast cancer.

Histone methylation is also known to play a key role in ERα-mediated activation of target genes. Recent studies found that histone demethylase KDM1 and ERα coregulator proline-, glutamic acid- and leucine-rich protein-1 (PELP1) plays a role in regulating histone methyl marks at ERα target genes [128]. PELP1 deregulation alters histone methylation at ERα target genes, contributing to hormone-driven tumor progression and resistance to treatment.

3.4.1. The synergistic role of HDACs and DNA methylation in breast cancer

Patients who have ER-negative breast cancer seldom respond to endocrine therapy. One of the mechanisms to explain the loss of estrogen receptors expression is the methylation of cytosine at the 5′ regulatory region of the gene at the CpG island [133]. CpG island in ERα genes is highly methylated in ER-negative breast cancer but remain unmethylated in normal breast tissue and many ER-positive tumors as well as ER-positive cancer cell lines. This abnormal methylation pattern could account for transcriptional inactivation of the ER gene and subsequent hormone resistance in some human breast carcinomas. The functional importance of this finding is demonstrated by the fact that treatment of ER-negative human breast cancer cells with the demethylating agent, 5-aza-2′-deoxycytidine (AZA), led to reactivation of *ER* mRNA and functional ER protein [129].

An abundant chromosomal methyl CpG-binding protein was the first protein identified to link methylated DNA and a HDAC-containing transcriptionally repressive complex for gene silencing. More recently, the well-known maintenance methyltransferase, DNMT1, was found to interact physically with HDAC through its N terminus, thereby leading to a transcriptionally inactive complex that represses transcription [130]. Thus, the loss of ER expression in some breast cancers is associated with transcriptional repression through HDAC activity on the methylated *ER* gene, linking HDAC activity closely to DNA methylation of *ERα* promoter and thereby helping in understanding the associated resistance to endocrine therapy.

Recent studies also demonstrated that combination therapy involving HDAC inhibitors with DNA methyltransferase-1 (DNMT1) inhibition is synergistically effective in inducing apoptosis, differentiation and/or cell growth arrest in many cancer types including breast cancer. The combination was also synergistic in inducing re-expression of *ERα* in ERα-negative breast cancer cells. Expression of ERα is induced by 5-aza-2′-deoxycytidine (DNMT1 inhibitor) and trichostatin A (HDAC inhibitor) in ER-negative breast cancer. Studies at the preclinical level indicate that sensitivity of ER-negative breast cancer cells could be restored to endocrine therapy by the use of AZA and TSA both *in vitro* and *in vivo*. When HDAC inhibitors such as vorinostat were used in combination with decitabine, the capacity of breast cancer cells to proliferate and to form colonies was inhibited significantly as compared to when either drug was used alone [146]. Histone methylation could also be a druggable target as some therapeutic benefits have been observed during the preclinical studies.

4. Coding and noncoding RNAs in breast cancer

4.1. Current techniques for detection of breast cancer

The genetic signature identified from gene expression arrays has been incorporated into five different breast cancer prognostic platforms. As an improvement over the classical ER/PR/HER2 status, a panel of eight genes has been identified to classify the different breast cancer subtypes [131]. This panel includes the genes *ER*, *PR*, *HER2*, CK5, CK14, *p53*, MKI67 and *EGFR*. Cytokeratin 5 (CK5) and cytokeratin 14 (CK14) genes expressed by basal/myoepithelial cells are used to characterize basal-like TNBC [132]. EGFR is frequently upregulated in TNBC cases with a basal phenotype and can be targeted for therapy. Ki-67 is a marker for proliferating cells. Ki-67 and *p53* expression can be used to distinguish Luminal A from Luminal B tumors. The different prognostic tests for breast cancer, namely, the 21-gene Oncotype DX® [133], 70-gene MammaPrint® [134], and 50-gene PAM50 [135] detect the presence of these various mRNA biomarkers in patient samples. The need for additional markers for breast cancer subtype classification and further treatment regime arises from the observation that while Oncotype Dx and MammaPrint are the only FDA-approved RNA-based assays, they only share one gene in common (*MKI67*), besides *ER* and *HER2*.

Less than 2% of the human genome is translated into proteins. However, around 97% of the genome is transcribed, indicating that most of transcripts are not translated. Initially described as "transcriptional noise," increasing evidence in the past few years has helped identify the regulatory functions of these "noncoding RNAs." Noncoding RNAs are classified as small noncoding RNAs and long noncoding RNAs (lncRNAs). Small noncoding RNAs include miRNAs, small-interfering RNAs (siRNAs) and piwi-interacting RNAs measuring <200 nt in length. LncRNAs as the name suggests are "long," ranging in length from 200 nt to 200 kb. Noncoding RNAs, both small and long, have been shown to regulate critical cellular functions such as transcriptional and posttranscriptional regulation which in turn modulate cell growth and differentiation [136]. Thus, it is no surprise that the aberrant expression of several noncoding RNAs has been observed and attributed to various diseases, including cancer.

Given that noncoding RNAs comprise the vast majority of the human transcriptome and evidence of their essential role in gene regulation, it is important that this largely unexplored class of molecules be studied in the cancer context more closely. Some miRNAs and lncRNAs implicated in breast cancer initiation, progression and metastasis have been summarized in **Figure 5**.

4.2. MiRNAs in breast cancer

MiRNAs are 18–24 nt in length noncoding RNA molecules that regulate gene expression by mRNAs degradation or inhibition of protein synthesis. MiRNAs have been shown to regulate numerous physiological processes such as differentiation, development and cell death as well as pathophysiological processes such as cancer biology, progression and prognosis. The aberrant expression of miRNAs in cancers can lead to an abnormal expression of their target genes thereby contributing to cancer etiology. Mounting evidence suggests a significant role of miRNAs in breast cancer classification, prognosis, as potential biomarkers for disease progression as well as treatment [137].

4.2.1. MiRNAs and breast tumor initiation

Mammary gland epithelia comprise different cells including mammary stem cells (MaSCs)/basal cells, luminal progenitors and mature luminal cells. Several subtypes have been described among breast cancers, including claudin-low, basal, luminal, normal-like and ERBB2-enriched subtypes. These distinct molecular subtypes derive from different "cells of origin," that is, cells that acquire the first oncogenic events in the initiation of breast tumorigenesis [138, 139]. The close association between cell lineage targeting and the resulting cancer phenotype suggests that lineage-restricted mechanisms that normally operate during the mammary gland development and homeostasis may contribute to tumorigenesis. Some miRNAs have been recently identified

http://dx.doi.org/10.5772/66888

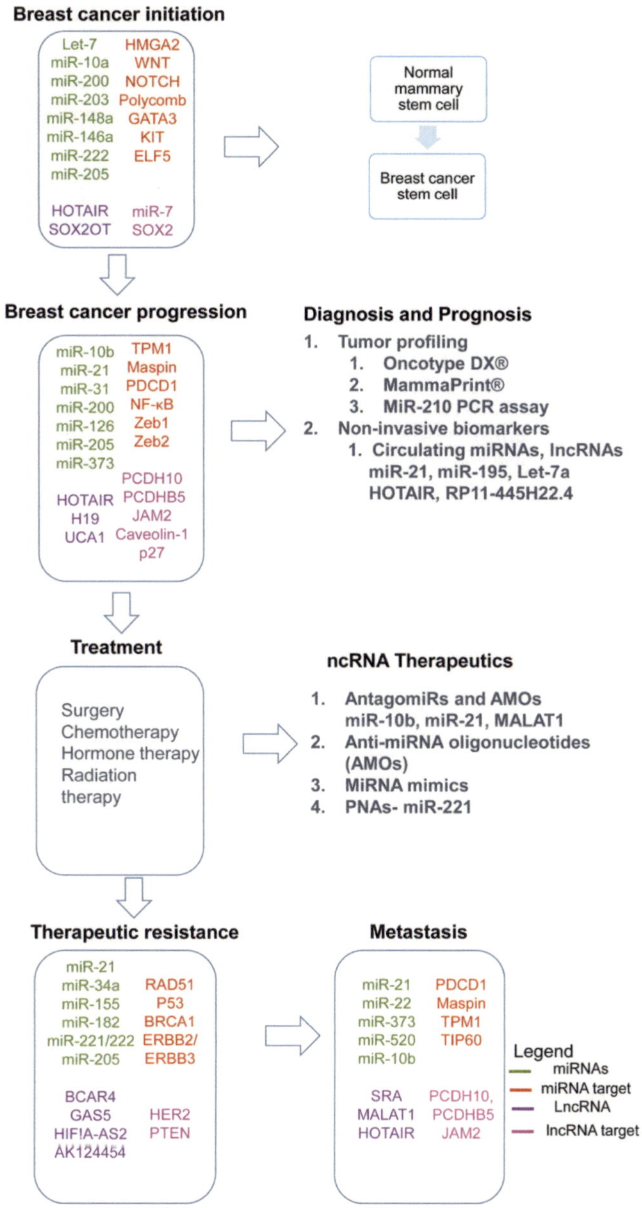

Figure 5. MiRNAs and lncRNAs implicated in breast cancer initiation, progression and metastasis. Several miRNAs and lncRNAs controlling key oncogenes such as *HMGA2* among others are downregulated in the breast cancer stem cells (BCSCs) leading to proliferation and self-renewal of these cells and breast cancer progression. Downregulation of tumor suppressor miRNAs such as the miR-200 family leads to an upregulation of the EMT markers *ZEB1* and *ZEB2*, thus aiding tumor proliferation and invasion. A number of mRNA markers are displayed by tumor cells at this stage aiding in their subtyping and prognosis. Additionally, several noncoding RNA biomarkers have also been identified including noninvasive circulating ncRNAs which closely correlate with patient prognosis. Further, several miRNAs and lncRNAs contribute to the hormonal resistance displayed by breast cancer cells *via* targeting tumor suppressors such as *PTEN*, cell cycle genes such as *p27* or members of the hormone signaling pathways such as ERα, thereby leading to more aggressive and metastasized cancer. Currently, a number of novel and safe therapeutic options are being researched to aid the conventional treatment options to help ameliorate breast cancer.

as potential "keepers" of this lineage-restricted identity. Thereby, aberrant expression of these miRNAs has been implicated in breast cancer molecular subtypes. Unique miRNA signatures characterize each step of the mammary differentiation hierarchy in the normal mammary gland (MaSCs/basal cells, luminal progenitors, mature luminal and stromal cells). MiRNA networks, also known as miRNome, are responsible for governing lineage commitment and cellular differentiation in the mammary tissue. MiRNAs act by targeting lineage-specific mRNAs thus regulating lineage-specific gene expression [140]. For example, the expression of miRNAs implied in MaSCs functions and pathways (WNT, NOTCH and Polycomb groups) such as miRNA-10a, miRNA-200a/b, miRNA-203 and miRNA-148a is restricted to the luminal subpopulation. Conversely, miRNA-146a, miRNA-221/222 and miRNA-205, known to regulate genes expressed in the luminal lineages (*BRCA1*, *GATA3*, *KIT* and *ELF5*), are restricted to the MaSCs population. Integrating these miRNA signatures with both transcriptomics and histone marks analysis has revealed that key developmental miRNAs are epigenetically regulated by global changes in histone methylation during differentiation [140]. By comparing miRNA signatures of normal breast epithelial cells with breast tumors, many miRNA-mRNA networks deregulated in cancer cells have been identified. Therefore, these miRNAs may potentially represent new biomarkers and targets. Furthermore, the miRNome of breast tumors allows the classification of tumors into molecular subtypes and can predict the patient's outcome [141–143].

4.2.2. Oncogenic and tumor suppressor-like miRNAs in breast cancer

Due to amplification of chromosomal regions of miRNAs, certain miRNAs may be overexpressed in cancer. If these miRNAs target TSGs, it would downregulate the TSGs leading to malignant growth. Hence, such potentially cancer-causing miRNAs are called oncomiRs. Conversely, oncosuppressor miRNA genes are frequently located in fragile loci, which are hotspots for deletions, mutations and promoter methylation. Genetic aberrations in such loci may result in downregulated miRNA expression and a concomitant increase in expression of oncogenes. These alternations of miRNA lead to tumor formation by inducing cell proliferation, invasion, loss of apoptosis, and angiogenesis. Thus, miRNAs can act both as oncogenes as well as TSGs [144, 145].

4.2.2.1. OncomiRs in breast cancer

MiR-21 is a prominent oncomiR which is upregulated in breast cancer. The targets of miRNA-21 include *BCL-2* (regulates apoptosis), *PTEN* (regulates cell survival) and *PDCD4*, *TPM1* and *MASPIN* (involved in tumor progression, invasion and metastasis). Thus, overexpression of miR-21 in breast cancer supports tumor growth [146, 147]. MiR-155 is an oncomiR, with an increase in expression in breast cancer, where it targets tumor suppressor gene *SOCS1* [148].

4.2.2.2. Tumor suppressor-like miRNAs in breast cancer

Let-7 is an important tumor suppressor miRNA with a decrease in expression in breast cancer. It targets the Ras pathway and regulates cell proliferation, adhesion and migration [149]. Targets of let-7 include *HMG2A* (responsible for maintenance of stemness of stem cells), *lin-28* and *PEBP1* (oncogenes involved in cancer progression and metastasis) [150, 151]. Thus, a loss of let-7 leads to an upregulation of these oncogenes resulting in breast cancer stem cell renewal and cancer progression.

4.2.3. MetastamiRs in breast cancer

Metastasis is a complex multistep process, which includes the formation of tumors at sites distant from the primary site of the cancer. The term 'metastamiR' refers to as a metastasis-associated miRNA [152]. Several miRNAs such as miR-10b, miR-21, miR-30a, miR-30e, miR-125b, miR-141, miR-200b, miR-200c and miR-205 have been implicated in controlling metastasis in breast cancer [152]. Different metastamiRs have been shown to both promote and inhibit metastasis and regulate key steps in the metastatic program. Key players of the miRNA biogenesis pathway are also targeted by miRNAs thereby controlling metastasis. For instance, in breast cancer patients, it was found that miR-103/107 family targets *Dicer1* to decrease its expression, and as a consequence, several miRNAs were downregulated [153].

4.2.3.1. MetastamiRs (metastasis-promoting miRNAs)

MiR-21 is a metastamiR targeting several TSGs in breast cancer. MiR-21 downregulates TSGs *PDCD4, TPM1* and *MASPIN* to increase breast cancer invasiveness and metastasis [146, 147, 154]. MiR-10b is an example of another oncomiR, which induces invasion and metastasis in breast cancer xenograft models when overexpressed in nonmetastatic breast tumors [33, 155–157]. MiR-373 and miR-520c are able to initiate breast cancer cell migration and invasion *in vitro* and *in vivo*, which implicates these miRNAs as metastasis-promoting miRNAs [158]. It has been shown that miR-22 targets *TIP60* (HIV-1 Tat interacting protein), a lysine acetyl transferase, in breast cancer and stimulates the expression of EMT genes. Furthermore, analysis of gene expression and survival data from the TCGA dataset and gene expression omnibus (GEO) database revealed that patients with high TIP60 and low miR-22 expression were associated with good survival, whereas patients with low TIP60 and high miR-22 levels showed poorer prognosis for survival. This suggests that TIP60 and miR-22 could act as prognostic marker in breast cancer disease progression and that targeting the TIP60–miR-22 axis could lead to an effective therapeutic strategy for metastatic breast cancer [159].

4.2.3.2. Metastasis-suppressing miRNAs

Tavazoie et al. [160] demonstrated that restoring the expression of those miRNAs whose expression is lost in malignant breast cancer cells suppresses lung and bone metastasis in metastatic breast cancer. Restoration of expression of miR-335 inhibited metastatic cell invasion while miR-126 restoration reduced overall tumor growth and proliferation. MiR-146a and b target *IRAK1* and *TRAF6* to down regulate NF-κB signaling and inhibit invasion and migration of breast cancer cells [161]. MiR-497, whose expression is downregulated in breast cancer samples, has been shown to induce apoptosis of breast cancer stem cells (BCSCs) by targeting Bcl-w. Additionally, its expression has been shown to be negatively correlated with tumor size, metastasis stage and HER2 status in breast cancer [162]. EMT is an important property of malignant cancer cells wherein the epithelial cells lose cell-cell contact allowing them to be motile and thus metastasize to distant organs. The miR-200 family is known to regulate EMT by targeting the EMT markers, *CDH1*or E-Cadherin, a marker for epithelial phenotype, *vimentin, ZEB1,* which regulates EMT as seen in *in vivo* studies by promoting metastasis of tumor cells in mouse model [163, 164] and *ZEB2,* which are expressed in mesenchymal cells and thus mark the mesenchymal phenotype [165]. Furthermore, it has been shown that *ZEB1* regulates EMT in human breast cancer by promoting metastasis of tumor cells in mouse model [163, 164]. The miR-200 family by targeting *ZEB1* and *ZEB2* downregulates their expression, thereby tipping the balance toward the epithelial phenotype [165, 166]. Gregory et al. Demonstrated that the miR-200b family is downregulated in response to the cytokine, transforming growth factor-β (TGF-β), which induces EMT. The authors further demonstrated that ectopic expression of the miR-200 family is able to inhibit EMT, thereby affecting breast cancer progression [167].

4.2.4. Regulation of signaling pathways by miRNAs in breast cancer

4.2.4.1. ER signaling

Among the two classes of estrogen receptors, the estrogen receptor-α (ERα) is overexpressed in approximately 75% of breast cancer cases. Increased signaling through ERα in mammary stem cell induces continuous replication of these cells, thereby increasing the risk of tumorigenesis. Tumor-suppressive miRNAs, such as miR-145 [168], miR-17/20 family, miR-193b, miR-206 and mir-302c, inhibit the ER signaling activated proliferation of mammary epithelia, by targeting either the ER receptor α or its coactivator AIB1 [169, 170]. MiR-206 is upregulated in ER-negative breast cancer but downregulated in ER-positive breast cancer [171]. MiR-17-5p targets AIB1, a coactivator of ERα [172]. The let-7 family of miRNAs is known to regulate the expression of both ERα66 and ERα36 (a novel short form of the ERα protein) in breast cancer. In breast cancer, let-7 is known to be downregulated, resulting in an upregulation of its targets, ERα66 and ERα36. ERα66 is predominantly nuclear in expression, where it regulates the transcription of *c-Myc, CCND1* and *pS2,* while ERα36 activates MAPK/ERK signaling pathway. Overexpression of let-7 miRNAs can negatively regulate these pathways by inhibiting the phosphorylation of ERK and Akt. Further, ERα36 protein levels were found to be upregulated in a tamoxifen-resistant MCF-7 breast cancer cell line, indicating that ERα36 might play a role in mediating resistance to tamoxifen therapy in breast cancer. However, overexpression of the let-7 family members in tamoxifen-resistant MCF-7 cells significantly decreased ERα36 protein level further increasing tamoxifen sensitivity in these cells [173]. These studies demonstrate the regulation of the ER signaling pathway and development of tamoxifen resistance in breast cancer by let-7 miRNAs, hence hinting at the possibility of developing novel therapeutic strategies.

4.2.4.2. HER2 (ERBB) signaling

In breast cancer, ERBB2/HER2 is found to be amplified and/or overexpressed in up to 30% of patients, correlating with poor prognosis. Further, abnormal HER signaling induces cell proliferation [174]. HER2 and HER3 are targeted by miR-125a/b thereby inhibiting breast cancer

http://dx.doi.org/10.5772/66888

growth [175]. HER3 receptor is also targeted by miR-205 inducing cell cycle arrest thereby inhibiting cell proliferation in breast cancer [176].

4.2.5. MiRNAs regulating breast cancer stem cells

Human breast cancer stem cells (BCSCs) were first isolated by Al-Hajj et al. [177] as cells displaying a different set of cell surface markers CD44þ/CD24/low as compared to normal mammary gland stem cells. Comparison of BCSCs with normal mammary stem cells revealed a differential expression of miRNAs. MiR-200c, let-7, miR-30 and miR-34 were observed to be downregulated, whereas miR-181 and miR-495 showed an increased expression in BCSCs. Let-7 inhibits the stem cell self-renewal in both normal and CSCs of breast and the downregulation of let-7 in breast cancer, thereby leading to the formation of BCSCs by unchecked self-renewal and undifferentiated status of mammary gland stem cells [60]. Moreover, let-7 is also known to target many oncogenes such as *HMGA2*, *k-Ras*, *p-RAS* and *ERK*, which are highly expressed in BCSCs [149, 150, 178]. These oncogenes further support the formation and maintenance of BCSCs *via* self-renewal and maintenance of undifferentiated status of BCSCs [178]. In BCSCs, miR-30 is downregulated 30 fold, leading to increased expression of its targets: ubiquitin conjugating enzyme 9 (*Ubc9*) and integrin β 3 (*ITBG3*), and promoting the self-renewal ability of BCSCs. Specific knockdown of miR-30 induced differentiation of BCSCs, suggesting that miR-30 regulates self-renewal and tumorigenicity of breast cancer [179]. Furthermore, three families of miRNAs, namely, miR-200c-141, miR-200b-200a-429, and miR-183-96-182 are known to be downregulated in human BCSCs, normal human and murine mammary stem/progenitor cells, and embryonal carcinoma cells. MiR-200c affects breast cancer proliferation by modulating the expression of *BMI1*, which regulates the self-renewal of stem cells. Furthermore, miR-200c has been shown to inhibit the development of normal mammary stem cells into mammary ducts as well as the ability of human BCSCs to form tumors *in vivo* [180].

4.2.6. MiRNAs resulting in breast cancer therapy resistance

Several miRNAs have been described as controlling genomic stability of breast cancer cells. DNA double-strand breaks are lesions induced by ionizing radiation (IR) and can be efficiently repaired by DNA homologous recombination, a system that requires RAD51 recombinase. Overexpression of miR-155 in human breast cancer cells reduces the level of *RAD51* and affects the cellular response to IR. Consequently, tumors overexpressing miR-155 are sensitive to radiation therapy. Furthermore, high miR-155 levels are associated with lower *RAD51* expression and with better overall survival of patients in a large series of triple-negative breast cancers [181]. Other miRNAs have also been shown to sensitize breast cancer cells to chemo/radio sensitivity. The tumor suppressor p53 whose expression is affected by DNA damage and oncogenic stress, is the direct inducer of miR-34a [182]. It has been observed that elevated expression of miR-34a in a HER-2 positive breast cancer cell line (UACC-812) contributes to increased resistance to ionizing radiation as opposed to MDA-MB-231 expressing low levels of miR-34a. Thus, while the mechanism is unknown, in p53-mutant breast cancers, inhibition of miRNA-34a enhances radio sensitivity [183]. Also, miRNA-182 controls DNA repair of breast cancer cells by targeting *BRCA1*, and inhibition of miRNA-182 leads to resistance to PARP inhibitors (poly ADP ribose polymerase) [184]. Because the BRCA pathway controls mammary stem cell fate, it is possible that overexpression of miR-182 in breast cancer stem cells would sensitize this radio-resistant cell population to radiation therapy. Anti-estrogen therapies are given to the patients with ER-positive breast tumors. Despite initial response, 25% of primary tumors and almost all metastatic tumors will develop resistance. MiRNA-221/222 are key regulators of hormonal resistance of breast cancer stem cells. MiRNA-221/222 act through diverse mechanisms by targeting ERα, by upregulating β-catenin and the TGF-β pathway [185] or by targeting the cell-cycle inhibitor *p27* [186]. Finally, 15–20% of breast tumors display an overexpression of the ERBB2 oncoprotein. ERBB2 overexpression promotes the expansion of the breast cancer stem cells through the activation of a PI3K/AKT/GSK3β/WNT signaling. ERBB2-positive tumors can be treated with several targeted therapeutics. MiRNA-21 plays a role in the resistance displayed by ERBB2-positive tumors to trastuzumab, by targeting the PTEN tumor suppressor. The authors further show that knockdown of miR-21 could restore PTEN levels thus sensitizing the cells to anti-HER-2 therapy [187]. MiRNA-205 regulates the ERBB3 receptor [188]. ERBB3 transactivates ERBB2, and both receptors trigger the PI3K/AKT signaling pathway. ERBB2/ERBB3 interaction could lead to anti-ERBB2 resistance of breast tumors. However, miR-205 is downregulated in breast cancer. Thus, restoration of miRNA-205 in breast tumors could help overcome resistance to anti-ERBB2 therapy.

4.2.7. Potential prognostic value of miRNAs

Several studies have evaluated the role of specific miRNAs in breast cancer spread and survival. A screen identified five upregulated miRNAs (miR-30b, miR-148a, miR-150, miR-450a and miR-155) and six downregulated miRNAs (miR-24, miR-99a, miR-99b, miR-125b, miR-130b and miR-205) in primary breast cancer tumors versus corresponding lymph nodes [189]. Further, miR-373 was identified as being overexpressed in lymph-node metastases as compared to primary tumors [158], indicating the prognostic value of these miRNAs. Other miRNAs such as miR-187 [190], miR-27b and miR-103/107 [191] have also been found to have a prognostic value in breast cancer. Moreover, in ER-positive lymph node-negative (LNN) breast cancer patients, 12 miRNAs have been identified with early relapse versus late relapse (miR-205, miR-22, miR-516-3p, miR-7, miR-34b, miR-151, miR-210, miR-193b, miR-489 miR-449, miR-145 and miR-128a). Indeed, four of these 12 miRNAs (miR-7, miR-128a, miR-210 and miR-516-3p) have been positively linked to breast cancer aggressiveness while miR-210 has also been associated with metastatic ability of TNBC [192].

4.2.8. MiRNAs as breast cancer biomarkers

4.2.8.1. MiRNA expression from tissue biopsies

MiRNAs can serve as biomarkers for breast cancer based on their expression profile from RNA sequencing or tissue microarray assays. This can be achieved by mapping the global mRNA and miRNA expression from tumor tissues using high-throughput platforms, such as microarray chips and deep sequencing. Also, other techniques such as in-situ hybridization

(ISH) can be used to detect mRNAs and miRNAs from fresh frozen or archived paraffin-embedded (FFPE) tumor tissue samples and protein expression can be evaluated using immunohistochemistry (IHC) [193]. The use of miRNA biomarkers has several advantages over protein coding genes: (1) miRNAs are more stable than mRNA and thus enable easier and reliable detection in FFPE samples (2) the presence of mere 1000 miRNAs makes the human miRNome much easier to screen and evaluate with less demanding bioinformatic analysis than the mRNA transcriptome [194]. The expression of a number of miRNAs closely correlates with the ER, PR and HER2 status in breast cancer, highlighting their use as biomarkers of disease progression and treatment response [141, 195]. MiR-210 has been validated as a prognostic biomarker in breast cancer since elevated miR-210 levels have been associated with poor outcome both in ER-positive and ER-negative cases [196]. Moreover, miR-210 has been developed to predict outcome in ER-positive cases that received adjuvant tamoxifen treatment for 5 years [197]. Other miRNA biomarkers include miR-205, which is used as a prognostic marker for the triple negative (TN) subtype since a positive correlation has been observed between miR-205 expression and favorable clinical outcome in TN cases [198].

4.2.8.2. Circulating miRNAs as breast cancer biomarkers

Circulating miRNAs are ideal for clinical use, since they are highly stable and can be detected by a noninvasive manner in a blood sample. Serum or plasma miRNAs have been shown to be resistant to RNases and DNases thus are more stable than their cellular counter parts as well as mRNAs. Serum and plasma miRNAs can be easily isolated and quantified by RT-qPCR analysis. Moreover, specific miRNAs have also been demonstrated as being indicative of the breast cancer stage and/or ER/PR status. Numerous studies have documented the presence and quantified serum miRNAs from breast cancer patient samples. Asaga et al. assayed circulating miR-21 of 102 breast cancer patients and 20 healthy controls and found higher concentrations in these patients, especially in metastatic cases [199]. A study that quantitatively profiled the expression of seven miRNAs by real-time PCR, in tissue and blood samples of patients with breast cancer at different clinical stages and age-matched healthy individuals found that, while the expression of two miRNAs, miR-195 and let-7a was significantly higher in blood samples of breast cancer patients in comparison to control subjects, their circulating levels remarkably decreased after surgical resection in a subset of 29 cases, reaching levels comparable with control subjects [200, 201]. 26 circulating miRNAs with two-fold differential expression have been identified from the plasma of early stage breast cancer patients as compared to healthy controls [202].

This mounting evidence generates the hypothesis for a signature of circulating miRNAs that could be a reliable biomarker for disease progression.

4.2.9. MiRNA therapeutics in breast cancer

4.2.9.1. AntagomiRs and anti-miRNA oligonucleotides targeting oncomiRs and metastamiRs

The most common miRNA therapeutic approach to inhibit the functions of miRNAs involve, targeting by using antisense miRNAs (antagomiRs) capable of knocking down these miRNAs. AntagomiRs are synthetic RNA molecules with favorable stability, resistance to RNase and pharmacologic properties that allow *in vivo* miRNA inhibition [203]. MiRNA knockdown therapy can be used in conjunction with chemotherapy to facilitate knockdown of oncomiRs along with concomitant targeting of the proliferating cells using anticancer drugs. Knockdown of miR-10b using sequence-specific antagomiRs led to an upregulation of its target mRNA *Hoxd10*. However, the use of miR-10b antagomiRs did not reduce primary mammary tumor growth in animal model but was successful in suppressing the formation of lung metastases. Furthermore, miR-10b antagomiR does not induce toxicity in healthy mice and thus can be a safe therapeutic option [204]. Moreover, knockdown of miRNAs by anti-sense approach also sensitizes cancer cells to chemotherapeutic drugs as in the case of miR-21, the knockdown of which sensitized MCF7 cells to the chemotherapeutic agent and topoisomerase inhibitor, topotecan [205].

Another approach of ablating miRNAs function is by using anti-miRNA oligonucleotides (AMOs) with 2-O-methyl groups and AMOs based on locked nucleic acid (LNA). AMOs are stable synthetic antisense oligonucleotides that can rapidly, selectively and irreversibly bind endogenous miRNAs, sequester and make them functionally inactive [206, 207]. Targeting oncomirs *via* either antagomiRs or AMOs has been demonstrated to reduce cancer cell proliferation and metastasis [79], sensitization to chemotherapeutic agents [80], hormone therapy [52] and anti-HER2 therapy [71] in breast cancer cell lines.

In addition to knocking down miRNAs, upregulating the expression and activity of tumor suppressor miRNAs has potential in ameliorating breast cancer. Tumor suppressor miRNAs can be upregulated using miRNA mimics, which are synthetic molecules with short double-stranded synthetic oligonucleotides with sequence similarity to the particular miRNA under consideration. Overexpression of TS miRNAs using miRNA mimics has been shown to decrease cancer cell proliferation as well as induce chemosensitivity in breast cancer cell lines [208, 209].

4.2.9.2. Peptide nucleic acids (PNA)

Peptide nucleic acid (PNA) is an artificially synthesized oligonucleotide similar to DNA and RNA with a backbone consisting of repeats of 2-aminoethylglycine units [210]. The absence of phosphate groups renders a neutral charge to the PNA resulting in stronger and specific bonds between complementary PNA/DNA and PNA/RNA as compared to DNA/DNA or RNA/RNA. Owing to its synthetic nature, PNA is resistant to degradation by DNases and proteases leading to increased intracellular stability. Inactivation of miR-221 with PNA has been successful in aggressive breast cancer cell lines where miR-221 is overexpressed [211]. An anti-miR-221 PNA (R8-PNA-a221) conjugated with polyarginine-peptide (R8) could inactivate miR-221 and upregulate its target mRNA, *p27/Kip1*. R8-PNA-a221 displayed efficient uptake within target cells without using transfection reagents. To assess the potential of PNA-anti-miR-221 on inhibition of breast cancer *in vivo*, MCF-7 cells treated with PNA-anti-221 or control PNAs were injected in nude mice [212]. Tumor formation was observed only in 60% of mice treated with anti-miR-221 therapy as compared to control. These studies highlight the potential of PNAs as anti-tumor therapeutics.

4.3. Long noncoding RNAs in breast cancer

Long noncoding RNAs are endogenous RNA molecules with a mature length of more than 200 bases that do not code for functional proteins [213]. LncRNAs are epigenetic regulators, and they control gene expression at both the transcriptional and posttranscriptional levels. LncRNAs utilize a variety of mechanisms to regulate gene expression. They can recruit chromatin modifiers to impair access to targeted genes, they can act as scaffolds to assemble complexes that do not have interacting domains, they can interact with transcription factors to directly regulate gene expression, and they can serve as 'miRNA sponges' to trap miRNAs and regulate translation. Moreover, lncRNAs can be involved in the regulation of the expression of either their neighboring genes in cis or more distant genes in trans. LncRNAs act as coactivators, binding to transcription factors and enhancing their transcriptional activity [214].

4.3.1. Oncogenic LncRNAs in breast cancer

H19 is among the first discovered lncRNAs and displays elevated expression in breast cancer [215]. This upregulation of expression is on account of increased binding of the transcription factor *E2F1* factor to H19 promoter. H19, in turn, promotes cell proliferation in MDA-MB-231 cells *in vitro* [216] and also accelerates tumor growth *in vivo* in animal model [217], possibly by repressing tumor suppressor genes such as *caveolin-1* [218].

HOTAIR is remarkably overexpressed in metastatic breast cancer. Upregulated HOTAIR in breast cancer cells provides a scaffold for *PRC2* and *LSD1-CoREST* (lysine-specific demethylase-1 with its corepressor protein CoREST (RE1 silencing transcription factor/neural-restrictive silencing factor)). *PRC2* binds to the 5′ region of HOTAIR while *LSD1-CoREST* binds to its 3′ region. This complex regulates the histone modifications H3K27me3 and H3K4me2 at the promoters of metastasis suppressing genes such as *PCDH10, PCDHB5* and *JAM2*. As a result, these metastasis suppressor genes are silenced; thereby contributing to HOTAIR-induced breast cancer metastasis. Indeed, overexpression of HOTAIR in breast cancer cell lines has been observed to increase their invasiveness both *in vitro* and *in vivo*. Furthermore, knockdown of HOTAIR has been shown to attenuate EZH2-induced invasion, in benign immortalized breast cells overexpressing *EZH2* [219]. Upregulated HOTAIR levels in primary breast tumor are an indicator of metastasis thus identifying HOTAIR as an important prognostic factor for breast cancer [220].

Urothelial cancer–associated 1 (UCA1) has been identified as an oncogene in breast cancer. Huang et al. demonstrated the oncogenic role of UCA1 in breast cancer, in part through suppression of *p27*. UCA1 competes with p27 mRNA to form a ribonucleoprotein complex with hnRNP I (heterogeneous nuclear ribonucleoprotein I) thereby increasing UCA1 stability and decreasing p27 protein levels, hence leading to increased proliferation of breast cancer cells [221]. Further, UCA1 has been shown to bind to and sequester miR-143 thus decreasing its expression in invasive breast cancer cell lines. MiR-143 is known to target and regulate the expression of ERBB3. Hence, it is possible that UCA1 increases breast cancer cell proliferation by deregulating miR-143–based ERBB3 repression [222].

MALAT1 (metastasis-associated lung adenocarcinoma transcript 1) or NEAT2 is a conserved nuclear noncoding RNA. The role of MALAT1 in breast cancer was controversial with reports indicating an oncogenic role by promoting cell proliferation, migration and invasion during breast cancer development [223] while a loss of MALAT1 was shown to promote EMT *via* phosphatidylinositide-3 kinase-AKT pathways on MALAT1 [224]. Recently, Arun et al. demonstrated an oncogenic role of MALAT1 in breast cancer where knockdown of MALAT1 using antisense oligonucleotides (ASOs) in a mouse model resulted in slower tumor growth and a reduction in metastasis. Thus, knockdown of MALAT1 using ASOs represents a viable therapeutic option in breast cancer [225].

SRA (steroid receptor RNA activator protein) gene generates both a coding as well as noncoding form of *SRA* RNA [226]. The noncoding (lnc) SRA RNA is significantly upregulated in breast cancer tumors [226], especially in PR-positive tumors [227] and in aggressive and invasive breast cancer cell lines (MDA-MB-231 and MDA-MB-468) [228]. LncSRA acts as a scaffold in assembling coregulator complexes by interacting with and coactivating several nuclear receptors (steroid and nonsteroid) and other transcription factors. This hints to a possibility of lncSRA aiding in the transcription of key oncogenes in breast cancer. Thus, it was no surprise that knockdown of SRA in MDA-MB-231 cells reduced cell invasion along with a downregulation of the genes associated with this phenotype. Moreover, depletion of lncSRA in MCF7 cells exhibited a similar response with a decrease in the genes responsible for invasion and metastasis [229].

Long stress-induced noncoding transcripts (LSINCTs) are a group of lncRNAs upregulated in breast cancer tumor tissues and cell lines. LSINCT5 has been shown to mediate cellular proliferation and is aided by lncNEAT-1 and *PSPC1* (Paraspeckle Component 1) in breast cancer [230, 231].

4.3.2. Tumor suppressor LncRNAs in breast cancer

The lncRNAs that are downregulated in cancer and whose enforced expression is associated with the suppression of cell proliferation or cell death are termed as tumor suppressor lncRNAs.

Maternally expressed gene 3 (MEG3) is a tumor suppressor lncRNA with a decrease in expression in breast cancer, especially in the most aggressive TNBC subtype [232, 233]. MEG3 forms a RNA-DNA triplex structure to regulate the TGF-β pathway genes in breast cancer cells [234]. Since TGF-β is an inducer of EMT and invasiveness in breast cancer, inhibition of this pathway *via* MEG3 could present a therapeutic opportunity to control breast cancer. MEG3 is also known to reduce breast cancer proliferation and invasion by indirectly modulating p53 activity. MEG3 regulates MDM2 (mouse double minute 2 homolog) leading to accumulation of p53 levels in breast cancer cell lines. This p53 could in turn bind to the promoters of its target genes and metastasis suppressors *p21, MASPIN* and *KAI1* inhibiting migration and invasion of MCF-7 breast cancer cells [232].

GAS5 (growth arrest specific 5), in breast cancer, the expression level of GAS5 has been shown to be significantly reduced in tumor samples as compared to surrounding normal breast epithelia [235]. This decrease in GAS5 expression was observed in grade I and II breast cancer patients, indicating that the GAS5 downregulation is an early event in breast cancer progression. Further, this observation also indicates that GAS5 expression may be used as a biomarker to predict cancer stage. GAS5 has additional roles in drug resistance and will be discussed in the next part.

NKILA (NF-κB interacting lncRNA) binds to the NF-κB/IKB complex masking the phosphorylation site on IKB. Thus, IKK is unable to phosphorylate IKB resulting in IKB remaining bound to NF-κB, rendering NF-κB inactive. Expression of NKILA was observed to increase apoptosis and reduce invasion in MDA-MB-231 cells. Moreover, ectopic expression of NKILA decreases invasion and metastasis in breast cancer mouse models. Also, low NKILA expression is associated with poor patient prognosis [236]. Thus, inhibiting NF-κB through NKILA may be a mechanism to suppress breast cancer metastasis.

4.3.3. LncRNAs and breast cancer stem cells

A number of lncRNAs have been implicated in maintaining stemness of breast cancer stem cells, thus promoting the spread of the cancer. The lncRNA HOTAIR has been shown to downregulate miRNA-7 associated with EMT and STAT3 activity [237]. The stemness factor SOX2 is upregulated by lncRNAs such as SOX2OT [238] and linc00617 [239]. Further, the self-renewal hedgehog (HH) pathway is activated by lncRNAs including lncRNA-Hh, which promotes CSCs maintenance through the activation of the HH-GLI1-SOX2 axis [240].

4.3.4. LncRNAs and drug resistance in breast cancer

The lncRNA BCAR4 (breast cancer antiestrogen resistance 4) was identified from a screen designed to find mechanisms of estrogen resistance in breast cancer. Ectopic expression of BCAR4 in tamoxifen-sensitive ZR-75-1 breast cancer cells inhibited the cancer cell death mediated by tamoxifen, thereby making *BCAR4* an important biomarker for tamoxifen resistant breast cancer. Since *BCAR4* expression has only been detected in human placenta apart from breast cancer epithelia, silencing of BCAR4 in breast cancer patients could be a potential anticancer therapy due to the limited number of side effects of diminishing BCAR4 expression in other healthy tissues [241].

Trastuzumab resistance is a major impediment in the clinical management of HER2-positive breast cancer. LncRNA GAS5 is downregulated in trastuzumab-treated breast cancer patient specimens, breast tumors in animal model *in vivo* and trastuzumab resistant breast cancer cell line, SKBR-3/Tr *in vitro*. GAS5 targets miR-21, resulting in a restoration of the levels of the miR-21 target, *PTEN*. Since *PTEN* is a tumor suppressor affecting cell proliferation, reactivation of this gene results in cell cycle arrest in breast cancer cells [242]. This identifies GAS5 as a novel prognostic marker and potential therapeutic target for HER-2 positive breast cancer. Also, GAS5 levels are significantly downregulated in TNBC cell line MDA-MB-231. Restoration of GAS5 levels in MDA-MB-231 sensitizes these cells to UV-C irradiation induced cell death. PI3K and mTOR inhibition could restore GAS5 levels [243]. Thus, reactivation of GAS5 using PI3K/mTOR inhibitors in TNBC may be a therapeutic option to sensitize this aggressive cancer to chemotherapy.

4.3.5. LncRNAs for breast cancer prognosis, diagnosis and therapy

LncRNAs are being evaluated to have potential as breast cancer biomarkers, for breast cancer subtype classification and developing diagnostics and therapies, owing to their cell-type specific expression and correlation with patient response to chemotherapy. In a recent study, more than 1300 lncRNAs and 2800 mRNAs were found to be enriched in HER-2-enriched subtype breast cancer as compared to normal tissue. *AFAP1-AS1* was identified as the most dysregulated lncRNA, whereas lncRNA *LOC100288637* displayed the highest positive correlation with HER-2 expression indicating the potential use of these lncRNAs as breast cancer biomarkers [244]. Furthermore, a transcriptomic analysis of triple negative (TN) breast cancer samples as compared to control identified a unique mRNA-lncRNA signature. The authors demonstrated that HIF1A-AS2 and AK124454 promoted cell proliferation and invasion in TNBC cells and contributed to paclitaxel resistance [245]. Such studies and many more in the future will help identify novel lncRNA biomarkers for breast cancer classification and disease progression.

Similar to miRNAs, circulating lncRNAs have been detected in plasma of cancer patients [246]. Recently, increased expression of lncRNA RP11-445H22.4 was detected in the plasma of breast cancer patients as compared to healthy individuals [247]. Further, HOTAIR DNA has been established as a potential biomarker for breast cancer as these patients displayed an upregulated expression of HOTAIR DNA as compared to healthy individuals. Moreover, the expression level of HOTAIR DNA correlated with the progress of the cancer [248].

In conclusion, noncoding RNAs including miRNAs and lncRNAs represent a significant resource of novel cancer biomarkers including noninvasive circulating noncoding RNAs, prognostic aids and potential therapeutic targets to be used in conjunction with chemotherapy and adjuvant therapy. However, significant research is required, especially in the lncRNA field, to take these RNA molecules from the bench to bedside.

5. Conclusion

In summary, due to the advances in sequencing techniques and novel methods to study chromatin organization, the repertoire of information about the significant role played by the chromatin architecture, and its dysregulation in cancer cells is slowly being uncovered. The knowledge that the epigenetic landscape shapes the underlying genetic information is revolutionizing the field of cancer biology, the organized chaos in the genome of cancer cells now can be attributed at least in part to the aberrant regulation of chromatin modifiers and remodelers. The way in which cell-signaling pathways interact with epigenetic elements in the genome appears to be wide spread and complex. Integrating both networks is important not only for the comprehension of complex processes such as development, cell differentiation, cell regulation and cell plasticity but also toward the study of the relationship between signal transduction pathways and its targeted effect over diverse epigenetic processes. The therapeutic implication of targeting the epigenetic regulators has been discussed in detail and is the focus of many ongoing clinical trials as well as research. An integrative research platform will help in curating the information and translating the current epigenetic discoveries into useful diagnostic and therapeutic tools.

http://dx.doi.org/10.5772/66888

Appendix

Abbreviation used	Full form
5caC	5-carboxylcytosine
5fC	5-formylcytosine
5hmC	5-hydroxymethylcytosine
AE	Antiestrogens
AI	Aromatase inhibitor
AIB1	Amplified in breast cancer 1
AKT1	AKT8 virus oncogene cellular homolog
AMO	Anti-miRNA oligonucleotides
APC	Adenomatous polyposis coli
ARID1A/ARID1B	AT-rich interactive domain-containing protein 1 A/B
ASOs	Antisense oligonucleotides
ATP	Adenosine triphosphate
Aza	5-aza-2′-deoxycytidine
BAF155/SMARCC1	*BRG1*-associated Factor 155/SWI/SNF related, matrix associated, actin dependent regulator of chromatin subfamily C member 1
BCAP31	B-cell receptor-associated protein 31
BCAR4	Breast cancer antiestrogen resistance 4
Bcl-2	B-Cell CLL/Lymphoma 2
BMI1	B lymphoma Mo-MLV insertion region 1 homolog
BRCA1	Breast cancer gene 1
BRG1	Brahma-related gene 1
BRM	Brahma
BRMS1	Breast cancer metastasis suppressor 1
CARM1	Coactivator associated arginine methyltransferase 1
CBP	Cyclic amp response element binding protein
CD44	Cluster of differentiation 44
CDH1	E-cadherin
cDNA	Complimentary deoxyribonucleic acid
CHD	Chromodomain helicase DNA-binding
ChIP	Chromatin Immunoprecipitation
CK5/CK14	Cytokeratin-5/14
CoREST	RE1-silencing transcription factor corepressor complex
CpG	Cytosine preceding Guanine
CSC	Cancer stem cells
CYP19A1	Cytochrome P450 family 19 subfamily A member 1
DNA	Deoxyribonucleic acid
DNMT	DNA methyltransferase

Abbreviation used	Full form
E2F1	Transcription factor activating adenovirus E2 gene
EED	Embryonic ectoderm development
EGFR	Epidermal growth factor receptor
ELF5	E74-like ETS transcription factor 5
EMT	Epithelial mesenchymal transition
ER	Estrogen receptor
ERBB2	Erb-B2 receptor tyrosine kinase 2
ERE	Estrogen-responsive elements
ERK1/2	Extracellular signal-regulated protein kinase 1/2
EZH2	Enhancer of zeste 2
FFPE	Formalin-fixed paraffin-embedded
FOXC1	Forkhead Box C1
GAS5	Growth Arrest Specific 5
GATA	Transcription factors that can bind to the DNA sequence (A/T)GATA(A/G).
GATA3	GATA binding protein 3
GLI1	Glioma-associated oncogene homolog 1 (Zinc Finger Protein)
GSK3B	Glycogen synthase kinase 3 Beta
HAT	Histone acetyltransferases
HDAC	Histone deacetylases
HER2	Human epidermal growth factor receptor 2
HH	Hedgehog
HMGA2	High mobility group AT-hook2
HMT	Histone methyl transferase
hnRNP I	Heterogeneous nuclear ribonucleoprotein I
HOXA	Homeobox A
HP1	Heterochromatin Protein 1
HRE	Hormone-responsive elements
IHC	Immunohistochemistry
IL-6	Interleukin 6
IR	Ionizing radiation
IRAK1	Interleukin 1 receptor-associated kinase 1
ISH	*In situ* hybridization
ITBG3	Integrin β 3
JARID1C	Jumonji, AT Rich Interactive Domain 1C
KDM/HDM	Lysine/histone demethylase
KIT	v-kit Hardy–Zuckerman 4 feline sarcoma viral oncogene homolog
LCOR	Ligand-dependent corepressor
LNA	Locked nucleic acid
lncRNAs	Long noncoding RNAs

http://dx.doi.org/10.5772/66888

Abbreviation used	Full form
LNN	Lymph node-negative
LSINCTs	Long stress-induced noncoding transcripts
LZTS1	Leucine zipper, putative tumor suppressor 1
MAL	MyD88-adapter-like
MALAT1	Metastasis associated lung adenocarcinoma transcript 1
MAPK	Mitogen-activated protein kinases
MaSCs	Mammary stem cells
MBD2/3	Methyl-CpG binding domain protein 2/3
MeCP2	Methyl-CpG binding protein 2
MEG3	Maternally expressed gene 3
miRNA	microRNA
MMP	Matrix metalloprotease
MOF	Male absent on the first
MORF	MOZ-related factor
MOZ	Monocytic leukemic zinc finger
mRNA	Messenger ribonucleic acid
MSK1	Mitogen and stress activated protein kinase 1
MTA	Metastasis-associated proteins
mTOR	Mammalian target of rapamycin
MYST	Moz, Ybf1, Sas2, TIP60
NCOR	Nuclear receptor corepressor
NEAT-1	Nuclear Paraspeckle Assembly Transcript 1
NFκB	Nuclear factor κB
NKILA	NF-κB interacting lncRNA
NOTCH1	Notch Homolog 1, translocation-associated
NSD3L	Nuclear SET domain-containing protein 3 long isoform
NuRD	Nucleosome remodeling and histone deacetylation
OHT	Hydroxytamoxifen
ORM2	Orosomucoid 2
p27	Cyclin-dependent kinase inhibitor 1B (p27, KIP1)
PARP	Poly (ADP-ribose) polymerase
PCAF	p300/CBP-associated factor
PCDH10	Protocadherin 10
PCDHB5	Protocadherin Beta 5
PCR	Polymerase chain reaction
PDCD4	Programmed cell death 4
PDXP	Pyridoxal phosphate phosphatase

Abbreviation used	Full form
PEBP1	Phosphatidylethanolamine binding protein 1
PELP1	Proline, glutamate and leucine-rich protein 1
PI3K	Phosphoinositide 3 kinase
piRNA	piwi-interacting RNA
Piwi	P-element induced WImpy testis in *Drosophila*
PKB	Protein kinase B
PKC	Protein kinase C
PNA	Peptide Nucleic Acids
PP1	Phosphoprotein phosphatase 1
PP2A	Phosphoprotein phosphatase 2A
PR	Progesterone receptor
PRC2	Polycomb repressive complex 2
pS2	Gene which codes for Trefoil factor 1 (TFF1)
PSPC1	Paraspeckle component 1
PTEN	Phosphatase and tensin homolog
RARβ	Retinoic acid receptor beta
RASSF1A	Ras association domain family member 1
RB1	Retinoblastoma 1
REA	Repressor of estrogen receptor activity
RNA	Ribonucleic acid
RUNX3	Runt related transcription factor 3
S6K1	Ribosomal protein S6 kinase beta-1
SAHA	Suberoylanilide hydroxamic acid
SAM	S-adenosyl methionine
SET domain	Suppressor of variegation 3-9 (Su(var)3-9), enhancer of zeste (E(z)), and trithorax (Trx) domain
SFRP1	Secreted frizzled-related protein 1
SHR	Steroid hormone receptors
siRNA	Small interfering RNA
SMARCD1	SWI/SNF related, matrix associated, actin dependent regulator of chromatin, subfamily D, member 1
SMRT	Silencing mediator of retinoid and thyroid hormone receptors
SOX-2	SRY (sex determining region Y)-box 2
SRA	Steroid receptor RNA activator protein
Src	Rous sarcoma oncogene cellular homolog
SRC	Steroid receptor coactivator
Suz12	Suppressor of zeste 12 protein homolog
SWI/SNF	Switch/sucrose nonfermentable
TET	Ten-eleven translocation
TGF-β	Transforming growth factor β

http://dx.doi.org/10.5772/66888

Abbreviation used	Full form
TIMP3	Tissue inhibitor of metalloproteinases 3
TIP60	TAT interactive protein 60 KDa
TNBC	Triple negative breast cancer
TNF-α	Tumor necrosis factor α
TP53	Tumor protein 53
TPM1	Tropomyosin 1
TRAF6	TNF receptor associated factor 6
TSA	Trichostatin A
TSG	Tumor suppressor gene
UBC9	Ubiquitin conjugating enzyme 9
UCA1	Urothelial cancer–associated 1
VA	Valproic acid
VEGFR2	Vascular endothelial growth factor receptor 2
Wnt	Wingless-type MMTV integration site family member
ZEB1/ZEB2	Zinc finger E-box binding homeobox 1/2

Abbreviations used in the text.

Author details

Sudhakar Jha[1, 2]*, Deepa Rajagopalan[1, 2], Shainan Hora[1, 2] and Shweta Pradip Jadhav[1]

*Address all correspondence to: csisjha@nus.edu.sg

1 Cancer Science Institute of Singapore, National University of Singapore, Singapore

2 Department of Biochemistry, Yong Loo Lin School of Medicine, National University of Singapore, Singapore

References

[1] Avgustinova, A. and S.A. Benitah, *The epigenetics of tumour initiation: cancer stem cells and their chromatin.* Curr Opin Genet Dev, 2016. 36: pp. 8–15.

[2] Bhattacharjee, D., S. Shenoy, and K.L. Bairy, *DNA methylation and chromatin remodeling: the blueprint of cancer epigenetics.* Scientifica (Cairo), 2016. 2016: p. 6072357.

[3] Lohrum, M., H.G. Stunnenberg, and C. Logie, *The new frontier in cancer research: deciphering cancer epigenetics.* Int J Biochem Cell Biol, 2007. 39(7–8): pp. 1450–61.

[4] Falkenberg, K.J. and R.W. Johnstone, *Histone deacetylases and their inhibitors in cancer, neurological diseases and immune disorders.* Nat Rev Drug Discov, 2014. 13(9): pp. 673–91.

[5] Locke, W.J., et al., *Coordinated epigenetic remodelling of transcriptional networks occurs during early breast carcinogenesis.* Clin Epigenetics, 2015. 7(1): p. 52.

[6] Schnitt, S.J., *Classification and prognosis of invasive breast cancer: from morphology to molecular taxonomy.* Mod Pathol, 2010. 23(Suppl 2): pp. S60–4.

[7] Malhotra, G.K., et al., *Histological, molecular and functional subtypes of breast cancers.* Cancer Biol Ther, 2010. 10(10): pp. 955–60.

[8] Vuong, D., et al., *Molecular classification of breast cancer.* Virchows Arch, 2014. 465(1): pp. 1–14.

[9] Weigelt, B., et al., *Refinement of breast cancer classification by molecular characterization of histological special types.* J Pathol, 2008. 216(2): pp. 141–50.

[10] Weigelt, B. and J.S. Reis-Filho, *Histological and molecular types of breast cancer: is there a unifying taxonomy?* Nat Rev Clin Oncol, 2009. 6(12): pp. 718–30.

[11] Ross, J.S., *Multigene classifiers, prognostic factors, and predictors of breast cancer clinical outcome.* Adv Anat Pathol, 2009. 16(4): pp. 204–15.

[12] Overdevest, J.B., D. Theodorescu, and J.K. Lee, *Utilizing the molecular gateway: the path to personalized cancer management.* Clin Chem, 2009. 55(4): pp. 684–97.

[13] Arrowsmith, C.H., et al., *Epigenetic protein families: a new frontier for drug discovery.* Nat Rev Drug Discov, 2012. 11(5): pp. 384–400.

[14] Ito, T., *Role of histone modification in chromatin dynamics.* J Biochem, 2007. 141(5): pp. 609–14.

[15] Bartova, E., et al., *Histone modifications and nuclear architecture: a review.* J Histochem Cytochem, 2008. 56(8): pp. 711–21.

[16] Stephens, P.J., et al., *The landscape of cancer genes and mutational processes in breast cancer.* Nature, 2012. 486(7403): pp. 400–4.

[17] Sotiriou, C. and L. Pusztai, *Gene-expression signatures in breast cancer.* N Engl J Med, 2009. 360(8): pp. 790–800.

[18] Elsheikh, S.E., et al., *Global histone modifications in breast cancer correlate with tumor phenotypes, prognostic factors, and patient outcome.* Cancer Res, 2009. 69(9): pp. 3802–9.

[19] Xiao, X.S., et al., *High expression of p300 in human breast cancer correlates with tumor recurrence and predicts adverse prognosis.* Chin J Cancer Res, 2011. 23(3): pp. 201–7.

[20] Gorrini, C., et al., *Tip60 is a haplo-insufficient tumour suppressor required for an oncogene-induced DNA damage response.* Nature, 2007. 448(7157): pp. 1063–7.

[21] Fraga, M.F., et al., *Loss of acetylation at Lys16 and trimethylation at Lys20 of histone H4 is a common hallmark of human cancer.* Nat Genet, 2005. 37(4): pp. 391–400.

http://dx.doi.org/10.5772/66888

[22] Pfister, S., et al., *The histone acetyltransferase hMOF is frequently downregulated in primary breast carcinoma and medulloblastoma and constitutes a biomarker for clinical outcome in medulloblastoma.* Int J Cancer, 2008. 122(6): pp. 1207–13.

[23] Muller, B.M., et al., *Differential expression of histone deacetylases HDAC1, 2 and 3 in human breast cancer--overexpression of HDAC2 and HDAC3 is associated with clinicopathological indicators of disease progression.* BMC Cancer, 2013. 13: pp. 215.

[24] Tryndyak, V.P., O. Kovalchuk, and I.P. Pogribny, *Loss of DNA methylation and histone H4 lysine 20 trimethylation in human breast cancer cells is associated with aberrant expression of DNA methyltransferase 1, Suv4-20h2 histone methyltransferase and methyl-binding proteins.* Cancer Biol Ther, 2006. 5(1): pp. 65–70.

[25] Kovalchuk, O., et al., *Estrogen-induced rat breast carcinogenesis is characterized by alterations in DNA methylation, histone modifications and aberrant microRNA expression.* Cell Cycle, 2007. 6(16): pp. 2010–8.

[26] Zhou, Z., et al., *The NSD3L histone methyltransferase regulates cell cycle and cell invasion in breast cancer cells.* Biochem Biophys Res Commun, 2010. 398(3): pp. 565–70.

[27] Angrand, P.O., et al., *NSD3, a new SET domain-containing gene, maps to 8p12 and is amplified in human breast cancer cell lines.* Genomics, 2001. 74(1): pp. 79–88.

[28] Kleer, C.G., et al., *EZH2 is a marker of aggressive breast cancer and promotes neoplastic transformation of breast epithelial cells.* Proc Natl Acad Sci U S A, 2003. 100(20): pp. 11606–11.

[29] Conway, E., E. Healy, and A.P. Bracken, *PRC2 mediated H3K27 methylations in cellular identity and cancer.* Curr Opin Cell Biol, 2015. 37: pp. 42–8.

[30] Trievel, R.C., et al., *Structure and catalytic mechanism of a SET domain protein methyltransferase.* Cell, 2002. 111(1): pp. 91–103.

[31] Fujii, S., et al., *Enhancer of zeste homologue 2 (EZH2) down-regulates RUNX3 by increasing histone H3 methylation.* J Biol Chem, 2008. 283(25): pp. 17324–32.

[32] Du, J., et al., *FOXC1, a target of polycomb, inhibits metastasis of breast cancer cells.* Breast Cancer Res Treat, 2012. 131(1): pp. 65–73.

[33] Yoo, K.H. and L. Hennighausen, *EZH2 methyltransferase and H3K27 methylation in breast cancer.* Int J Biol Sci, 2012. 8(1): pp. 59–65.

[34] Holm, K., et al., *Global H3K27 trimethylation and EZH2 abundance in breast tumor subtypes.* Mol Oncol, 2012. 6(5): pp. 494–506.

[35] Gonzalez, M.E., et al., *EZH2 expands breast stem cells through activation of NOTCH1 signaling.* Proc Natl Acad Sci U S A, 2014. 111(8): pp. 3098–103.

[36] Wang, Q., et al., *Histone demethylase JARID1C promotes breast cancer metastasis cells via down regulating BRMS1 expression.* Biochem Biophys Res Commun, 2015. 464(2): pp. 659–66.

[37] Berry, W.L. and R. Janknecht, *KDM4/JMJD2 histone demethylases: epigenetic regulators in cancer cells.* Cancer Res, 2013. 73(10): pp. 2936–42.

[38] Wade, M.A., et al., *The histone demethylase enzyme KDM3A is a key estrogen receptor regulator in breast cancer.* Nucleic Acids Res, 2015. 43(1): pp. 196–207.

[39] Cohen, I., et al., *Histone modifiers in cancer: friends or foes?* Genes Cancer, 2011. 2(6): pp. 631–47.

[40] Prenzel, T., et al., *Estrogen-dependent gene transcription in human breast cancer cells relies upon proteasome-dependent monoubiquitination of histone H2B.* Cancer Res, 2011. 71(17): pp. 5739–53.

[41] Clapier, C.R. and B.R. Cairns, *The biology of chromatin remodeling complexes.* Annu Rev Biochem, 2009. 78: pp. 273–304.

[42] Zinzalla, G., *A new way forward in cancer drug discovery: inhibiting the SWI/SNF chromatin remodelling complex.* Chembiochem, 2016. 17(8): pp. 677–82.

[43] Fujita, N., et al., *MTA3, a Mi-2/NuRD complex subunit, regulates an invasive growth pathway in breast cancer.* Cell, 2003. 113(2): pp. 207–19.

[44] Zhang, X., et al., *Frequent low expression of chromatin remodeling gene ARID1A in breast cancer and its clinical significance.* Cancer Epidemiol, 2012. 36(3): pp. 288–93.

[45] Bedford, M.T. and S.G. Clarke, *Protein arginine methylation in mammals: who, what, and why.* Mol Cell, 2009. 33(1): pp. 1–13.

[46] Wang, L., et al., *CARM1 methylates chromatin remodeling factor BAF155 to enhance tumor progression and metastasis.* Cancer Cell, 2014. 25(1): pp. 21–36.

[47] Wu, Q., et al., *The SWI/SNF ATPases are required for triple negative breast cancer cell proliferation.* J Cell Physiol, 2015. 230(11): pp. 2683–94.

[48] Bochar, D.A., et al., *BRCA1 is associated with a human SWI/SNF-related complex: linking chromatin remodeling to breast cancer.* Cell, 2000. 102(2): pp. 257–65.

[49] Pfister, N.T., et al., *Mutant p53 cooperates with the SWI/SNF chromatin remodeling complex to regulate VEGFR2 in breast cancer cells.* Genes Dev, 2015. 29(12): pp. 1298–315.

[50] Mazzio, E.A. and K.F. Soliman, *Basic concepts of epigenetics: impact of environmental signals on gene expression.* Epigenetics, 2012. 7(2): pp. 119–30.

[51] Ellis, L., P.W. Atadja, and R.W. Johnstone, *Epigenetics in cancer: targeting chromatin modifications.* Mol Cancer Ther, 2009. 8(6): pp. 1409–20.

[52] Baylin, S.B., et al., *Aberrant patterns of DNA methylation, chromatin formation and gene expression in cancer.* Hum Mol Genet, 2001. 10(7): pp. 687–92.

[53] Narayan, A., et al., *Hypomethylation of pericentromeric DNA in breast adenocarcinomas.* Int J Cancer, 1998. 77(6): pp. 833–8.

[54] Dumitrescu, R.G., *DNA methylation and histone modifications in breast cancer.* Methods Mol Biol, 2012. 863: pp. 35–45.

[55] Sharma, G., et al., *Prognostic relevance of promoter hypermethylation of multiple genes in breast cancer patients.* Cell Oncol, 2009. 31(6): pp. 487–500.

[56] Wong, E.M., et al., *Constitutional methylation of the BRCA1 promoter is specifically associated with BRCA1 mutation-associated pathology in early-onset breast cancer.* Cancer Prev Res (Phila), 2011. 4(1): pp. 23–33.

[57] Stefansson, O.A., et al., *A DNA methylation-based definition of biologically distinct breast cancer subtypes.* Mol Oncol, 2015. 9(3): pp. 555–68.

[58] Ateeq, B., et al., *Pharmacological inhibition of DNA methylation induces proinvasive and prometastatic genes in vitro and in vivo.* Neoplasia, 2008. 10(3): pp. 266–78.

[59] Chik, F. and M. Szyf, *Effects of specific DNMT gene depletion on cancer cell transformation and breast cancer cell invasion; toward selective DNMT inhibitors.* Carcinogenesis, 2011. 32(2): pp. 224–32.

[60] Pakneshan, P., et al., *Reversal of the hypomethylation status of urokinase (uPA) promoter blocks breast cancer growth and metastasis.* J Biol Chem, 2004. 279(30): pp. 31735–44.

[61] Scourzic, L., E. Mouly, and O.A. Bernard, *TET proteins and the control of cytosine demethylation in cancer.* Genome Med, 2015. 7(1): pp. 9.

[62] Tahiliani, M., et al., *Conversion of 5-methylcytosine to 5-hydroxymethylcytosine in mammalian DNA by MLL partner TET1.* Science, 2009. 324(5929): pp. 930–5.

[63] Ficz, G. and J.G. Gribben, *Loss of 5-hydroxymethylcytosine in cancer: cause or consequence?* Genomics, 2014. 104(5): pp. 352–7.

[64] Langemeijer, S.M., et al., *Acquired mutations in TET2 are common in myelodysplastic syndromes.* Nat Genet, 2009. 41(7): pp. 838–42.

[65] Delhommeau, F., et al., *Mutation in TET2 in myeloid cancers.* N Engl J Med, 2009. 360(22): pp. 2289–301.

[66] Yang, H., et al., *Tumor development is associated with decrease of TET gene expression and 5-methylcytosine hydroxylation.* Oncogene, 2013. 32(5): pp. 663–9.

[67] Kudo, Y., et al., *Loss of 5-hydroxymethylcytosine is accompanied with malignant cellular transformation.* Cancer Sci, 2012. 103(4): pp. 670–6.

[68] Wielscher, M., et al., *Cytosine 5-hydroxymethylation of the LZTS1 gene is reduced in breast cancer.* Transl Oncol, 2013. 6(6): pp. 715–21.

[69] Sun, M., et al., *HMGA2/TET1/HOXA9 signaling pathway regulates breast cancer growth and metastasis.* Proc Natl Acad Sci U S A, 2013. 110(24): pp. 9920–5.

[70] Wu, M.Z., et al., *Hypoxia drives breast tumor malignancy through a TET-TNFalpha-p38-MAPK signaling axis.* Cancer Res, 2015. 75(18): pp. 3912–24.

[71] Paska, A.V. and P. Hudler, *Aberrant methylation patterns in cancer: a clinical view.* Biochem Med (Zagreb), 2015. 25(2): pp. 161–76.

[72] Szyf, M., *DNA methylation signatures for breast cancer classification and prognosis.* Genome Med, 2012. 4(3): pp. 26.

[73] Tinoco, G., et al., *Treating breast cancer in the 21st century: emerging biological therapies.* J Cancer, 2013. 4(2): pp. 117–32.

[74] Connolly, R. and V. Stearns, *Epigenetics as a therapeutic target in breast cancer.* J Mammary Gland Biol Neoplasia, 2012. 17(3–4): pp. 191–204.

[75] Lustberg, M.B. and B. Ramaswamy, *Epigenetic therapy in breast cancer.* Curr Breast Cancer Rep, 2011. 3(1): pp. 34–43.

[76] Hatzimichael, E. and T. Crook, *Cancer epigenetics: new therapies and new challenges.* J Drug Deliv, 2013. 2013: p. 529312.

[77] Bug, G., et al., *Valproic acid stimulates proliferation and self-renewal of hematopoietic stem cells.* Cancer Res, 2005. 65(7): pp. 2537–41.

[78] Arzate-Mejia, R.G., D. Valle-Garcia, and F. Recillas-Targa, *Signaling epigenetics: novel insights on cell signaling and epigenetic regulation.* IUBMB Life, 2011. 63(10): pp. 881–95.

[79] Li, Y., et al., *Comparative epigenetic analyses reveal distinct patterns of oncogenic pathways activation in breast cancer subtypes.* Hum Mol Genet, 2014. 23(20): pp. 5378–93.

[80] Nelson, L.R. and S.E. Bulun, *Estrogen production and action.* J Am Acad Dermatol, 2001. 45(3 Suppl): pp. S116–24.

[81] Hall, J.M. and D.P. McDonnell, *Coregulators in nuclear estrogen receptor action: from concept to therapeutic targeting.* Mol Interv, 2005. 5(6): pp. 343–57.

[82] Kawai, H., et al., *Overexpression of histone deacetylase HDAC1 modulates breast cancer progression by negative regulation of estrogen receptor alpha.* Int J Cancer, 2003. 107(3): pp. 353–8.

[83] Chen, H., et al., *Regulation of hormone-induced histone hyperacetylation and gene activation via acetylation of an acetylase.* Cell, 1999. 98(5): pp. 675–86.

[84] Heldring, N., et al., *Estrogen receptors: how do they signal and what are their targets.* Physiol Rev, 2007. 87(3): pp. 905–31.

[85] Kumar, P., A. Kamat, and C.R. Mendelson, *Estrogen receptor alpha (ERalpha) mediates stimulatory effects of estrogen on aromatase (CYP19) gene expression in human placenta.* Mol Endocrinol, 2009. 23(6): pp. 784–93.

[86] Mazumdar, A., et al., *Transcriptional repression of oestrogen receptor by metastasis-associated protein 1 corepressor.* Nat Cell Biol, 2001. 3(1): pp. 30–7.

[87] Delcuve, G.P., D.H. Khan, and J.R. Davie, *Roles of histone deacetylases in epigenetic regulation: emerging paradigms from studies with inhibitors.* Clin Epigenetics, 2012. 4(1): p. 5.

[88] Jene-Sanz, A., et al., *Expression of polycomb targets predicts breast cancer prognosis.* Mol Cell Biol, 2013. 33(19): pp. 3951–61.

[89] Hwang, C., et al., *EZH2 regulates the transcription of estrogen-responsive genes through association with REA, an estrogen receptor corepressor.* Breast Cancer Res Treat, 2008. 107(2): pp. 235–42.

[90] Kumar, R., et al., *The clinical relevance of steroid hormone receptor corepressors.* Clin Cancer Res, 2005. 11(8): pp. 2822–31.

[91] Palijan, A., et al., *Function of histone deacetylase 6 as a cofactor of nuclear receptor coregulator LCoR.* J Biol Chem, 2009. 284(44): pp. 30264–74.

[92] Yang, X., et al., *Synergistic activation of functional estrogen receptor (ER)-alpha by DNA methyltransferase and histone deacetylase inhibition in human ER-alpha-negative breast cancer cells.* Cancer Res, 2001. 61(19): pp. 7025–9.

[93] Bird, A.P., *CpG-rich islands and the function of DNA methylation.* Nature, 1986. 321(6067): pp. 209–13.

[94] Chow, C.W. and R.J. Davis, *Proteins kinases: chromatin-associated enzymes?* Cell, 2006. 127(5): pp. 887–90.

[95] Vicent, G.P., et al., *Minireview: role of kinases and chromatin remodeling in progesterone signaling to chromatin.* Mol Endocrinol, 2010. 24(11): pp. 2088–98.

[96] Beato, M., P. Herrlich, and G. Schutz, *Steroid hormone receptors: many actors in search of a plot.* Cell, 1995. 83(6): pp. 851–7.

[97] Wang, W., *The SWI/SNF family of ATP-dependent chromatin remodelers: similar mechanisms for diverse functions.* Curr Top Microbiol Immunol, 2003. 274: pp. 143–69.

[98] Zafar, A., et al., *Chromatinized protein kinase C-theta directly regulates inducible genes in epithelial to mesenchymal transition and breast cancer stem cells.* Mol Cell Biol, 2014. 34(16): pp. 2961–80.

[99] Gervasi, M., et al., *JunB contributes to Id2 repression and the epithelial-mesenchymal transition in response to transforming growth factor-beta.* J Cell Biol, 2012. 196(5): pp. 589–603.

[100] Shin, S. and R. Janknecht, *Activation of androgen receptor by histone demethylases JMJD2A and JMJD2D.* Biochem Biophys Res Commun, 2007. 359(3): pp. 742–6.

[101] Berry, W.L., et al., *Oncogenic features of the JMJD2A histone demethylase in breast cancer.* Int J Oncol, 2012. 41(5): pp. 1701–6.

[102] Li, B.X., et al., *Effects of RNA interference-mediated gene silencing of JMJD2A on human breast cancer cell line MDA-MB-231 in vitro.* J Exp Clin Cancer Res, 2011. 30: p. 90.

[103] Li, B.X., et al., *Effects of siRNA-mediated knockdown of jumonji domain containing 2A on proliferation, migration and invasion of the human breast cancer cell line MCF-7.* Exp Ther Med, 2012. 4(4): pp. 755–61.

[104] Fagnocchi, L., S. Mazzoleni, and A. Zippo, *Integration of signaling pathways with the epigenetic machinery in the maintenance of stem cells.* Stem Cells Int, 2016. 2016: p. 8652748.

[105] Losel, R. and M. Wehling, *Nongenomic actions of steroid hormones.* Nat Rev Mol Cell Biol, 2003. 4(1): pp. 46–56.

[106] Madak-Erdogan, Z., et al., *Genomic collaboration of estrogen receptor alpha and extracellular signal-regulated kinase 2 in regulating gene and proliferation programs.* Mol Cell Biol, 2011. 31(1): pp. 226–36.

[107] Li, C., et al., *Essential phosphatases and a phospho-degron are critical for regulation of SRC-3/AIB1 coactivator function and turnover.* Mol Cell, 2008. 31(6): pp. 835–49.

[108] Smith, C.L., *A shifting paradigm: histone deacetylases and transcriptional activation.* Bioessays, 2008. 30(1): pp. 15–24.

[109] Margueron, R., et al., *Histone deacetylase inhibition and estrogen receptor alpha levels modulate the transcriptional activity of partial antiestrogens.* J Mol Endocrinol, 2004. 32(2): pp. 583–94.

[110] Spiegel, S., S. Milstien, and S. Grant, *Endogenous modulators and pharmacological inhibitors of histone deacetylases in cancer therapy.* Oncogene, 2012. 31(5): pp. 537–51.

[111] Sharma, D., et al., *Release of methyl CpG binding proteins and histone deacetylase 1 from the Estrogen receptor alpha (ER) promoter upon reactivation in ER-negative human breast cancer cells.* Mol Endocrinol, 2005. 19(7): pp. 1740–51.

[112] Margueron, R., et al., *Histone deacetylase inhibition and estrogen signalling in human breast cancer cells.* Biochem Pharmacol, 2004. 68(6): pp. 1239–46.

[113] Dillon, R.L., D.E. White, and W.J. Muller, *The phosphatidyl inositol 3-kinase signaling network: implications for human breast cancer.* Oncogene, 2007. 26(9): pp. 1338–45.

[114] Citro, S., et al., *PI3K/mTOR mediate mitogen-dependent HDAC1 phosphorylation in breast cancer: a novel regulation of estrogen receptor expression.* J Mol Cell Biol, 2015. 7(2): pp. 132–42.

[115] Fingar, D.C. and J. Blenis, *Target of rapamycin (TOR): an integrator of nutrient and growth factor signals and coordinator of cell growth and cell cycle progression.* Oncogene, 2004. 23(18): pp. 3151–71.

[116] Creighton, C.J., et al., *Proteomic and transcriptomic profiling reveals a link between the PI3K pathway and lower estrogen-receptor (ER) levels and activity in ER+ breast cancer.* Breast Cancer Res, 2010. 12(3): p. R40.

[117] Yang, X., et al., *Transcriptional activation of estrogen receptor alpha in human breast cancer cells by histone deacetylase inhibition.* Cancer Res, 2000. 60(24): pp. 6890–4.

[118] Demirpence, E., et al., *An estrogen-responsive element-targeted histone deacetylase enzyme has an antiestrogen activity that differs from that of hydroxytamoxifen.* Cancer Res, 2002. 62(22): pp. 6519–28.

http://dx.doi.org/10.5772/66888

[119] Mann, M., V. Cortez, and R.K. Vadlamudi, *Epigenetics of estrogen receptor signaling: role in hormonal cancer progression and therapy.* Cancers (Basel), 2011. 3(3): pp. 1691–707.

[120] Widschwendter, M. and P.A. Jones, *DNA methylation and breast carcinogenesis.* Oncogene, 2002. 21(35): pp. 5462–82.

[121] Klarmann, G.J., A. Decker, and W.L. Farrar, *Epigenetic gene silencing in the Wnt pathway in breast cancer.* Epigenetics, 2008. 3(2): pp. 59–63.

[122] Serman, L., et al., *Epigenetic alterations of the Wnt signaling pathway in cancer: a mini review.* Bosn J Basic Med Sci, 2014. 14(4): pp. 191–4.

[123] Bafico, A., et al., *An autocrine mechanism for constitutive Wnt pathway activation in human cancer cells.* Cancer Cell, 2004. 6(5): pp. 497–506.

[124] Katoh, M., *Expression and regulation of WNT1 in human cancer: up-regulation of WNT1 by beta-estradiol in MCF-7 cells.* Int J Oncol, 2003. 22(1): pp. 209–12.

[125] Ying, J., et al., *WNT5A is epigenetically silenced in hematologic malignancies and inhibits leukemia cell growth as a tumor suppressor.* Blood, 2007. 110(12): pp. 4130–2.

[126] Shu, J., et al., *Silencing of bidirectional promoters by DNA methylation in tumorigenesis.* Cancer Res, 2006. 66(10): pp. 5077–84.

[127] Jaiswal, A.S., R. Balusu, and S. Narayan, *Involvement of adenomatous polyposis coli in colorectal tumorigenesis.* Front Biosci, 2005. 10: pp. 1118–34.

[128] Nair, S.S., et al., *PELP1 is a reader of histone H3 methylation that facilitates oestrogen receptor-alpha target gene activation by regulating lysine demethylase 1 specificity.* EMBO Rep, 2010. 11(6): pp. 438–44.

[129] Ottaviano, Y.L., et al., *Methylation of the estrogen receptor gene CpG island marks loss of estrogen receptor expression in human breast cancer cells.* Cancer Res, 1994. 54(10): pp. 2552–5.

[130] Rountree, M.R., K.E. Bachman, and S.B. Baylin, *DNMT1 binds HDAC2 and a new co-repressor, DMAP1, to form a complex at replication foci.* Nat Genet, 2000. 25(3): pp. 269–77.

[131] Cheang, M.C., et al., *Basal-like breast cancer defined by five biomarkers has superior prognostic value than triple-negative phenotype.* Clin Cancer Res, 2008. 14(5): pp. 1368–76.

[132] Cheang, M.C., et al., *Ki67 index, HER2 status, and prognosis of patients with luminal B breast cancer.* J Natl Cancer Inst, 2009. 101(10): pp. 736–50.

[133] Paik, S., et al., *A multigene assay to predict recurrence of tamoxifen-treated, node-negative breast cancer.* N Engl J Med, 2004. 351(27): pp. 2817–26.

[134] Weigelt, B., et al., *Molecular portraits and 70-gene prognosis signature are preserved throughout the metastatic process of breast cancer.* Cancer Res, 2005. 65(20): pp. 9155–8.

[135] Parker, J.S., et al., *Supervised risk predictor of breast cancer based on intrinsic subtypes.* J Clin Oncol, 2009. 27(8): pp. 1160–7.

[136] Peschansky, V.J. and C. Wahlestedt, *Non-coding RNAs as direct and indirect modulators of epigenetic regulation.* Epigenetics, 2014. 9(1): pp. 3–12.

[137] van Schooneveld, E., et al., *Dysregulation of microRNAs in breast cancer and their potential role as prognostic and predictive biomarkers in patient management.* Breast Cancer Res, 2015. 17: p. 21.

[138] Visvader, J.E., *Cells of origin in cancer.* Nature, 2011. 469(7330): pp. 314–22.

[139] Blanpain, C., *Tracing the cellular origin of cancer.* Nat Cell Biol, 2013. 15(2): pp. 126–34.

[140] Pal, B., et al., *Integration of microRNA signatures of distinct mammary epithelial cell types with their gene expression and epigenetic portraits.* Breast Cancer Res, 2015. 17: p. 85.

[141] Blenkiron, C., et al., *MicroRNA expression profiling of human breast cancer identifies new markers of tumor subtype.* Genome Biol, 2007. 8(10): p. R214.

[142] Dvinge, H., et al., *The shaping and functional consequences of the microRNA landscape in breast cancer.* Nature, 2013. 497(7449): pp. 378–82.

[143] de Rinaldis, E., et al., *Integrated genomic analysis of triple-negative breast cancers reveals novel microRNAs associated with clinical and molecular phenotypes and sheds light on the pathways they control.* BMC Genomics, 2013. 14: pp. 643.

[144] Tang, J., A. Ahmad, and F.H. Sarkar, *The role of microRNAs in breast cancer migration, invasion and metastasis.* Int J Mol Sci, 2012. 13(10): pp. 13414–37.

[145] Calin, G.A., et al., *Human microRNA genes are frequently located at fragile sites and genomic regions involved in cancers.* Proc Natl Acad Sci U S A, 2004. 101(9): pp. 2999–3004.

[146] Qi, L., et al., *Expression of miR-21 and its targets (PTEN, PDCD4, TM1) in flat epithelial atypia of the breast in relation to ductal carcinoma in situ and invasive carcinoma.* BMC Cancer, 2009. 9: p. 163.

[147] Song, B., et al., *MicroRNA-21 regulates breast cancer invasion partly by targeting tissue inhibitor of metalloproteinase 3 expression.* J Exp Clin Cancer Res, 2010. 29: p. 29.

[148] Jiang, S., et al., *MicroRNA-155 functions as an OncomiR in breast cancer by targeting the suppressor of cytokine signaling 1 gene.* Cancer Res, 2010. 70(8): pp. 3119–27.

[149] Johnson, S.M., et al., *RAS is regulated by the let-7 microRNA family.* Cell, 2005. 120(5): pp. 635–47.

[150] Lee, Y.S. and A. Dutta, *The tumor suppressor microRNA let-7 represses the HMGA2 oncogene.* Genes Dev, 2007. 21(9): pp. 1025–30.

[151] Sakurai, M., et al., *LIN28: a regulator of tumor-suppressing activity of let-7 microRNA in human breast cancer.* J Steroid Biochem Mol Biol, 2012. 131(3–5): pp. 101–6.

[152] Hurst, D.R., M.D. Edmonds, and D.R. Welch, *Metastamir: the field of metastasis-regulatory microRNA is spreading.* Cancer Res, 2009. 69(19): pp. 7495–8.

http://dx.doi.org/10.5772/66888

[153] Martello, G., et al., *A MicroRNA targeting dicer for metastasis control.* Cell, 2010. 141(7): pp. 1195–207.

[154] Weinrich, S.L., et al., *Reconstitution of human telomerase with the template RNA component hTR and the catalytic protein subunit hTRT.* Nat Genet, 1997. 17(4): pp. 498–502.

[155] Gee, H.E., et al., *MicroRNA-10b and breast cancer metastasis.* Nature, 2008. 455(7216): pp. E8–9; author reply E9.

[156] Liu, Y., et al., *MicroRNA-10b targets E-cadherin and modulates breast cancer metastasis.* Med Sci Monit, 2012. 18(8): pp. BR299–308.

[157] Ma, L., J. Teruya-Feldstein, and R.A. Weinberg, *Tumour invasion and metastasis initiated by microRNA-10b in breast cancer.* Nature, 2007. 449(7163): pp. 682–8.

[158] Huang, Q., et al., *The microRNAs miR-373 and miR-520c promote tumour invasion and metastasis.* Nat Cell Biol, 2008. 10(2): pp. 202–10.

[159] Pandey, A.K., et al., *TIP60-miR-22 axis as a prognostic marker of breast cancer progression.* Oncotarget, 2015. 6(38): pp. 41290–306.

[160] Tavazoie, S.F., et al., *Endogenous human microRNAs that suppress breast cancer metastasis.* Nature, 2008. 451(7175): pp. 147–52.

[161] Bhaumik, D., et al., *Expression of microRNA-146 suppresses NF-kappaB activity with reduction of metastatic potential in breast cancer cells.* Oncogene, 2008. 27(42): pp. 5643–7.

[162] Shen, L., et al., *miR-497 induces apoptosis of breast cancer cells by targeting Bcl-w.* Exp Ther Med, 2012. 3(3): pp. 475–80.

[163] Tania, M., M.A. Khan, and J. Fu, *Epithelial to mesenchymal transition inducing transcription factors and metastatic cancer.* Tumour Biol, 2014. 35(8): p. 7335–42.

[164] Zhang, P., Y. Sun, and L. Ma, *ZEB1: at the crossroads of epithelial-mesenchymal transition, metastasis and therapy resistance.* Cell Cycle, 2015. 14(4): pp. 481–7.

[165] Paterson, E.L., et al., *The microRNA-200 family regulates epithelial to mesenchymal transition.* Sci World J, 2008. 8: pp. 901–4.

[166] Burk, U., et al., *A reciprocal repression between ZEB1 and members of the miR-200 family promotes EMT and invasion in cancer cells.* EMBO Rep, 2008. 9(6): pp. 582–9.

[167] Gregory, P.A., et al., *The miR-200 family and miR-205 regulate epithelial to mesenchymal transition by targeting ZEB1 and SIP1.* Nat Cell Biol, 2008. 10(5): pp. 593–601.

[168] Spizzo, R., et al., *miR-145 participates with TP53 in a death-promoting regulatory loop and targets estrogen receptor-alpha in human breast cancer cells.* Cell Death Differ, 2010. 17(2): pp. 246–54.

[169] Leivonen, S.K., et al., *Protein lysate microarray analysis to identify microRNAs regulating estrogen receptor signaling in breast cancer cell lines.* Oncogene, 2009. 28(44): pp. 3926–36.

[170] Castellano, L., et al., *The estrogen receptor-alpha-induced microRNA signature regulates itself and its transcriptional response.* Proc Natl Acad Sci U S A, 2009. 106(37): pp. 15732–7.

[171] Adams, B.D., D.M. Cowee, and B.A. White, *The role of miR-206 in the epidermal growth factor (EGF) induced repression of estrogen receptor-alpha (ERalpha) signaling and a luminal phenotype in MCF-7 breast cancer cells.* Mol Endocrinol, 2009. 23(8): pp. 1215–30.

[172] Hossain, A., M.T. Kuo, and G.F. Saunders, *Mir-17–5p regulates breast cancer cell proliferation by inhibiting translation of AIB1 mRNA.* Mol Cell Biol, 2006. 26(21): pp. 8191–201.

[173] Zhao, Y., et al., *let-7 microRNAs induce tamoxifen sensitivity by downregulation of estrogen receptor alpha signaling in breast cancer.* Mol Med, 2011. 17(11–12): pp. 1233–41.

[174] Slamon, D.J., et al., *Studies of the HER-2/neu proto-oncogene in human breast and ovarian cancer.* Science, 1989. 244(4905): pp. 707–12.

[175] Guo, X., Y. Wu, and R.S. Hartley, *MicroRNA-125a represses cell growth by targeting HuR in breast cancer.* RNA Biol, 2009. 6(5): pp. 575–83.

[176] Iorio, M.V., et al., *microRNA-205 regulates HER3 in human breast cancer.* Cancer Res, 2009. 69(6): pp. 2195–200.

[177] Al-Hajj, M., et al., *Prospective identification of tumorigenic breast cancer cells.* Proc Natl Acad Sci U S A, 2003. 100(7): pp. 3983–8.

[178] Shimono, Y., et al., *MicroRNA regulation of human breast cancer stem cells.* J Clin Med, 2015. 5(1).

[179] Yu, F., et al., *Mir-30 reduction maintains self-renewal and inhibits apoptosis in breast tumor-initiating cells.* Oncogene, 2010. 29(29): pp. 4194–204.

[180] Shimono, Y., et al., *Downregulation of miRNA-200c links breast cancer stem cells with normal stem cells.* Cell, 2009. 138(3): pp. 592–603.

[181] Gasparini, P., et al., *Protective role of miR-155 in breast cancer through RAD51 targeting impairs homologous recombination after irradiation.* Proc Natl Acad Sci U S A, 2014. 111(12): pp. 4536–41.

[182] Yamakuchi, M. and C.J. Lowenstein, *MiR-34, SIRT1 and p53: the feedback loop.* Cell Cycle, 2009. 8(5): pp. 712–5.

[183] Kato, M., et al., *The mir-34 microRNA is required for the DNA damage response in vivo in C. elegans and in vitro in human breast cancer cells.* Oncogene, 2009. 28(25): pp. 2419–24.

[184] Moskwa, P., et al., *miR-182-mediated downregulation of BRCA1 impacts DNA repair and sensitivity to PARP inhibitors.* Mol Cell, 2011. 41(2): pp. 210–20.

[185] Rao, X., et al., *MicroRNA-221/222 confers breast cancer fulvestrant resistance by regulating multiple signaling pathways.* Oncogene, 2011. 30(9): pp. 1082–97.

[186] le Sage, C., et al., *Regulation of the p27(Kip1) tumor suppressor by miR-221 and miR-222 promotes cancer cell proliferation.* EMBO J, 2007. 26(15): pp. 3699–708.

http://dx.doi.org/10.5772/66888

[187] Gong, C., et al., *Up-regulation of miR-21 mediates resistance to trastuzumab therapy for breast cancer.* J Biol Chem, 2011. 286(21): pp. 19127–37.

[188] Wu, H., S. Zhu, and Y.Y. Mo, *Suppression of cell growth and invasion by miR-205 in breast cancer.* Cell Res, 2009. 19(4): pp. 439–48.

[189] Baffa, R., et al., *MicroRNA expression profiling of human metastatic cancers identifies cancer gene targets.* J Pathol, 2009. 219(2): pp. 214–21.

[190] Mulrane, L., et al., *miR-187 is an independent prognostic factor in breast cancer and confers increased invasive potential in vitro.* Clin Cancer Res, 2012. 18(24): pp. 6702–13.

[191] Shen, S., et al., *A prognostic model of triple-negative breast cancer based on miR-27b-3p and node status.* PLoS One, 2014. 9(6): p. e100664.

[192] Foekens, J.A., et al., *Four miRNAs associated with aggressiveness of lymph node-negative, estrogen receptor-positive human breast cancer.* Proc Natl Acad Sci U S A, 2008. 105(35): pp. 13021–6.

[193] Matos, L.L., et al., *Immunohistochemistry as an important tool in biomarkers detection and clinical practice.* Biomark Insights, 2010. 5: pp. 9–20.

[194] Lu, J., et al., *MicroRNA expression profiles classify human cancers.* Nature, 2005. 435(7043): pp. 834–8.

[195] van Schooneveld, E., et al., *Expression profiling of cancerous and normal breast tissues identifies microRNAs that are differentially expressed in serum from patients with (metastatic) breast cancer and healthy volunteers.* Breast Cancer Res, 2012. 14(1): p. R34.

[196] Jung, E.J., et al., *Plasma microRNA 210 levels correlate with sensitivity to trastuzumab and tumor presence in breast cancer patients.* Cancer, 2012. 118(10): pp. 2603–14.

[197] Rothe, F., et al., *Global microRNA expression profiling identifies MiR-210 associated with tumor proliferation, invasion and poor clinical outcome in breast cancer.* PLoS One, 2011. 6(6): p. e20980.

[198] Berber, U., et al., *miR-205 and miR-200c: predictive micro RNAs for lymph node metastasis in triple negative breast cancer.* J Breast Cancer, 2014. 17(2): pp. 143–8.

[199] Asaga, S., et al., *Direct serum assay for microRNA-21 concentrations in early and advanced breast cancer.* Clin Chem, 2011. 57(1): pp. 84–91.

[200] Heneghan, H.M., N. Miller, and M.J. Kerin, *Circulating microRNAs: promising breast cancer biomarkers.* Breast Cancer Res, 2011. 13(1): p. 402; author reply 403.

[201] Heneghan, H.M., et al., *Circulating microRNAs as novel minimally invasive biomarkers for breast cancer.* Ann Surg, 2010. 251(3): pp. 499–505.

[202] Zhao, H., et al., *A pilot study of circulating miRNAs as potential biomarkers of early stage breast cancer.* PLoS One, 2010. 5(10): p. e13735.

[203] Krutzfeldt, J., et al., *Silencing of microRNAs in vivo with 'antagomirs'*. Nature, 2005. 438(7068): pp. 685–9.

[204] Ma, L., et al., *Therapeutic silencing of miR-10b inhibits metastasis in a mouse mammary tumor model*. Nat Biotechnol, 2010. 28(4): pp. 341–7.

[205] Si, M.L., et al., *miR-21-mediated tumor growth*. Oncogene, 2007. 26(19): pp. 2799–803.

[206] Meister, G., et al., *Sequence-specific inhibition of microRNA- and siRNA-induced RNA silencing*. RNA, 2004. 10(3): pp. 544–50.

[207] Hutvagner, G., et al., *Sequence-specific inhibition of small RNA function*. PLoS Biol, 2004. 2(4): p. E98.

[208] Gao, S., et al., *miRNA oligonucleotide and sponge for miRNA-21 inhibition mediated by PEI-PLL in breast cancer therapy*. Acta Biomater, 2015. 25: pp. 184–93.

[209] Gong, Y., et al., *The role of miR-100 in regulating apoptosis of breast cancer cells*. Sci Rep, 2015. 5: pp. 11650.

[210] Dean, D.A., *Peptide nucleic acids: versatile tools for gene therapy strategies*. Adv Drug Deliv Rev, 2000. 44(2–3): pp. 81–95.

[211] Brognara, E., et al., *Peptide nucleic acids targeting miR-221 modulate p27Kip1 expression in breast cancer MDA-MB-231 cells*. Int J Oncol, 2012. 41(6): pp. 2119–27.

[212] Yan, L.X., et al., *Knockdown of miR-21 in human breast cancer cell lines inhibits proliferation, in vitro migration and in vivo tumor growth*. Breast Cancer Res, 2011. 13(1): pp. R2.

[213] Ponting, C.P., P.L. Oliver, and W. Reik, *Evolution and functions of long noncoding RNAs*. Cell, 2009. 136(4): pp. 629–41.

[214] Wang, K.C. and H.Y. Chang, *Molecular mechanisms of long noncoding RNAs*. Mol Cell, 2011. 43(6): pp. 904–14.

[215] Adriaenssens, E., et al., *H19 overexpression in breast adenocarcinoma stromal cells is associated with tumor values and steroid receptor status but independent of p53 and Ki-67 expression*. Am J Pathol, 1998. 153(5): pp. 1597–607.

[216] Berteaux, N., et al., *H19 mRNA-like noncoding RNA promotes breast cancer cell proliferation through positive control by E2F1*. J Biol Chem, 2005. 280(33): pp. 29625–36.

[217] Lottin, S., et al., *Overexpression of an ectopic H19 gene enhances the tumorigenic properties of breast cancer cells*. Carcinogenesis, 2002. 23(11): pp. 1885–95.

[218] Matouk, I.J., et al., *The oncofetal H19 RNA connection: hypoxia, p53 and cancer*. Biochim Biophys Acta, 2010. 1803(4): pp. 443–51.

[219] Gupta, R.A., et al., *Long non-coding RNA HOTAIR reprograms chromatin state to promote cancer metastasis*. Nature, 2010. 464(7291): pp. 1071–6.

http://dx.doi.org/10.5772/66888

[220] Lu, L., et al., *Association of large noncoding RNA HOTAIR expression and its downstream intergenic CpG island methylation with survival in breast cancer.* Breast Cancer Res Treat, 2012. 136(3): pp. 875–83.

[221] Huang, J., et al., *Long non-coding RNA UCA1 promotes breast tumor growth by suppression of p27 (Kip1).* Cell Death Dis, 2014. 5: p. e1008.

[222] Tuo, Y.L., X.M. Li, and J. Luo, *Long noncoding RNA UCA1 modulates breast cancer cell growth and apoptosis through decreasing tumor suppressive miR-143.* Eur Rev Med Pharmacol Sci, 2015. 19(18): pp. 3403–11.

[223] Zhao, Z., et al., *17beta-Estradiol treatment inhibits breast cell proliferation, migration and invasion by decreasing MALAT-1 RNA level.* Biochem Biophys Res Commun, 2014. 445(2): pp. 388–93.

[224] Xu, S., et al., *Downregulation of long noncoding RNA MALAT1 induces epithelial-to-mesenchymal transition via the PI3K-AKT pathway in breast cancer.* Int J Clin Exp Pathol, 2015. 8(5): pp. 4881–91.

[225] Arun, G., et al., *Differentiation of mammary tumors and reduction in metastasis upon Malat1 lncRNA loss.* Genes Dev, 2016. 30(1): pp. 34–51.

[226] Leygue, E., et al., *Expression of the steroid receptor RNA activator in human breast tumors.* Cancer Res, 1999. 59(17): pp. 4190–3.

[227] Cooper, C., et al., *Increasing the relative expression of endogenous non-coding Steroid Receptor RNA Activator (SRA) in human breast cancer cells using modified oligonucleotides.* Nucleic Acids Res, 2009. 37(13): pp. 4518–31.

[228] Hube, F., et al., *Alternative splicing of the first intron of the steroid receptor RNA activator (SRA) participates in the generation of coding and noncoding RNA isoforms in breast cancer cell lines.* DNA Cell Biol, 2006. 25(7): pp. 418–28.

[229] Foulds, C.E., et al., *Research resource: expression profiling reveals unexpected targets and functions of the human steroid receptor RNA activator (SRA) gene.* Mol Endocrinol, 2010. 24(5): pp. 1090–105.

[230] Silva, J.M., et al., *LSINCT5 is over expressed in breast and ovarian cancer and affects cellular proliferation.* RNA Biol, 2011. 8(3): pp. 496–505.

[231] Silva, J.M., et al., *Identification of long stress-induced non-coding transcripts that have altered expression in cancer.* Genomics, 2010. 95(6): pp. 355–62.

[232] Sun, L., Y. Li, and B. Yang, *Downregulated long non-coding RNA MEG3 in breast cancer regulates proliferation, migration and invasion by depending on p53's transcriptional activity.* Biochem Biophys Res Commun, 2016. 478(1): pp. 323–9.

[233] Zhou, Y., X. Zhang, and A. Klibanski, *MEG3 noncoding RNA: a tumor suppressor.* J Mol Endocrinol, 2012. 48(3): pp. R45–53.

[234] Mondal, T., et al., *MEG3 long noncoding RNA regulates the TGF-beta pathway genes through formation of RNA-DNA triplex structures.* Nat Commun, 2015. 6: p. 7743.

[235] Mourtada-Maarabouni, M., et al., *GAS5, a non-protein-coding RNA, controls apoptosis and is downregulated in breast cancer.* Oncogene, 2009. 28(2): pp. 195–208.

[236] Liu, B., et al., *A cytoplasmic NF-kappaB interacting long noncoding RNA blocks IkappaB phosphorylation and suppresses breast cancer metastasis.* Cancer Cell, 2015. 27(3): pp. 370–81.

[237] Zhang, H., et al., *MiR-7, inhibited indirectly by lincRNA HOTAIR, directly inhibits SETDB1 and reverses the EMT of breast cancer stem cells by downregulating the STAT3 pathway.* Stem Cells, 2014. 32(11): pp. 2858–68.

[238] Askarian-Amiri, M.E., et al., *Emerging role of long non-coding RNA SOX2OT in SOX2 regulation in breast cancer.* PLoS One, 2014. 9(7): p. e102140.

[239] Li, H., et al., *Long noncoding RNA linc00617 exhibits oncogenic activity in breast cancer.* Mol Carcinog, 2015. 56(1): pp. 3–17.

[240] Zhou, M., et al., *LncRNA-Hh strengthen cancer stem cells generation in twist-positive breast cancer via activation of hedgehog signaling pathway.* Stem Cells, 2016. 34(1): pp. 55–66.

[241] van Agthoven, T., et al., *Breast cancer anti-estrogen resistance 4 (BCAR4) drives proliferation of IPH-926 lobular carcinoma cells.* PLoS One, 2015. 10(8): p. e0136845.

[242] Li, W., et al., *Downregulation of LncRNA GAS5 causes trastuzumab resistance in breast cancer.* Oncotarget, 2016. 7(19): pp. 27778–86.

[243] Pickard, M.R. and G.T. Williams, *Regulation of apoptosis by long non-coding RNA GAS5 in breast cancer cells: implications for chemotherapy.* Breast Cancer Res Treat, 2014. 145(2): pp. 359–70.

[244] Yang, F., et al., *Expression profile analysis of long noncoding RNA in HER-2-enriched subtype breast cancer by next-generation sequencing and bioinformatics.* Onco Targets Ther, 2016. 9: pp. 761–72.

[245] Jiang, Y.Z., et al., *Transcriptome analysis of triple-negative breast cancer reveals an integrated mRNA-lncRNA signature with predictive and prognostic value.* Cancer Res, 2016. 76(8): pp. 2105–14.

[246] Qi, P., X.Y. Zhou, and X. Du, *Circulating long non-coding RNAs in cancer: current status and future perspectives.* Mol Cancer, 2016. 15(1): p. 39.

[247] Xu, N., et al., *Clinical significance of high expression of circulating serum lncRNA RP11–445H22.4 in breast cancer patients: a Chinese population-based study.* Tumour Biol, 2015. 36(10): pp. 7659–65.

[248] Zhang, L., et al., *Circulating DNA of HOTAIR in serum is a novel biomarker for breast cancer.* Breast Cancer Res Treat, 2015. 152(1): pp. 199–208.

Chapter 24

Immune Regulation in Breast Cancer Metastasis and Immunotherapy

Ming-Shen Dai

Additional information is available at the end of the chapter

http://dx.doi.org/10.5772/66991

Abstract

There are significant alterations in the tumor surrounding stromal cells in addition to the cancer cells in tumor microenvironment. Tumor cells can metastasize by acquiring the ability to escape immune control and surveillance. A decline in the ability of the immune cells to recognize and kill the tumor leads to tumor relapse or metastasis after primary treatment. Comprehensive review in this chapter will be conducted to further investigate into the mechanism of immune evasion in metastatic tumor microenvironment. The immune cells, stromal cells, extracellular matrix protein/component, and their interaction will be reviewed and summarized. Breast cancer has not been previously viewed as a particularly immunogenic type of tumor. Nevertheless, immune parameters have been increasingly studied in breast cancer, and accumulating data show that they are relevant for the development and progression of this tumor type. Consequently, immunotherapies of breast cancer are now tested in different clinical trials. The prospect of immunotherapy in metastatic breast cancer will be introduced. The importance of host-targeted modulation/therapy will be increased in addition to cancer-targeted strategies. We have to better define subpopulations of breast cancer patients to optimize the immunological way to overcome the cancer metastasis.

Keywords: oncology, breast cancer, immunotherapy, microenvironment, stroma

1. Introduction

The innate and adaptive immune responses are crucial for combating pathogen infection, repairing damaged tissue, and maintaining immune homeostasis. The immune system is composed mainly of macrophages and lymphocytes, including B-cells, CD4+ T-cells, CD8+ cells, and natural killer (NK) cells [1, 2]. The innate immune response is a nonspecific general response to infection used mainly by macrophages and natural killer cells, while the adaptive immune system is a more developed system in which certain lymphocytes "recall" specific pathogen-antigenic patterns and alert the immune system when activated. The macrophage plays an important role in the innate immune system to help the adaptive immune system. In the lung alveoli, these macrophages phagocytize apoptotic cells and debris and digest them in lysosomes [1]. Binding of antigens presented by major histocompatibility complex (MHC-I/II) to antigen-presenting cells' (APCs') Toll-like receptors can help to avoid an autoimmune response by having a system for recognizing cells that are native to the host body. The APCs then express the MHC/antigen complex and a co-stimulatory molecule to the naïve T-cells to suppress their activation against the normal tissue cells, preventing autoimmune damage [3]. An essential factor in the adaptive immune system is the recognition of antigens. All microbes, cells, cancer cells, and other pathogens possess antigens. As explained earlier, MHC complexes present cell antigens for APCs to copy and express themselves. The APCs then present this MHC/antigen complex with a co-stimulatory molecule to activate or suppress naïve T-cells, depending on the nature of the antigens [3]. Although derived from normal cells, cancer cells have significant mutations to alter their antigenic peptide sequences and become immunogenic [4]. If the antigen can be recognized as pathogenic, the T-cells release cytokines to allow themselves to differentiate into cytotoxic phenotypes and then secrete chemokines to recruit more immune cells from the circulation. B-cells also produce complementary antibodies to help target the pathogen for destruction if its antigens are previously recognized from past infections [5]. Many of the antigen-presenting functions are dysregulated in cancer environment. Tumor cells secrete factors that induce immunological tolerance (e.g., lactic acid, indoleamine 2,3-dioxygenase (IDO), and various cytokines), recruit immunosuppressive immune cells such as M2 macrophages, alter their cell attributes to avoid recognition (e.g., by suppressing antigen presentation or becoming elusive mesenchymal-like cells), and skew immune cell function by triggering immunosuppressive pathways. Additionally, they constitutively proliferate by activating signaling pathways that promote growth (e.g., the estrogen-induced growth pathway in breast cancer). Consequently, there are many interacting factors that have to be considered in breast cancer therapy in order to better improve tumor treatment response and survival.

The tumor microenvironment consists of not only a stroma composed of fibroblasts, adipocytes, endothelial, and resident immune cells but also an insoluble extracellular matrix (ECM). The ECM itself is composed by a complex mixture of components, including proteins, glycoproteins, proteoglycans, and polysaccharides [6, 7]. Breast cancer-associated alterations in the amount and organization of extracellular components have been demonstrated in previous studies. These changes lead to tumor metastasis progression and treatment resistance through dysregulated biochemical and physical properties of tumor-associated ECM and subsequently affecting peri-tumoral stromal cells, including immune, endothelial, and other stromal cells in promoting oncogenesis (e.g., evolution of ductal carcinoma in situ to invasive disease). Although many ECM components have been identified as relevant factors in breast cancer progression, evaluation and targeting of a single molecule appears to have limited usefulness in predicting therapeutic response. This might attribute to the large number of ECM components, which, even if likely redundant, collectively contribute to distinctive physical, biochemical, and biomechanical properties of the tumor microenvironment [8]. In gene expression, profiles of breast cancer-associated fibroblasts identify distinct stromal patterns with prognostic implication, and the expression profiles of some extracellular matrix genes provide prognostic information of patients at risk of clinical progression and/or predictive significance for treatment efficacy. It needs to define function and composition of the distinct stromal components, and integrated by proteomic studies to compose and clarify the complex interactions between tumor cells and their surrounding microenvironment.

2. Tumor-associated immune stroma and immunosuppressive cells in the tumor microenvironment

Immune cells can functionally suppress cancer or become dysregulated with immune suppression in the tumor-associated microenvironment. Dendritic cells, macrophages, natural killer cells, regulatory T cells (Tregs), and myeloid-derived suppressor cells (MDSCs) all have been demonstrated to participate in the tumor-promoting microenvironment because of their functional characteristics within the tumor niche. Especially, M2-polarized macrophage populations in the tumor-associated macrophages (TAMs) promote pro-angiogenesis, immune suppression/evasion, and tumor cell migration and invasion [9]. TAMs-targeted strategy may lead to reduced angiogenesis, tumor cell invasion, and metastasis, as well as enhance the antitumor activity of chemotherapeutics [10]. Upon tumor progression, MDSCs could differentiate into dendritic cells and TAMs and lead to tumor immune suppression/evasion, extracellular matrix remodeling, and epithelial-mesenchymal transition (EMT) [11]. Dysfunctional dendritic cell activity within cancer leads to lower number of mature dendritic cells. Inefficient maturation of dendritic cell may contribute to tolerogenic effect and immunosuppression [12]. Two specific NK subpopulations have been demonstrated in tumor microenvironment: tumor-infiltrating natural killer cells (TINKs) and tumor-associated natural killer cells (TANKs) [13]. These NK subpopulations represent distinct cytokine profiles leading to enhanced angiogenesis and tumor progression [14]. Additionally, Tregs have been shown to play a crucial role in tumor progression via infiltration of tumor tissue and mitigation of the antitumor immune response [15]. Furthermore, it is reported that Tregs may enhance angiogenesis in a mouse model of ovarian cancer [16]. Taken together, this evidence suggests that contextual responses of immune cells within the tumor stroma help to modulate tumor progression. Given the complicated crosstalk between tumor cells, local endogenous stroma, and tumor-associated stroma, personalized multimodal therapeutic strategies should be developed that target not only the tumor bulk but also the tumor-associated immunosuppressive stromal compartment and associated cell-derived factors.

3. Overcoming the immunosuppression

Proper T-cell activation will require two signals regulating T-cell survival, proliferation, and/or responsiveness to antigens. The first signal is initiated by the T-cell receptor (TCR) through antigen recognition, while the second one is mediated by an interaction between receptors and ligands of co-stimulatory and/or co-inhibitory signals, also known as immune checkpoints, in particular the B7 family [17, 18]. Under physiologic conditions, there exists a counterbalance between co-inhibitory and co-stimulatory signals, which is essential for the maintenance of self-tolerance and immune homeostasis, thereby protecting the host from unnecessary damage upon the clearance of the pathogen by the immune system [19]. In tumors following oncogenic transformation, immune inhibitory molecules are overexpressed resulting in the attenuation of adapted immune reactions and immune resistance. T-cells are able to control diverse effector responses by integrating both adaptive and innate immune mechanisms. Therefore, agonists of co-stimulatory receptors or antagonists of inhibitory receptors might enhance antigen-specific T-cell response [20]. The blockade of immune checkpoints monoclonal antibodies has been demonstrated to trigger effective antitumor responses not only in classical "immunogenic" tumor types, such as melanoma and renal cell carcinoma [21, 22], but also in many other solid cancers, such as lung [23], colorectal [24], ovarian [25], gastric [26], esophageal [27], bladder [28], and more recently breast cancer [29]. In addition to anti-CTLA4, mAbs directed against PD1 and PD-L1 are emerging as important therapeutic strategies in the treatment of cancer patients. These drugs are characterized by a better safety profile and more effective antitumor activity. PD1 is an immune inhibitory receptor mainly expressed on activated T-cells, B-cells, and monocytes, but also on Tregs. Following interaction with its ligands (i.e., PD-L1 and/or PD-L2), PD1 induces T-cell anergy, leading to immune escape [30–32]. PD-L1 is the best characterized of the two known PD1 ligands and can be expressed by tumor cells as well as by T- and B-cells, macrophages, and dendritic cells [33, 34]. Food and Drug Administration (FDA) has approved the use of anti-PD1 mAbs nivolumab and pembrolizumab in metastatic melanoma (in 2014) and non-small cell lung cancer (in 2015), while anti-PD-L1 has demonstrated similar antitumor activities and is currently in a glowing stage of development [35, 36].

In breast cancer, PD-L1 transcript expression positively correlates with that of interferon (IFN)-γ and other inflammatory genes [37] and in 12 of 41 triple-negative breast cancer (TNBC) found the same chromosomal amplification, which is associated with higher expression of PD1 ligands compared to estrogen receptor (ER)-positive or human epidermal growth factor receptor 2 (HER2)-positive breast cancer tissues [38]. The largest immunohistochemical evaluation evaluating almost 4000 breast cancer tissues detected PD-L1 expression (cutoff at 1%) in 1.7% of all tumors and in 19% of the 302 TNBC samples [39]. However, among the tumor-infiltrating lymphocytes (TILs), PD-L1 expression was present in 6% overall and in 39% of TNBCs. Luminal A and luminal B subtypes are the major breast cancer tumors. However, PD-L1 expression is rather less common in luminal subtypes given their high prevalence, they still represent a considerable proportion of PD-L1-positive tumors (i.e., 44% of all PD-L1-positive tumors in the study by Ali et al. [39]). This subgroup of luminal PD-L1-expressed patients might benefit from immunotherapy [40]. A transcriptomic meta-analysis of 5454 breast cancer tissues demonstrated a highly variable frequency of PD-L1 mRNA expression [39]. Expression was most prevalent in basal tumors, followed by HER2, and then luminal subtypes. High PD-L1 expression levels were associated with poor clinical prognostic factor such as larger tumor size, higher grade, triple negative, and higher proliferative activity [39]. Recently, PD-L1 expression was detected in circulating tumor cells (CTCs) in the blood

http://dx.doi.org/10.5772/66991

of hormone receptor-positive, HER2-negative breast cancer patients [41]. Thus, PD-L1 expression of circulating tumors cells or soluble form detection can be plausible for stratification and monitoring of tumor patients undergoing immune checkpoint blockade. The influence of confounding variables is less strong in the therapeutic setting where the expression of PD-L1, which is in turn associated with the expression of ICR genes, is correlated with responsiveness to neoadjuvant breast cancer chemotherapy [42, 43]. The predictive role of PD-L1 in the metastatic setting is completely unknown.

4. Immunotherapy in breast cancer

Breast cancer has been considered as non-immunogenic tumor, and therefore immunotherapies play a limited role in breast cancer patients. In the metastatic setting, vaccination therapies have shown some signs of activity [44, 45], but results have been overall disappointing with lower objective response (OR) and clinical benefit. NeuVax, which is composed of the human epidermal growth factor receptor 2 (HER2)-derived peptide E75 (nelipepimut-S) combined with granulocyte-macrophage colony-stimulating factor (GM-CSF) as an immunoadjuvant, appears to have clinical efficacy in early phase I/II trials [46, 47]. It is now the only breast cancer vaccine being evaluated in a phase III trial [48, 49]. Adoptive therapy with TILs is relatively active in melanoma patients [50]. However, this approach has not yet been applied in breast cancer due to the difficulty to generate sufficiently effective TIL cultures against the original tumor [51]. A phase I/IIa study in metastatic breast cancer by Domschke et al. [52] and Stefanovic et al. [53] demonstrated promising results in terms of immunological response, disease control, and survival by using bone marrow-derived tumor-reactive memory T-cells. An intriguing median overall survival (OS) of 34 months was achieved with three (20%) patients alive at last follow-up and more than 7 years after treatment. Interestingly, the survival rate correlates with the immunological response in the peripheral blood. They are now testing this approach in combination with cyclophosphamide to counteract the response to Tregs in a phase II study [54].

The first study employing checkpoint inhibitors tested the anti-CTLA4 mAb tremelimumab in combination with endocrine therapy (examestane) in metastatic ER-positive breast cancer patients. No significant clinical response was observed by treatment although 42% of patients achieved stable disease for more than 3 months [55]. The anti CTLA4 mAb ipilimumab is now being tested in patients with earlier stage or lower tumor burden. Based on the predictive and/or prognostic role of TILs [56, 57] and immune signatures [37] in breast cancers, and in view of the encouraging activity of PD1 blockade among multiple tumors, this strategy is now actively studied in breast cancer.

In general, TNBCs have a higher density of TILs, more active expression of inflammatory-related genes, and considering that the prognostic role of TILs is more prominent in TNBC than in other subtypes, the efficacy of PD1 inhibition has so far been evaluated in this setting [58, 59]. Results from two studies assessing the anti-PD1 mAb pembrolizumab and the anti-PDL1 atezolizumab were recently presented. The pembrolizumab phase Ib KEYNOTE-012 trial recruited 32 metastatic TNBC patients, most of whom had previously received at least three lines of chemotherapy for metastatic disease [60]. Only patients with PD-L1 staining in the stroma or in ≥1% of tumor cells (evaluated by IHC) in archived samples were eligible. Satisfactory response rate of 19% was obtained with one complete and four partial responders. The atezolizumab phase Ia expansion trial enrolled 54 TNBC patients [61]. Even with previous chemotherapy heavily pretreated patients (85% had received four or more lines of chemotherapy), a similar overall response rate of 24% was reported with three partial and two complete responses in the 21 studied patients [62]. The efficacy of single-agent immunotherapy soon led to combination strategies and showed better efficacies with the combination of anti-PD1 mAb nivolumab and ipilimumab in melanoma [63]. Some combinatorial trials have been initiated to evaluate the activity of these and other anti-PD1/PD-L1 mAbs in multiple tumors, including breast cancer. These trials include combinations with co-stimulatory molecules, different checkpoint inhibitors, p53 vaccine, HER2-targeted monoclonal antibodies, histone deacetylase inhibitors, less cytotoxic chemotherapy or tyrosine kinase inhibitor (nab-paclitaxel, eribulin, PLX3397), poly I:C (a Toll-like receptor agonist), bevacizumab (an anti-angiogenic mAb), and radiotherapy [29].

5. Conclusions/perspectives

Over the last 20 years, we have learned more about the correlation of solid tumors and the immune system. By understanding the interactions has come a renaissance in cancer therapy, as immunotherapeutic interventions, which augment tumor-specific responses and inhibit the suppressive pathways maintaining cancer cells' immune privilege, have shown increasing efficacy in the clinical practice. However, despite the advancement we have made in understanding these mechanisms, we have just started to translate this knowledge into therapeutic implications.

Trastuzumab was the first antibody that could induce an antigen-specific antitumor immune response [64]. It remains to be investigated whether the main effect of trastuzumab is related to immunological mechanisms or to synergistic activity with chemotherapy [65]. Meanwhile, many antibodies have been approved for treating solid tumors including breast cancer. However, tumor-targeted antibodies represent only a small part of the immunotherapeutic strategies.

The treatment or prevention of metastatic breast cancer remains challenging. Targeting the immune checkpoint molecules in the tumor microenvironment, to modulate antitumor immune response with manageable toxicity, is an attractive and promising therapeutic strategy for breast cancer. Nevertheless, only the minority of breast cancer patients with metastatic disease has responded to an anti-PD-1 therapy (18% with the antibody pembrolizumab). Future in-depth research is urgently needed to identify the predictive biomarkers in those responders before starting the treatment. These therapies may represent the future standards of care but "one size doesn't fit all" is a dictum reflecting the wide range of immune treatments. We need to define the susceptible subpopulations (with predictive biomarkers) and to apply those treatments as monotherapy, combined with standard therapies, in a more optimized sequence of therapy, or at the optimal timing of therapy (adjuvant vs. metastatic setting).

http://dx.doi.org/10.5772/66991

Understanding the pathological mechanisms of different checkpoint molecules involved in cancer progression, immune-related toxicities, and the mechanisms of immunologic resistance to checkpoint modulation may further enhance the efficacy of cancer immunotherapies with its potential clinical applications.

Conflict of interest

The author declares no financial or commercial conflict of interest.

Author details

Ming-Shen Dai

Address all correspondence to: dms1201@gmail.com

Hematology/Oncology, Tri-Service General Hospital, Department of Medicine, National Defense Medical Center, Taipei, Taiwan

References

[1] Torroella-Kouri M, Rodriguez D, Caso R. Alterations in macrophages and monocytes from tumor-bearing mice: evidence of local and systemic immune impairment. Immunol Res. 2013;57(1–3):86–98.

[2] Ruffell B, DeNardo DG, Affara NI, Coussens LM. Lymphocytes in cancer development: polarization towards pro-tumor immunity. Cytokine Growth Factor Rev. 2010;21(1):3–10.

[3] Medzhitov R, Janeway CA, Jr. Decoding the patterns of self and nonself by the innate immune system. Science. 2002;296(5566):298–300.

[4] Gajewski TF, Schreiber H, Fu YX. Innate and adaptive immune cells in the tumor microenvironment. Nat Immunol. 2013;14(10):1014–22.

[5] Vivier E, Raulet DH, Moretta A, Caligiuri MA, Zitvogel L, Lanier LL, et al. Innate or adaptive immunity? The example of natural killer cells. Science. 2011;331(6013):44–9.

[6] Lu P, Weaver VM, Werb Z. The extracellular matrix: a dynamic niche in cancer progression. J Cell Biol. 2012;196(4):395–406.

[7] Pickup MW, Mouw JK, Weaver VM. The extracellular matrix modulates the hallmarks of cancer. EMBO Rep. 2014;15(12):1243–53.

[8] Giussani M, Merlino G, Cappelletti V, Tagliabue E, Daidone MG. Tumor-extracellular matrix interactions: Identification of tools associated with breast cancer progression. Semin Cancer Biol. 2015;35:3–10.

[9] Medrek C, Ponten F, Jirstrom K, Leandersson K. The presence of tumor associated macrophages in tumor stroma as a prognostic marker for breast cancer patients. BMC Cancer. 2012;12:306.

[10] DeNardo DG, Brennan DJ, Rexhepaj E, Ruffell B, Shiao SL, Madden SF, et al. Leukocyte complexity predicts breast cancer survival and functionally regulates response to chemotherapy. Cancer Discov. 2011;1(1):54–67.

[11] Yu J, Du W, Yan F, Wang Y, Li H, Cao S, et al. Myeloid-derived suppressor cells suppress antitumor immune responses through IDO expression and correlate with lymph node metastasis in patients with breast cancer. J Immunol. 2013;190(7):3783–97.

[12] Steinman RM, Hawiger D, Nussenzweig MC. Tolerogenic dendritic cells. Annu Rev Immunol. 2003;21:685–711.

[13] Bruno A, Ferlazzo G, Albini A, Noonan DM. A think tank of TINK/TANKs: tumor-infiltrating/tumor-associated natural killer cells in tumor progression and angiogenesis. J Natl Cancer Inst. 2014;106(8):dju200.

[14] Bruno A, Focaccetti C, Pagani A, Imperatori AS, Spagnoletti M, Rotolo N, et al. The proangiogenic phenotype of natural killer cells in patients with non-small cell lung cancer. Neoplasia. 2013;15(2):133–42.

[15] Curiel TJ, Coukos G, Zou L, Alvarez X, Cheng P, Mottram P, et al. Specific recruitment of regulatory T cells in ovarian carcinoma fosters immune privilege and predicts reduced survival. Nat Med. 2004;10(9):942–9.

[16] Facciabene A, Peng X, Hagemann IS, Balint K, Barchetti A, Wang LP, et al. Tumour hypoxia promotes tolerance and angiogenesis via CCL28 and T(reg) cells. Nature. 2011;475(7355):226–30.

[17] Ceeraz S, Nowak EC, Noelle RJ. B7 family checkpoint regulators in immune regulation and disease. Trends Immunol. 2013;34(11):556–63.

[18] Chen L, Flies DB. Molecular mechanisms of T cell co-stimulation and co-inhibition. Nat Rev Immunol. 2013;13(4):227–42.

[19] Jung K, Choi I. Emerging co-signaling networks in T cell immune regulation. Immune Netw. 2013;13(5):184–93.

[20] Sanmamed MF, Pastor F, Rodriguez A, Perez-Gracia JL, Rodriguez-Ruiz ME, Jure-Kunkel M, et al. Agonists of co-stimulation in cancer immunotherapy directed against CD137, OX40, GITR, CD27, CD28, and ICOS. Semin Oncol. 2015;42(4):640–55.

[21] Robert C, Long GV, Brady B, Dutriaux C, Maio M, Mortier L, et al. Nivolumab in previously untreated melanoma without BRAF mutation. N Engl J Med. 2015;372(4):320–30.

[22] Hodi FS, O'Day SJ, McDermott DF, Weber RW, Sosman JA, Haanen JB, et al. Improved survival with ipilimumab in patients with metastatic melanoma. N Engl J Med. 2010;363(8):711–23.

[23] Rizvi NA, Hellmann MD, Snyder A, Kvistborg P, Makarov V, Havel JJ, et al. Cancer immunology. Mutational landscape determines sensitivity to PD-1 blockade in non-small cell lung cancer. Science. 2015;348(6230):124–8.

[24] Le DT, Uram JN, Wang H, Bartlett BR, Kemberling H, Eyring AD, et al. PD-1 Blockade in Tumors with Mismatch-Repair Deficiency. N Engl J Med. 2015;372(26):2509–20.

[25] Ojalvo LS, Nichols PE, Jelovac D, Emens LA. Emerging immunotherapies in ovarian cancer. Discov Med. 2015;20(109):97–109.

[26] Muro K, Chung HC, Shankaran V, Geva R, Catenacci D, Gupta S, et al. Pembrolizumab for patients with PD-L1-positive advanced gastric cancer (KEYNOTE-012): a multicentre, open-label, phase 1b trial. Lancet Oncol. 2016;17(6):717–26.

[27] Shah MA. Update on metastatic gastric and esophageal cancers. J Clin Oncol. 2015;33(16):1760–9.

[28] Bracarda S, Altavilla A, Hamzaj A, Sisani M, Marrocolo F, Del Buono S, et al. Immunologic checkpoints blockade in renal cell, prostate, and urothelial malignancies. Semin Oncol. 2015;42(3):495–505.

[29] Bedognetti D, Maccalli C, Bader SB, Marincola FM, Seliger B. Checkpoint inhibitors and their application in breast cancer. Breast Care (Basel). 2016;11(2):108–15.

[30] Fife BT, Pauken KE, Eagar TN, Obu T, Wu J, Tang Q, et al. Interactions between PD-1 and PD-L1 promote tolerance by blocking the TCR-induced stop signal. Nat Immunol. 2009;10(11):1185–92.

[31] Francisco LM, Salinas VH, Brown KE, Vanguri VK, Freeman GJ, Kuchroo VK, et al. PD-L1 regulates the development, maintenance, and function of induced regulatory T cells. J Exp Med. 2009;206(13):3015–29.

[32] Latchman Y, Wood CR, Chernova T, Chaudhary D, Borde M, Chernova I, et al. PD-L2 is a second ligand for PD-1 and inhibits T cell activation. Nat Immunol. 2001;2(3):261–8.

[33] Pardoll DM. The blockade of immune checkpoints in cancer immunotherapy. Nat Rev Cancer. 2012;12(4):252–64.

[34] Sponaas AM, Moharrami NN, Feyzi E, Standal T, Holth Rustad E, Waage A, et al. PDL1 Expression on plasma and dendritic cells in myeloma bone marrow suggests benefit of targeted anti PD1-PDL1 Therapy. PLoS One. 2015;10(10):e0139867.

[35] Adachi K, Tamada K. Immune checkpoint blockade opens an avenue of cancer immunotherapy with a potent clinical efficacy. Cancer Sci. 2015;106(8):945–50.

[36] Anagnostou VK, Brahmer JR. Cancer immunotherapy: a future paradigm shift in the treatment of non-small cell lung cancer. Clin Cancer Res. 2015;21(5):976–84.

[37] Bedognetti D, Hendrickx W, Marincola FM, Miller LD. Prognostic and predictive immune gene signatures in breast cancer. Curr Opin Oncol. 2015;27(6):433–44.

[38] Barrett MT, Anderson KS, Lenkiewicz E, Andreozzi M, Cunliffe HE, Klassen CL, et al. Genomic amplification of 9p24.1 targeting JAK2, PD-L1, and PD-L2 is enriched in high-risk triple negative breast cancer. Oncotarget. 2015;6(28):26483–93.

[39] Ali HR, Glont SE, Blows FM, Provenzano E, Dawson SJ, Liu B, et al. PD-L1 protein expression in breast cancer is rare, enriched in basal-like tumours and associated with infiltrating lymphocytes. Ann Oncol. 2015;26(7):1488–93.

[40] Shiao SL, Ganesan AP, Rugo HS, Coussens LM. Immune microenvironments in solid tumors: new targets for therapy. Genes Dev. 2011;25(24):2559–72.

[41] Mazel M, Jacot W, Pantel K, Bartkowiak K, Topart D, Cayrefourcq L, et al. Frequent expression of PD-L1 on circulating breast cancer cells. Mol Oncol. 2015;9(9):1773–82.

[42] Bertucci F, Finetti P, Colpaert C, Mamessier E, Parizel M, Dirix L, et al. PDL1 expression in inflammatory breast cancer is frequent and predicts for the pathological response to chemotherapy. Oncotarget. 2015;6(15):13506-–19.

[43] Denkert C, von Minckwitz G, Brase JC, Sinn BV, Gade S, Kronenwett R, et al. Tumor-infiltrating lymphocytes and response to neoadjuvant chemotherapy with or without carboplatin in human epidermal growth factor receptor 2-positive and triple-negative primary breast cancers. J Clin Oncol. 2015;33(9):983–91.

[44] Emens LA, Tuohy VK, Stanton SE, Clarke E. Immunotherapy for breast cancer: is it feasible? Immunotherapy. 2015;7(11):1135–43.

[45] Emens LA. Breast cancer immunobiology driving immunotherapy: vaccines and immune checkpoint blockade. Expert Rev Anticancer Ther. 2012;12(12):1597–611.

[46] Murray JL, Gillogly ME, Przepiorka D, Brewer H, Ibrahim NK, Booser DJ, et al. Toxicity, immunogenicity, and induction of E75-specific tumor-lytic CTLs by HER-2 peptide E75 (369-377) combined with granulocyte macrophage colony-stimulating factor in HLA-A2+ patients with metastatic breast and ovarian cancer. Clin Cancer Res. 2002;8(11):3407–18.

[47] Mittendorf EA, Clifton GT, Holmes JP, Schneble E, van Echo D, Ponniah S, et al. Final report of the phase I/II clinical trial of the E75 (nelipepimut-S) vaccine with booster inoculations to prevent disease recurrence in high-risk breast cancer patients. Ann Oncol. 2014;25(9):1735–42.

[48] Peoples GE, Gurney JM, Hueman MT, Woll MM, Ryan GB, Storrer CE, et al. Clinical trial results of a HER2/neu (E75) vaccine to prevent recurrence in high-risk breast cancer patients. J Clin Oncol. 2005;23(30):7536–45.

[49] Peoples GE, Holmes JP, Hueman MT, Mittendorf EA, Amin A, Khoo S, et al. Combined clinical trial results of a HER2/neu (E75) vaccine for the prevention of recurrence in high-risk breast cancer patients: U.S. Military Cancer Institute Clinical Trials Group Study I-01 and I-02. Clin Cancer Res. 2008;14(3):797–803.

[50] Rosenberg SA, Yang JC, Sherry RM, Kammula US, Hughes MS, Phan GQ, et al. Durable complete responses in heavily pretreated patients with metastatic melanoma using T-cell transfer immunotherapy. Clin Cancer Res. 2011;17(13):4550–7.

http://dx.doi.org/10.5772/66991

[51] Hinrichs CS, Rosenberg SA. Exploiting the curative potential of adoptive T-cell therapy for cancer. Immunol Rev. 2014;257(1):56–71.

[52] Domschke C, Ge Y, Bernhardt I, Schott S, Keim S, Juenger S, et al. Long-term survival after adoptive bone marrow T cell therapy of advanced metastasized breast cancer: follow-up analysis of a clinical pilot trial. Cancer Immunol Immunother. 2013;62(6):1053–60.

[53] Stefanovic S, Schuetz F, Sohn C, Beckhove P, Domschke C. Adoptive immunotherapy of metastatic breast cancer: present and future. Cancer Metastasis Rev. 2014;33(1):309–20.

[54] Domschke C, Schneeweiss A, Stefanovic S, Wallwiener M, Heil J, Rom J, et al. Cellular immune responses and immune escape mechanisms in breast cancer: determinants of immunotherapy. Breast Care (Basel). 2016;11(2):102–7.

[55] Vonderheide RH, LoRusso PM, Khalil M, Gartner EM, Khaira D, Soulieres D, et al. Tremelimumab in combination with exemestane in patients with advanced breast cancer and treatment-associated modulation of inducible costimulator expression on patient T cells. Clin Cancer Res. 2010;16(13):3485–94.

[56] Savas P, Salgado R, Denkert C, Sotiriou C, Darcy PK, Smyth MJ, et al. Clinical relevance of host immunity in breast cancer: from TILs to the clinic. Nat Rev Clin Oncol. 2016;13(4):228–41.

[57] Salgado R, Denkert C, Demaria S, Sirtaine N, Klauschen F, Pruneri G, et al. The evaluation of tumor-infiltrating lymphocytes (TILs) in breast cancer: recommendations by an International TILs Working Group 2014. Ann Oncol. 2015;26(2):259–71.

[58] Mittendorf EA, Philips AV, Meric-Bernstam F, Qiao N, Wu Y, Harrington S, et al. PD-L1 expression in triple-negative breast cancer. Cancer Immunol Res. 2014;2(4):361–70.

[59] Anders CK, Abramson V, Tan T, Dent R. The evolution of triple-negative breast cancer: from biology to novel therapeutics. Am Soc Clin Oncol Educ Book. 2016;35:34–42.

[60] Nanda R, Chow LQ, Dees EC, Berger R, Gupta S, Geva R, et al. Pembrolizumab in patients with advanced triple-negative breast cancer: phase Ib KEYNOTE-012 Study. J Clin Oncol. 2016;34(21):2460–7.

[61] Cha E, Wallin J, Kowanetz M. PD L1 inhibition with MPDL3280A for solid tumors. Semin Oncol. 2015;42(3):484–7.

[62] Markham A. Atezolizumab: first global approval. Drugs. 2016;76(12):1227–32.

[63] Larkin J, Chiarion-Sileni V, Gonzalez R, Grob JJ, Cowey CL, Lao CD, et al. Combined nivolumab and ipilimumab or monotherapy in untreated melanoma. N Engl J Med. 2015;373(1):23–34.

[64] Slamon DJ, Leyland-Jones B, Shak S, Fuchs H, Paton V, Bajamonde A, et al. Use of chemotherapy plus a monoclonal antibody against HER2 for metastatic breast cancer that overexpresses HER2. N Engl J Med. 2001;344(11):783–92.

[65] Moasser MM. Two dimensions in targeting HER2. J Clin Oncol. 2014;32(19):2074–7.

Chapter 25

Felt Needs for Rehabilitation After Breast Cancer Treatment in Mexico

Viveka Hammelin, Luz María Tejada-Tayabas,
Dulce María Galarza-Tejada and
Joel Monárrez-Espino

Additional information is available at the end of the chapter

http://dx.doi.org/10.5772/66436

Abstract

Breast cancer (BC) is the most frequent type of malignancy among women worldwide and the most common cause of mortality, particularly in low and middle-income countries. As detection and treatment have improved, a larger number of surviving women need adequate rehabilitation after treatment. However, awareness among affected patients remains low. Thus, the aim of this study was to explore the needs and expectations concerning rehabilitation among Mexican women after breast surgery. An ethnographic approach was used. Eight focus groups were conducted in the north-central state of San Luis Potosí, Mexico, in 2014, in which women under treatment and survivors participated. Results showed that women had insufficient and misleading information concerning the need for rehabilitation from health care authorities. Women seemed to focus more on survival than on quality of life after treatment even though impairments limiting their daily life activities caused frustration and feelings of uselessness. In conclusion, many women perceived the need for rehabilitation, but information was largely lacking. Public health services fail to provide rehabilitation services, which are now partially covered by private organizations. Treatment for breast cancer should be accompanied by rehabilitation. Awareness, availability and access to physiotherapy services need to be put in place.

Keywords: breast cancer, physiotherapy, Mexico, postsurgery care, rehabilitation

1. Introduction

Breast cancer (BC) is one of the most common malignancies in the world [1]. In Mexico, it is the most frequent cancer among women, with incidence and mortality rates of 25 and 14 cases per 100,000 person-years, respectively [2]. Between 2007 and 2014, the incidence of BC has been increasing steadily reaching 29 cases per 100,000 women [3] with a large proportion being diagnosed in stages III and IV, which are associated with a more complex treatment and a lower survival probability [4].

The central-northern state of San Luis Potosí (SLP), where this study was carried out, is one of the most affected areas by this tumor [5]. During 2013, BC was the main cause of hospital discharge among women aged 20 years or more and it accounted for 24.6% of all reported malignancies, becoming the first cause of hospital morbidity with 55% of all registered cases of women aged 40–59 years old [5].

Timely diagnosis remains a major concern, especially in poor and marginalized women, due to the limited availability and access to preventive health services [6, 7]. Therefore, when women are detected with BC, it is often at an advanced stage when surgery is the primary treatment modality [8].

Mastectomy [9], but also chemo and radiotherapy [10, 11], often results in decreased motion of the affected extremity and along with pain and edema impairs the mobility and reduces the strength of the upper limb [10] affecting the women's quality of life (QoL) [10, 12]. The occurrence of these conditions can vary depending on who is assessing them (e.g., physiotherapist or self-reported), the treatment modality (e.g., surgery with or without chemo/radiotherapy) and the time elapsed since the surgery [11, 13].

Some relatively common consequences derived from the operation are difficult to deal with, especially if physiotherapy is lacking. For instance, lymphedema arising from the resection of lymph nodes can develop in 15–25% of the women after 1–5 years of surgery [13]. In such cases, physiotherapy can decrease edema by using manual lymph drainage or by compressing garments. Pain, another complaint affecting up to 50% of women surviving cancer [14], can also be relieved through physical means. Thus, postsurgical care should involve physical rehabilitation to help women recover the motion of her upper limbs and to reduce the edema and pain associated [15].

However, many women from low- and middle-income countries, who undergo a mastectomy, do not receive physiotherapy [16, 17]. This could be due to various reasons, including the fact that women are not aware of the existence and relevance of physical therapy after surgery [17], or because availability and access to rehabilitation services is constrained [18, 19].

In Mexico, health care services offered for BC patients include those provided by social security institutions, those covered by the people's health insurance (PHI) run by the Ministry of Health and the costly private medical care [20]. One of the free public programs prioritized by the national health system is the "specific action program for BC," which covers both diagnosis and treatment, but pays little attention to rehabilitation care [21].

As detection and treatment have improved during the last decades, a larger number of women now survive who need adequate physiotherapy after treatment [22, 23]. However, awareness among affected patients still remains low, especially among poor women [13, 24].

So far, there is limited knowledge and understanding of the importance and use of physiotherapy after BC treatment in Mexican women [25]. Thus, this study aims at filling this gap by exploring the needs and expectations concerning rehabilitation after surgery. This information could be of value to better design and implement rehabilitation programs that can translate into a better QoL.

2. Methodology

The study presented here was part of a larger evaluation of the BC program in SLP, Mexico [26]. An ethnographic approach was used [27] with a purposive sample [28] of women diagnosed with BC who were either receiving or had received treatment at a public facility, though few family members were also included. Participants were contacted through the group RETO (i.e., total recovery in Spanish, but also means "challenge"), a nongovernmental organization (NGO) that provides social assistance to women with BC at SLP public Central Hospital. Eight focus groups (FGs) [29] comprising four to twelve participants were conducted (**Table 1**). FGs took place at the Faculty of Nursing and Nutrition of SLP Autonomous University between February and March 2014 by one of the coauthors trained and skilled in FG interviews (LMTT) until saturation was reached [30, 31]. Sessions lasted between 29 and 110 min and followed an interview guide that covered various themes dealing with experiences, limitations, strategies, needs and expectations concerning rehabilitation. FGs were audio-taped with the consent of participants. In some cases, family members also participated (this was differentiated in the transcriptions).

ID	Participants (relative)[1]	Duration in min	Age mean (min-max)
FG1	11 (2F)	82	51 (33–69)
FG2	4 (1F)	57	58 (49–76)
FG3	7	110	48 (27–74)
FG4	4 (2F)	51	57 (48–62)
FG5	4 (2M)	46	51 (45–57)
FG6	5 (1F)	36	53 (29–75)
FG7	12	29	44 (34–60)
FG8	5 (1F)	47	41 (36–50)

[1]Number and sex of family member(s) who participated in the group.

Table 1. Description of the focus groups.

Prior to the FGs, women filled in a questionnaire to obtain socio-demographic data. The disability of arm shoulder hand (DASH) questionnaire, a self-reported function validated and reliable instrument was used to determine the women's upper limb motion after surgery [32]. Thereafter, a clinical examination was carried out by one of the authors (VH), a professional physiotherapist, to examine the functional status of the shoulder and arm to identify the presence of limitations that hamper mobility among these women.

Women were examined in a sitting position where the active range of motion (ROM) of the shoulder was measured using a goniometer [33]. The arm volume was determined using the circumference of the arm to compute the volume of a cone [34]. Impaired ROM was defined as an inter-limb difference of more than 10° [35]. Observations made during the clinical examinations were recorded as field notes [36] and used in order to understand the context during the data analysis.

FG data was examined using content analysis, interpreting both manifest and latent content in order to understand both the context and subjectivity in the material [37]. Systematic codification and categorization were made using an inductive approach.

The full process included the following steps: (1) verbatim transcriptions of the FGs, (2) translation from Spanish into English, (3) systematic codification, (4) grouping into categories, (5) second codification of the segments to identify narrative consistency and variability and (6) final discussion among authors to reach consensus about the findings. The software ATLAS.ti 5.2 was used for the analytical process.

Ethical principles were followed concerning self-determination, anonymity and confidentiality. All participants signed an informed consent form using standard practices.

3. Findings

Women included in the study were between the ages of 26 and 76 years with a mean age of 50. Their overall socioeconomic status was low. Most were married, were housewives and had one or more children. About half of them went to secondary school and one in four completed college. Most women were affiliated to the PHI (the free public medical service for the lower-income segment of the population), but still reported having made personal payments for the health care received. The average time elapsed from the surgery to the survey date was nearly 3 years, ranging from 1 month to 23 years.

More than half of the women had impaired flexion and abduction and almost one-third of women had impaired lateral rotation of the shoulder. One in four had lymphedema and nearly all reported difficulties in performing tasks in daily life to a more or less severe extent.

The following sections present the findings using five relevant categories that arose from the data analyses: (1) functional limitations in daily life, (2) reasons for limitations and discomfort, (3) strategies to deal with impairments, (4) felt needs for information and (5) expectations of rehabilitation from the health care services.

3.1. Functional limitations in daily life

The limitations the women referred to after treatment included problems moving their arm and the lack of strength on the affected side, which hindered them from lifting and carrying heavy objects. This problem occurred in various degrees depending on the time elapsed since the breast surgery, being more severe the shorter the time elapsed. For instance, from 3 to 4 weeks after surgery, the limitation was complete resulting in difficulties even to perform basic personal hygiene actions, which made them rely on others. Yet, many household chores, such as doing the laundry or squeezing the mop, which are commonly performed by hand by these relatively poor women, were still constrained even after 6 months of treatment.

> *"For me it was very difficult. At first I couldn't do anything, like for half a year, I couldn't for example squeeze the mop [by hand]. I couldn't, it hurt in this hand and it hurt in the whole arm. It took me half a year until I had the strength to squeeze it, to be able to really squeeze it." (Woman FG 1)*

The impact of the limitation depended upon the specific context of every woman; while some received support from family members, others felt obliged to fulfill their household duties on their own in whatever way possible. For instance, a mother with young children was forced to move her arm to be able to care for her family.

> *"For me personally, I have my little girls, I need to move on, to continue doing things, that's why you do it, for the girls really, for the girls and the husband, you have to move on." (Woman FG 6)*

3.2. Reasons for limitations and discomfort

The women ascribed their limitations to both direct and indirect causes, which can be grouped into medical, emotional and idiosyncratic. While some described the limitations in medical terms, others referred them more simply as pain or weakness. Emotional reasons included the fear of moving the arm or unawareness of impairment. The role of culture and the perception of impairment in the Mexican context were also referred to by some women.

Sometimes the limitations were explained as a result of the extraction of lymph nodes and/or muscles and nerves being cut off. The bottom line was that these provided a logical explanation for the experienced sensations and difficulties. Women seemed to have obtained this information from their doctors, from members of the RETO group, or by reading educational materials.

> *"…because they take out the lymph nodes the circulation is insufficient, unlike it was before; they take out muscles, arteries and veins. For me it was a radical mastectomy, they took all the breast out, so it makes sense what I feel because some muscles and nerves die…" (Woman FG 4)*

The main discomforts mentioned by the women included pain, numbness, weakness, swelling of the arm and the feeling of having a heavy arm. Both women working at home and those with professional careers emphasized the impact that these problems had on their ability to perform daily tasks. Activities such as lifting heavy objects or working in the computer for various hours resulted in pain and exhaustion leading to feelings of incompetence.

> *"I felt incapable, I felt incapable of not being able to, like use a pen, an eraser…" (Woman FG 5)*

Some women reported being reluctant to move their arm out of fear that the wound would open, potentially damaging the neighboring anatomic structures and others were worried about the chance that the movement could increase the pain. Thus, the lack of information regarding the motion possibilities of their upper extremities resulted in fear, making some women overly cautious and over protective of their arms.

> *"…I was scared, mostly regarding the exercises. I thought that maybe they [the doctors] told me not to move the arm, as I might hurt myself and the wound could open… I was scared." (Woman FG 5)*

Another reason for the limitations faced was the acceptance of the impairment; a sense of normality concerning the discomfort, which they assumed would not require any therapeutic measure. Some women were not even aware of their inability to lift their arms until they were about to receive radiotherapy, as this was a requirement to get such treatment. Until then, some women had not even tried to improve their arms' mobility.

> *"I have gone every week [to the doctor] since February 10, but the doctor didn't tell me that I had to move my arm. I had the first radiation session yesterday, but I couldn't lift the arm; now I have to go next Tuesday to see if I can lift it for the radiation, otherwise I will have to wait week after week." (Woman FG 7)*

The local idiosyncrasy also seemed to play a role for preventing women from recognizing impartments as disabilities at least until they are completely unable to perform conventional tasks. Some discomfort and/or limitations were often seen as natural and justified as part of the normal healing process by both patients and doctors themselves.

> *"My arm has been fine; it hasn't hurt at all. I can lift it perfectly, like I don't feel anything. I only feel it when I'm carrying something. But if I forget and carry something heavy, then later I feel it; it's normal." (Woman FG 2)*

Fear of recurrence and feelings of loss of femininity due to the removal of the breast were heavy burdens to women. Consequently, many women expressed the need for psychological assistance and ascribed psychological rehabilitation more value than to physiotherapy.

> *"…we need information, but also psychological care; we need it a lot, really, because we women are very strong, but sometimes it knocks you down, really, it does." (Woman FG 2)*

3.3. Strategies to deal with impairments

Women used various strategies to decrease their impairment. While few used the available medical services, for the majority, this was not a feasible option due to financial constraints and geographic difficulties accessing rehabilitation services. For those unable to receive professional medical therapy, the alternative was to perform exercises at home and to adjust their daily tasks to their condition. Women also discussed about the relevance of keeping a good attitude toward recovery and the importance of being motivated to do so.

The use of medical services varied and ranged from the utilization of compression garments, manual lymphatic drainage and physiotherapy to the use of prosthetic devices and medications such as diuretics. Those using a prosthesis saw it more as an aesthetic device rather than as a functional implement; thus, women tended to use just the cloth without weight or nothing at all. Many women got in contact with the providers of these services through RETO or received help directly from this organization.

> *"...at RETO they gave me advice and a lot of help; they told me how to do many exercises. They sent me to lymphatic drainage because my arm had started to get swollen and heavy, but this drainage helped me a lot. They [RETO] also teach you how to do the massage." (Woman FG 3)*

In order to decrease the sense of impairment, many women made adjustments in their life. For instance, they would modify the way in which they use to perform a task or would just remove such activity from the agenda. Occasionally, women would receive help from their family or from close acquaintances, but this was rather exceptional. As a rule, women were responsible to take care of their children and other family members. Thus, to fulfill their chores they mentioned that they tried to plan their activities according to what could be done considering their limitations.

> *"... I have constant pain in my arm. This is because of the physical activities I do when I work at home with all my chores. I have to plan according to what my arm allows. If it goes well one day I sweep and I mop. But I always do the dishes and fix the food. I know that I have to do the daily tasks, but I plan for doing the laundry and to sweep because these are the things that cause most trouble; it's very heavy to mop." (Woman FG 2)*

Being able to manage household chores, work and to a smaller extent to perform recreational activities were often reasons for moving or exercising. Some women emphasized that their children and spouses provided motivation to continue fighting and to overcome their limitations.

> *"...I was 40 years old, so I still had a life, I had to fight for my kids, for my husband..." (Woman FG 4)*

Some women mentioned that feeling like a disabled person that has to cope with her reality worked as a motivator to become more active. For many, there was no alternative but to help themselves improve, as they have to support their families, which were already living on scarce means. Therefore, recovery became a necessity.

> *"...my doctor told me that I was going to have like a disability, well, he didn't say it like that and then I thought 'how will I make a living?'" (Woman FG 4)*

3.4. Felt needs for information

Women described functional limitations as a consequence of the lack of adequate information, exercise, or movement. Limited knowledge was often a source of insecurity. However, they also emphasized the value of the help received from RETO and highlighted the importance of the assistance of such NGOs for women during the course of treatment and thereafter.

After surgery many women left the hospital with bandages attaching their affected arm to the torso without knowing what they could or could not do. Some of them were actually told not to move their arm, even after the bandages had been taken off to avoid the opening of the wound, which resulted in fear and insecurity.

> *"... I liked to have the arm here [attached to the body]. I didn't move it and until today; I still cannot lift it very high, because I liked to walk with the arm here. The doctor said: 'leave it like that' [laughs]; I was scared to lift it."* (Woman FG 1)

Some women mentioned that few doctors and nurses gave them good and adequate information and advice. Yet, for the most part, it was lacking, contradictory, or failed to sufficiently clarify things for them and to provide full understanding of the issues involved. Consequently, the fear and insecurity persisted.

> *"I get scared of getting close to the stove because, who knows what could happen to me? I never got a clear explanation, not at any point after the operation. They never explained to me at any stage what kind of things I could do or not."* (Woman FG 4)

The most frequent support for rehabilitation was the instructions provided by RETO, which contained general information and guidelines for exercise and for the lymphatic drainage. These instructions were generally given in the form of a brochure that was handed out when leaving the hospital after the surgery. In fact, the support of RETO was often the only organization providing some kind of rehabilitation information for women.

> *"I went looking for information; I had to know what was going to come after [the surgery]. I took the little brochure and then at RETO they explained everything to you: how to do the exercises, how to start, how many days and all, everything. I got the information about that from them."* (Woman FG 5)

However, the presence of RETO at the hospital somehow also prevented the public health services to offer additional information and support concerning rehabilitation.

> *"...apart from the RETO group, I think that the doctors, well, here at the hospital it's like they think, or I don't know, that if the RETO group is helping us to survive then they are taking care of our needs."* (Woman FG 1)

3.5. Expectations of rehabilitation from the health care services

Women's views regarding the care that they believe BC patients should be given were also explored along with suggestions on how to do this. The presence of family members in the discussions shed additional light in topics such as the unequal access to care.

http://dx.doi.org/10.5772/66436

While the medical and surgical treatment for BC was covered by the popular health insurance, women mentioned financial and logistic obstacles to access adequate and comprehensive care that included rehabilitation. For instance, one spouse commented on the possible effect of not paying for services could have affected the coverage and quality of care of his wife.

> *"…well, I don't know, maybe it's because one doesn't pay, because it's given for free (…) and I guess it's that, because for the most part I don't contribute with anything economically that they leave you like that. You get your surgery and that's enough for you to be satisfied and then the rest is up to God to help you (…) because if one could pay, I guess they would say 'come on, let's go'."(Male relative, FG 5)*

Conversely, posttreatment care, including physical therapy, lymphatic drainage and the provision of assistive devices (e.g., prosthesis) are not covered by the PHI. Thus, since for most women were unable to pay out of their pocket for rehabilitation care, then they just had to rely on charitable assistance such as the one provided by RETO or simply receive no care whatsoever.

> *"…I didn't have the possibility [to get rehabilitation]; in fact, they didn't say anything to me about rehabilitating exercises, nothing, even though I wanted that. At that time, that year, my husband was out of work and God knows, you have to eat, so for one, paying rehabilitation, was impossible for one, we had to pay rent (…) it's impossible." (Woman FG 3)*

The financial problems were paired with the logistic access to rehabilitation services. This was particularly relevant for those women living in marginalized or rural areas where means of transportations became the main concern.

> *"…the truth is that I didn't, I didn't have rehabilitation of my arm. Yes, the oncologist sent me to rehabilitation, but it was very difficult for me because I lived two hours from Tampico [a major city where the service was available]. I needed to go every day and so this was one of the things that I couldn't do, thank you very much, but I couldn't do it." (Woman FG 2)*

Most women suggested additional public clinics and doctors that can spend more time with each patient. However, since women were not informed about the treatment procedures and the consequences thereof, they did not have a clear picture of what kind of care they could ask for. Some suggested seminars to inform and guide patients and their families about BC treatment and posttreatment care.

> *"We have to become people who demand and ask for better care, like 'you are going to take care of me because it's your job and I pay you for it and you have to do it'." (Woman FG 7)*

4. Discussion

This study aimed to explore the needs and expectations concerning rehabilitation among Mexican women after BC surgery. Due to insufficient and sometimes misleading information from the health care services, the actual need for posttreatment care is neither met nor acknowledged. However, the positive attitude found among women toward rehabilitation is an important resource for future interventions. How these women perceive their right to comprehensive health care seems to be affected by the structure of the health care services and the Mexican idiosyncrasy.

The study provides in-depth information about the rehabilitation needs and expectations of BC survivors from a middle-size central Mexican city. Various themes emerged that underlie factors associated with the lack of rehabilitation care for most women such as the absence of free- or low-cost public facilities that provide such services, as previously observed [18].

A relevant issue was the lack of knowledge concerning the various aspects of treatment and posttreatment care. There was a general unawareness of the impairments as such or a belief that the discomforts were part of the normal healing process. Contrary to previous findings showing that the needs and complications reported by patients tend to be greater than those reported by clinicians [38], the women in this study seemed to give less importance to the functional limitations than to what their actual clinical assessment revealed (nearly all women included in this study had significant functional motion restrictions as assessed by a physiotherapist; data not presented). Yet, most of those experiencing limitations after surgery did not even try to seek rehabilitation care in agreement with others studies reporting that just few women are aware of the importance of posttreatment rehabilitation, especially in poor settings [17, 39, 40].

The findings of this study are also added to the evidence that there is a dissatisfaction regarding the information and support given by physicians and health care personnel after BC surgery. Fear, insecurity and confusion are generated by absent or misleading information [16, 39] which makes women have an overtly protective attitude toward the movement of their affected arms. Advice to keep the arm still and to avoid heavy lifting led to the belief that strenuous activity can have a negative effect on movement and volume, when studies suggesting the opposite [41, 42]. The motion restrictions advised by the health care personnel seemed to derive from outdated information concerning the effects of arm movement after surgery [41] which points to the need to update physicians and health professionals on the current physiotherapy guidelines for BC patients.

Most women were not informed about the procedures or the consequences that the treatment entailed. In particular, they were neither told nor they themselves requested for rehabilitation care for the experienced discomfort. In accordance with previous studies [43, 44], many women tried to handle their bothers either by changing the usual way in which they carried out an activity, by modifying their work schedule, or by eliminating tasks considered too difficult to perform. The relatively lack of assistance from spouse, family members, or friends to carry out daily activities also needs to be considered, as it can affect the interaction of this women with their family and social environment [43].

Cancer brings negative consequences associated with both the disease and the medical and surgical treatment [45]. As women experience the cancer process, some of them develop a fatalist attitude with a loss of hope that results in less energy and motivation to continue

http://dx.doi.org/10.5772/66436

fighting the disease [46, 47]. This can in turn prevent women from trying to improve their welfare while alive, which partially explains why they do not prioritize their rehabilitation. However, the disease can also result in a positive proactive attitude [48], as it was observed among many of the women interviewed here whereby they try to keep themselves alive in optimal conditions for their children and husbands. A positive mindset and the will to fight the disease with the hope to survive are also part of the survival strategies used by BC women [49]. Unfortunately, these women still lack the information and support needed to face their physical limitations and many end up prioritizing the needs of others at the expense of their physical rehabilitation.

While taking care of the close family can grow in relevance among BC women [50] becoming a key issue to face the disease, it seems that there can also have a negative effect when it comes to paying attention to their physical rehabilitation.

One must also consider the importance of providing social support to these women during this stage of the disease [51], including that of spouse, grown-up children and other family members, which is crucial to take appropriate decisions with respect to rehabilitation [52].

It is important that the public health services pay attention to the rehabilitation needs of BC women after surgery by designing and implementing follow-up programs that have been proven successful [53] involving family members that provide support [54] and optimizing the resources and offering benefits that translate into a better quality of life.

Since the survival rate for BC is increasing, so it is the importance of posttreatment care. As it is the case in many other low- and middle-income countries, there is no institutional public program available in Mexico that provides free coverage for rehabilitation services to BC women after surgery [55]. At present, the health system mainly focuses on survival, namely, on primary and adjuvant treatment [56, 57] whereby posttreatment care is left to NGOs such as the RETO group that provide information, exercise programs, lymphatic drainage and other activities to support women during the rehabilitation period. Yet, this study and others [16, 17, 39, 40] illustrate the need of rehabilitation and psychological therapy in addition to surgical treatment and radiotherapy for BC women.

During the discussions, economic and logistic issues were brought up as reasons limiting the access to comprehensive care. Those few women referred for rehabilitation found significant barriers to access those services either because of the high cost involved and/or due to distance and transportation difficulties. Differential accessibility to health services has been acknowledged in Mexico by health authorities who have even called for strong patients' advocacy groups to improve cancer care [58]. Unfortunately, the notion that survival is the main and almost only goal of treatment seems to prevail among both, patients and health personnel and so far little attention is being paid to the provision of better care after BC surgery [57].

The structure and recent evolution of the Mexican health system has had an impact on how the right to health care is looked upon by the population. The PHI, implemented in 2003 with the aim of providing comprehensive health care to those uninsured, entitled nearly 50 million Mexicans to a regulated and structured health care service. Thus, it is important to considered that many of the women interviewed here would have received an even more limited health care service prior to the inclusion of BC treatment in the insurance policies of 2007 [8, 55, 56]. However, the inclusion of posttreatment rehabilitation is yet to be part of such insurance to achieve a more humane comprehensive care for these women.

It is worth noting that while the public health services in SLP have insufficient human resources and infrastructure to rehabilitate BC women after surgery, the health authorities fail to even provide women with relevant information concerning the benefits of motility and physical exercise after surgery and during chemo and radiotherapy; instead, women have to rely upon the support and guidance of a NGO for that purpose [18]. Governmental authorities must be aware of this and as a result take a more active role rehabilitating these women. The same logic applies to the psycho-emotional support, which is commonly overlooked, as both BC women and health professionals are mostly focused on survival, but far less on the women's quality of life.

Altogether the findings of this study stress the pain and difficulties of BC women have to go through, which affect their quality of life significantly, including their social interaction with those dearest and nearest to them. However, the positive attitude of most women in their will to improve their functionality after surgery should be seen as an opportunity to design and implement effective rehabilitation programs with high adherence to its guidelines.

5. Conclusion

Many women perceived the need for rehabilitation, but information is still largely lacking. At present, public health services fail to provide rehabilitation services, which are now partially covered by private organizations. Treatment for BC should be accompanied by adequate rehabilitation. Therefore, awareness, availability and access to physiotherapy services need to be put in place.

Abbreviation list

BC	Breast cancer
DASH	Disability of arm shoulder hand
FG	Focus groups
NGO	Nongovernmental organization
PHI	People's health insurance
RETO	Recuperación total (total recovery)
ROM	Range of motion
SLP	San Luis Potosí

http://dx.doi.org/10.5772/66436

Author details

Viveka Hammelin, Luz María Tejada-Tayabas, Dulce María Galarza-Tejada and Joel Monárrez-Espino*

*Address all correspondence to: joel.monarrez-espino@ki.se

Department of Public Health Sciences, Karolinska Institutet, Stockholm, Sweden

References

[1] Torre L, Bray F, Siegel R, Ferlay J, Lortet-Tieulent J, Jemal A. Global cancer statistics, 2012. CA: A Cancer Journal for clinicians 2015, 65(2):87–108. Available from: http://onlinelibrary.wiley.com/doi/10.3322/caac.21262/epdf

[2] Soto-Perez-de-Celis E, Chavarri-Guerra Y. National and regional breast cancer incidence and mortality trends in Mexico 2001–2011: Analysis of a population-based database. *Cancer Epidemiol*, 2016. 41: 24–33. DOI: http://dx.doi.org/10.1016/j.canep.2016.01.007

[3] Ministry of Health. Statistical information. Statistics on Breast Cancer and Uterine Cervical Cancer [internet]. Available from: http://www.gob.mx/salud/acciones-y-programas/informacion-estadistica

[4] Caplan L. Delay in breast cancer: Implications for stage at diagnosis and survival. *Front PublicHealth*, 2014. 2: 87.

[5] National Institute of Statistics and Geography (INEGI). Statistics on the international day against breast cancer, 2013. Available from: http://www.inegi.org.mx/saladeprensa/aproposito/2016/mama2016_0.pdf

[6] Cruz-Castillo AB, Hernández-Valero MA, Hovick S, Campuzano-González ME, Karam-Calderón MA. Bustamante-Monte P. A study on the knowledge, perception and use of breast cancer screening methods and quality of care among women from central Mexico. *J Cancer Educ*, 2015. 30(3): 453–459.

[7] Lee CI, Bogart A, Germino J, et al. Availability of advanced breast imaging at screening facilities serving vulnerable populations. *J Med Screen*, 2016. 23: 24–30.

[8] Chavarri-Guerra, Y, Villarreal-Garza C, Liedke P, et al. Breast cancer in Mexico: A growing challenge to health and the health system. *Lancet Oncol*, 2012. 13(8): 335–343.

[9] Inger-Lise N, Alv AD, Løkkevik E, Mengshoel AM, fosså SD. Arm and shoulder morbidity in breast cancer patients after breast-conserving therapy versus mastectomy, Acta Oncologica, 2008. 47(5): 835–842. Available from: http://dx.doi.org/10.1080/02841860801961257

[10] Campbell KL, Pusic KL, Zucker D, et al. A prospective model of care for breast cancer rehabilitation: Function. *Cancer*, 2012. 118: 2300–2311. Available from: http://onlinelibrary.wiley.com/doi/10.1002/cncr.27464/pdf

[11] Lee TS, Kilbreath S, Refshauge K, et al. Prognosis of the upper limb following surgery and radiation for breast cancer. *Breast Cancer Res Treat*, 2008. 110: 19–37.

[12] Rietman JS, Dijkstra PU, Hoekstra HJ, et al. Late morbidity after treatment of breast cancer in relation to daily activities and quality of life: a systematic review. *Eur J Surg Oncol*, 2003. 29(3): 229–238.

[13] Ewertz M, & Jensen AB. Late effects of breast cancer treatment and potentials for rehabilitation. *Acta Oncol*, 2011. 50(2): 187–193.

[14] Kurita GP, & Sjogren P. Pain management in cancer survivorship. *Acta Oncol*, 2015. 54(5): 629–634.

[15] Van Dijck S, Nelissen P, Verbelen H. et al. The effects of physical self-management on quality of life in breast cancer patients: A systematic review. *The Breast*, 2016. 28: 20–28.

[16] Binkley JM, Harris SR, Levangie P, et al. Patient perspectives on breast cancer treatment side effects and the prospective surveillance model for physical rehabilitation for women with breast cancer. *Cancer*, 2012. 118(Suppl 8): 2207–2216. Available from: http://onlinelibrary.wiley.com/doi/10.1002/cncr.27469/pdf

[17] Ganz PA, Yip Ch, Gralow J, et al. Supportive care after curative treatment for breast cancer (survivorship care): Resource allocations in low- and middle-income countries. A Breast Health Global Initiative 2013 consensus statement. *The Breast*, 2013. 22: 606–615.

[18] Tejada-Tayabas, L.M., Amell, L., Monárrez-Espino, J. Medical therapeutic itineraries of women with breast cancer diagnosis affiliated to the people's health insurance in San Luis Potosí, central Mexico. *Cad Saúde Pública*, 2015. 31(1): 60–70. Available from:http://www.scielo.br/pdf/csp/v31n1/0102-311X-csp-31-01-00060.pdf

[19] Borman P, Yaman A, Yasrebi S, et al. The importance of awareness and education in patients with breast cancer-related lymphedem. *J Canc Educ*, 2016. Apr 6 [Epub ahead of print]. Available from: http://link.springer.com/article/10.1007/s13187-016-1026-1/fulltext.html

[20] Pauwels, EE. Charlier C, De Bourdeaudhuij I, Lechner L, Van Hoof E. Care needs after primary breast cancer treatment. Survivors' associated sociodemographic and medical characteristics. *Psychooncology*, 2013, 22(1): 125–132.

[21] Gómez-Dantes, O., Sesma, S., Becerril, V.M., Knaul, F.M., Arreola, H., Frenk, J. Sistema de salud de México. *Salud Publica Mex*, 2011. 53(Suppl 2): 220–232. Available from: http://www.scielosp.org/pdf/spm/v53s2/17.pdf

[22] Ministry of Health. Specific Action Program for the Prevention and Control of Breast Cancer 2013–2018. 1st ed. 2014. Mexico City. National Health System. Available from:

http://cnegsr.salud.gob.mx/contenidos/descargas/cama/PrevencionyControldelCancerdelaMujer_2013_2018.pdf

[23] Anaya-Ruiz M, Vallejo-Ruiz V, Flores-Mendoza L, Perez-Santos M. Female breast cancer incidence and mortality in Mexico, 2000–2010. *Asian Pac J Cancer Prev*, 2014. 15(3): 1477–1479. Available from: http://ocean.kisti.re.kr/downfile/volume/apocp/POCPA9/2014/v15n3/POCPA9_2014_v15n3_1477.pdf

[24] Schmitz KH, Stout NL, PT andrews A, et al. Prospective evaluation of physical rehabilitation needs in breast cancer survivors. *Cancer*, 2012. 118(Suppl 58): 2187–2190. Available from: http://onlinelibrary.wiley.com/doi/10.1002/cncr.27471/pdf

[25] Systematization of the Navigation´s Experience (support) of Breast Cancer Patients. 2012, Heredia, National University of Costa Rica. Available from: http://www.kerwa.ucr.ac.cr/handle/10669/1408

[26] Tejada-Tayabas LM, Castillo T, Monarrez-Espino J. Qualitative evaluation, a interpretive and critical approach to improving programs and health services. *Int J Qualitative Stud Health Well-Being*, 2014, 9: 24417. http://dx.doi.org/10.3402/qhw.v9.24417

[27] Cook KE. Using critical ethnography to explore issues in health promotion. *Qual Health Res*, 2005. 15: 129–138.

[28] Suri H. Purposeful sampling in qualitative research synthesis. *Qual Res J*, 2011. 11(2): 63–75. Available from: http://www.emeraldinsight.com/doi/pdfplus/10.3316/QRJ1102063

[29] Morgan DL, Krueger RA. Planning focus groups. Focus group Kit 2. United States of America: SAGE publications India Pvt. Ltd, 1998.

[30] Guest G, Bunce A, & Johnson L. How many interviews are enough? An experiment with data saturation and variability. *Field methods*, 2006. 18: 59–82.

[31] Kerr C, Nixon A, & Wild D. Assessing and demonstrating data saturation in qualitative inquiry supporting patient-reported outcomes research. *Expert Rev Pharmacoecon Outcomes Res*, 2010. 10(3): 269–281.

[32] Gummesson C, Ward MM, Atroshi I. The shortened disabilities of the arm, shoulder and hand questionnaire (QuickDASH): validity and reliability based on responses within the full-length DASH. *BMC Musculoskelet Disord*, 2006. 7: 44. Available from: http://bmcmusculoskeletdisord.biomedcentral.com/articles/10.1186/1471-2474-7-44

[33] Muir SW, Corea CL, Beaupre L. Evaluating change in clinical status: Reliability and measures of agreement for the assessment of glenohumeral range of motion. *N Am J Sports Phys Ther*, 2010. 5(3): 98–110.

[34] Brorson H, & Hoijer P. Standardised measurements used to order compression garments can be used to calculate arm volumes to evaluate lymphoedema treatment. *J Plast Surg Hand Surg*, 2012. 46(6): 410–415.

[35] Thomas-Maclean RL, Thomas H, Winkle K, et al. Arm morbidity and disability after breast cancer: New directions for care. *Oncol Nurs Forum*, 2008. 35(1): 65–71.

[36] Emerson, R.M., Fretz, R.I. & Shaw, L.L. Writing ethnographic fieldnotes. Chicago: University of Chicago Press, 1995.

[37] Graneheim UH, & Lundman B. Qualitative content analysis in nursing research: concepts, procedures and measures to achieve trustworthiness. *Nurse Educ Today*, 2004. 24(2): 105–112.

[38] Cheville AL, Beck LA, Petersen TL, Marks RS. The detection and treatment of cancer-related functional problems in an outpatient setting. *Support Care Cancer*, 2009. 17(1): 61–67.

[39] Ridner S, Rhoten B, Radina E, et al. Breast cancer survivors' perspectives of critical lymphedema self-care support needs. Supportive Care in Cancer, 2016, 24(6): 2743–2750. Available from: http://link.springer.com/article/10.1007/s00520-016-3089-2

[40] Keast DH, Despatis M, Allen JO, Brassard A. Chronic edema/lymphoedema: Under-recognised and under-treoated. *Int Wound*, 2015. 12(3): 328–333.

[41] Lee TS. Kilbreath S, Sullivan G. et al. Factors that affect intention to avoid strenuous arm activity after breast cancer surgery. *Oncology nursing forum*, 2009. 36(4): 2454–2462.

[42] McNeely ML, Binkley M, Pusic AL, et al. A prospective model of care for breast cancer rehabilitation: Postoperative and postreconstructive issues. *Cancer*, 2012. 118: 2226–2236. Available from: http://onlinelibrary.wiley.com/doi/10.1002/cncr.27468/pdf

[43] Thomas–MacLean R, et al. "This is a kind of betrayal": A qualitative study of disability after breast cancer. *Curr Oncol*, 2009. 16(3): 26–32.

[44] Tiedtke, C. Dierckx B, Rijkc A et al. Breast cancer treatment and work disability: Patient perspectives. *Breast*, 2011. 20(6): 534–538.

[45] Khan F, Amatya B, Pallant JF, Rajapaksa I. Factors associated with long-term functional outcomes and psychological sequelae in women after breast cancer. *The Breast*, 2012. 21(3): 314–320.

[46] Curtis R, Groarke A, McSharry J, Kerin M. Experience of breast cancer: burden, benefit, or both? *Cancer Nurs*, 2014. 37(3): E21-E30.

[47] Nakatani Y, Iwamitsu Y, Kuranami M, Okazaki S, Yamamoto K, Watanabe M, Miyaoka H. Predictors of psychological distress in breast cancer patients after surgery. *Kitasato Med J*, 2013. 43: 49–58.

[48] Scheffold K, Mehnert A, Muller V, Koch U, Harter M, Vehling S. Sources of meaning in cancer patients—influences on global meaning, anxiety and depression in a longitudinal study. *Eur J Cancer Care*, 2014. 23(4): 472–480.

[49] Rotegard AK, Fagermoen MS, Ruland CM. Cancer patients' experiences of their personal strengths through illness and recovery. *Cancer Nurs*, 2012, 35(1): E8–E17.

[50] Salander P, Lilliehorn S, Hamberg K, Kero A. The impact of breast cancer on living an everyday life 4.5-5 years post-diagnosis — A qualitative prospective study of 39 women. *Acta Oncol*, 2011. 50(3): 399–407.

[51] Drageset S, Lindstrom TC, Giske T, Underlid K. "The support I need": Women's experiences of social support after having received breast Cancer diagnosis and awaiting surgery. *Cancer Nurs*, 2012. 35(6): E39-E47.

[52] Jensen CG, Elsass P, Neustrup L, et al. What to listen for in the consultation. Breast cancer patients' own focus on talking about acceptance-based psychological coping predicts decreased psychological distress and depression. *Patient Educ Couns*, 2014. 97(2): 165–172.

[53] Stanley S, Arriola KJ, Smith S, Hurlbert M, Ricci C, Escoffery C. Reducing barriers to breast cancer care through a patient navigation programs. *J Public Health Manag Pract*, 2013. 19(5): 461–467.

[54] Marshall CA, Badger TA, Curran MA, Koerner SS, Larkey LK, Weihs KL, et al. Un abrazo para la familia: Providing low-income Hispanics with education and skills in coping with breast cancer and caregiving. *Psychooncology*, 2013. 22(2): 470–474.

[55] Kaul FM. et al. The quest for universal health coverage: achieving social protection for all in Mexico. *The Lancet*, 2012. 380(9849): 1259–1279

[56] Gonzalez-Robledo MC, Wong R, Arreola H, Knaul F. Costs of breast cancer care in Mexico: analysis of two insurance coverage scenarios. *Ecancermedicalscience*, 2015. 9: 587.

[57] Yip CH. Cazap E anderson B, et al. Breast cancer management in middle-resource countries (MRCs): Consensus statement from the breast health global initiative. *The Breast*, 2011. 20(2): 12–19.

[58] Chertorivski S. Planning cancer control — A Mexican perspective. *The lancet oncol*, 2013. 14(5): 386–387.

Chapter 26

Naringenin Inhibits Proliferation and Survival of Tamoxifen-Resistant Breast Cancer Cells

Joseph Ramos, Talia Hatkevich, Lauren Eanes,
Idalys Santos-Sanchez and Yashomati M. Patel

Additional information is available at the end of the chapter

http://dx.doi.org/10.5772/66698

Abstract

The majority of breast cancers are estrogen receptor positive (ER+) and utilize estrogen to promote cell proliferation. Thus, the ER has been the target of many therapies. While this strategy has been successful, the long-term use of antiestrogen therapies, such as tamoxifen (Tam), frequently results in Tam resistance (Tam-R). Tam-R cells may proliferate due to the activation of the phosphatidylinositol-3 kinase (PI3K) and the mitogen-activated protein kinase (MAPK) pathways. Targeting these proliferation and survival pathways after the development of resistance is critical for the treatment of drug-resistant cancers. We have identified the flavanone Naringenin (Nar) as an inhibitor of both the PI3K and MAPK pathways. Here, we show that Nar impairs cell proliferation and induces apoptosis of Tam-R MCF-7 breast cancer cells. We also demonstrate that Nar treatment reduced the levels of both ERK and AKT in Tam-R cells. Furthermore, Nar treatment localized ERα to a perinuclear region in Tam-R cells. Nar may function by inhibiting both the PI3K and MAPK pathways as well as localizing ERα to the cytoplasm to impair cell proliferation of Tam-R MCF-7 cells. These studies provide insight into the molecular mechanisms involved in cell proliferation of Tam-R breast cancer cells.

Keywords: naringenin, tamoxifen-resistant, breast cancer, proliferation, MAPK

1. Introduction

The majority of breast cancers are estrogen receptor positive (ER+) and depend on estrogen for cell proliferation [1]. The majority of ER+ breast cancers respond to antiestrogen therapies such as tamoxifen (Tam) [2]. Unfortunately, the long-term use of Tam frequently results in Tam resistance. Tam resistance is often accompanied by the activation of other proliferation promoting pathways such as growth factor receptor pathways and their downstream signaling molecules such as phosphatidylinositol 3-kinase (PI3K) and mitogen-activated protein kinase (MAPK) [3]. Endocrine resistance and activation of growth promoting signaling molecules are indicative of a poor prognosis and increased mortality [4]. Thus, the identification of therapeutic compounds that regulate proliferation in Tam-resistant cancers could lead to more effective treatment options.

In order to impair proliferation in ER+ breast cancer cells, antiestrogen therapies such as Tam are utilized to target the ER [2]. Normally, estrogen binds the ER that results in dimerization, translocation into the nucleus, and regulation of gene transcription [5–8]. The estrogen-ER complex regulates numerous genes that affect cell proliferation and survival [5–8]. Tam acts as an agonist or antagonist to the ER depending on the cell type [9]. In breast tissue, Tam functions mainly as an antagonist to the ER. It does so by binding the ER and preventing it from transcribing estrogen-responsive genes [2, 9–11]. Inhibiting transcription of these genes impairs cell proliferation and survival. Previous studies have shown that overactivation of the MAPK and PI3K pathways during Tam treatment may be involved in Tam resistance via ligand-independent activation of the ER, decreasing the overall rate of ER+ breast cancer survival [6]. Both the MAPK and PI3K pathways regulate cellular growth and survival [12]. These pathways have also been shown to activate the ER via phosphorylation in a ligand-independent manner [13, 14]. Conversely, the ER can activate both the MAPK and PI3K pathways by a nongenomic mechanism [13, 14]. Taken together, these findings suggest that Tam resistance may be the result of complex interactions between the ER and components of kinase signaling pathways. Therefore, identification of compounds that inhibit the activity of the PI3K or MAPK pathways may restore growth arrest to Tam resistant cells. Chemical inhibitors of MEK and PI3K are currently being investigated as promising new strategy for breast cancer patients [15, 16].

Previous studies have identified the grapefruit flavanone, Naringenin (Nar) as an inhibitor of both the MAPK and PI3K pathways [15, 17–20]. Flavanones have low toxicity compared to other plant compounds and can function to impair cell proliferation, angiogenesis, and signaling cascades [21–26]. Previous studies have shown that Nar hinders cell proliferation and motility by interfering with the PI3K and MAPK pathways [26, 27]. Nar has also been shown to bind directly to the estrogen receptor and function as an ER antagonist [26, 27]. The ability of Nar to impair the MAPK and PI3K pathways as well as function as an antagonist to the ER suggests that Nar has the potential to growth arrest Tamoxifen-resistant cells (Tam-R). In this study, we show that Nar inhibits cell proliferation of Tam-R MCF-7 cells. Furthermore, we demonstrate that Nar impairs both the MAPK and PI3K pathways by reducing the levels of ERK and AKT. Nar treatment results in relocalization of ERα to a perinuclear location in Tam-R cells. Thus, Nar acts by impairing both the MAPK and PI3K pathways as well as functioning as an antagonist to the ER.

http://dx.doi.org/10.5772/66698

2. Materials and methods

2.1. Cell culture

MCF-7 cells were maintained in Dulbecco's modified Eagle medium (DMEM)/10% fetal bovine serum (FBS), supplemented with insulin, or phenol red-free DMEM (PRF-DMEM) supplemented with 10% charcoal-stripped fetal bovine serum (CS-FBS). Cells were maintained at 37°C with 5% CO_2. Media was changed every 2 days and cells were passaged at 80% confluency.

2.2. Generation of Tam-R cells

Tam-R cells were generated by culturing MCF-7 cells in DMEM supplemented with 100 U/mL penicillin/streptomycin, 0.01 mg/mL bovine insulin, 10% FBS, and 10^{-6} M of 4-OH-tamoxifen for 10 months [28–30].

2.3. Naringenin treatment

Naringenin was purchased from Sigma Aldrich. Cells were treated with Naringenin (2,3-Dihydro-5,7-dihydroxy-2-(4-hydroxyphenyl)-4*H*-1-benzopyran-4-one, 4′,5,7-Trihydroxyflavanone) (Nar) or treated with a vehicle DMSO alone. Cells were treated with Nar (at the indicated concentration) a few hours after plating. Cells were treated for the indicated times and then assayed for a variety of parameters.

2.4. Cell density assays

Cells either treated with the vehicle DMSO alone or Nar (at the indicated concentrations and the indicated time points) were washed twice with 1×PBS, trypsinized and then centrifuged at 5000 × *g* for 5 min. Pelleted cells were resuspended in 1×PBS. Cells (1:20 dilution) were incubated in ViaCount Reagent for 5 min in the dark and analyzed by Guava easy-Cyte™ flow cytometry (Millipore) using the ViaCount software. The ViaCount Reagent determines cells density (a measure of all cells) as well as viable, apoptotic, and dead cells by using two dyes. The nuclear dye stains only nucleated cells and the viability dye stains only dying cells. Levels of the stains allows for accurate assessment of viable, apoptotic, and dead cells.

2.5. Immunoblot analysis

Cells either treated with the vehicle DMSO alone or Nar (250 μM) for 7 days were washed once with 1×PBS and lysed. Cell lysates were rocked for 20 min and then centrifuged for 20 min at 4°C. Proteins (30 μg) were subjected to 10% SDS-PAGE and Western blot analysis protein were immunostained with the indicated antibody and detected using ECL and a Bio-Rad ChemiDoc XRS system. Protein bands were analyzed using Quantity One software.

2.6. Immunofluorescence

Cells were cultured on sterilized glass coverslips for 7 days. Cells were either treated with the vehicle DMSO alone or Nar (250 μM) for 7 days. After treatment, cells were washed with 1×PBS, fixed with 3.7% paraformaldehyde for 15 min, and then permeabilized in 0.25% Triton. Cells were incubated with an ERα antibody (1:100) for 1 h and then a secondary antibody for 45 min. Cells were incubated with DAPI (1:1000) for 5 min and then washed with 1×PBS. Cells were visualized using an Olympus iX81 Motorized Inverted Confocal Microscope equipped with Fluoview FV500 software. To determine the effect of Nar on apoptosis, cells were stained with DAPI and cells containing condensed and fragmented nuclei (presented as punctate DAPI staining) were counted. Cells in 5–7 different fields/slides were counted and averaged. The experiment was performed three times.

2.7. Quantification of ERα

ERα levels were quantified by fluorescence intensity in both the cytoplasm and nucleus. The ratio of nuclear/cytoplasmic signal was measured for 5–7 fields under various conditions and averaged. The experiment was performed three times.

2.8. Nuclear and cytoplasmic fractionation

Cells either treated with the vehicle DMSO alone or Nar (250 μM) for 7 days were washed with 1×PBS and centrifuged at 8000 rpm for 2 min. The supernatant was removed and cells were resuspended in 1 mL of Hank's balanced salt solution. Cells were then centrifuged at 4000 rpm for 2 min. The supernatant was removed and the cells were resuspended in 100 μL of CE buffer (10 mM Hepes pH7.6, 60 mM KCl, 1 mM EDTA, 1 mM DTT, 0.7% NP-40). They were placed on ice for 5 min, and then centrifuged at 4000 rpm for 4 min. The supernatant was collected as the cytoplasmic extract. The remaining pellet was resuspended in 500 μL of CE buffer without NP-40 and then centrifuged at 10,000 rpm for 4 min. The supernatant was removed and the remaining pellet was the nuclear extract.

2.9. Statistical analysis

Results are the means ± SEM of three independent experiments ($^*p < 0.05$). The significance was assessed by two-way analysis of Student's *t*-test (StatPlus, AnalystSoft).

3. Results

3.1. Characterization of Tam-R MCF-7 cells

Previous studies have shown that growth factor pathways are upregulated in Tam-R cells [3]. Since Nar targets the MAPK and PI3K pathways, we wanted to determine the effect of Nar on Tam-R cells. In order to do this, we first had to establish a Tam-R cell line. Previous studies have shown that MCF-7 cells can become tamoxifen-resistant through prolonged exposure to 4-OH-tamoxifen [28–30]. We cultured MCF-7 cells in the presence of 4-OH-tamoxifen for 10 months as described in Section 2. After 10 months of 4-OH-tamoxifen treatment, cells were assayed for proliferation and compared to Tamoxifen-sensitive MCF-7 cells (Tam-S). Cells were grown in either full medium (10% FBS) or medium containing charcoal-stripped serum. Since

http://dx.doi.org/10.5772/66698

MCF-7 cell proliferation is primarily driven by estrogen, the untreated wild-type Tam-S cells had a 462% increase in cell density when grown in full medium and a low rate of proliferation in the charcoal-stripped serum compared to cells grown in full medium. The cell density of Tam-S cells cultured in charcoal-stripped serum only increased 37% over 7 days (**Figure 1A**). Furthermore, Tam-S cells treated with tamoxifen also had a low rate of proliferation. In contrast, cell density of Tam-R cells increased by 378% in full medium and 287% in the presence of charcoal-striped medium in 7 days. Additionally, tamoxifen treatment had no effect on cell density. Thus, the level of cell proliferation observed in the presence of Tam indicated that the cells were Tam-resistant. In all treatments the vehicle control (EtOH) had no effect when compared to untreated cells.

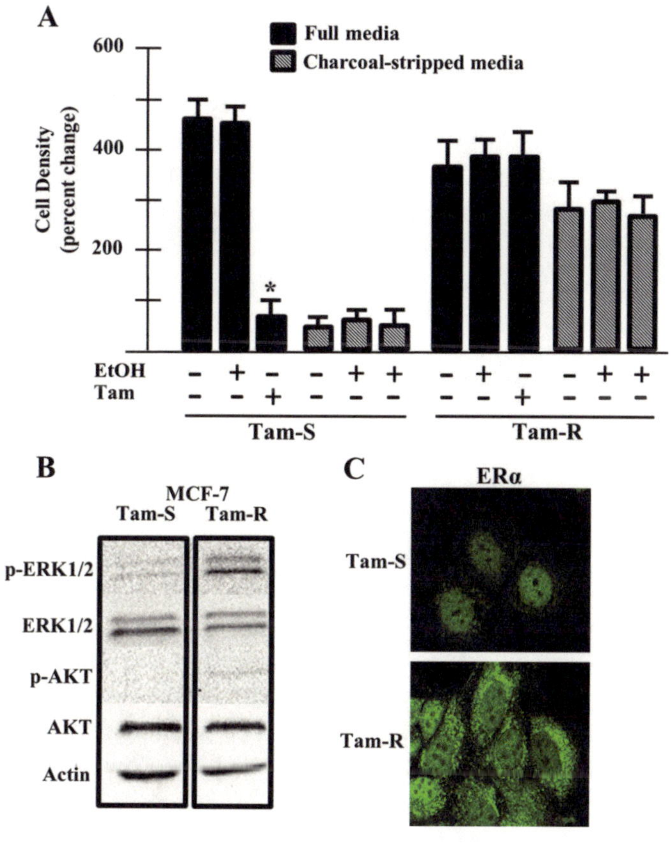

Figure 1. Characterization of Tam-R MCF-7 cells. Tam-S (MCF-7 wild-type) and Tam-R cells were cultured in phenol red free media containing FBS (Full media) or charcoal-stripped FBS and either left untreated or treated with the vehicle (ethanol) or 4-OH-tamoxifen (100 nM) for 7 days. (A) Cell densities (cells/ml) were determined and compared to initial counts to calculate percent change. Results are the means ± SEM of three independent experiments. Differences between Full media and Charcoal-stripped media were tested for statistical significance (*$p < 0.05$). (B) Cell lysates were collected and proteins were subjected to SDS-PAGE. Proteins were immunoblotted using antibodies against p-ERK1/2, ERK1/2, p-AKT, AKT, and actin. Results are representative of five independent experiments. (C) Cells were fixed and stained for ERα and visualized using confocal microscopy. The results are representative of three independent experiments.

Previous studies have suggested that cell proliferation in Tam-R cells may be due to the activation of growth factor pathways [3]. In order to determine if the change in growth rate was associated with a change in the protein levels and/or phosphorylation of ERK1/2 and/or AKT, we assayed p-ERK1/2, ERK1/2, p-AKT, AKT, and actin. Tam-S MCF-7 cells express both ERK1/2 and AKT and low levels of both p-ERK1/2 and p-AKT were detected. Tam-R cells also express both ERK1/2 and AKT at similar levels when normalized to actin levels. In agreement with previous studies, we observed an increase in p-ERK1/2 in the Tam-R cells when compared to Tam-S (**Figure 1B**) [31]. Surprisingly, Tam resistance did not stimulate the phosphorylation of AKT when normalized to actin levels in our cells (**Figure 1B**).

Another observed difference present in Tam-R cells is the redistribution of ERα to the cytoplasm upon tamoxifen resistance [31]. We wanted to determine whether our Tam-R cells exhibited any alteration in ERα localization when compared with Tam-S cells. To investigate the localization pattern of ERα, both Tam-S and Tam-R MCF-7 cells were assayed for ERα localization by confocal microscopy (**Figure 1C**). In Tam-S cells, ERα was localized primarily to the nucleus (72 ± 4 of total ERα) with lower levels present in the cytoplasm (28 ± 7 of total ERα). In contrast, Tam-R cells exhibited increased levels of ERα in the cytoplasm (47 ± 6 of total ERα) compared to Tam-S cells. This increased level of ERα was evenly distributed throughout the cytoplasm. ERα was still present in the nucleus of Tam-R cells although at lower levels (53 ± 7 of total ERα) then that observed in Tam-S cells.

3.2. Nar impairs cell density of Tam-R MCF-7 cells

Next we wanted to determine if Nar could inhibit cell proliferation in Tam-R MCF-7 cells. Previous studies suggested that Tam-R cells utilize PI3K and/or MAPK pathways for cell proliferation. Since Nar inhibits both these pathways, it should result in impaired growth of Tam-R cells. We first wanted to determine the time- and concentration-dependent effects of naringenin on Tam-R cells. As shown in **Figure 2A**, Nar treatment decreased cell density within 2 days when compared to untreated cells and cell density further declined at 4 and 7 days. There was a significant difference in cell density at day 4 and 7, so we conducted all of our studies on day 7. We then wanted to determine the effect of Nar concentration on cell density (**Figure 2B**) and viability (**Figure 2C**) of Tam-R cells. While Nar treatment (at all concentrations) decreased both the cell density and viability of Tam-R cells in 7 days only a Nar concentration of 250 μM had a significant effect on both cell density and cell viability when compared to untreated Tam-R cells. In our studies, we determined that Nar inhibited cell proliferation of both Tam-S and Tam-R cells with an IC_{50} value of 237 μM. While previous studies have shown that lower concentrations of Nar impaired the proliferation and viability of MCF-7 cells, our studies here demonstrate that Tam-R MCF-7 cells require higher concentrations of Nar to impair proliferation and viability [15, 17]. Higher concentration of Nar in cell culture as well as in animal studies have been employed in other studies and may reflect the specific sensitivities of the targets of Nar to elicit specific physiological effects [32–35].

http://dx.doi.org/10.5772/66698

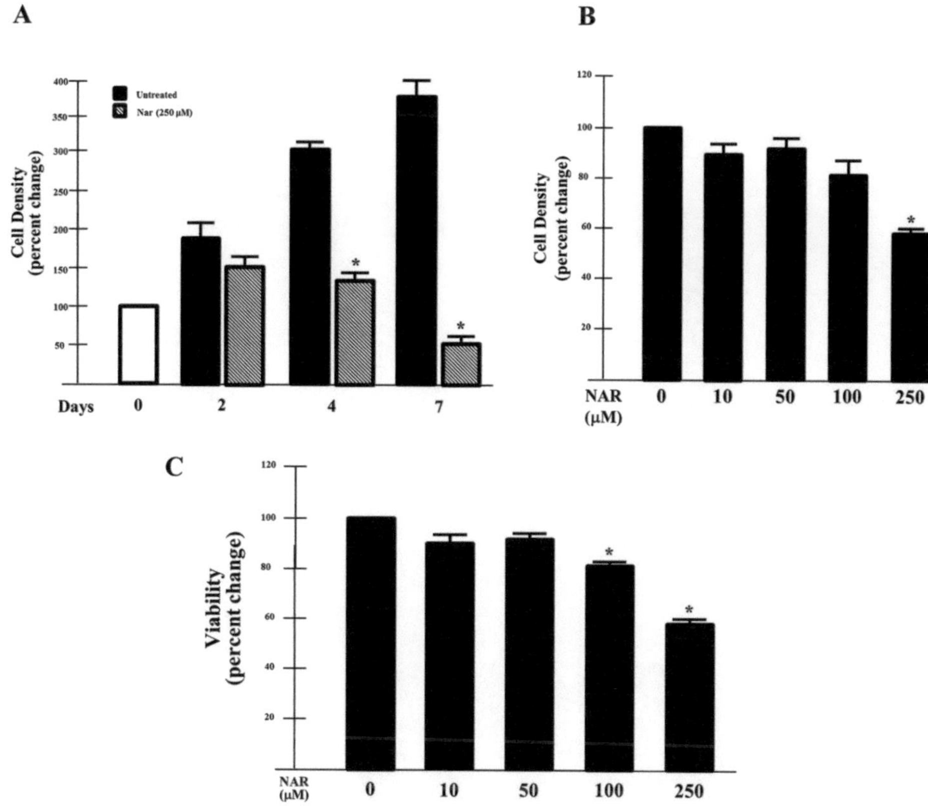

Figure 2. Nar inhibits cell proliferation in a concentration- and time-dependent manner. Tam-R cells were cultured in phenol red free media containing charcoal-stripped FBS with 4-OH-tamoxifen (100 nM). (A) Cell densities (cells/ml) were determined in the presence or absence of Nar (250 μM) for the indicated time points. (B) Cell density (cells/ml) and (C) cell viability were determined at various Nar concentrations and compared to initial counts to calculate percent change. Results are the means ± SEM of three independent experiments. Differences between untreated and Nar treated were tested for statistical significance (*$p < 0.05$).

3.3. Nar induces apoptosis in Tam-R cells.

To determine whether the potential effect of Nar on cell proliferation were similar in Tam-S and Tam-R cells, both cell types were grown in media containing Tam in the presence or absence of Nar [34–37]. As shown previously, Tam impaired the proliferation of Tam-S cells. Nar treatment of Tam-S cells not only further impaired cell proliferation it also decreased viability (**Figure 3A**). As expected the Tam-R cells exhibited increased proliferation in the presence of Tam when compared to Tam-S cells (**Figure 3A**). However, the increase in proliferation was completely reversed by the addition of Nar. Nar impaired viability of Tam-R cells to a similar extent as that seen in Tam-S MCF-7 cells (**Figure 3A**). Next, we assayed for apoptotic and dead cells upon Nar treatment of Tam-R cells (**Figure 3B** and **C**). There was an increase in both apoptotic and dead cells in Nar treated cells over 7 days when compared to untreated cells. In complementary studies, we assayed for condensed and fragmented nuclei by DAPI staining (**Figure 3D** and **E**). Nar treatment of Tam-R cells resulted in a 16% increase in nuclear apoptosis when compared to untreated cells.

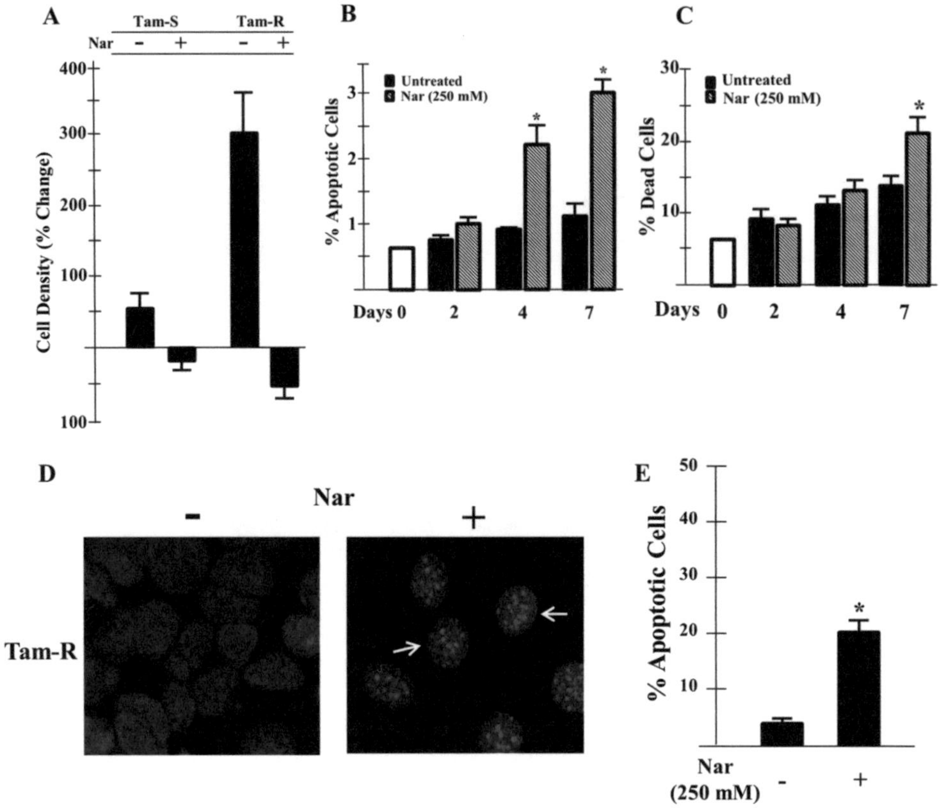

Figure 3. Nar is cytotoxic to Tam-R cells. (A) Tam-S and Tam-R cells were cultured in phenol red free media plus charcoal-stripped FBS (PRF-DMEM + CS-FBS) containing 4-OH-tamoxifen (100 nM) in the presence or absence of Nar (250 μM). After 7 days, cells were collected, cell densities quantified, and growth rate calculated. Results are the means ± SEM of five independent experiments. Tam-R cells were cultured in the presence or absence of Nar for the indicated time points and assayed for (B) apoptotic and (C) dead cells. Percent apoptosis and percent dead cells were determined by flow cytometry. Results are the means ± SEM of three independent experiments. Differences between untreated and Nar treated at the indicated time points were tested for statistical significance (*$p < 0.05$). (D) Tam-R cells were cultured in the presence or absence of Nar for 7 days and then stained with DAPI and visualized by confocal microscopy. Condensed and fragmented nuclei are indicated by arrows. (E) Quantification staining is expressed as % apoptotic cells in Nar treated cells compared to untreated cells. Results are the means ± SEM of three independent experiments. *$p < 0.05$.

3.4. Nar decreases the levels of ERK and AKT protein in Tam-R cells

Previous studies have shown that short-term exposure to Nar reduces both AKT and ERK1/2 phosphorylation in MCF-7 cells. Our recent studies demonstrated that long-term (days) exposure to Nar decreased the protein levels of ERK1/2 and AKT in Tam-S MCF-7 cells [20]. We wanted to determine whether Nar had similar effects on ERK1/2, and AKT in Tam-R MCF-7 cells. To determine if Nar altered the levels and/or the phosphorylation of ERK1/2 and AKT, we incubated Tam-R cells with Tam alone, Nar alone, or a combination of Nar and Tam. While Tam-R MCF-7 cells expressed both AKT and ERK1/2, as shown previously, the addition of Nar in the presence or absence of Tam in Tam-R cells resulted in significantly lower levels (30–40%) of both ERK1/2 and AKT (**Figure 4A** and **B**). Next, we examined the effect of Nar on the phosphorylation status of ERK1/2 and AKT in Tam-R cells. Our findings show that Tam-R cells have increased levels of p-ERK1/2 but unchanged levels of p-AKT when compared to Tam-S cells as seen in **Figure 1B**. As shown in **Figure 4A**, Nar alone and in combination with Tam resulted in undetectable levels of p-ERK1/2 in Tam-R cells. This may be due in part to the reduced levels of total ERK1/2. Phosphorylated AKT was undetectable in all samples.

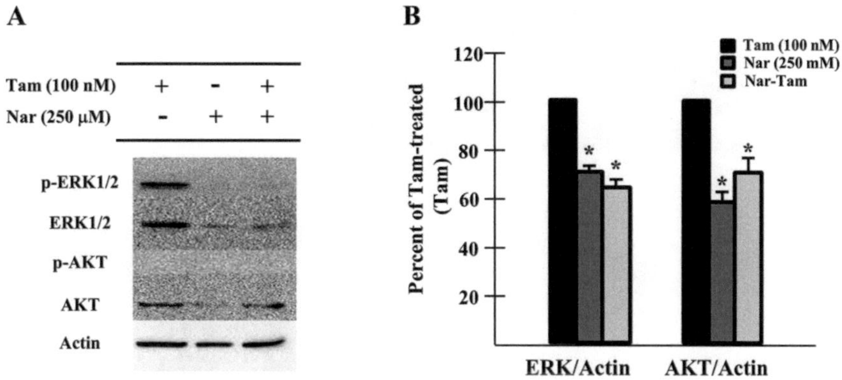

Figure 4. Nar impairs the expression of ERK1/2 and AKT. Tam-R MCF-7 cells were grown in phenol red free media plus charcoal-stripped FBS (PRF-DMEM + CS-FBS) in the presence of 4-OH-tamoxifen (100 nM), Nar (250 μM), or a combination of the two. (A) Following 7 days of treatment, cells lysates were collected. Proteins were subjected to SDS-PAGE and immunoblotted using antibodies against p-ERK1/2, ERK1/2, p-AKT, AKT, and actin. (B) Protein levels were quantified using densitometry. Results are the means ± SEM of three independent experiments. Differences between Tam-treated and Nar or Nar-Tam treated were tested for statistical significance (*$p < 0.05$).

3.5. Nar alters ERα localization in Tam-R MCF-7 cells

Since ER localization changes upon tamoxifen resistance and Nar is known to bind ERα, we wanted to determine whether Nar had an effect on ERα localization in Tam-R cells [31]. To investigate the localization pattern of ERα, Tam-R MCF-7 cells were cultured in the presence or absence of Nar and ERα localization was determined by confocal microscopy. Cells were also stained with DAPI. In untreated Tam-R cells, ERα was uniformly distributed in the cytoplasm (**Figure 5A** and **B**). ERα was also present although at lower levels in the nucleus when compared to levels present in the cytoplasm. Surprisingly, Nar treatment resulted in a redistribution of ERα to a perinuclear localization in Tam-R MCF-7 cells. Significantly, lower levels of ERα were present in the nucleus (19%) as well as throughout the cytoplasm in Nar treated cells when compared to untreated cells. In complimentary studies, we fractionated Tam-R cells incubated in the presence or absence of Nar into cytosolic and nuclear fractions and assayed for ERα localization (**Figure 5C**). In untreated Tam-R cells there was a relatively even distribution of ERα and in contrast, Nar treatment reduced the levels of ERα in the nucleus. Since our fractionation studies do not distinguish region of the cytoplasm, the total cytoplasmic ERα levels include the perinuclear ERα levels and thus higher total cytoplasmic ERα levels.

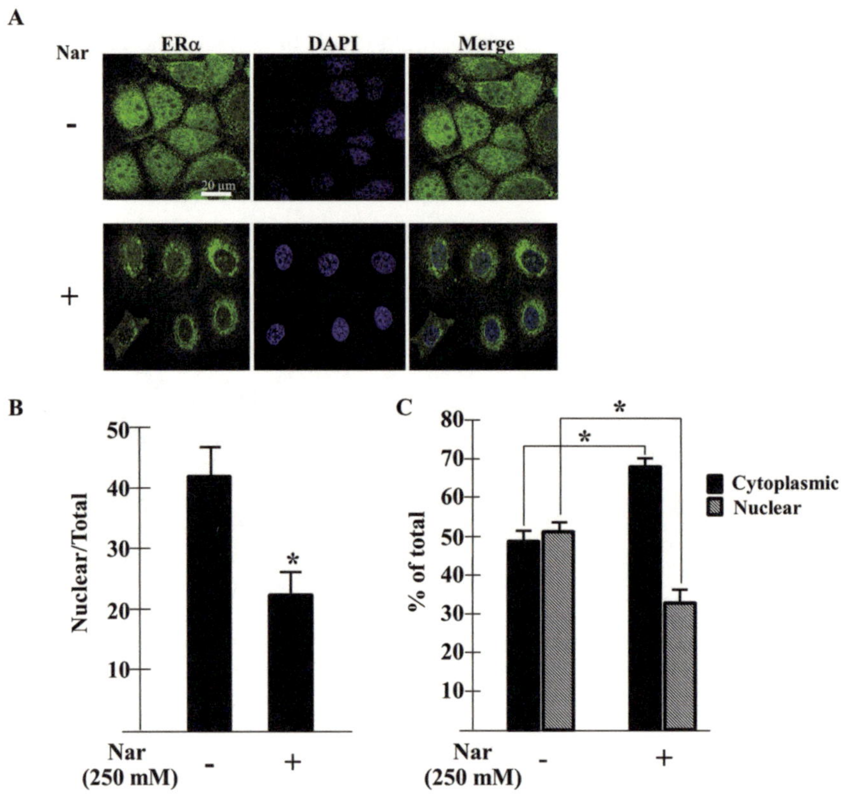

Figure 5. Effect of Nar on ERα localization in Tam-R cells. Tam-R MCF-7 cells were grown in phenol red free media plus charcoal-stripped FBS containing 4-OH-tamoxifen (100 nM) in the presence or absence of Nar (250 μM) for 7 days. (A) Cells were fixed, stained for ERα and DAPI and visualized using confocal microscopy. The results are representative of three independent experiments. (B) Quantification of ERα nuclear localization. Results are the means ± SEM of three independent experiments. $^{*}p < 0.05$. (C) Cells were fractionated into nuclear and cytosolic fractions and assayed for ERα by Western blot analysis. ERα levels were quantified and expressed as % of total ERα. Results are the means ± SEM of three independent experiments. $^{*}p < 0.05$.

4. Discussion

Since ER+ breast cancers utilize estrogen to promote proliferation, pharmaceutical treatments have targeted the ER. One of the most widely used and successful breast cancer treatments is the antiestrogen, Tam. The optimal Tam treatment duration needed to decrease recurrence and improve survival is 5 years. Unfortunately, prolonged Tam treatment leads to Tam resistance. Resistance may in part be due to the activation of other proliferation promoting pathways.

Tam-R cells activate signal kinase pathways to promote cellular proliferation. Currently, the use of Tam in conjunction with multiple kinase inhibitors is being investigated for the treatment of breast cancers [38]. Since Nar also has been shown to have antiproliferative effects, we investigated the ability of Nar to impair cell proliferation of Tam-R breast cancer cells. Our findings suggest that Nar targets both ERK1/2 and ERα to impair cell proliferation of Tam-R MCF-7 cells.

While initially Tam binds to the ER and acts in an antagonist to prevent the ER from interacting with coactivators on the promoters of estrogen responsive genes that regulate cell proliferation and survival, eventually with prolonged treatment cells become Tam resistant [10, 11]. Previous studies have implicated the overactivation of the MAPK and PI3K pathways as contributors of acquired Tam resistance [4]. The ER is able to activate both the MAPK and PI3K pathways [3, 13, 31, 39–43]. In turn, the MAPK and PI3K pathways activate the ER in a ligand-independent manner [3, 13, 31, 39–43]. In order to determine the effects of Nar, we first generated a Tam-R MCF-7 cell line by culturing MCF-7 cells in the presence of 4-OH-tamoxifen for 10 months [28–30]. We monitored the cells for changes in growth rate, ERK1/2 and AKT and ERα localization. Following 10 months of treatment with Tam, the proliferation rate of the treated cells began to increase. These cells were classified as Tam-R. Since the cells were cultured in charcoal-stripped serum, the Tam-R cells appear to be mediating their proliferation through pathway(s) other than the estrogen requiring pathway. Previous studies have shown the activation of both the MAPK and PI3K pathways in Tam-R cells [44–47]. Since Nar impairs both MAPK and PI3K pathways, we wanted to determine whether Nar could reduce Tam-R cell proliferation. Nar treatment caused a complete reversal of proliferation in our Tam-R cell line. Not only did Nar abolish cell proliferation, but it also resulted in a lower cell density then was initially plated. We further show that Nar decreased viability and increased levels of apoptotic and dead cells. In complementary studies, we show that Nar treatment resulted in fragmented and condensed nuclei suggesting apoptotic cell death. Previous studies have documented the ability of Nar to fragment and condense nuclei [32]. These results demonstrate that Nar induces cell death in Tam-R cells.

Since a possible mechanism promoting cell proliferation and survival in the Tam-R cells is the MAPK and PI3K pathways, we investigate the effect of Nar treatment on ERK1/2 and AKT. Previous studies have shown that both the MAPK and PI3K pathways can facilitate proliferation in MCF-7 cells following estrogen deprivation [3, 48]. Furthermore, PI3K and MAPK pathways are upregulated in Tam-R cells [3]. While previous studies have shown that Nar treatment reduced the phosphorylation of both AKT and ERK1/2, our studies show that Nar significantly reduced the levels of both AKT and ERK1/2 in Tam-R cells [15, 17]. Our studies examined the effects of Nar over longer time periods and thus examined the longer term effects of Nar. We have similar effects of Nar on ERK1/2 and AKT levels in MCF-7 cells [20]. Reduced levels of ERK1/2 and AKT activation have been shown to contribute to impaired proliferation and survival of cells. These findings suggest that inhibition of the MAPK and PI3K pathways by Nar may contribute to the impairment of cell proliferation and survival in Tam-R cells.

In Tam-R cells ERα is relocalized from the nucleus to the cytoplasm [31]. This relocalization of ERα may allow for its interaction with kinase signaling pathways such as the PI3K and

MAPK pathways [31]. Both the MAPK and PI3K pathways in these cells may be activated by ERα and in turn ERK1/2 and AKT may activate ERα in the cytosol. This may support the idea that the ERα is more active in the cytosol in the Tam-R cells exhibiting nongenomic effects by interacting with the kinase signaling pathways. In addition, p-ERK1/2 has been shown to activate ERα by direct phosphorylation allowing ERα to resume transcription of estrogen-responsive genes [13, 39]. In this way, ERα would be active in both the cytoplasm and the nucleus. These data suggest that Tam-R cells increase cell proliferation not only through effects on estrogen-responsive genes, but also through activation of the MAPK and/or the PI3K pathways. While the Tam-R cells exhibited an even distribution of ERα throughout the cytoplasm, the addition of Nar localized ERα to a perinuclear region of the cell with significantly lower levels in the nucleus. One interpretation of the mechanism of Nar action is that the Tam-ERα complex that may have been activating components of the MAPK and PI3K signaling pathways in the cytosol was now ineffective because Nar treatment results in reduced levels of ERK1/2 and AKT. Conversely, reduced levels of ERK1/2 and AKT decrease the levels of phosphorylated ERα and thus decrease the transcriptional activity of ERα. Nar may also function by competing with Tam for the ER and unlike the Tam-ERα complex which can translocate into the nucleus the Nar-ERα complex may be unable to enter the nucleus as seen in the perinuclear localization of ER in Nar treated Tam-R cells.

5. Conclusion

In summary, our studies demonstrate that Nar inhibits cellular proliferation and induces apoptosis in Tam-R MCF-7 cells. We show that Nar treatment reduced the levels of ERK1/2 and AKT and resulted in a perinuclear localization pattern of ERα in Tam-R cells. Since Nar can reduce the protein levels of ERK1/2 and AKT as well as reduce the levels of ERα in the nucleus in Tam-R cells, this may explain the reduced cell proliferation/survival. These studies also suggest that Nar may be a potential candidate therapy for Tam-R ER+ breast cancers.

Author details

Joseph Ramos, Talia Hatkevich, Lauren Eanes, Idalys Santos-Sanchez and Yashomati M. Patel*

*Address all correspondence to: ympatel@uncg.edu

Department of Biology, University of North Carolina at Greensboro, Greensboro, North Carolina, USA

References

[1] DeSantis C, Ma J, Bryan L, Jemal A (2014) Breast cancer statistics, 2013. CA Cancer J Clin 64: 52–62.

[2] Baum M (1998) Tamoxifen – the treatment of choice. Why look for alternatives? Br J Cancer 78(Suppl 4): 1–4.

[3] Ghayad SE, Vendrell JA, Ben Larbi S, Dumontet C, Bieche I, et al. (2010) Endocrine resistance associated with activated ErbB system in breast cancer cells is reversed by inhibiting MAPK or PI3K/Akt signaling pathways. Int J Cancer 126: 545–562.

[4] Ali S, Coombes RC (2002) Endocrine-responsive breast cancer and strategies for combating resistance. Nat Rev Cancer 2: 101–112.

[5] Deroo BJ, Korach KS (2006) Estrogen receptors and human disease. J Clin Invest 116: 561–570.

[6] Kumar V, Green S, Stack G, Berry M, Jin JR, et al. (1987) Functional domains of the human estrogen receptor. Cell 51: 941–951.

[7] Safe S, Kim K (2008) Non-classical genomic estrogen receptor (ER)/specificity protein and ER/activating protein-1 signaling pathways. J Mol Endocrinol 41: 263–275.

[8] Sommer S, Fuqua SA (2001) Estrogen receptor and breast cancer. Semin Cancer Biol 11: 339–352.

[9] Shang Y, Brown M (2002) Molecular determinants for the tissue specificity of SERMs. Science 295: 2465–2468.

[10] Lavinsky RM, Jepsen K, Heinzel T, Torchia J, Mullen TM, et al. (1998) Diverse signaling pathways modulate nuclear receptor recruitment of N-CoR and SMRT complexes. Proc Natl Acad Sci U S A 95: 2920–2925.

[11] Shang Y, Hu X, DiRenzo J, Lazar MA, Brown M (2000) Cofactor dynamics and sufficiency in estrogen receptor-regulated transcription. Cell 103: 843–852.

[12] Driggers PH, Segars JH (2002) Estrogen action and cytoplasmic signaling pathways. Part II: the role of growth factors and phosphorylation in estrogen signaling. Trends Endocrinol Metab 13: 422–427.

[13] Migliaccio A, Di Domenico M, Castoria G, de Falco A, Bontempo P, et al. (1996) Tyrosine kinase/p21ras/MAP-kinase pathway activation by estradiol-receptor complex in MCF-7 cells. EMBO J 15: 1292–1300.

[14] Razandi M, Pedram A, Levin ER (2000) Estrogen signals to the preservation of endothelial cell form and function. J Biol Chem 275: 38540–38546.

[15] Bulzomi P, Bolli A, Galluzzo P, Acconcia F, Ascenzi P, et al. (2012) The naringenin-induced proapoptotic effect in breast cancer cell lines holds out against a high bisphenol a background. IUBMB Life 64: 690–696.

[16] Kurokawa H, Nishio K, Fukumoto H, Tomonari A, Suzuki T, et al. (1999) Alteration of caspase-3 (CPP32/Yama/apopain) in wild-type MCF-7, breast cancer cells. Oncol Rep 6: 33–37.

[17] Galluzzo P, Ascenzi P, Bulzomi P, Marino M (2008) The nutritional flavanone naringenin triggers antiestrogenic effects by regulating estrogen receptor alpha-palmitoylation. Endocrinology 149: 2567–2575.

[18] Harmon AW, Patel YM (2003) Naringenin inhibits phosphoinositide 3-kinase activity and glucose uptake in 3T3-L1 adipocytes. Biochem Biophys Res Commun 305: 229–234.

[19] Harmon AW, Patel YM (2004) Naringenin inhibits glucose uptake in MCF-7 breast cancer cells: a mechanism for impaired cellular proliferation. Breast Cancer Res Treat 85: 103–110.

[20] Hatkevich T, Ramos J, Santos-Sanchez I, Patel YM (2014) A naringenin-tamoxifen combination impairs cell proliferation and survival of MCF-7 breast cancer cells. Exp Cell Res 327: 331–339.

[21] Coelho RC, Hermsdorff HH, Bressan J (2013) Anti-inflammatory properties of orange juice: possible favorable molecular and metabolic effects. Plant Foods Hum Nutr 68: 1–10.

[22] Doostdar H, Burke MD, Mayer RT (2000) Bioflavonoids: selective substrates and inhibitors for cytochrome P450 CYP1A and CYP1B1. Toxicology 144: 31–38.

[23] Miksicek RJ (1993) Commonly occurring plant flavonoids have estrogenic activity. Mol Pharmacol 44: 37–43.

[24] Robak J, Gryglewski RJ (1988) Flavonoids are scavengers of superoxide anions. Biochem Pharmacol 37: 837–841.

[25] Ruh MF, Zacharewski T, Connor K, Howell J, Chen I, et al. (1995) Naringenin: a weakly estrogenic bioflavonoid that exhibits antiestrogenic activity. Biochem Pharmacol 50: 1485–1493.

[26] Virgili F, Acconcia F, Ambra R, Rinna A, Totta P, et al. (2004) Nutritional flavonoids modulate estrogen receptor alpha signaling. IUBMB Life 56: 145–151.

[27] Totta P, Acconcia F, Leone S, Cardillo I, Marino M (2004) Mechanisms of naringenin-induced apoptotic cascade in cancer cells: involvement of estrogen receptor alpha and beta signalling. IUBMB Life 56: 491–499.

[28] Farabegoli F, Papi A, Orlandi M (2011) (-)-Epigallocatechin-3-gallate down-regulates EGFR, MMP-2, MMP-9 and EMMPRIN and inhibits the invasion of MCF-7 tamoxifen-resistant cells. Biosci Rep 31: 99–108.

[29] Knowlden JM, Hutcheson IR, Jones HE, Madden T, Gee JM, et al. (2003) Elevated levels of epidermal growth factor receptor/c-erbB2 heterodimers mediate an autocrine growth regulatory pathway in tamoxifen-resistant MCF-7 cells. Endocrinology 144: 1032–1044.

[30] Oyama M, Nagashima T, Suzuki T, Kozuka-Hata H, Yumoto N, et al. (2011) Integrated quantitative analysis of the phosphoproteome and transcriptome in tamoxifen-resistant breast cancer. J Biol Chem 286: 818–829.

[31] Fan P, Wang J, Santen RJ, Yue W (2007) Long-term treatment with tamoxifen facilitates translocation of estrogen receptor alpha out of the nucleus and enhances its interaction with EGFR in MCF-7 breast cancer cells. Cancer Res 67: 1352–1360.

[32] Ahamad MS, Siddiqui S, Jafri A, Ahmad S, Afzal M, et al. (2014) Induction of apoptosis and antiproliferative activity of naringenin in human epidermoid carcinoma cell through ROS generation and cell cycle arrest. PLoS One 9: e110003.

[33] Maggioni D, Nicolini G, Rigolio R, Biffi L, Pignataro L, et al. (2014) Myricetin and naringenin inhibit human squamous cell carcinoma proliferation and migration in vitro. Nutr Cancer 66: 1257–1267.

[34] Nahmias Y, Goldwasser J, Casali M, van Poll D, Wakita T, et al. (2008) Apolipoprotein B-dependent hepatitis C virus secretion is inhibited by the grapefruit flavonoid naringenin. Hepatology 47: 1437–1445.

[35] Yamagishi N, Yamamoto Y, Noda C, Hatayama T (2012) Naringenin inhibits the aggregation of expanded polyglutamine tract-containing protein through the induction of endoplasmic reticulum chaperone GRP78. Biol Pharm Bull 35: 1836–1840.

[36] Pellegrini M, Bulzomi P, Galluzzo P, Lecis M, Leone S, et al. (2014) Naringenin modulates skeletal muscle differentiation via estrogen receptor alpha and beta signal pathway regulation. Genes Nutr 9: 425.

[37] Yoshida H, Watanabe H, Ishida A, Watanabe W, Narumi K, et al. (2014) Naringenin suppresses macrophage infiltration into adipose tissue in an early phase of high-fat diet-induced obesity. Biochem Biophys Res Commun 454: 95–101.

[38] Chappell WH, Steelman LS, Long JM, Kempf RC, Abrams SL, et al. (2011) Ras/Raf/MEK/ERK and PI3K/PTEN/Akt/mTOR inhibitors: rationale and importance to inhibiting these pathways in human health. Oncotarget 2: 135–164.

[39] Bunone G, Briand PA, Miksicek RJ, Picard D (1996) Activation of the unliganded estrogen receptor by EGF involves the MAP kinase pathway and direct phosphorylation. EMBO J 15: 2174–2183.

[40] Campbell RA, Bhat-Nakshatri P, Patel NM, Constantinidou D, Ali S, et al. (2001) Phosphatidylinositol 3-kinase/AKT-mediated activation of estrogen receptor alpha: a new model for anti-estrogen resistance. J Biol Chem 276: 9817–9824.

[41] Fox EM, Arteaga CL, Miller TW (2012) Abrogating endocrine resistance by targeting ERα and PI3K in breast cancer. Front Oncol 2: 145.

[42] Harmon AW, Paul DS, Patel YM (2004) MEK inhibitors impair insulin-stimulated glucose uptake in 3T3-L1 adipocytes. Am J Physiol Endocrinol Metab 287: E758-766.

[43] Sun M, Paciga JE, Feldman RI, Yuan Z, Coppola D, et al. (2001) Phosphatidylinositol-3-OH Kinase (PI3K)/AKT2, activated in breast cancer, regulates and is induced by estrogen receptor alpha (ERα) via interaction between ERα and PI3K. Cancer Res 61: 5985–5991.

[44] Normanno N, Di Maio M, De Maio E, De Luca A, de Matteis A, et al. (2005) Mechanisms of endocrine resistance and novel therapeutic strategies in breast cancer. Endocr Relat Cancer 12: 721–747.

[45] Riggins RB, Schrecengost RS, Guerrero MS, Bouton AH (2007) Pathways to tamoxifen resistance. Cancer Lett 256: 1–24.

[46] Tokunaga E, Kataoka A, Kimura Y, Oki E, Mashino K, et al. (2006) The association between Akt activation and resistance to hormone therapy in metastatic breast cancer. Eur J Cancer 42: 629–635.

[47] Tokunaga E, Kimura Y, Mashino K, Oki E, Kataoka A, et al. (2006) Activation of PI3K/Akt signaling and hormone resistance in breast cancer. Breast Cancer 13: 137–144.

[48] Martin LA, Farmer I, Johnston SR, Ali S, Marshall C, et al. (2003) Enhanced estrogen receptor (ER) alpha, ERBB2, and MAPK signal transduction pathways operate during the adaptation of MCF-7 cells to long term estrogen deprivation. J Biol Chem 278: 30458–30468.